PRINCIPLES OF RISK MANAGEMENT AND PATIENT SAFETY

Edited by
Barbara J. Youngberg, JD, MSW, BSN, FASHRM
Visiting Professor of Health Law and Policy
Loyola University Chicago
College of Law
Beazley Institute for Health Law and Policy
Chicago, Illinois

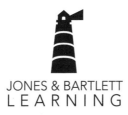

JONES & BARTLETT
LEARNING

World Headquarters
Jones & Bartlett Learning
5 Wall Street
Burlington, MA 01803
978-443-5000
info@jblearning.com
www.jblearning.com

Jones & Bartlett Learning books and products are available through most bookstores and online booksellers. To contact Jones & Bartlett Learning directly, call 800-832-0034, fax 978-443-8000, or visit our website, www.jblearning.com.

Substantial discounts on bulk quantities of Jones & Bartlett Learning publications are available to corporations, professional associations, and other qualified organizations. For details and specific discount information, contact the special sales department at Jones & Bartlett Learning via the above contact information or send an email to specialsales@jblearning.com.

This publication is designed to provide accurate and authoritative information in regard to the Subject Matter covered. It is sold with the understanding that the publisher is not engaged in rendering legal, accounting, or other professional service. If legal advice or other expert assistance is required, the service of a competent professional person should be sought.

Production Credits
Publisher: Michael Brown
Associate Editor: Catie Heverling
Editorial Assistant: Teresa Reilly
Production Manager: Tracey Chapman
Associate Production Editor: Kate Stein
Senior Marketing Manager: Sophie Fleck
Manufacturing and Inventory Control Supervisor: Amy Bacus
Composition: Shepherd, Inc.
Cover Design: Scott Moden
Cover Image: **Main image:** © Dewayne Flowers/ShutterStock, Inc. **Bottom images, from left to right:** © Ambient Ideas/ShutterStock, Inc.; © Angela Luchianiuc/ShutterStock, Inc.; © beerkoff/ShutterStock, Inc.
Printing and Binding: Edwards Brothers Malloy
Cover Printing: Edwards Brothers Malloy

Library of Congress Cataloging-in-Publication Data
Youngberg, Barbara J.
   Principles of risk management and patient safety / Barbara J. Youngberg.
      p. ; cm.
   Includes bibliographical references and index.
   ISBN-13: 978-0-7637-7405-9 (pbk.)
   ISBN-10: 0-7637-7405-7 (pbk.)
   1. Health facilities—Risk management. 2. Medication errors—Prevention. 3. Hospitals—Safety measures. I. Title.
   [DNLM: 1. Malpractice. 2. Medical Errors—prevention & control. 3. Delivery of Health Care—organization & administration. 4. Quality Assurance, Health Care—organization & administration. 5. Risk Management—methods. 6. Safety Management—methods. WB 100 Y78p 2011]
   RA971.38.Y68 2011
   610.289—dc22
                                    2010010518

6048

Printed in the United States of America
18 17 16 15 14   10 9 8 7 6 5

This book is dedicated to my beautiful daughter, Anie, who has changed my life in a thousand ways and who patiently suffered through lost weekends and holidays while I finished this book.

CONTENTS

PREFACE

An earlier edition of this book, originally titled *The Risk Manager's Desk Reference*, was released in the same year that the Institute of Medicine (IOM) released its groundbreaking report titled "To Err Is Human: Building a Safer Health Care System." The authors began that report with some startling data regarding the number of preventable medical errors that occur within the U.S. healthcare system every year. The report cited many reasons for this, among them a punitive culture that punishes individuals when they are involved in mistakes, a level of complexity (both as related to the patients receiving care and the environment in which care is provided) that is now the norm in health care and that makes errors more likely to occur, and the fact that we fail to learn from our errors or to openly discuss the systemic vulnerabilities that manifest every day and predispose individuals to err.

For me as a risk manager, much in the report was not a surprise, but it was, in my mind, an accurate statement about the lack of sustainable success that we have been able to achieve as healthcare risk managers, clinicians, and healthcare administrators. I recalled the early days when I began my career as a lawyer managing medical-malpractice claims and being struck with how seldom organizations and providers asked about what could be learned from the claim. Once a claim was resolved, the risk manager, the clinicians, and the administrators were already involved in something else, usually the next bad claim. In addition, I was struck by how often in the debate around healthcare reform, which occurred almost 20 years ago and seems to be repeating itself now, there seemed to be a desire to blame the legal system for the malpractice problems when, in truth, many of the problems are ours alone to fix.

Although the initial plan was to merely do a third edition of the *Desk Reference*, it soon became apparent that a more full-scale revision was required. Much has changed since the release of the IOM report 10 years ago. Many risk managers have been courageous enough to acknowledge specific aspects of the traditional risk management approach that were flawed and not yielding the desired results, and to embrace a new way of thinking about risk, error, transparency, and safety. The most successful risk managers realize that incorporating patient safety principles into risk management is about more than just changing the name of the department or adding an additional job responsibility to their business card. In fact, in many cases, it requires a reassessment of the long-held practices.

Risk managers often found it difficult to reconcile traditional principles of risk management, which frequently focused on protecting the financial assets of the organization through vigorous defense of all claims asserted against it, to limiting the sharing of information so that it could be shielded from discovery, to focusing more on the aftermath of a claim than on the development of why the claim occurred in the first place and, more importantly, how it might have been prevented. There was lack of synergy between departments that often resulted in duplicate or fragmented work, or work that never achieved its potential. In addition, even when results seemed positive, they were often isolated to the area where the problem arose and not applied across the organization.

There remains in some organizations a healthy debate about where risk management ends and patient safety begins. In addition, patient safety, although a concept now better understood, is still in need of operational traction. Many departments and individuals in healthcare organizations have tried to claim patient safety as their singular responsibility, artificially segmenting the activities in ways that make little sense and yield diminished results. Also, at a time when many healthcare employees attempt to justify their own existence and positions, it may be threatening to think that the best organizations decentralize both risk management and patient safety so that everyone in the organization feels that keeping patients and colleagues safe and keeping the environment free of risks is their job. When this happens, the role of the risk manager is not diminished, but certainly it does change. This book lays out the ways in which a risk manager thinks to conform to this new reality and, ideally, bring about the changes associated with patient safety that 10 years of research have identified as necessary.

Readers familiar with the first and second editions of *The Risk Manager's Desk Reference* will notice a number of things. Firstly, this text is clearly divided into the three domains that remain a part of most risk managers' job responsibility: claims management, risk financing, and proactive risk reduction or patient safety. In the first two domains there have been some changes, as certainly discussions about transparency, disclosure, and early-offer programs has dramatically changed the manner in which many risk managers now respond to errors. The most significant changes, however, are noted in the final section of the book where, instead of characterizing risks as unique in light of the clinical specialty where they originate, I organized the section based on what I have learned over the past 10 years as a result of analyzing patient safety and risk management data, that is, that regardless of the department where the error occurs, the root cause of the problem is often identified as a systemic problem often caused by workplace complexity, pressure within the system to do more with less, and a lack of focus on simple human interaction between provider and patient or provider and colleague. Indeed, problems such as poor communication, inadequate handoffs, and fatigue often appear as a root cause of the majority of problems that continue to occur. There is still a great deal of research done that, in the years to come, will continue to advance our knowledge about the etiology of risk and, more importantly, the best manner in which to intervene to reduce and ultimately eliminate the risks that are identified. It will be our job to acknowledge what is learned and apply it to our current practice. Our knowledge base, our style of collaboration, and our way of seeing our work will change, and I am hopeful that this book will help to prepare both, the risk managers working today and people who seek risk management as a profession, for the challenges of the future.

CONTRIBUTORS

Diana L. Alvarez, MT, (ASCP)^{CM}
Medical Laboratory Scientist—Transfusion
  Services
Exempla–St. Joseph's Hospital
Denver, Colorado

Deb Ankowicz, BSN, RN, CPHQ, CPHRM
Director of Risk Management
University of Wisconsin Hospital and Clinics
Madison, Wisconsin

S. Joseph Austin, JD, LLM
Regulatory Coordinator
Institutional Review Board for Human
  Subject Research (IRBMED)
University of Michigan Medical School
Ann Arbor, Michigan

Margaret L. Begalle, JD
Compliance Manager
Office of Ethics & Compliance for
  Pharmaceutical Products Group
Abbott Laboratories
Abbott Park, Illinois

Renée Bernard, JD
Director of Risk Management
Stanford University Medical Center
Palo Alto, California

Roberta Carroll, MBA, ARM, CPCU
Senior Vice President
AON Healthcare
Odessa, Florida

Caroline Chapman, JD
Staff Attorney
Legal Assistance Foundation of Metropolitan
  Chicago
Chicago, Illinois

Stacey A. Cischke, JD
Partner
Cassiday Schade, LLP
Chicago, Illinois

Barbara A. Connelly, RN, MJ
Director of Risk Management
Medical College of Wisconsin Affiliated
  Hospitals (MCWAH)
Milwaukee, Wisconsin

Krista M. Curell, JD, BSN
Associate Vice President
Quality and Risk Management
University of Chicago Hospital and Clinics
Chicago, Illinois

Sherri DeVito, JD, BA
Assistant Legal Counsel
Illinois State Medical Society
Chicago, Illinois

Jeffrey F. Driver, MBA, JD
Executive Vice President
Stanford University Medical Indemnity
    and Trust
Chief Risk Officer
Stanford University Medical Center
Palo Alto, California

Thomas V. Ealy, MBA
National Partner of the Midwest Region
Willis Group Holdings
Chicago, Illinois

Alice L. Epstein MHA, CPHRM, CPHQ, CPEA
Director Risk Control Consulting
CNA Financial Corp

David M. Gaba, MD
Associate Dean for Immersive and
    Simulation-Based Learning
Professor of Anesthesia
Stanford University
Staff Anesthesiologist and Director
Patient Simulation Center of Innovation
VA Palo Alto Health Care System
Palo Alto, California

Michelle M. Garvey, MEd, BA
Loyola University Chicago
College of Law
Beazley Institute for Health Law and Policy
Chicago, Illinois

Kristopher Goetz, MA
Manager, Performance and Innovation
Northwestern Memorial Hospital
Chicago, Illinois

Josephine Goode-Evans, MA, BSN
Corporate Vice President
SSM Healthcare
St. Louis, Missouri

Gary H. Harding BS, BMET
Director, Technical Services
GP, LLC

Nancy Hill-Davis, MJ, MA, BA, BSN
Vice President
Human Resources and Risk Management
Mercy Hospital and Medical Center
Chicago, Illinois

Mahendr S. Kochar, MD, MS, MBA, MACP, FACC, FRCP (London)
Professor of Medicine, Pharmacology, and
    Toxicology
Executive Director, Medical College of
    Wisconsin Affiliated Hospitals
Senior Associate Dean for Graduate Medical
    Education
Medical College of Wisconsin
Milwaukee, Wisconsin

A. Michelle Kuhn, BA
Senior Vice President, Risk Management
Chart Services, Inc.

Geoffrey K. Lighthall, MD, PhD
Associate Professor
Anesthesia and Critical Care
Department of Anesthesia
Stanford University School of Medicine
Stanford, California

Drew McCormick, MA, BA
Loyola University Chicago
College of Law
Beazley Institute for Health Law and Policy
Chicago, Illinois

Terence McMahon, MBA
Senior Director Financial Operations
Blue Cross/Blue Shield of Illinois
Chicago, Illinois

Patricia Meersman, MBA, MJ, BA
American Hospital Association
Chicago, Illinois

Judith Napier, MSN, BSN
VP System Safety and Risk Prevention
Allina Hospitals and Clinics
Minneapolis, Minnesota

Stephen Pavkovic, MPH, JD, BSN
Risk Manager
Northwestern Memorial Hospital
Chicago, Illinois

Amit Prachand, MEng
Administrator
Division of Hospital Medicine
Northwestern Memorial Hospital
Chicago, Illinois

Jennifer Ruocco, PhD, CIP
Deputy Compliance Officer
Cincinnati Children's Hospital Medical
   Center
Cincinnati, Ohio

Lisa Saar, JD, MSN
Lieutenant Commander Nurse Corps
   Officer—Retired
U.S. Navy
Silverdale, Washington

Mark G. Schneider, MBA
Director of Insurance
Loyola University Medical Center
Maywood, Illinois

Katherine V. Schostok, JD, LLM
Social Security Administration
Attorney Advisor at the Chicago National
   Hearing Center
Office of Disability, Adjudication, and Review
Chicago, Illinois

Michael Sheppard, MBA
Vice President
Beecher Carlson
Chicago, Illinois

Scott Stanley, JD, BSN
Risk Manager
Northwestern Memorial Hospital
Chicago, Illinois

Sara Greening Truss, MBA
Director of Programs and Education
Vital Rehabilitation
Chicago, Illinois

Jayne Westendorp-Holland, JD, BA
Loyola University Chicago
College of Law
Beazley Institute for Health Law and Policy
Chicago, Illinois

**Barbara J. Youngberg, JD, MSW, BSN,
   FASHRM**
Visiting Professor of Health Law and Policy
Loyola University Chicago
College of Law
Beazley Institute for Health Law and Policy
Chicago, Illinois

ABOUT THE AUTHOR

Barbara Youngberg, JD, BSN, MSW, FASHRM has over 25 years experience helping academic medical centers and other complex healthcare organizations restructure quality, risk management, and patient safety programs to meet current needs and challenges. During her 20-year career at University HealthSystem Consortium (UHC) she analyzed malpractice data and trends, quality and patient safety data, and best practice information to assist members in finding creative solutions to difficult risk and patient safety problems. As the Vice President of Insurance, Risk, Quality, and Legal Services and co-leader of UHC's Patient Safety Net (PSN), Ms. Youngberg helped to develop a Web-based reporting tool utilizing standardized language to allow of analysis of events and their root causes and worked to help members integrate patient-safety activities into existing quality and risk-management structures. Often these efforts include helping members understand the way in which the legal climate could help or hinder them in their efforts.

Ms. Youngberg is a graduate of DePaul University College of Law (JD), University of Illinois–Jane Addams School of Social Work (MSW), and Illinois Wesleyan University (BSN). She is presently a Visiting Professor of Law at Loyola University Chicago, Beazley Health Law Institute and helps to develop online curriculum for online health law MJ and LL.M degrees. She is also a professor of Law for Concord Kaplan University School of Law and serves on the Board of Directors of the National Patient Safety Foundation. She is the author of numerous articles and textbooks on quality management, risk management, and patient safety.

THE INTEGRATION OF RISK MANAGEMENT AND PATIENT SAFETY

Risk Management and Patient Safety: The Synergy and the Tension

Judith Napier, MSN, BSN
Barbara J. Youngberg, JD, MSW, BSN, FASHRM

INTRODUCTION

There is a great deal of confusion about both the differences and the similarities between risk management and patient safety. Many healthcare organizations and providers have sought to demonstrate their support for patient safety merely by changing the name of either the risk management or quality department to the patient safety department, often without changing the nature or focus of the work. It is important as a risk manager to not only understand the distinction but also to recognize how it might impact the manner in which risk is addressed in one's organization.

Historically, risk management in health care evolved from programs that existed in other industries and were focused primarily on the transferring of risk through the purchase of insurance. Risk managers, even those in health care, often came out of the insurance industry and reported to the finance department. Their job was to buy the best coverage,

the correct limits, and to make certain that claims, once they appeared, were reported to the appropriate carrier who would then assume responsibility for them. This complete transfer of risk became more difficult as medical malpractice cases became more frequent and more costly. The risk manager then required additional knowledge and skill to understand a more complex transaction instead of merely transferring all of the risk to a carrier. The role evolved to allow for the risk manager to assess the organization's total potential risk, determine the organization's risk appetite (or ability to fund and finance some of their own risk), and then select partners to assist them in structuring a program that would combine self-insurance, co-insurance, and excess insurance. This process is described in detail in the chapters in this book specifically associated with risk financing.

The second aspect of the risk manager's role, claims management, generally revolved around the management and defense of malpractice claims. Physicians, hospital employees, and the hospital itself historically became familiar with the risk manager after a patient had sustained an injury or when a lawsuit was filed requiring defense. The risk manager's job description often included protecting the assets of the organization as well as supporting and defending providers who were named in these suits. The relationship with the patient was secondary to protecting the assets of the organization or the provider's malpractice carrier, so resolving a claim by paying as little as possible was the goal.

The injury or suit historically triggered a detailed investigation of the factors that gave rise to the claim. The focus of this investigation was often on developing a strategy for defending the organization or the care provider. Due to the fact that the legal system is by nature adversarial, those named in suits often felt shame, anger, a sense of punishment, and often a sense of isolation, all of which limited the amount of discussion surrounding the claim and tended to put the focus on the individual who had provided care rather than on the system that might have contributed to the harm. Seldom were claims viewed as learning opportunities, and generally each claim was viewed as an isolated case, even though factors similar to those of other cases might have been present. The initial response to a claim was to "hunker down," sequester the information, prepare to aggressively defend and/or contain the loss, admit to nothing, and leave it to the attorneys to resolve. Resolution of claims often involved the hiring of outside counsel, who learned many things about the claim but seldom were asked to share that information with the organization or the provider. By the time one claim ended, the organization, the providers involved, and the risk manager had moved on to other claims and new issues.

The third component of a risk manager's role prior to the introduction of patient safety was loss control. This aspect of the job was not initially part of the risk manager's job but

emerged as malpractice costs rose and as individuals became aware of specific clinical issues that often were giving rise to increasingly costly claims. At that point many nurses entered the field of risk management because they were familiar with the nuances of clinical care and were better able to work effectively with clinicians. This more proactive and clinically focused approach actually was encouraged initially in the specialties of obstetrics, anesthesia, and emergency medicine where losses were increasing in frequency and were often catastrophic in severity. Risk managers began to identify both patterns of behavior that gave rise to claims and changes to make in practice that could allow the practitioner to avoid costly lawsuits. The motivation for much of the activity was the injury or loss suffered by a patient, so in many cases it still did not serve to prevent an injury but rather to contain or prevent future injuries.

In 1998, the Institute of Medicine (IOM) report[1] contained information that surprised the public. The information about the alarming numbers of preventable medical errors was not a surprise to most risk managers or to clinicians who continued to face rising malpractice premiums due to continued catastrophic injuries sustained by patients. Many people recognized that current activities had been unsuccessful in preventing harm to patients, and that the approach of blaming individuals who were involved in harmful events suppressed any potential for learning. The challenge to healthcare providers and administrators was to develop a culture of learning, to become more transparent and open in hopes of advancing knowledge, and to create systemic mindfulness that focused more on the situations and conditions in which individuals work rather than on the individuals themselves. This new approach served to challenge risk managers to think differently about the work they were doing, which, given the number of preventable errors that continued to be reported, suggested that the approaches being taken were having only limited success in actually preventing harm to patients.

The changes can be described best by revisiting the functions of risk management. As related to the function of risk financing, the underlying job responsibilities remain the same, though perhaps they are more complex given the cyclical nature of the insurance industry and the desire for insurance providers to move further away from the risk, forcing the organization and often individual providers or groups of providers to either pay more or assume a deductible. (See Chapter 11, which covers enterprise risk management and details the new levels of sophistication now required to not only better understand the true nature of risk but also to design a program that protects the organization from catastrophic financial loss while creating incentives for aggressive loss control.)

The second function of risk management, which is claims management, changes when principles of patient safety are applied. Though a risk manager still will work hard to defend their organization or a provider from frivolous lawsuits or claims where there has been no negligence, when preventable errors or errors caused by negligence are identified a different approach is generally taken. Under principles that are at the core of patient safety, transparency becomes imperative and involves providers being honest with patients about the cause of their injury. In addition, the investigation and resolution process is viewed as a learning experience, and sharing what is learned with all stakeholders in a manner that maintains privacy and confidentiality of patient and provider occurs so that the underlying issues can be fully understood and resolved. Though risk management can do little to change the adversarial nature of the legal process under principles of patient safety, risk managers can reorient their investigation to be more about understanding the systemic vulnerabilities that caused the event, as opposed to merely looking at the behaviors of the caregiver. In addition, under principles of patient

safety every attempt is made to preserve the patient–provider relationship. When errors are made and injuries result, both parties can speak about them freely, discuss how to compensate the patient for their loss, share the learning that was extracted, and if desired, maintain the relationship into the future. Other chapters in this book (e.g., Chapter 19) deal with disclosure and early-offer programs and describe in great detail not only how these programs should be structured but the benefits that organizations are already seeing from this approach.

What has changed most dramatically following the IOM report is the manner in which the third aspect of risk management, loss control, is influenced by applying principles of patient safety. Whereas in the past a patient injury or sentinel event was often the trigger for a risk management investigation, now, under a concept known as "systemic mindfulness," risk managers, guided by patient safety principles, continually assess the environment in which care is given to identify potentially harmful practices, processes, or failure modes, and then modify them before an injury can occur. The focus is less on the error operator (or the individual involved in the error) and more on the myriad factors that endangered the individual and caused or contributed to the error. In addition, focus is not only given to actual events but also to near-miss events, the latter being an attempt to better understand how errors get intercepted due to caregiver vigilance, technology, or improved processes. As an organization attempts to create an overarching culture of safety, the risk manager's role changes from being the person responsible for investigation and problem resolution to the aggregator of information that allows for the identification of trends and patterns as well as for improved prioritization. This information comes from everyone in the organization who are encouraged and empowered to speak up when they notice a potential problem or weakness in the system. Achieving the goal of systemic mindfulness, as this increased awareness is termed in patient safety parlance, requires that everyone in the organization (including physicians) become a risk manager or, at the very least, a risk identifier. Their knowledge of what is required of them relative to the care they provide, as well as how best to achieve an appropriate and sustainable solution once problems are identified, improves the likelihood of success relative to the solution applied to the problem. Furthermore, this knowledge, coupled with the widespread dissemination of what is learned, improves the likelihood that all of the goals of risk management, decreased insurance costs, fewer liability claims, and safer systems resulting in fewer injured patients will be achieved. Because this aspect of the risk manager's job has changed dramatically, the remainder of this chapter addresses how a risk manager perceives the synergy between their role and that of others in the organization who also contribute to patient–provider safety.

Figure 1–1 shows business-strategy decisions with regard to redesigning a healthcare system in order to expand a clinical service line such as obstetrics. This may be done to meet a changing demand in the community and to increase revenue and market share.

The finances are devised with appropriate budgets, only to later see erosion due to adverse outcomes and claims. This occurs when the strategic decision is not reached with a full understanding of the necessary clinical and professional demands that will be needed to meet the standard of care.

THE RISK-INTELLIGENT ENTERPRISE

Figure 1-1 also illustrates the direction of risk management beyond clinical risk. Moving beyond insurance and the obvious clinical risks associated with professional liability in the day-to-day delivery of health care, the expanding risk management model highlights what some people call risk intelligence.[1] The risk-intelligent enterprise develops a full-spectrum vision of risk. It entails developing an enlightened approach to risk management that spans the entire organization, with a leader who is capable of applying the following four functions of risk management to current and future organizational risks:[2]

- Oversight of the organization's ability to meet the regulatory requirements

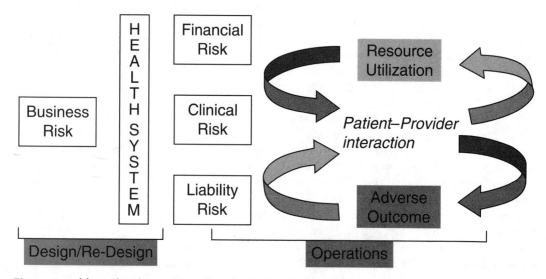

Figure 1–1 Managing Interrelated Risks in the Healthcare Setting
By permission of Anna Marie Hajek.

- Working with business units to assist the leaders in understanding risk in business transactions
- Advising staff and leaders on the best approach to manage the new or emerging risk for the organization
- Providing leadership to maintain an understanding of the organization's mission and goals, and defining who is able to provide direction

It is important to have expertise that includes a deep understanding of the various components of risk, whether it is billing and compliance relative to a Recovery Audit Contractors (RAC) audit, risk associated with regulatory compliance with Stark laws, or professional liability exposure with clinical care. No one person can cover the level of detail required in all areas; however, the risk-intelligent enterprise builds bridges between risk "silos" to open lines of communication and share information. Having someone who is able to work across these lines and have a broad understanding of the full portfolio of risks that the organization faces, and an ability to influence direction of the management of the risks, is critical for value-added risk management rather than risk avoidance or risk transfer.

Risk is defined as the chance of loss. Risk analysis is the process used by the person or the person's assigned risk management functions to determine the potential severity of the loss from an identified risk, the probability that the loss will happen, and alternatives for dealing with the risk.[3] The key here is the alternatives for managing the risk. The decision to retain the risk, transfer the risk to the organization, or attempt to modify the risk is part of the responsibility of the "enlightened" risk manager. Using multiple avenues to understand the degree of the risk, and then using knowledge and experience to modify that risk, is part of the responsibility. A person can only do this with a complete understanding of the risk.

VALUE PROTECTION OR VALUE CREATION

Unrewarded risk is defined as the prerequisites: Occupational Safety and Health Administration (OSHA) requirements with health and safety standards, Joint Commission standards, Centers for Medicare and Medicaid Services (CMS) requirements, etc. We could perform all of the regulatory requirements in a timely and competent manner and might still have a bad outcome that results in a claim or legal filing. These activities just meet the baseline expectations. The primary reason to address these risks is for value protection, not value creation. We must meet the baseline in order to secure accreditation with Joint Commission survey or CMS standards of participation. The standards have indeed been developed to improve patient care, but that will not move us up the innovation scale or assist us in developing new models of care delivery until we build the processes into the daily lexicon, practices, and culture of our organization.

Rewarded risks, on the other hand, are those that you undertake to spur value creation.[4] New business acquisitions, new models of care, new clinical services—all are designed to add value, not to sustain the status quo. In a risk-intelligent enterprise, assuming risk is part of the equation for growth; how that risk is assumed and managed is up to the organization, which must determine the direction and level of analysis, the risk appetite for the organization, and how the leaders will choose to offset or manage the risk beyond the obvious exposure.

The American Society of Healthcare Risk Managers (ASHRM) defines domains that highlight the interconnectedness of risk in health care.[3] These domains include:

- Strategic
- Operational
- Financial
- Human capital

- Legal and regulatory
- Technology

Risks do not exist or behave in "isolation" but instead can be identified, grouped, and catalogued in risk domains. These domains assist organizations to not only identify risk across the spectrum but also to develop mitigating strategies that interface across business lines. Risk management continues to evolve as a process to identify practice concerns from quality data, clinical indicators, and outcomes, and to develop various strategies to mitigate the risk (reduce or eliminate) through risk management techniques such as practice modification, insurance transfer, or risk avoidance such as when we eliminate the risk by closing of an obstetrics unit or mental health services or reducing the privileges of a specific provider who may not have the requisite skill to safely perform a specific procedure. Risk management expands beyond the clinical setting to the organization at large as health care begins to look at risk in the broader context for the organization.

PATIENT SAFETY

Some people would argue that risk management and patient safety are one in the same discipline. Risk management has always had an element of prevention; however, due to the day-to-day risks, management of the prevention has often gone unattended. In 1999, with the advent of the IOM report, which stated that 48,000–98,000 people are injured or die each year at the hands of health professionals, the focus on prevention became targeted. This launched work from professionals outside of the healthcare industry who began to look beyond the individual-practice issues and analyze why the injuries and deaths were occurring. What in the system was allowing the repeated problems to happen, and how could we analyze in a systematic manner the practices, behaviors, and outcomes that were causing these problems?

James Reason introduced his book, "Managing the Risks of Organizational Accidents," which focuses on the risks of hazardous technologies, to the healthcare community.[5] This book prompted the healthcare industry to begin looking at errors and accidents differently, and led healthcare leaders to begin to understand how accidents occurred and, more importantly, to look at accidents and patient events from a systems perspective rather than a case-by-case perspective. The "swiss cheese" model as defined by Reason[5] is a dynamic process with moving "holes" that break down the defenses established to maintain a safety net in the organization. The holes allow the "risk" to penetrate and at times reach the patient. These holes are failures in the system. Because the conditions are ever changing, the system has built-in defenses that do not allow the holes in the system to line up and create an avenue for the error to reach a patient; instead, the defenses, both active and latent, are designed to:[5]

- Create understanding and awareness of the local hazards
- Provide clear guidelines on how to operate safely
- Provide alarms and warnings when danger is imminent
- Restore the system to a safe state in an abnormal situation
- Interpose safety barriers between the hazards and the potential losses
- Contain and eliminate the hazards should they escape this barrier
- Provide the means to escape and rescue should hazard containment fail

The purpose of patient safety is to provide a safe environment, to explore the possibility of failure, and to create "defenses" that will change the current system of operation in order to reduce the potential for failure. One of the fundamental differences between risk management and patient safety is the difference between fixing problems and driving change toward creating a safer environment.

Risk Management	Patient Safety
It's about the organizational tactics to fix problems.	*It's about the culture of the organization that will drive change.*
• Focus is on *individual case*	• Focus is on *system failures*
• Post-event investigation	• Recovering from error to reduce harm
• Implement *tactics* to address the event rather than the system failures	• Relationship with human factors that impact failures in system
• Relationship with legal standard of care	• System *themes and patterns* identified
• Unexpected outcomes drive the process	• Good Catches and AWTH focus the efforts
• *Reactive*	• *Proactive*

Figure 1–2 Risk Management Versus Patient Safety

Change management includes a host of processes that may or may not come to light in one case but will, over time, shine through from patterns, themes, and archetypes that resonate in many events (Figure 1–2).

Patient safety is more about changing the work culture than about the problem itself. Developing a resilient organization that is able to respond to the changing environment, rather than developing individual policies and procedures to solve all of what may come up in the course of a work day, is the goal of patient safety. The latter task is impossible and would result in failure over time. The point is to use knowledge learned in other high-risk industries where they have come to understand system failure in their environment, and to apply this knowledge to the health care delivery system. Such organizations are termed highly reliable organizations (HROs) because of the success rates that they are able to achieve repeatedly under pressure. Karlene Roberts[6] studied these organizations to understand the processes and practices that have impacted their ability to respond to unexpected problems and to overcome those problems without significant failure. The HROs have some common characteristics. They typically do the following:[6]

• Track small failures

• Resist oversimplification
• Remain sensitive to operations
• Maintain capability for resilience
• Take advantage of shifting locations of expertise

As previously stated, risk managers tend to rely on lessons learned from past mistakes, which they apply to the case at hand in order to "defend" the actions of those involved. Because of the continued volume of events, risk management has not been able to evolve quickly enough in terms of developing prevention models. Risk managers have relied on legal findings, large claim settlements, as well as verdicts and legal theories to implement change through fear rather than attacking the problem at the root–the culture and environment.

Patient safety has the ability to support the risk management efforts through new ways of understanding how things go wrong and applying new models to the problems. Defining teamwork and communication in ways that address how individuals communicate across disciplines, departments, and organizational expectations relative to the caregivers' role in this work begins to anchor the safety agenda for an organization. Developing a better understanding of situational awareness and applying knowledge learned through human-factors theories, to gain a broader understanding of why the failures occur, has been the progress in safety that risk management has not yet been able to reach.

Patient safety is designed to create an environment whereby everyone operates from the same set of principles and the organizational design conforms with what Weick and Sutcliffe refer to as the seven properties of sense making.[7,8] Think of the questions that address the seven principles relative to the time-out process with universal protocol in the operating suite:

- *Social context:* Does the process encourage conversation? Is it open and does it allow for questions and clarification?
- *Identification:* Does the process give people a distinct, stable sense of who they are and what they represent? In other words, what is their role?
- *Retrospect:* Does the process preserve elapsed data and legitimate use of the data? Do we study our flaws and work toward performance and process improvement?
- *Salient cues:* Does the process enhance the visibility of cues? Do we rely on memory or do we use human-factors knowledge to trigger with visual cues and forcing functions?
- *Ongoing projects:* Does the process enable people to be resilient in the face of interruptions? In health care, do we teach situational awareness and how to recognize when colleagues have lost situational awareness?
- *Plausibility:* Does the process encourage people to accumulate and exchange plausible accounts? Do we allow staff time to brief and debrief following critical exchange of information and/or actions such as surgery or a cardiac-arrest response?
- *Enactment:* Does the process encourage action or hesitation? Do we recognize the behavior we want versus reprimanding the behavior we do not want?

CONCLUSION

Patient safety and comprehension of the science of safety are not only expectations in the healthcare industry but also a cause for continual struggle internally with regard to who is responsible for patient safety and what patient safety strives to do. Is it designed to establish a culture that is responsive to safety issues? Is it designed to monitor and measure outcomes of core policies, national patient safety goals, or other regulatory requirements that address safety? Is patient safety designed to understand the system failures that are impacting the outcomes and design models of care in order to support the caregivers and providers in a more reliable way? Is the purpose of patient safety to redesign the system of care in a way that is more responsive to new technologies, accounts for human factors that impact outcomes and create system failures, and makes it possible to reduce harm to patients and staff through the new models?

The reality is that patient safety is all of the above. The work of patient safety spans the entire system and begins to embrace much of the risk-intelligent-enterprise model. The work crosses multiple "silos" and needs to be addressed from a systems approach. It needs to be embedded throughout all that we do in health care beyond the regulatory requirements and the individual sentinel events, and it must begin to penetrate to the most fundamental levels in the organization: how we think and act toward each other; how we include patients and families in decision making relative to care and treatment; and when a failure occurs, how we respond. All of these factors influence the organization's effectiveness in implementing a patient safety culture.

Patient safety is the outcome. The work is in designing a system of care that applies the principles learned from highly reliable organizations, and the properties of sense making, in an environment that is highly complex, rapidly changing with technology, and dependent on people and staff to adhere to the appropriate principles and rules in the face of production pressures. Designing a culture that recognizes these flaws and, more importantly, begins to piece together in a systems approach the principles outlined in this chapter, for both risk management and patient safety, will move us closer to understanding these two worlds.

ADDITIONAL RESOURCES

Coffin, B. (April, 2009). The way forward: Rethinking enterprise risk management. *Risk Management (RIMS) 56*.

Porto, G., & Lauve, R. (2006). *Disruptive clinical behavior: A persistent threat to patient safety.* http://www.qrshealthcare.com/PDFs/PSQH3%204_Porto%20Preprint3.pdf. Accessed April 14, 2008.

The Joint Commission. (2008). *Behaviors that undermine a culture of safety.* http://www.jointcommission.org/sentinelevents/sentineleventalert/sea_40.htm. Sentinel Event Alert #40, July 9, 2008. Accessed February 12, 2009.

References

1. Kohn, L., Corrigan, J., & Donaldson M.S. (Eds.). (2000). *To err is human: Building a safer health care system.* Committee on Quality of Health Care in America, Institute of Medicine. Washington, DC: National Academy Press.
2. Ristuccia, H., & Epps, D. (2009, April). Becoming risk intelligent. *Risk Management (RIMS) 56*, 88.
3. Wagner, S., & Layton, M. (2007, August). The two faces of risk. *Deloitte Review*, 71–75.
4. Carroll, R., et al. (2006). *Risk management handbook for health care organizations*, American Hospital Publishing, Edition 5, 1.
5. Reason, J. (1997). *Managing the risks of organizational accidents* (p. 7). Burlington, VA: Ashgate Publishing Company.
6. Roberts, K.H., Madsen, P.M., Desai, V.M., & Van Stralen, D. (2005). A case of the birth and death of a high reliability healthcare organization. *Quality and Safety in Health Care 14*: 216–220.
7. Weick, K.E., & Sutcliffe, K.M. (Eds.). (2007). *Managing the unexpected: What business can learn from high-reliability organizations* (2nd ed.). San Francisco: Wiley & Sons.
8. Weick, K. (2001). *Making sense of the organization.* Malden, MA: Blackwell Publishing.

2

Integrating Risk Management, Quality Management, and Patient Safety into the Organization

Krista M. Curell, JD, BSN

INTRODUCTION

Since the 2000 publication of the Institute of Medicine's report, "To Err Is Human: Building a Safer Health System,"[1] healthcare organizations have recognized the need for robust programs to manage risk and improve the safety and quality of patient care. Because of differences in the underlying culture and the availability of resources, strategies vary widely among institutions. Some organizations, especially larger academic medical centers, have assimilated risk management and quality into their patient safety program, while many others maintain distinct departments. Regardless of the organizational structure, successful institutions encourage close collaboration of all three programs.

Clinicians and administrators from all areas are turning to their quality and risk management departments for assistance in improving clinical practice and organizational systems. External pressures from regulators, payers, and the public are inducing organizations to broaden the scope and complexity of their quality and safety programs and are virtually requiring the incorporation of quality, risk, and safety analyses into all aspects of professional practice. In addition, many national organizations, such as the Agency for Healthcare Research and Quality (AHRQ), and the National Quality Forum (NQF), have specifically focused on projects that demonstrate continued focus on patient safety and quality. Since 2003, The Joint Commission (TJC) has endorsed many specific safe practices (such as use of patient identifiers, use of standardized abbreviations, and improving and standardizing handoff communications) as further defined under their National Patient Safety Goals program and have incorporated them into their accreditation process. TJC continues to expand its requirements related to quality and now also includes broader physician competency and credentialing criteria under its agenda.

Due to these external requirements and the continued threat of discoverability related to peer-review analysis and quality improvement, risk and quality managers remain valuable assets within organizations. The integration and collaboration of risk and quality activities with various key departments will improve patient care and help guarantee implementation of external compliance requirements, while also shielding the institution from discovery requests related to protected documents and data. In addition, recent implementation of the Patient Safety and Quality Improvement Act of 2005[2] also allows for an extension of protection of information gathered in pursuit of patient safety. This act specifically addresses how an organization can utilize a federally qualified external patient safety organization (PSO) both to foster the advancement of knowledge related to patient safety and also to extend the protection of that information. Chapter 8 describes the current thinking regarding how to best use this law to further enhance protection of information gathered in the pursuit of patient safety.

RISK AND QUALITY: THE REQUIRED ALLIANCE AND THE PEER-REVIEW PRIVILEGE

The patient safety movement continues to strengthen the collaboration between risk and quality. Risk managers can ensure a steady flow of information between departments to improve patient care while protecting their institutions from exposure to liability by ensuring applicability of their state's peer-review-privilege statutes. Some states do not have statutes defining a peer-review privilege or refrain from applying existing statutes to medical-malpractice claims;[3] however, if the privilege exists within a jurisdiction, its application to quality and safety analysis is critical to the success of a risk management and patient safety program. Protecting confidential, peer-review data allows an organization to foster a culture that embraces the open exchange of infor-

mation and analysis without fear of medical-malpractice litigation.

The rationale for states' peer-review privilege statutes is to improve healthcare systems and define best-practice recommendations for clinical providers by promoting and protecting candid review of patient care.[4] In many jurisdictions, the documents associated with such a review are shielded from discovery if created, obtained, or used by an applicable committee under the statute, such as a medical-staff quality assurance committee.[4] This review process is routinely recorded for the courts in the form of a privilege log or a signed affidavit, typically drafted by the author of the reports.[3] The organization must also be able to show the date on which the peer-review or quality-assurance activities were initiated.[3] By working closely with their colleagues in the quality department, risk managers can use this peer-review privilege to shield from discovery the results of the quality and safety reviews conducted as part of their investigations into adverse patient-care events.

The medical staff must also be familiar with the privilege statutes and conduct their morbidity and mortality conferences and intradepartmental peer-review analyses in a manner that is covered by the privilege. Specifically, they must understand that merely designating a document as "confidential" or "prepared for quality committee" does not afford protection.[3]

It is imperative that risk and quality managers maintain vigilance throughout the organization to guarantee that processes be conducted within the framework defined by their jurisdiction's peer-review statutes. For example, occurrence reports, intake forms, and patient-complaint letters may not be protected by the peer-review privilege, so the risk manager may want to limit the narrative section on occurrence reports and intake forms and design a parallel process for review and analysis of patient complaints.[5]

COLLABORATION WITH OTHER DEPARTMENTS FOR MONITORING PHYSICIAN COMPETENCY AND CREDENTIALING

Medical Staff and Quality Monitoring

TJC and other national quality and safety organizations have placed stricter requirements on hospitals to include a greater emphasis on physician competency, thereby ensuring safe, quality care. TJC recently expanded several standards governing medical-staff organization to help guide physician practice and credentialing procedures within healthcare organizations. Case law in certain states has reinforced this move and recently expanded the legal risk to a hospital charged with negligence in physician credentialing.[6]

TJC requires the medical staff to be active participants in an organization's quality-monitoring initiatives. Under certain performance-improvement standards, the medical-staff organization is charged with conducting ongoing professional-practice quality evaluations and actively participating in "the measurement, assessment, and improvement" of a variety of quality-care metrics.[7] These metrics include blood utilization, surgical-case review, morbidity and mortality statistics, and operative-procedure outcomes.[7] The specific data-collection requirements compel close coordination between the departments of risk, quality, and medical staff. In addition to these historic standards, TJC now requires a much more vigorous analysis of each provider's care at the time of credentialing and privileging. Organizations are charged with reviewing data and compiling reports specific to individual provider performance for the various credentialing and privileging committees.

Credentialing

To demonstrate that a physician is competent and should be granted certain privileges during the credentialing process, hospitals are now required to collect a more robust set of data focusing on evidence-based guidelines and standards. TJC requires hospitals to demonstrate a physician's competency by looking at key core competencies coupled with requirements for ongoing and focused professional-practice review.[8] To demonstrate general physician competency, TJC encourages accredited organizations to utilize current standards for competency measurement such as those promulgated by the Accreditation Council for Graduate Medical Education in its General Competency requirements (see Table 2–1).

To demonstrate competency, healthcare organizations should focus on common activities and utilize data already collected. Some examples of core-competency criteria are listed in Table 2–2.

According to the Centers for Medicare and Medicaid Services (CMS) and TJC, "core" or "bundled" privileges may be used by a medical-staff organization during the credentialing process; however, the core or bundled privilege must specifically define those activities considered part of the core versus those activities that fall outside of the bundle.[9] The core activities must also reflect activities that are being performed by a majority of the clinicians at the specific organization. Criteria for what constitutes a more specialized privilege should also be defined.[10] The core privilege must be tailored to an individual clinician if issues of competency arise.

To better understand the role that "core privileges" and "bundled privileges" can play in helping to streamline the demand for data now a necessary component of the privilege delineation and recredentialing process, consider the case of a family physician for whom the complicated multipage recredentialing process may be mostly irrelevant to his or her practice. In standard credentialing each item on the form requires a predefined criteria that establishes the qualifications for each item on the list. This process can be overly

Table 2–1 General Competencies

Core Competency	Definition
Patient care	Residents must be able to provide patient care that is compassionate, appropriate, and effective for the treatment of health problems and the promotion of health
Medical/clinical knowledge	Residents must demonstrate knowledge of established and evolving biomedical, clinical, epidemiological, and social-behavioral sciences, as well as the application of this knowledge to patient care.
Practice-based learning and improvement	Residents must demonstrate the ability to investigate and evaluate their care of patients, to appraise and assimilate scientific evidence, and to continuously improve patient care based on constant self-evaluation and lifelong learning. Residents are expected to develop skills and habits to be able to meet the following goals: • identify strengths, deficiencies, and limits in one's knowledge and expertise; • set learning and improvement goals; • identify and perform appropriate learning activities; • systematically analyze practice using quality improvement methods, and implement changes with the goal of practice improvement; • incorporate formative evaluation feedback into daily practice; • locate, appraise, and assimilate evidence from scientific studies related to their patients' health problems; • use information technology to optimize learning; and • participate in the education of patients, families, students, residents and other health professionals.
Interpersonal and communication skills	Residents must demonstrate interpersonal and communication skills that result in the effective exchange of information and collaboration with patients, their families, and health professionals. Residents are expected to: • communicate effectively with patients, families, and the public, as appropriate, across a broad range of socioeconomic and cultural backgrounds; • communicate effectively with physicians, other health professionals, and health-related agencies; • work effectively as a member or leader of a healthcare team or other professional group; • act in a consultative role to other physicians and health professionals; and • maintain comprehensive, timely, and legible medical records, if applicable.

(continues)

Table 2–1 (Continued)

Core Competency	Definition
Professionalism	Residents must demonstrate a commitment to carrying out professional responsibilities and an adherence to ethical principles. Residents are expected to demonstrate: • compassion, integrity, and respect for others; • responsiveness to patient needs that supersedes self-interest; • respect for patient privacy and autonomy; • accountability to patients, society, and the profession; and • sensitivity and responsiveness to a diverse patient population, including but not limited to diversity in gender, age, culture, race, religion, disabilities, and sexual orientation.
Systems-based practice	Residents must demonstrate an awareness of and responsiveness to the larger context and system of health care, as well as the ability to call effectively on other resources in the system to provide optimal health care. Residents are expected to: • work effectively in various healthcare delivery settings and systems relevant to their clinical specialty; • coordinate patient care within the healthcare system relevant to their clinical specialty; • incorporate considerations of cost awareness and risk-benefit analysis in patient and/or population-based care as appropriate; • advocate for quality patient care and optimal patient care systems; • work in interprofessional teams to enhance patient safety and improve patient care quality; and • participate in identifying system errors and implementing potential systems solutions.

Used with permission of Accreditation Counsel for Graduate Medical Education © ACGME 2009 American College of Graduate Medical Education (ACGME) http://www.acgme.org/outcome/comp/General CompetenciesStandards21307.pdf (Accessed March 23, 2010).

complicated and unduly burdensome. Furthermore it may fail to reflect the type of work being performed by the specific provider. In core privileging, the items on the recredentialing list are bundled to reflect those activities commonly performed by the family physician, which is reflective of how family physicians are trained in their accredited residency and more accurately describes what family physicians do. In the case of a family medicine provider, the core privilege might be "to admit, diagnose, and treat children and adults for most injuries and illnesses and to promote health and wellness." The specific activities would then be bundled under this competency. In addition the specific qualification to hold this core of privileges would be the completion of an approved family medicine residency. This would eliminate the need to identify the

Table 2–2 Core-Competency Criteria

Core Competency	Example
Patient care	Peer-review-analysis data
Medical/clinical knowledge	Continuing medical education
Practice-based learning and improvement	Author a book chapter; analyze and report Physician Quality Reporting Initiative (PQRI) data (PQRI is a voluntary program that provides a financial incentive to physicians and other eligible professionals who successfully report quality data related to services provided under the Medicare Physician Fee Schedule [MPFS]).
	The eligible professional should gather three approved measures on at least 80% of appropriate patients and submit the specified quality-data codes for services paid under the MPFS and provided during the reporting period. (Eligible professionals may earn an incentive payment of up to 1.5% of their total allowed charges for MPFS covered professional services furnished during the reporting period.) Participate in teaching rounds. Demonstrate interpersonal and communication skills.
	Participate in Performance Improvement (PI) of a multidisciplinary institutional review board-approved study; serve on a clinical committee; lead a Failure Mode and Effects Analysis (FMEA) or PI project.
Professionalism	Actively participate in a professional society.
Systems-based practice	Participate in annual safety rounds; comply with specific regulatory standards; complete mandatory training programs (e.g., electronic-medical-record training).

hundreds of specific procedures and treatments that might fall under this more general description.

TJC-accredited organizations are also required to complete ongoing and focused professional-practice evaluations to demonstrate that a requesting physician is competent to perform the privilege(s) requested. This requirement applies to new physicians and currently privileged physicians who are requesting new or expanded privileges.[11] The medical-staff organization must also define criteria that trigger further, focused monitoring when questions related to competency or quality of care arise.[12] Often these issues will be flagged by the risk management department conducting their adverse-event case reviews, or by the quality department working with various clinical sections on their

morbidity and mortality case conferences. The criteria for review should be well defined in the organization's bylaws, policies and procedures, or quality plan. Examples of such "focused privileging triggers" can include (1) the incidence of malpractice claims within a defined time period, (2) the required reporting to a state's department of professional regulations, (3) an involvement in a sentinel event, and/or (4) a high incidence of adverse events.

To mitigate the risk of the healthcare organization being sued for negligent credentialing because of these new standards, risk managers are encouraged to work with their medical staff office or entity responsible for granting privileges to providers to ensure that their credentialing and appointment processes meet these new regulatory requirements.

Doctrine of Corporate Negligence

Plaintiffs have put forth the doctrine of corporate negligence to argue their theory of liability against healthcare organizations. To prove this theory, plaintiffs must demonstrate the basic tenets of a negligence claim: duty, breach of duty, causation, and injury. Plaintiffs raising a negligent-credentialing allegation will likely suggest that a hospital failed to follow its credentialing and privileging procedures, defined in its bylaws or applicable policies and procedures, and/or negligently credentialed or granted privileges to an unqualified physician.[13]

Duty

According to the doctrine, a hospital and its medical staff have a duty to exercise reasonable care to confirm that physicians are qualified to perform the privileges requested at the time of hire, during the recredentialing process, and/or when new privileges are requested. If the hospital knew or should have known that a physician was not qualified, and the physician injures a patient through an act of negligence, the hospital can be found separately liable for the negligent credentialing of the physician.[14] To demonstrate that this duty has been met, hospitals should evaluate how their medical staff organization determines privileges and whether they are using core, rather than specialized, privileges.

Breach of Duty

Plaintiffs will argue that a hospital has breached its duty by failing to adopt state licensing requirements and/or accreditation standards, or by failing to follow its own medical-staff bylaws, rules and regulations, or policies and procedures.[15] Examples include reappointing a physician without evaluating quality or performance data related to that physician's practice or the physician's failure to meet the criteria defined for specialized privilege requests. Hospitals also have a duty to review the past malpractice and disciplinary-action data and to monitor more closely physicians who have a "dirty file." These types of files should be referred to the organization's peer-review committee. If the physician is permitted to practice, he or she should undergo a period of focused, professional-practice review.

Causation

Causation may be more difficult to demonstrate in a negligent-credentialing case than in a malpractice claim that asserts negligence. The plaintiff must still prove negligence and that the patient's injury was directly related to the negligence. The plaintiff must also demonstrate that if the hospital had met its duty to perform a proper credentialing review, the physician would not have been granted privileges to perform the type of care that led to the adverse outcome.

Unlike a medical-negligence case, it is difficult to defend against a corporate negligence claim when peer-review data cannot be used to demonstrate compliance with the peer-review analysis conducted as part of the credentialing process.[16] The risk management and legal departments determine whether the jurisdiction's peer-review statutes allow an organization to waive the privilege and produce certain documents normally shielded from discovery in malpractice litigation.[17] Risk managers may consider working jointly with the medical-staff office to develop credentialing documents that are completely transparent, accessible, and separate from for-cause peer-review analysis. Risk managers and attorneys may also consider developing a "red flag" system for use during the credentialing process. These criteria would alert the credentials committee that a physician has a high number of malpractice claims, criminal convictions, sanctions from the department of professional regulation, and/or patient or staff complaints.[17] These "flags" should trigger higher scrutiny of the physician's practice and may appropriately result in a period of focused, professional-practice review. Legal counsel can help hospitals decide whether to make this review process transparent to discovery or perform the type of peer-review analysis typically covered under peer-review privilege statutes.

To avoid a negligent-credentialing claim and demonstrate compliance with regulatory standards during accreditation surveys, it is imperative that an organization's risk and quality departments work closely with the medical-staff office to ensure that the current credentialing process meets these requirements.

EARLY WARNING SIGNS OF POSSIBLE LIABILITY

Patient and family dissatisfaction is often an early indicator of potential litigation or adverse media attention. Ongoing communication between certain departments within an organization may reveal a subtle problem that will prompt the review of a patient's care. A close, collaborative relationship between the risk and quality departments, as well as other departments, such as patient relations/advocacy, billing, the HIPAA office, and medical records, will provide opportunities for quick problem identification and allow for early interventions with patients and family members.

Patient Complaints

A proactive and responsive patient relations office can often intervene early during a patient's hospital stay to counter negative patient, friend, or family impressions of care. Many times, a simple explanation or help in quickly resolving a problem experienced by a patient may be all that is needed to change perceptions and resolve a negative patient experience. Patient-relations specialists are often instrumental in coordinating patient–family conferences with the healthcare team. Such conferences provide open lines of communication between a physician and the patient, helping to adjust unrealistic patient expectations and allay criticism related to patient care. Dissatisfaction can often be

resolved prior to a patient's discharge, but occasionally a patient's or family member's expectations will not be met. Patient or family dissatisfaction is an early indicator of potential liability, regardless of the presence or absence of evidence of negligence.[18] Data sharing between the patient relations office and the risk manager is essential to early liability analysis and possible prevention of litigation.

An organization's billing office is another outlet for patients to voice their concerns related to patient care. Requests for bill adjustments are typically coupled with allegations of inadequate or substandard care. Such complaints should be referred to the risk or quality departments for quality and/or peer-review analysis to trigger the peer-review privilege. Final recommendations related to bill adjustments may be made, but an organization may wish to check with their legal counsel or compliance officer to determine if such recommendations are discoverable under their state peer-review statutes, or subject to different billing practices.

Many hospitals now track patient complaints and trend this data for each healthcare provider. This tactic allows an organization to implement strategies to improve physician–patient relations and strengthen the communication skills of those providers who generate a high number of patient complaints. Early intervention and physician mentoring may help reduce the incidence of malpractice claims.[18]

Medical Records

One of the strongest allies of the risk management department is the medical records department. It supplies the raw material (i.e., the medical-record documentation), and risk and quality managers turn to this department regularly for support and services. Charts are routinely requested for case-review analysis and abstraction, with expedited requests made during times of accreditation surveys and on-site inspections.

The role of this department in identifying adverse events and quality-of-care concerns increased exponentially with the implementation of the CMS "Never Events" legislation in October 2008, which focuses on many hospital-acquired conditions (HAC). Also known as "The Deficit Reduction Act of 2005," it "authorized the Secretary of the Department of Health and Human Services to select conditions that are: (1) high cost, high volume, or both; (2) identified through ICD-9-CM coding for billing purposes as complicating conditions or major complicating conditions that, when present as secondary diagnoses on claims, result in a higher-paying reimbursement code and (3) reasonably preventable through the application of evidence-based guidelines," and refuse to pay for the associated care.[19] The specific conditions that have been identified as preventable and therefore are subject to reduced reimbursement are listed in Table 2–3.

These conditions must be acquired during a patient's hospital stay for the rules related to condition of payment to apply. If an HAC is documented as having been present on admission, the healthcare facility may still apply the secondary billing code to that diagnosis, placing the admission into a higher category of reimbursement. The intent of the new rules is to advance the quality- and safety-improvement initiatives related to these conditions. Coders working in a medical-records department often identify these HACs and initiate a report to the risk and quality departments for peer review and quality analysis

Another early indicator for a potential claim against an institution is a request for medical records, especially by an attorney. Medical-records staff should notify their risk management department upon receipt of such requests.

POST-EVENT MANAGEMENT AND MEDIA RELATIONS

Plaintiffs' attorneys, patients, and family members use public media outlets to voice their dissatisfaction or anger toward individ-

Table 2–3 Selected Healthcare-Acquired Conditions

Foreign object retained after surgery
Air embolism
Blood incompatibility
Pressure ulcers (stages III and IV)
Falls and traumas
Fracture
Dislocation
Intracranial injury
Crushing injury
Burn
Electric shock
Catheter-associated urinary tract infection
Vascular catheter-associated infection
Manifestations of poor glycemic control

ual healthcare providers or institutions. If an institution is provided with an opportunity to respond to an article or media report, the time frame to submit a response can be limited to as little as 30 minutes, and some reporters may ask for an immediate comment. The healthcare organization must be ready to respond immediately. If a risk manager or clinical provider has reason to believe an adverse patient-care event may become a media event, the media relations team should review the details and consider drafting an appropriate response. The risk manager can assist the media relations team by ensuring that the response follows Health Insurance Portability and Accountability Act (HIPAA) rules and regulations. A well-drafted response based on in-depth knowledge of the event is critical.

CONCLUSION

Risk and quality professionals have been key drivers in the national patient safety movement. They have witnessed and embraced the increasing emphasis on patient safety and provider accountability and have incorporated the tenets of this reform into their professional practice. They coordinate their organizations' endeavors to create a culture of safety and collaboration throughout their institutions to implement safety-systems analysis, data collection, and proactive risk-reduction strategies. Through their efforts, organizations will achieve the best practices resulting in innovative and effective safety, quality, and risk management programs.

References

1. Kohn, L., Corrigan, J., & Donaldson, M. (Eds.). (2000). *To err is human: Building a safer health care system.* Committee on Quality of Health Care in America, Institute of Medicine. Washington, DC: National Academy Press.
2. Patient Safety and Quality Improvement Final Rule, 73 Fed. Reg. 70,732 (November 21, 2008) (to be codified at 42 C.F.R. pt. 3). Retrieved March 22, 2010 from http://www.pso.ahrq.gov/regulations/regulations.htm/.
3. Bremer, W.D. (2009). Scope and extent of protection from disclosure of medical peer review proceedings relating to claim in medical malpractice action. Westlaw; 69 American Law Reports 5th 559, p. 18.
4. Ibid, p. 16.
5. Ibid, p. 17.
6. Illinois Hospital Association White Paper. (2009, February). Legal Department. Eliminating negligence in physician credentialing. Frigo v. Silver Cross Hospital and Medical Center, 377 Ill. App. 3d 43, 876 N.E. 2d 697 (1st Dist. 2007); Larson v. Wasemiller (Minnesota Supreme Court, 2007).
7. The Joint Commission. (n.d.). Comprehensive office manual for hospitals: The official handbook. CAMH Refreshed Core, Standard MS.05.01.01, MS-11, 12.
8. The Joint Commission. (n.d.). Comprehensive office manual for hospitals: The official handbook. CAMH Refreshed Core, Standard MS.06.01.01, MS-13 to MS-16.
9. Department of Health and Human Services. (2004, November 12). Ref: S&C-05-04. http://www.jointcommission.org/Accreditation Programs/Hospitals/Standards/09_FAQs/MS/Core_Bundled_Privileges.htm/. Accessed May 23, 2009.
10. Callahan, M. (2008). Negligent credentialing developments: Impact of recent cases and new Joint Commission medical staff standards. Katten, Muchin, Rosenman, LLP, Webinar presentation, April 16, 2008, p. 8.
11. The Joint Commission. (n.d.). Comprehensive office manual for hospitals: The official handbook. CAMH Refreshed Core, Standard MS.08.01.01, MS-22; MS.08.01.03, MS-23.
12. The Joint Commission. (n.d.). Comprehensive office manual for hospitals: The official handbook. CAMH Refreshed Core, MS.08.01.01, MS-23.
13. Illinois Hospital Association White Paper. (February, 2009). Legal Department. Eliminating negligence in physician credentialing. Frigo v. Silver Cross Hospital and Medical Center, 377 Ill. App. 3d 43, 876 N.E. 2d 697 (1st Dist. 2007); Larson v. Wasemiller (Minnesota Supreme Court, 2007), p. 4.
14. Ibid, p. 3; Darling v. Charleston Memorial Hospital, 33 Ill. 2d 326 (1965).
15. Illinois Hospital Association White Paper. (2009, February). Legal Department. Eliminating negligence in physician credentialing. Frigo v. Silver Cross Hospital and Medical Center, 377 Ill. App. 3d 43, 876 N.E. 2d 697 (1st Dist. 2007); Larson v. Wasemiller (Minnesota Supreme Court, 2007), p. 5.
16. Ibid, p. 7.
17. Ibid, p. 10.
18. Hickson, G., Federspiel, C., Pichert, J., Miller, C., Gauld-Jaeger, J., & Bost, P. (2002). Patient complaints and malpractice risk. *Journal of the American Medical Association, 287*(22), 2951–2957.
19. The Deficit Reduction Act of 2005. Retrieved May 28, 2010 from http://edocket.access.gpo.gov/2008/pdf/E8-17914.pdf/.

3

BENCHMARKING IN RISK MANAGEMENT

Barbara J. Youngberg, JD, MSW, BSN, FASHRM

INTRODUCTION

More and more healthcare administrators are demanding accountability for the work performed by department and programmatic managers. As budgets shrink in healthcare organizations, it becomes increasingly important to attempt to quantify the value of the service that each department contributes to the organization. This phenomenon is as true for risk management as it is for any other department within the organization. As risk managers work to quantify the value that they bring to an organization, they must be careful to do so only through the appropriate use of data and by finding effects with clearly attributable causes. As many risk managers are aware, benchmarking can be very difficult in the work they do, because all too often one of the key indicators of risk management success, reduced malpractice costs, can be related more to external factors such as (1) the volatility of the venue or the existence of tort reform where a claim arises, (2) ran-

dom factors, such as whether a claim might be settled due to fear of adverse publicity or fear of a jury failing to understand the legal and medical issues and thus reacting to the emotional issues, or (3) other factors that often make a claim or event unique and likely to not recur.

Developing and maintaining a risk management benchmarking program does not have to cost a lot of money, nor does it need to take a significant amount of time. It does, however, require some preplanning, careful development of the data-collection instrument, and knowledge about what data can and cannot provide in terms of meaningful information. It is also advisable to attempt to determine how the organization believes it will use the information learned from the benchmarking project. In addition, the risk manager and the organization should determine if both internal and external benchmarking projects are likely to provide value, and if external benchmarking is also desired, the risk manager should attempt to find organizations with similar profiles so that the data collected is comparable.

WHAT IS BENCHMARKING?

Many definitions exist for the process of benchmarking. Basically, the risk manager should think of benchmarking as the process of collecting and analyzing data to identify trends in performance and, when compared with other collectors of the same data, identifying best performers and determining if interventions that were introduced to address identified problems yielded the desired results. Risk management benchmarking can be internal or external. The value of each form of benchmarking is different, but so are, in the minds of some people, the risks.

INTERNAL BENCHMARKING

When risk managers use internal benchmarking, they collect only data elements from within their own organization. The data can be analyzed after the first data collection to identify best performers at the unit or department levels. After multiple data-collection cycles, the risk manager can also begin to see trends within the organization indicative of either improvement or deterioration of the risk environment. For many healthcare organizations, internal benchmarking is a low-risk way to analyze what is occurring in the organization and what type of trends are developing. These trends can be linked to the organization changes, such as reengineering or work redesign, which may have an impact on risk. For those risk managers working within a healthcare system, it can provide a way to focus on best performers without risk of exposing the perceived weaknesses of an organization to key competitors. A weakness of this type of benchmarking is that if the organization is doing poorly (or extremely well), there is no way to determine that when there is no comparative data from similar organizations or key com-

petitors. It is possible, however, to set up an internal benchmarking program modeled after another local, regional, or national project by collecting the same data elements. If the results of the other initiatives are published or otherwise available, you can then compare your results with others.

EXTERNAL OR COMPETITIVE BENCHMARKING

External or competitive benchmarking allows risk managers or healthcare organizations to look outside their own setting to identify best performers in the industry. When processes are to be evaluated (e.g., scheduling or billing systems), healthcare organizations may wish to look outside the healthcare industry to identify other service providers who have excelled at the same or similar function (e.g., the hotel industry may be able to provide some insight into the scheduling of guests).

Many organizations are very reluctant to externally benchmark in risk management because of the sensitive nature of much of the information that is to be shared. It is also essential in this form of benchmarking that there be clear definition of all the data elements that are to be collected. From organization to organization, words that seem clear may take on very different meanings, which can distort the results of the benchmarking initiative (e.g., What is a claim? What is a potentially compensable event? What is an incident?). Although there are ways to protect the anonymity of the information, some organizations are still reluctant for fear that their organization may be reflected in a less-than-favorable light. If this is a significant concern, benchmarking participants may wish to have all participants sign confidentiality agreements prior to any data collection or to submit the data anonymously. (It is noteworthy, however, that anonymous data collection can thwart the ability to gain valuable information from those identified as best performers.) In addition, the cost of external benchmarking may be greater than that of internal benchmarking, and the time required to participate may be greater. Notwithstanding these factors, the benefits from external benchmarking can be many, enabling risk managers to look beyond their own environment or style of management to gain new insight.

SELECTING WHAT TO BENCHMARK

It is often difficult for risk managers to select areas to benchmark, particularly when they attempt, through benchmarking, to establish a causal relationship between the proactive strategies practiced by the risk manager (e.g., focused risk management education or proactive risk assessments) and a reduction in claims or lawsuits or dollars paid out to patients for injuries that they may have sustained. Many administrators believe that there should be a relationship between items, and indeed ideally there should be; however, the legal system for malpractice, as it is currently structured, often allows for the recovery of damages in the absence of negligence. Careful removal of outliers (which could be defined as claims in which money was paid in the absence of negligence or awards in excess of an agreed-on amount that might be considered a one-time event) may help to make the comparison more meaningful, but it is the present author's belief that risk managers must take great care in attributing their efforts in education or risk assessment as the reason for a reduction in malpractice claims.

WHAT CAN RISK MANAGERS BENCHMARK?

What can risk managers benchmark? This seems like a fairly simple question, and perhaps the simple answer would be "anything." The reality, however, is that although much of what risk managers do can be evaluated, measured, and compared through systematic data collection and benchmarking, care must

be taken to not collect disparate data elements and draw conclusions from them. Some examples of benchmarking projects in risk management follow.

COMPARATIVE-CLAIMS BENCHMARKING

A number of organizations have designed annual-claims benchmarking initiatives that have grown out of a concern, primarily from medical staff, that they had no meaningful data to help them understand how they (and their organizations) compared with other similar organizations in the area of malpractice claims. The first responsibility in designing the data-collection instrument is to identify important demographic characteristics that enable benchmarking participants to select organizations that truly mirror their own. Having the data also allowed the calculation of mean, median, and average numbers, which for some organizations is useful. Organizations such as the University Health System Consortium in Oak Brook, Illinois, and the insurance brokerage AON working in conjunction with the American Society for Healthcare Risk Management (ASHRM), gather the following types of information to perform their annual analysis:

- Location of organization. (These data were needed to allow for geographic adjustment of financial information collection, which was necessary due to the variability of jurisdictional venues.)
- Number of occupied inpatient beds.
- Number of annual inpatient and outpatient admissions.
- Number of employees (non-physician).
- Number of insured faculty physicians.
- Number of insured residents or house staff.
- General information about the venue, such as existence of tort reform, legislative damage caps, etc., that could influence the ultimate payout for any particular event reported.

Great care must be taken to define terms that are to be used for the purpose of gaining an understanding of the claims activity at each organization. It should be recognized that the definitions agreed on by the benchmarking committee might not be the same as those used by the organizations in their daily work. Organizations must be able to submit data using the agreed-upon definition in order to make the data comparisons meaningful. The claims data collected as part of the benchmarking process are often aggregated to establish rates for the following:

- Number of incidents per year. An incident can be defined as any written or verbal communication to the risk manager that an event has occurred that warrants further investigation. A year could be defined as a fiscal or calendar year but should always represent 12 months of data.
- Number of potentially compensable events. This is defined as incidents that, following a review, the risk manager determines warrant the posting of a reserve.
- Number of claims per year. A claim means simply a demand for money. This demand can come from a patient, family member, or any other person.
- Number of lawsuits per year. This is defined as a case in litigation.
- Number of lawsuits closed per year without a payment made.
- Number of lawsuits closed with a payment made.
- Total dollars reserved and paid for indemnity, which is defined as dollars that might ultimately be paid to the injured party.
- Total dollars reserved and paid for expense, which is defined as any money paid to investigate, develop, or defend a case.
- Number of cases currently reserved or paid, in excess of $1 million, during the

year. The total amount of reserves and/or payments made in these cases is also separately identified. This allows the organization sponsoring the benchmarking initiative to note when an outlier situation skewed the data of a particular organization. (For example, a single claim that may have settled for $10 million when added to the annual totals would greatly skew the data and indeed might not represent activity likely to appear in subsequent claim years. One might want to add the $10 million in with an asterisk that it represented a single claim. Some organizations leave these outlier claim out of the annual totals and note them separately.)

With the collection of those fairly simple data elements, organizations are able to learn a great deal. With a single year of data, all participants should be provided with a summary track and trend for medical-malpractice claims, including the average cost per claim, the percentage of total dollars paid to lawyers as opposed to plaintiffs, and numbers of claims per occupied bed and per insured person. These data, once adjusted, can be very useful to all those who participated and can also help an organization demonstrate the value of their risk management and patient safety programs to external underwriters and actuaries. With multiple-years data analysis, benchmarking organizations can also provide longitudinal data, attempting to track frequency and severity of claims over time. This information is important as the organization develops a long-term strategic risk financing plan.

As with all data-collection projects, it is important for risk managers to understand the importance of "de-identifying" the data in order to protect the privacy of the patients involved. In addition, names of providers should also be removed so as not to make these benchmarking activities appear punitive.

AON is a worldwide insurance brokerage with a large health practice and also partners with ASHRM to produce an annual benchmarking report that utilizes actuarial data drawn from AON's healthcare clients. This benchmarking study is intended to be a way for systems to use the power of aggregated data to provide industry insights and points of comparison for hospital professional liability (HPL) claim costs, whether retained or insured.[1] In 2009 this annual benchmarking study presented the following key findings:

- After seven consecutive years of decreasing frequency, the frequency of HPL claims is increasing.
- Claim severity continues to increase at a consistent 4% annual rate.
- For the 2010 accident year, the study analysts project that hospitals will experience an annual loss cost of $3,170 per occupied-bed equivalent.
- One of every four claims and 24% of total HPL costs are associated with five specific hospital-acquired conditions.
- Frequency, severity, and loss-cost benchmark statistics vary significantly by state.[1]

The drafters of the final report then went into great detail in describing the specific factors that contributed to each of these key findings, and they provided valuable strategic information to assist risk managers not only regarding their claims-management responsibilities but also in terms of where to focus patient safety efforts.

ROLE OF PROACTIVE RISK MANAGEMENT IN EARLY IDENTIFICATION OF CLAIMS

In this type of benchmarking analysis, the risk managers may wish to identify which claims or suits they knew about before there was an actual demand for money by an injured person. The presumption is that if risk managers learn early about a potential claim or suit immediately after the potential

incident giving rise to injury occurs, they can investigate while the information is fresh and intervene perhaps by developing strategies such as bill write-offs. It is believed by many people that using these strategies can decrease the likelihood that a claim or suit will ever be filed. Although this intuitively seems to be correct, it is noteworthy that even early intervention can result in enormous verdicts and/or settlements. In one of the key findings of the AON benchmarking study, it was noted that five specific hospital-acquired conditions contributed to roughly 25% of the events and 25% of dollars spent on claims. These hospital-acquired conditions were identified as follows:[1]

- Hospital-acquired infections
- Hospital-acquired injuries (fractures, burns, intracranial injury, crushing injuries, etc.)
- Medication errors in hospital
- Objects left in surgery
- Pressure ulcers

It is easy to see how a risk manager, by utilizing this type of information from a claims benchmarking study, can begin to focus on strategically important patient safety initiatives.

ROLE OF RISK MANAGEMENT EDUCATION AS A STRATEGY TO MINIMIZE CLAIMS

Although risk managers would like to be able to show that their efforts in fostering risk management education throughout the organization will have a positive impact on claims, often those staff who willingly attend risk management education programs might not be those responsible for the greatest number or most significant claims; thus, by attempting to prove that individuals who receive risk management education are less likely to be sued, one might only be capturing data on the already low-risk populations. In addition, attendance at an educational program does not guarantee incorporation of the knowledge gained into actual practice, so ideally, the risk manager should attempt to tie education efforts to actual change in practice patterns that had previously been identified as problematic. This will be a far better measure of risk management success than merely presenting the number of educational sessions held or the numbers of those in attendance.

BEGINNING THE BENCHMARKING PROJECT

Once an acceptable data-collection instrument has been developed, it should be distributed to all people who express an interest in participating. If there is the need for confidentiality agreements to be signed, they should be sent out with the data-collection instrument. A specified due date should be set so that analysis of data can be performed following assurance that all people who wish to participate have submitted their data.

The Data

The person analyzing the data should initially evaluate the data by using a series of edit checks, which can assist in identifying data that seem incorrect. Any concerns in this area should be checked with the persons submitting the data to determine their correct interpretation of the question and the correctness of the data.

Aggregating and Analyzing the Results

Prior to beginning the analysis, the analysts should have an understanding of the type of report or analysis that the participants expect. An agreement should be established regarding the types of graphics and relationships, if any, that will be established, and conclusions, if any, that will be drawn. A sample report may be provided to some or all members of the project to confirm that the analysis is proceeding as anticipated.

Applying the Results

If the project incorporates data from many different sites, it might also be helpful to ask the best performers to include examples of the operational policies in place or the changes they made in a process that led to their achievement. These types of examples can be very helpful in demonstrating the type of changes that might be necessary to yield the desired results. These follow-up activities can often be more valuable than the data-intensive reports themselves.

PREREQUISITES FOR SUCCESS

Organizational Support

As with any other labor- and data-intensive initiative, members of the organization must be interested in the project and be convinced that the results will assist them in gaining a better understanding of their own operations. Going into a benchmarking study with the organizational leadership already convinced that their organization is so different from others that data comparability will be impossible will probably not result in much value. Also, having the organization's guarantee in advance that they will commit the leadership required to initiate and support changes that are deemed necessary will ensure that the benchmarking initiative will yield more than academic interest—an important factor for the already overworked risk manager.

Preexisting Commitment to Change

It is helpful to know that the organization is willing and able to make the changes that might be identified. Define the objectives and the actions, as well as the financial commitment, that might be necessary to address problems. In addition, gaining support from all key personnel who might be affected by the changes will also help to ensure that the time committed to the benchmarking initiative yields valuable results.

CONCLUSION

Benchmarking in risk management can be both a challenging and exciting activity, yielding valuable information that can provide important direction to the organization's risk managers as they attempt to prioritize the many activities that are part of their role. Learning from others about strategies that have yielded favorable results elsewhere can also eliminate the trial-and-error method of achieving and sustaining positive results.

Reference

1. Johnson, E., & Coleianne, C. (2009). *2009 Aon/ASHRM hospital professional liability benchmark analysis.* ASHRM conference, Denver, October 22–25, 2009.

4

RISK MANAGEMENT STRATEGIC PLANNING FOR A CHANGED HEALTHCARE DELIVERY SYSTEM

A. Michelle Kuhn, BA
Barbara J. Youngberg, JD, MSW, BSN, FASHRM

INTRODUCTION

Strategic planning is an organized process that is used to define long-term goals and methods for achieving those goals. Lewis Carroll, in his classic book, *Alice in Wonderland,* wrote that "if you don't know where you're going, any road will get you there." This might be true in fantasy, but in health care it is essential that the risk manager attempt to understand the past, define the future, and then capitalize on the skills already developed to move the organization or system in the direction of success and prosperity.

The risk management professional must know how healthcare reform and healthcare financing is proceeding in order to map out a strategy for risk management and patient safety. With the changes in the healthcare field and the current focus on patient safety, the field of healthcare risk management must also change, and the risk management professional should consider this transition and move with it or, optimally, lead the way. To develop a strategic plan, risk managers must consider what changes have occurred and/or are projected for the organization or system in which they work. Next, the risk manager needs to carefully evaluate existing strengths and weaknesses within the organization and determine how those factors will impact the changes that must be made in order to successfully manage the new challenges.

Probably the most significant change in health care is the change in focus that has occurred following the release of the Institute of Medicine (IOM) report, "To Err Is Human: Building a Safer Health System,"[1] which has forced healthcare organizations to acknowledge the many systemic causes of error and to create a new culture for addressing them. In addition, the government's focus on quality and the need to better manage hospital-acquired conditions—or suffer adverse economic consequences—has created a challenge for leaders to see quality, error reduction, and patient safety in a new business light. Because this current delivery system includes affiliations, alliances, and various other legal relationships with physician groups, community hospitals, extended-care facilities, durable medical equipment manufacturers and suppliers, home health agencies, and clinics, the need to also manage this care across the continuum has become essential but complex. These specific changes make it necessary for risk management to look at an expanded number of risk management issues and to shift the focus from the individuals involved in errors to the complex and often chaotic systems in which those individuals work. The risk manager, who possesses technical skills as well as conceptual skills, can use the same processes that were used to assess the traditional individual-generated error in the inpatient setting in order to gain an understanding of the systemic risks across the continuum, and can model new tools after existing tools that have proven effectiveness. The process, once developed, should be shared with all components of the healthcare delivery system and all members of the team who must come together to provide safe and effective care. This might include administration, physicians, nurses, allied health professional staff, consumers, and the governing board.

The risk manager must change the focus of the risk management process from reactive to proactive and from individual to systems focused if it is to survive. In the *Essentials of Managed Health Care* handbook, Kongstvedt states that "ideally, risk management should be concerned with identifying and eliminating potential risks. In the reality of everyday crises, however, its function has been to minimize undesirable consequences of already identified adverse occurrences. . . . As such, although its contribution to reducing legal and marketing exposure is clear, its contribution to quality assurance is too little and too late."[2] In addition, reports about the continued prevalence of errors in health care would suggest that our current strategies for managing risk and successfully integrating its

concepts into those advanced by performance improvement and patient safety have yet to achieve maximum effectiveness.

In an effort to respond to market needs to manage care (and risks) across the continuum, organizations must begin to recognize the substantial benefit that risk management can contribute. Risk managers' already well-honed technical skills in risk identification, risk finance, and risk transfer, as well as their well-developed interpersonal and communication skills, position them well to contribute to this new type of delivery model and to this enhanced understanding of the systemic vulnerabilities giving rise to errors.

DEVELOPING A PLANNING MODEL

In this chapter we provide a methodological approach to developing a road map for risk management success and, ultimately, organizational success. We develop a conceptual model (Figure 4–1) that builds on critical factors for success and that will enable the organization to plan for changes in staffing, thinking, and prioritization relative to the risks that could be created as different delivery models emerge. We provide a model strategic plan, which we believe is appropriate for the types of organizations in which many risk managers work. We encourage readers, given the following definitions, to revise the plan to make it more appropriate for their organizations. The plan, once developed, should be shared with administrators and clinicians for approval, and each should understand not only the goals of risk management but also the strategies that will enable those goals to be achieved.

To facilitate the planning process, it is important to understand the following terms:

- Critical success factor is an activity or focus that, if achieved, would significantly improve the prospects for organizational success. Critical success factors are the foundation of the goals, objectives, and strategic initiatives. Although

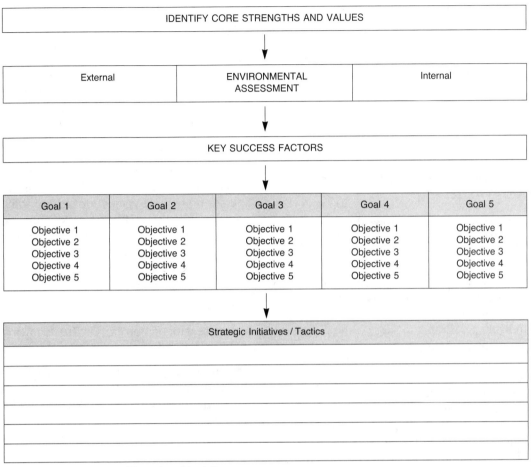

FIGURE 4–1 Strategic Planning Model

they should be developed to reflect the risk management role in organizational success, they should dovetail with the mission, values, and strategic plan for the organization, and with the patient safety and quality goals that the organization has established to comply with external mandates and to demonstrate best practice to competitors. In this chapter we select organizational critical success factors for risk management, recognizing that the risk management strategic plan will only be of value if it identifies organizational, as opposed to departmental, issues and solutions.

- Goals are defined as statements that describe what the risk manager wants to achieve or create. The intent is to work toward the achievement of the goals, recognizing that fully achieving them might be impossible. It might be necessary to work as a team with other departments to achieve goals or to maximize their effectiveness.
- Objectives are statements that help to measure movement toward or away from a goal during a specific time frame. They are directly linked to measuring progress on a specific goal and to the outcomes of implementing various strategies.

- Strategic initiatives help to achieve a critical success factor in a way that fits with multiple goals and objectives. Tactics are specific, easily identified activities that support the strategic initiatives. Each of these elements can be shared by multiple professionals in the organization or can be specifically related to a particular facility, department, or discipline.

IDENTIFICATION OF CORE STRENGTHS AND VALUES

Analysis of Departmental Strengths and Weaknesses

Prior to beginning any strategic planning process, the risk manager should carefully and honestly evaluate the current strengths and weaknesses of the department and the individuals working to support the risk management program in the organization. The commitment of the senior leadership team to the risk management process should also be assessed. Since patient safety is such an essential component of risk management, the risk manager should determine if and where other safety-oriented functions are occurring and how the risk department can work collaboratively to maximize the effectiveness of all patient safety efforts. The reporting structure of risk management in the organization and the departments that work collaboratively with risk management must also be evaluated. We provide a sample analysis of the strengths, weaknesses, opportunities, and threats for a risk management department (Figure 4–2). The risk manager, on completing the departmental review, should also identify where else in the organization activities occur that support the risk management and patient safety functions. This will be helpful as the process moves forward, as it will enable the developer of the plan to determine if the current department or organizational structure will indeed be able to make the

changes necessary to ensure desired results. although risk managers possess many unique and beneficial skills, it might be necessary that they learn new skills (such as those related to human factors and organizational development) in order to maximize their success.

Analyzing the current risk manager's function and the core strengths and values of the profession allowed us to identify some core sets of skills currently well developed within the healthcare risk management profession. The strengths and values most commonly used by today's healthcare risk manager, although they may not be present in every risk management department, include risk assessment, risk finance, and risk or loss control.

Risk Assessment

Risk assessment comprises the following abilities:

1. To assess particular environments and situations that pose a threat of risk to patients, healthcare providers, or the organization
2. To understand the root-cause-analysis process in order to identify the true systemic components contributing to risk
3. To use data to estimate the economic value to the risks assessed, and to minimize existing risks

Risk Finance

Risk finance comprises the following abilities:

1. To evaluate a variety of commercial insurance products to determine which is most appropriate for the risks assessed
2. To analyze the capability of the organization to assume some of the financial risk and transfer the rest in a manner that allows for the most sound financial portfolio for the organization

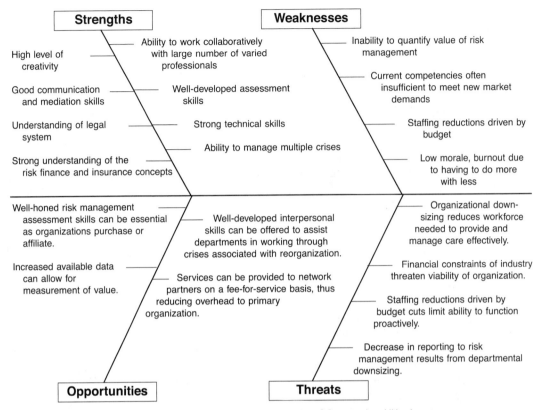

FIGURE 4–2 Risk Management Department—Analysis of Strengths, Weaknesses, Opportunities, and Threats

Risk Control

Risk control comprises the following abilities:

1. To design unique and creative approaches to minimizing the risks that are identified
2. To relate to multiple persons through education to ensure that all who contribute to the organization understand key risk management and patient safety concepts
3. To understand the legal process and to assist in achieving the most favorable resolution of a claim or incident

ASSESSING THE ENVIRONMENT

As the risk manager continues with the strategic planning process, it should be rec-ognized that past and present skills and services may not fully meet the needs of the organization in the future healthcare environment. Assessing the environment should be the next process, prior to beginning to formulate the actual plan. When performing this assessment, the risk manager should focus on both the external and internal environments; both will be essential in understanding the future challenges, and both are also in a period of enormous change.

Analysis of the Internal Environment

There are profound changes taking place, which already have fundamentally altered the way healthcare services are provided in the United States, and there is little disagreement that more changes are on the way.

Some people believe that the healthcare reform bill, which was signed by President Obama, will result in transformational change not only as related to issues of access and finance, but also as pertains to quality, efficiency, and safety. Other people would argue that discussion of healthcare reform might have accelerated change, but that change was inevitable and was already occurring in a number of settings and through the implementation of a number of organizational changes, particularly following the release of the IOM report.

In the late 1980s, healthcare administrators began studying the methods that industry had used to reduce operational over-head. Total quality management and continuous quality-improvement methods, which included a detailed analysis of the process of care and the variability in providing care, led a number of organizations to restructure themselves. Through this process, an array of customers were identified, each presenting with unique needs and challenges. As revenue plummeted in the early 1990s, restructuring of the organization included (1) reduction of the many layers of management previously found in the healthcare organization and (2) the mandate that departments be able to collect and analyze data showing the contribution that their efforts made to the hospital bottom line.

In the late 1990s a series of groundbreaking reports released from the Institute of Medicine[1,3] suggested not only that the delivery of health care was inherently unsafe, but also that the systems in which care was been delivered needed to be dramatically changed in order to deliver on the promise of quality health care into the future. These reports challenged providers and administrators to think differently about the environment in which care was delivered and the culture that often served to thwart innovation, accountability, and change.

Acute-care hospitals, the foundation of the traditional healthcare delivery system (and generally self-sufficient entities), began to question their ability to safely provide the full range of services requested by payers across the continuum and began to explore becoming either a "hub" or a "spoke" of an integrated delivery network. This expansion activity has created many new risks for the organization. In addition, it has moved the risk management function from one that was centralized and well defined to one that is decentralized and requires the delegation of duties and the education and training of all persons to recognize and manage risks and advance a culture of safety in their own environments.

Many risk managers struggled as they attempted to quantify the value of the service they provided, while many others, lacking the skill to process and analyze data and to uncover the true root cause of an event, were having an even more difficult time forecasting the future. In addition, risk managers had to determine how, and if, to protect data that they were collecting from payers and the public.

Exhibit 4–1 lists the major changes that might be evident in the internal environment.

Analysis of the External Environment

The external healthcare environment is also undergoing profound changes. Many of the changes most obvious to the healthcare risk manager can be addressed and managed with the skills that risk managers currently use to handle risks in the internal environment. Some of the risks created by managing complex care across the continuum are the same as those posed in the hospital setting. The challenge that risk managers face is identifying the potential for risk as delivery systems take shape, and making changes so that there are no adverse occurrences. This risk identification must take place (1) before there is a patient injury or patient-related incident, (2) definitely before the risk manager receives notice of a lawsuit, or (3) when the risk manager learns that a lawsuit has

Exhibit 4–1 Internal Environmental Assessment

From:	*To:*
Focus on acute-care hospital	Part of an integrated delivery system or network
Focus on clinical risk	Increasingly complicated with diverse risks
Focus on patients as customers	Many customers identified
Risks contained within single entities	Risks extremely varied and increasingly complex
Reactive approach	Proactive approach
Multiple managers with autonomy	Streamlined individual management with shared responsibility
Focus on individual incidents and the individuals involved in the incidents	Focus on systemic failures as the root cause of error and of the accountability of individuals working in those complex, vulnerable systems
Data generated for internal use	Risk management data provided to payers and consumers
Risk management activities centralized and well defined	Risk management activities shared or delegated
Monopolistic	Focus on free market
Volume-driven staffing	Organization streamlined by function
Internal stability	Chaotic environment with multiple changes
Physician driven	Market driven
Professional roles clearly defined	Roles of healthcare professionals blurred by multi-disciplinary and cross-function training

been filed against an entity now owned or managed by the risk manager's organization, for which there is no coverage. This proactive approach has been evolving in risk management, but it must now be accelerated to keep pace with the rapidly evolving environments where complex care is provided.

In addition, emerging financial pressures arise from the restricted payment now being offered by payers for the hospital-acquired conditions frequently referred to as "never events." The Center for Medicare and Medicaid Services (CMS) has now devised a policy whereby hospitals will no longer be reimbursed for so-called never events. Never events are rare medical errors such as surgery performed on the wrong body part, leaving a foreign object inside a patient after surgery, or an infant discharged to the wrong

person. They are clearly identifiable, largely preventable, and serious in their consequences. Many such events have, coincidentally, long been on the risk manager's radar screen, and they often require immediate notification to the liability insurance carrier.[4] This program is described in greater detail in Chapter 7. Risk managers should be familiar with the list of never events, because these types of occurrences, when managed correctly, can demonstrate the business case for risk management and patient safety.

Exhibit 4–2 lists the major changes evident in the external environment.

Other chapters in this book address specific and significant root causes of error that have been identified as significant systemic issues that are often present when errors are classified as equally often identifiable in

Exhibit 4–2 External Environmental Assessment

From:	To:
Managing episodes of care	Managing care across the continuum
Managing illness	Promoting health
Primary risk of clinical exposure	Organizations at significant financial risk due to changes in payment, including denial of payment for "never events"
Appropriate care determined and quality defined by providers	Reimbursable care and definition of quality determined by payers and legislators
Ethical decisions regarding health care made by hospitals and providers	Ethical standards set by consumers and various legislators
"Hospital-contained" risks	Risks prevalent in many settings, varied, and unique
Risk management reliant on conceptual and philosophical skills	Risk management requiring enhanced technical and theoretical skills while retaining interpersonal and communication skills
Privileged data not shared	Data widely shared

almost every aspect of our healthcare delivery system. We suggest that these chapters be reviewed prior to beginning the organization's strategic plan.

KEY SUCCESS FACTORS FOR RISK MANAGEMENT

Key success factors for risk management in the new healthcare environment, for organizations seeking to provide care across the continuum, include the following:

- Develop a systematic process for proactively identifying the nature and severity of risks created or acquired through the expansion into diverse healthcare services that manage a patient population well beyond the inpatient experience
- Determine the risk tolerance of the organization, and design the most advantageous risk-transfer and risk-sharing program to minimize dependence of fragile insurance and financial markets
- Develop a strategy for managing and controlling the systemic clinical, administrative, and contractual liabilities aris-

ing out of delivering care in the changing healthcare environment
- Develop and provide innovative strategies and tools that will contribute to improvement of patient care and service
- Develop a system for collecting risk management information in a manner that will be beneficial for benchmarking and strategic planning

GOALS

Goals that have been identified as supporting the critical success factors for healthcare organizations to provide care to patients across the continuum include the following:

- To develop a comprehensive methodology for identifying and managing the multiple systemic factors that cause or contribute to risks associated with managing patient care across the continuum
- To be positioned to accept appropriate levels of financial risk and become less reliant on the turbulent financial and insurance markets

- To have achieved a leadership position within the healthcare delivery system through development of creative and comprehensive risk management programs and services that focus on system support and provider accountability
- To foster systemic mindfulness by creating a nonpunitive accountable culture where information about errors is shared to enhance learning and drive change
- To set the standard for defining rational, ethical, and safe use of all technology and service

Goal 1

Goal 1 is to develop a comprehensive methodology for identifying and managing the multiple systemic risks associated with managing complex care across the continuum. The objectives of goal 1 are as follows:

1. The number of members in the organization that have access to a risk-assessment tool, enabling the members to understand the nature of the risk associated with their specific operation, increases.
2. The number of proactive risk assessments performed on specific aspects of the healthcare enterprise increases annually.
3. The number of consults requested of the risk manager by department heads and chiefs of service increases.
4. The number of lawsuits received by risk management without prior notice from the healthcare organization of a potential problem annually decreases.
5. The number of contracts reviewed by the risk manager prior to their being signed increases.

Goal 2

Goal 2 is to be positioned to accept appropriate levels of financial risk and become less reliant on the turbulent financial and insurance markets. The objectives of goal 2 are as follows:

1. The risk manager identifies appropriate external service providers and drafts a clear risk financing strategy prior to beginning the annual renewal process.
2. The risk manager works with the chief financial officer to determine the level of loss that the organization can comfortably retain.
3. The maximum potential loss per year is greater than the actual loss.
4. The risk manager completes a due diligence to determine the risk potential of all new and anticipated business ventures prior to the annual renewal period.

Goal 3

Goal 3 is to achieve a leadership position within the healthcare delivery system through development of creative and comprehensive risk management programs and services that focus on system support and provider accountability. The objectives of goal 3 are as follows:

1. The number of physicians actively engaged in risk management and patient safety activities increases.
2. Systemic mindfulness is evident by an increase in near-miss events, which detail the active recovery of staff intervention that served to intercept the potential error, reported to risk management.
3. The number of early-resolution strategies implemented increases as the number of adverse occurrences decreases.
4. Systems to measure numbers of actions taken and the effectiveness of those actions reveal a decrease in claims (both frequency and severity) when early interventions occur.

Goal 4

Goal 4 is to foster systemic mindfulness by creating a nonpunitive accountable culture where information about errors is shared to enhance learning and drive change. The objectives of goal 4 are as follows:

1. The number of entities within the healthcare system that are provided with risk-benchmarking data increases annually.
2. The organization willingly participates in external-benchmarking collaboratives and increasingly is identified as a "best performer."

Goal 5

Goal 5 is to promote a process that supports and monitors rational, ethical, and safe practices, as well as the appropriate use of technology. The objectives of goal 5 are as follows:

1. The number of ethical consults in which risk management participates increases annually.
2. The number of protocols that define rational usage of new technology prior to the purchase of new equipment increases annually.
3. The number of denials for inappropriate use of technology decreases annually.
4. The number of lawsuits that include allegations of unethical, inequitable treatment or denial of care based on a patient's gender, race, or ability to pay decreases annually (or stays at zero).

RISK MANAGEMENT STRATEGIC INITIATIVES AND TACTICS

The actions described in this section will assist risk managers in accomplishing the previously defined goals, objectives, and critical success factors.

First Strategic Initiative

The first strategic initiative is to develop and implement a set of services that will support the organization's ability to manage the risks of patients across the continuum. The tactics are as follows:

- Hire appropriate staff or train existing staff to ensure that they will be effective in their new roles and with the addition of new areas of responsibility in their understanding of human factors and systemic factors that contribute to error.
- Provide services or develop "how to" manuals to help all partners of the healthcare system to proactively identify and manage the risks associated with their individual settings.
- Design and offer educational opportunities for all health system participants to help avoid activities that would place the entire organization at risk.
- Design a system that monitors the involvement of risk management and patient safety prior to the addition of new risks to the organization, and that issues alerts to those who proceed to add new risks prior to completion of a risk assessment.
- Develop a system for benchmarking the best practices for managing risk and advancing safe practices, as developed by participants of the healthcare organization.

Second Strategic Initiative

The second strategic initiative is to assist the organization in its ability to collect, analyze, and report information that will enable it to identify, analyze, quantify, and control risk, and to advance a culture of safety. The tactics are as follows:

- Develop an understanding of the reports currently produced, and identify those that will assist in the assessment of financial risk to the healthcare organization
- Identify outside firms or consultants who can provide expertise and identify benchmarks for financial performance and assumption of risk

Third Strategic Initiative

The third strategic initiative is to assist the organization in identifying the appropriate markets and products that can be used to transfer the risks associated with the healthcare organization's business to a third-party partner. The tactics are as follows:

- Develop a set of criteria for determining appropriate companies to which the organization's financial risk might be transferred.
- Work with the hospital finance department to determine patient-care services that might be impacted by the payer's "never events" policy and determine the amount of dollars "at risk."
- Analyze current insurance agreements and determine if terms and conditions are appropriate, given the risks assumed by the healthcare organization.
- Negotiate with the carrier to automatically add new risks to the contract, with the understanding that an additional premium can be assessed later, if necessary.
- Develop a relationship with the carrier that allows the health system to recognize economies of scale by designing an insurance program that is tailored to the needs of the entire enterprise.
- Continually assess the risk tolerance of the healthcare organization and determine the appropriate amount of risk to be assumed versus the amount to be transferred.

Fourth Strategic Initiative

The fourth strategic initiative is to expand programs and services that help to identify new areas of risk created by all aspects of the healthcare system's operation. The tactics are as follows:

- Monitor legislative and regulatory changes that could impact the organization, and design educational programs that alert staff to these changes and teach them how to stay in compliance.
- Meet regularly with staff at various healthcare system partners to determine what their assessment and educational needs are relative to risk management and patient safety.

Fifth Strategic Initiative

The fifth strategic initiative is to develop and implement a set of services that assist members of the healthcare organization to manage clinical and financial risk. The tactics are as follows:

- Hire appropriate staff or offer additional training to existing personnel, as needed, to support risk management and patient safety across all aspects of the healthcare system.
- Invest responsibilities in existing personnel to support risk management and patient safety initiatives.
- Acquire appropriate risk management information systems to support tracking and trending of risk management data and analysis of financial exposures associated with those risks identified. Segregate patient safety data from risk management data as appropriate to maximize protection of information.
- Develop tools or "how to" manuals to help members of the healthcare system to recognize and manage their unique risks.
- Evaluate existing insurance clauses included in managed-care contracts, identify coverage triggers, and assist integrated delivery system (IDS) members in development of a system to increase claims reporting.

CONCLUSION

In this period of turbulence in health care in general and risk management and patient safety in particular, it is critically important for the risk manager to determine how the well-developed strengths of risk management can be integrated with principles of patient safety to guide the organization into the future. The model presented in this chapter for planning for the future can be used as a general guide, and many of the key success factors, goals, objectives, initiatives, and tactics may be transferable to a number of environments. They should not, however, be universally adopted until there has been a determination that they are consistent with the thorough assessment of the environment as described in this chapter.

References

1. Kohn, L., Corrigan, J., & Donaldson, M. (Eds.). (2000). *To err is human: Building a safer health care system.* Committee on Quality of Health Care in America, Institute of Medicine. Washington, DC: National Academy Press.
2. Kongstvedt, P.R. (1995). *Essentials of managed health care.* Gaithersburg, MD: Aspen Publishers.
3. Institute of Medicine. (2001). *Crossing the quality chasm: A new health system for the 21st century.* Committee of Quality of Healthcare in America, Institute of Medicine. Washington, DC: National Academy Press.
4. The Leapfrog Group. (2006). *Call for hospitals to commit to new policy on health care "never events."* Retrieved from http://www.leapfrog group.org/media/file/never_events_release _final.pdf/.

5

SETTING UP A RISK MANAGEMENT DEPARTMENT

Barbara J. Youngberg, JD, MSW, BSN, FASHRM
Thomas V. Ealy, MBA

INTRODUCTION

Much has been written about the necessity of analyzing carefully the needs of an institution or healthcare organization before determining the configuration, goals, and organizational structure of a risk management department and the services that the department will offer. Important considerations, such as the role the risk manager will play in the institution or system, the interface and support the risk manager will receive from other organization departments, the integration the risk management department will have with patient safety and performance improvement efforts, and the outside support provided to the risk manager and staff, will influence hiring requirements, program support, and program design.

RISK MANAGEMENT IDENTIFICATION

The purpose of this chapter is (1) to assist the reader in identifying activities that are typi-

cally considered part of the risk management function and are aligned to the three primary functions of risk management as already discussed in previous chapters, (2) to assist in organizing a risk management department that will appropriately interface with the organization, and (3) to determine how best to communicate the risk management function to senior leadership.

In determining the functions that should come under the purview of a risk management department, it is essential to analyze each suggested function and ask the following questions:

- Is this a function necessary or appropriate for the successful control of risk and advancement of safe practices at this organization or system?
- Is this function already being handled by another department within the organization or system? If so, which department is most appropriate for handling this responsibility?

- Are outside consultants performing any or all of the work described in this function?
- If outside firms or consultants are being used, is this the most effective, efficient, and cost-effective method for providing this service?
- What would be the possible negative repercussions of placing this function under the risk management program?
- What would be the benefits of placing this function under risk management?
- What type of risk management staff is needed to support this function?

FUNCTIONS OF RISK MANAGEMENT

Insurance Purchasing and Risk Financing

The early theories of risk management are derived from an insurance framework in which risks are transferred through the purchase of insurance or the self-funding of a trust or other risk financing vehicle. Risk managers were often assigned the responsibility of working with insurance brokers to identify and analyze the available commercial products that would best meet the needs of their organizations. In addition, they also worked with actuaries, financial analysts, and underwriters to assure that the structure selected by the organization protected the organization from an unanticipated catastrophic loss. Risk managers also had the responsibility of presenting the risks of the organization in such a way that the underwriter could correctly analyze the risks to be insured. With changes in the insurance marketplace, many risk managers now also have been required to analyze the alternatives to the purchase of commercial insurance, strategize with the organization's chief financial officer, and work with independent actuaries to determine which structural alternatives are best suited to the organization and its risks and the level of risk to retain to provide the greatest protection at the least cost to the insured. Often, a large hospital with formal self-insurance and off-shore captive programs may find that it needs additional staff to run what is in essence a small insurance company for the organization or system.

The risk manager is often expected to analyze the exposures (and the dollars associated with them) for each of the high-risk clinical specialties within the hospital and must be familiar with its historical loss-payout data. Risk financing requires much more than a retrospective cost analysis. At the very least, an active risk management program should have input into financial decisions as they relate to the funding of risk. The risk manager's insight into faculty and staff, high-risk procedures, and claims history is an invaluable addition to this process.

In addition, the risk manager must receive input from others to assess the potential of financial risk associated with other exposures more closely related to management of the organization. These exposures include workers' compensation, directors' and officers' liability, errors and omissions, property insurance, and auto and aircraft coverage. Securing coverage for these exposures may also be part of the risk manager's responsibility.

A healthcare organization or system that follows the more traditional approach of purchasing commercial insurance should evaluate the services supplied by a carrier or broker and hire risk management staff to support, but not duplicate, the services required. These services may include the following:

- Computer support and data and benchmarking services
- Technical coverage and policy determinations
- Assistance with allocation of premium across all insured entities
- Management of trust assets
- Investment or financial modeling of assets and potential liabilities
- Solvency review of carriers

The functions identified require a high level of specialized skill and many of them are best handled through a partnership between the financial officer and the risk manager of the organization and external service providers.

The section that follows in this book describes the risk financing process and the partnership with external service providers in detail.

Claims Handling

The handling of actual and potential lawsuits is frequently assigned to the organization's risk management department. If in-house legal counsel is employed by the organization, they may also perform or share this responsibility. Although these services are often available through the organization's liability carrier, there are many advantages to having this function managed within the organization. They include the following:

- The level of comfort among staff members involved in actual or potential lawsuits is generally greater when they deal with familiar persons who have the best interests of the organization and its staff in mind when managing claims; thus, an organization or system risk manager may be able to elicit more candid and forthright comments about the care rendered than an outside claims adjuster.
- Clinical staff involved in the claims process can conduct a more thorough evaluation of issues that are related to the standard of medical and nursing care rendered in a case and can better understand the systemic factors that may have given rise to the injury.
- The organization's staff is generally committed to fostering the concept of transparency and recognizing the importance of early investigation to determine if an error was made and, if so, to acknowledging it and working to resolve the matter fairly and in a non-adversarial manner.

- Internal staff may also be in a better position to support the caregivers involved in error and to make certain that they get the help they need to overcome the anxiety of being involved in a harmful event.
- The costs of evaluation and defense are generally less if the bulk of investigations and evaluations occur internally and if the organization supports early intervention when an investigation reveals negligence.

Efficient claims handling requires considerable staff expertise. If risk management is in charge of this function, the staff must have a thorough knowledge of the legal environment in which claims will be managed. Staff members also should have a working knowledge of the clinical issues relating to alleged injuries so that they can interpret the standard of care and proximate causation. When the risk manager does not have this information, he or she must have access to a committee or list of practitioners within the hospital who can provide this assistance. The risk manager also must be familiar with the legal system and understand the process that takes place when a lawsuit is filed. This part of the function may be assumed by outside adjusters or defense counsel or performed by a claims-handling service; however, the organization's administration must carefully weigh the costs against the benefits if claims handling is not one of the risk manager's responsibilities.

Proactive Clinical Risk Management and Patient Safety Support

Risk management programs often take a more proactive approach to the risk environment and focus both on the individuals involved with delivering care and the systems in which they work. Integrating various aspects of risk management with those of quality assurance or performance improvement, patient safety, and credentialing has allowed risk managers to identify and manage the environment of the clinical areas where losses occur and to analyze specific behaviors (human factors) and practices (task factors) that frequently result in injury and litigation. The risk manager can then develop educational programs that will increase sensitivity to risk and more readily enable the staff to identify potential threats to the hospital and its personnel and to actively work to remediate them. (The final section of this book provides in great detail the many specific aspects of this function and the skills needed to create high reliability and to promote a culture of safety.)

A proactive risk management program looks at safety-related issues and works diligently with physicians and other clinicians to help them understand the risk management process and methods of interacting with staff, patients, and their families to minimize the risk of becoming involved in litigation. In addition, ideally the risk manager also works with staff to create systemic mindfulness, which allows everyone in the organization to recognize an unsafe environment or practice and to intervene in reducing or eliminating it. The types of services and skills required for proactive risk management mandate that their development receive support from within the hospital leadership. Outside consultants are often helpful in identifying problem areas or performing environmental assessments but are seldom able to operate this type of program successfully, because the hospital staff usually relates more favorably when it deals with in-house risk management personnel.

Patient-and-Guest Relations

The operation of a patient/guest relations or hospital ombudsman program is often assigned to the risk management department. Because it is generally true that individuals do not sue persons they like,

healthcare administrators are starting to recognize the importance of a system that listens to and supports patients and their families when questions arise about the quality or adequacy of care. If this service is not directly under the risk management department, there should at least be a mechanism in place to allow for the sharing of information between the two departments. (Section 3 of this book addresses specific strategies for claims management, the importance and mechanics of transparency, and the role of the risk manager in leading this initiative.) When the risk manager learns that a patient has been injured, the patient's representative can begin working with family members to allow them to vent their frustration and request answers to their questions. Conversely, when a patient's representative speaks with a disgruntled patient, he or she can notify the risk manager of the actual or perceived problem; this enables the risk manager to intervene and investigate the situation more fully. Developing a system for aggregating these data to enable the tracking and trending of repetitive behaviors is essential to the optimal management of potential risk.

Quality Management

Smaller hospitals may wish to establish a single department to handle quality management and risk management. (See sample organizational and flow charts for this combined activity in Figures 5–1 and 5–2.) This can be more readily accomplished if the right staff person is chosen. Obviously, the ideal person has a clinical background as well as the knowledge and ability to deal with issues related to claims investigation and evaluation. This individual must also possess the ability to relate well with physicians and nurses, because the major focus of an organization-wide quality-management program involves quality-of-care issues.

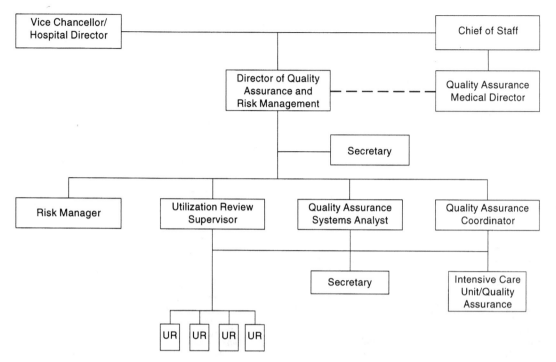

UR = Utilization Review

Figure 5–1 *Sample Organizational Chart of a Quality Assurance/Risk Management Department*

Other responsibilities of a quality management department frequently include the following:

- Utilization review and management
- Medical-staff credentialing and reappointment
- Infection control
- Discharge abstracting
- Concurrent diagnosis and diagnosis-related-group (DRG) coding
- Severity indexing
- DRG case-mix analysis
- Medical records
- External quality reporting

It may be difficult to find someone with expertise in all these areas. In that case, the hospital may establish a better program by dividing the various responsibilities among several individuals.

Other responsibilities of a quality-management department may include facilitating clinical benchmarking projects to identify best practices and making staff aware of practice guidelines that have been proven to be effective in reducing variability in care and improving outcomes. Once an organization adopts the use of evidence-based practice, the quality-management or performance-improvement staff measure clinicians' compliance with these guidelines. In addition, quality-management staff are often also responsible for external reporting to agencies that want to assess clinical outcomes and quality performance.

Patient Safety

Many organizations struggle with where to structure their patient safety activities, and

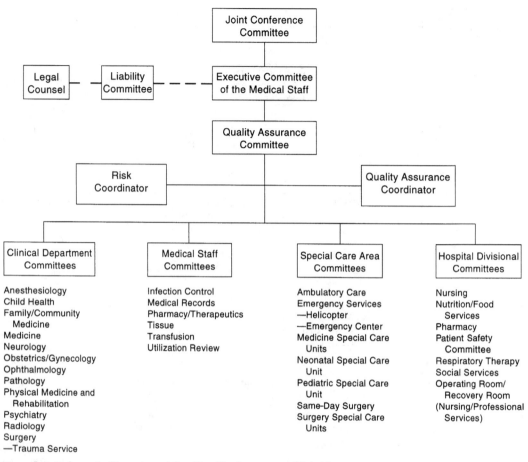

Figure 5–2 Sample Flowchcart for Quality Assurance/Risk Management

many even choose to have a separate department that focuses only on patient safety. As many chapters in this book illustrate, however, a clear and logical separation of patient safety activities from risk- or quality-management activities is often illogical and does not optimize the skills developed by those already working in risk- and quality-management departments. Patient safety activities might best be thought of as those that specifically relate to how the environment in which care is provided is optimized so that care can be delivered in a safe and effective manner. Patient safety principles also aggressively promote the concept of systemic mindfulness, which requires open and honest discussion about the root causes of problems within the organization and the commitment of leadership to resolve them. Patient safety is generally focused on the internal vulnerabilities of the organization and attempts to learn from other industries and from other best-practice healthcare providers about how to effectively reduce the potential for patient or staff harm. Patient safety staff often generally recognize the value of using data to understand the true impact of human error on a system, in all aspects of the hospital operation, and focus on solving problems centrally so that all units and departments can learn and benefit. This is better than using a more episodic approach, which historically addressed each problem as a single, isolated event. The study of human factors, team and task factors, transparency, and accountability are all aspects of the patient safety movement that have not yet been fully developed into risk- or quality-management programs, but in a truly integrated organization, they should be at least closely aligned.

Education

A significant part of the risk manager's job should focus on education. Other organization departments also play important roles in staff education, but the role of the risk manager in this process cannot be underestimated. The risk manager should interface with the staff-education department to coordinate educational programs and determine the topics most relevant to individual staff groups. Whenever possible, the risk manager should participate in new-employee orientation and be a part of all staff continuing education.

PHYSICIAN SUPPORT FOR RISK MANAGEMENT

Many risk managers have complained about physicians' traditional lack of interest in the risk management effort. Risk management also has been viewed negatively by some physicians who associate it only with litigation, placing blame, and technical insurance-related issues. With the change in focus of risk management, physician involvement is no longer a luxury—it is a necessity. Clinically based programs will be endorsed only by departments that have been given the opportunity to assist in their development and to identify risk management factors significant to them. Their active and ongoing involvement in department-specific programs can help to determine potential problems and make necessary changes before patients are injured. When selling the concepts of risk management to physicians, the risk manager must stress that the discipline has changed and that the integration of risk management with patient safety should

reduce errors to patients and thus litigation for physicians. Although the focus is now on offering safe and effective care through recognition of system faults, rather than seeing each error as an individual or personal fault, physicians (as well as all staff) must understand the concept of personal accountability. Physicians also should understand the aspect of risk management that addresses the defense of lawsuits and the evaluation of claims, and how their involvement in the early investigative stage and their honest and fully transparent discussions with patients may actually prevent a suit and aid in a favorable resolution of a claim.

It is often easier to engage physicians who are employees of the organization in the risk management process, especially when they are appointed to various risk management committees by the chief executive officer or by the chief of staff; however, physicians who have staff privileges at the organization but are not employees may need to have the values of risk management and their involvement in it "personalized" so that the benefits become more apparent to the individual practitioners. For example, the risk manager may be able to provide these physicians with information from professional-liability insurers who offer premium credits to physicians who are actively engaged in risk management programs. The risk manager also should explain that the program focuses on patient safety issues and helping physicians to identify types of behaviors and practices, as well as systemic frailties, that have historically resulted in malpractice claims and litigation.

Stressing the educational components of risk management may attract physicians to the program. In-service seminars specifically related to issues that concern physicians (how to avoid malpractice litigation is a popular item), as well as copies of relevant articles and other printed material, may also help risk managers to gain credibility. If physicians perceive the program as useful and important, they are more likely to become involved in it.

A number of important risk management functions can be identified and earmarked for direct physician involvement. Examples of such functions include:

- Establishment of department-specific standards of care for treatment provided by practitioners within their specialties.
- Identification of the tools or technologies used in care of specific patients that might require additional training or proof of competency in order to operate safely.
- Design and monitoring of a rigorous peer-review process and required follow-up and monitoring when physicians fail to meet the standards.
- Initial review of hospital records when a lawsuit is filed or when the risk manager or physician believes that a suit may address standards of care, in order to identify and support care that was rendered and colleagues who can provide expert testimony on the physician's behalf. (Leaving litigation solely in the hands of defense counsel can result in a defense much weaker than one in which the physician provides input.)

Developing a Physician's Handbook

A handbook or manual for physicians that specifically describes the types of issues and concerns under the purview of risk management can be beneficial to the healthcare organization. By engaging physicians in the process of working with the risk management department on the project and distributing the handbook to all physicians, a constant risk management "presence" can be enforced and the concept of systemic mindfulness can be introduced and explained.

The following suggestions are typical of the contents that would be helpful to physicians:

- The handbook should be small enough to fit easily into a laboratory coat pocket or be readily available on all hospital units in case of an emergency. The handbook should also be available online via

the organization's intranet and should be searchable through use of key words, common problems, or challenges.
- Information that includes important hospital telephone extensions, the year's calendar, normal laboratory values for common tests, a list of routine preoperative tests, and other practical data increases the likelihood that physicians will refer to the handbook on a daily basis.
- Brief summary data, rather than extensive didactic information, makes the manual user friendly.
- Emergency and information telephone numbers that can be reached 24 hours a day should be included.

The following risk management subjects can make the handbook even more informative:

- The hospital's malpractice insurance program, if it covers a physician's practice
- The risk management department's system for identifying and reporting actual and potential losses and patient injuries
- A physician's response to receipt of a subpoena or a summons and complaint
- A physician's response to a call from an attorney about a specific patient or case
- The importance of physician communication and documentation in the care of patients
- The medical–legal issues surrounding informed consent, including the hospital's position on the subject
- The medical–legal issues surrounding the "do-not-resuscitate" order and the care and treatment of terminally ill patients, including the hospital's position on these matters
- A brief checklist of issues related to medical records, such as confidentiality, access to records, and disclosure of information
- Various state legal requirements related to statutory reporting, testing, and treat-

ment (e.g., reporting of communicable diseases, reporting of injuries from violent crimes, and reporting of suspected child, spouse, or elder abuse)

- A brief discussion of a physician's responsibility in dealing with an impaired colleague
- A list of risk management education programs scheduled for the coming year

Obviously, this list can be altered in any manner, according to the perceived needs of the physicians who practice within the organization. Their input into the contents of the handbook can make it a useful and valuable product.

CREATING MEANINGFUL RISK MANAGEMENT REPORTS

When the organization's risk management program becomes effective, the risk manager must collect and measure data to show the value of the risk management effort. This data collection also enables the risk manager to identify areas in need of additional risk management support and recognize aspects of care that may require modification, additional resources, or termination. A mechanism is required that will enable the risk manager to communicate the program's statistics in a meaningful way. The development of a good reporting format will greatly enhance the risk manager's ability to prove the value of risk management to the administration and the governing board. This device can also help the risk manager gain the necessary support to make important changes in the program, even if they are not initially endorsed or supported by physicians and hospital staff. If the risk manager also has responsibility for patient safety, he or she may wish to segment what is being presented (separate the report detailing claims and litigation events from the report detailing patient safety trends and concerns and root-cause-analysis summaries). This might be neces-

sary to gain the greatest protection and mirror external reporting requirements.

Before developing appropriate reports, it is necessary to identify a number of factors. Firstly, the risk manager must decide for whom a specific report is intended. Risk management reports may vary in type of information provided, depending on the groups that will receive them. Generally, risk management reports are reviewed by the following:

- Board of trustees
- Hospital executive committee
- Medical staff
- Joint conference committee
- Unit or department managers

Secondly, the risk manager should determine the purpose of the report. Answers to the following questions may be helpful:

- Has the report been prepared in compliance with a regulatory or licensure agency?
- Is the purpose of the report to introduce the goals and functions of the risk management program to the board?
- Is the purpose of the report to alert managers of specific units or departments about issues of concern that require their attention, to advise them of improvement or deterioration of performance on their unit, or to highlight specific successful strategies?
- Is the purpose of the report to demonstrate the value of the risk management program or of a specific action taken by unit staff?
- Is the report presented to provide the board with financial information associated with the organization's professional-liability exposure?
- Is the report prepared to enable the board to comply with its public duty and legal obligation to the organization?
- Is the purpose of the report to assist the organization's marketing effort, or does it focus on its particular strengths and weaknesses?

• Is systematic, regular reporting by the risk manager to the governing body and administration required by the organization's policy?

Thirdly, the risk manager should evaluate the background and function of the group who will receive the information. For example, if the report is being prepared for administrative officers, they usually require less background information about the day-to-day operation of the risk management program than the governing board. Directors or trustees, however, may need information related not only to the role of risk management within the organization but also to their legal responsibilities as they relate to quality of care. This aspect of risk management has emerged with landmark legal decisions such as (1) Darling v. Charleston Community Memorial Hospital, 211 N.E.2d 253 (Ill. 1665), cert. denied, 383 U.S. 646 (1666); and (2) Johnson v. Misericordia, 301 N.W.2d 156 (Wis. 1681). These cases established the concept of corporate liability, which allows courts to hold a healthcare organization independently negligent for failing to ensure that appropriate policies and practices are in place and being monitored to assure that patients will receive high-quality, safe care.

Reports should be prepared in a manner that allows recipients to gain necessary information without becoming overburdened by unnecessary details. Graphics are appropriate when presenting statistical data and information showing changes over time. There is limited value in providing raw-number data (e.g., the number of claims per quarter) to board members without also providing total numbers or denominator data (e.g., admissions without incident). It is also helpful to provide the board with data that indicate changes (e.g., Is the organization improving its care or is it getting worse?). Reports that demonstrate changes and improvements are more actionable than those that merely provide numerical information. (More issues associated with the responsibility of the board and how information can best be conveyed to them is given in Chapter 6.)

Following a basic introduction describing the purpose and goals of the risk management and patient safety programs and its interface with the organization's mission, the risk manager may wish to include the following information:

• The number of incident reports filed during the quarter (include figures for the number of incidents during the prior quarter and during the same quarter of the prior year, if available).
• A breakdown of figures to identify incidents that occurred in "high-risk" areas or those that the risk manager believes to be meritorious or likely to result in a claim. (These incidents also should be compared with prior-quarter and prior-year statistics.)
• The number of active lawsuits and the dollars reserved for these cases.
• The number of claims and suits closed during the quarter with a brief narrative as to how they were resolved (e.g., settled, dismissed, or tolling of statute).
• The portion of the organization's budget spent on payment of claims and lawsuits (with comparison figures for prior quarter and year).

To maximize the ability to protect information, it is suggested that a separate report be prepared to discuss near-miss events, root-cause analysis, and information relevant to patient safety but unrelated to liability or the litigation process. (See Chapter 8 for a more detailed discussion of this topic as articulated under the Patient Safety and Quality Improvement Act.)

Some boards or administrators may wish to see data that compare their organization with other similar organizations. The risk manager should stress that such comparative data can be misleading unless the other organizations (1) offer similar services, (2) have the same patient mix and case mix, (3) have a similar incident tracking, reporting, and reserving philosophy, and (4) are located in the same or similar geographic area. It is usually more beneficial to compare the organization against itself by providing statistical data broken down by quarters and compared with previous years. (See Chapter 3 for a discussion about the benefits and limitations of benchmarking of risk management and patient safety data.)

The risk manager may wish to highlight specific problem areas or significant improvements that have occurred during the quarter. This type of information helps the board to understand the dynamics of a risk management process and also should help to maintain the board's interest in the program.

COMMUNICATING RISK MANAGEMENT INFORMATION TO SENIOR LEADERSHIP

The stakes in healthcare risk management have never been higher. With healthcare spending continuing to rise, consuming an ever-greater share of the gross domestic product, focus has shifted to the healthcare delivery system and those who provide care within that system. Providing higher-quality care at a lower cost and getting individuals out of the hospital faster places higher demands on providers and exposes them to potentially greater risks. Compounding the challenges faced by risk managers is the higher potential risk of injury to patients resulting from elimination of support services, dwindling staffs, and shrinking healthcare budgets.

With organizational and personal stakes so high and resources so precious, it is more important than ever for a risk manager to have a well-defined risk management strategy that articulates to the senior management team the vital role played by risk management in helping the organization meet its goals. The challenge is not so much in crafting a risk management strategy that anticipates and advances the organization's objectives and public responsibility to pro-

vide quality health care, but rather in communicating the strategy with data that grab senior management's attention and drive home risk management's acute importance.

One way to express the vitality of healthcare risk management (and thereby ensure that protecting the organization's assets and revenues, while at the same time providing high-quality care, is foremost in the minds of senior managers) is to tightly link the risk management and patient safety strategies to the organization's mission and strategic vision. This linkage might be best understood by demonstrating risk management's relationship to the organization in the following three key areas:

1. Competitive strategy, i.e., enabling the organization to compete successfully with other providers in its marketplace by developing a system that collects data and analyzes it to proactively address issues related to the quality and efficiency of service
2. Operating strategy, i.e., ensuring that a process is in place to satisfy both internal and external customers in the areas of quality and value
3. Financial strategy, i.e., ensuring continued financial viability in an era when healthcare spending is tightly controlled and when the costs of malpractice, patient injury, and customer dissatisfaction are substantial

The benefits of intertwining risk management strategy and organizational strategy are many. For the healthcare risk manager, linking the two provides an architecture for designing a risk management strategy that is comprehensive, cohesive, and consistent. It also elevates risk management's importance by grounding it in concepts and thought patterns that are second nature to senior managers. Meanwhile, the organization benefits because potentially crippling exposures to loss are more widely understood and better managed, and as a direct result, the quality of service improves.

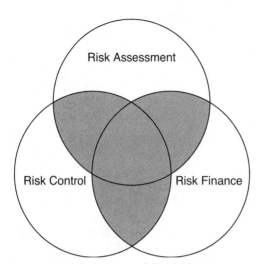

Figure 5–3 Interplay of Risk Management Disciplines

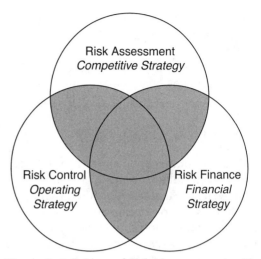

Figure 5–4 Pairing of Risk Management with the Organizational Mission

The remainder of this chapter describes a framework that will enable a risk manager to unite a healthcare organization's risk management and corporate strategies effectively and communicate the union to senior managers by using persuasive logic and familiar language.

Although there are many possible definitions for risk management strategy, the framework for linking it with the organizational strategy defines it as the sum of the choices risk managers and companies make with respect to (1) risk assessment, (2) risk control, and (3) risk finance. It is the interplay of these three disciplines that determines risk management strategy (Figure 5–3). No longer can the risk manager view his or her job as merely identifying financing mechanisms to pay for losses once they occur; instead, risk management must be part of an aggressive collaborative team effort that continually identifies potential problems and makes necessary modifications before an injury occurs.

The significance of this definition is illuminated by pairing each risk management discipline with the organization's mission and long-term strategic vision:

- Risk assessment with competitive strategy
- Risk control or patient safety with operating strategy
- Risk finance with financial strategy (Figure 5–4)

RISK MANAGEMENT STRATEGY

Competitive Strategy and Risk Assessment

Risk management strategy begins with risk assessment. In turn, risk assessment—identifying, analyzing, and quantifying the risks of financial loss that can result from patient/visitor/employee injury or a deterioration in the quality of service—is rooted in the organization's mission and competitive strategy. In the healthcare setting, because risk is often closely linked to patient injury or harm, the need to identify and correct risks is extremely important and should be grounded in the patient safety principles given in the final section of this book. To persuasively communicate risk assessment's relationship to the organization's competitive strategy, a risk manager must strive first to develop a thorough understanding of the organization's mission and strategic vision. Every healthcare organization consciously seeks to occupy a place in its market that will maximize its value to the community by providing high-quality service while maintaining financial viability. Its policies, statements, and actions that contribute to attaining or preserving this place define the mission and competitive strategy. Michael Porter, in his book *Competitive Strategy,* identifies five forces that influence competitive strategy:[1]

1. The threat of new entrants to the industry
2. The threat of substitute products or services
3. The bargaining power of suppliers
4. The bargaining power of customers
5. The intensity of rivalry among the industry's existing competitors

An organization's response to these five forces can take one or a combination of three basic strategic forms:

1. Cost leadership. The healthcare organization must become increasingly cognizant of the need to provide value as well as quality service to customers. Although in today's market low cost seems to be of paramount importance (especially when negotiating contracts with third-party payers), quality is also considered. Furthermore, when quality suffers, not only might a hospital find itself unable to compete with other hospitals in the area, it might also experience the additional financial pressures associated with a rise in (1) insurance costs, (2) the dollars spent to settle claims (if the hospital self-insures), and (3) costs associated with defensive medicine, which may not be reimbursed by payers.

2. Differentiation. Instead of striving to achieve cost leadership, the healthcare organization must set a competitive price for its services and distinguish the institution in the marketplace through superior product features and outcomes as well as outstanding customer service. Many risk managers are now expected to collect data that can show how proactive risk management initiatives positively affect the quality of care, the volume of lawsuits or patient complaints, and the dollars required to resolve claims or lawsuits. Achieving superior outcomes through quality service at a competitive price is the key to survival of hospitals today, and this can only be achieved through the collaborative efforts of risk management, quality services, hospital administration, and clinicians.

3. Focus. The healthcare organization may choose a specific product line, often referred to as a center of excellence. This product line may be targeted toward a particular healthcare need of the community (e.g., a cancer center or hypertension clinic) or a service that is unique and not available in other local hospitals. The role of risk management in assisting with the proactive analysis of the risks inherent in particular services offered should be stressed.

An organization's competitive strategy and mission must drive the assessment of its risks. The central question facing a risk manager when linking competitive strategy and risk assessments is: Given the organization's strategic focus and corporate mission, what exposures to loss or quality problems are likely to significantly affect its ability to manage its operations? Its earnings? Its assets? Its continued growth? Failing to ask these questions could lead a risk manager to an incomplete assessment of the organization's risks and potentially an inability to adequately fund and cover liabilities should they arise.

This could place the entire organization in financial peril.

Some examples will help to show how a hospital's competitive strategy influences the assessment of risk. One example is the organization that seeks to offer a new, technologically superior procedure that requires additional staff training and costly equipment. Although the procedure may be viewed as being very desirable to patients (and to the organization, if the procedure is not offered elsewhere), the cost of providing the service or the risks associated with it (when staff is improperly trained or when equipment malfunctions or is used improperly) may lead to a decision not to offer the service. A risk assessment based on this company's competitive strategy would concentrate on issues of competitiveness and need for the service but would also focus on quality, safety, and liability issues that could arise if the service is performed.

Operating Strategy and Risk Control

The second element of a risk management strategy is risk control. After bringing to senior management's attention the magnitudes and probabilities of loss implicit in the organization's competitive strategy, a risk manager should strive to ensure that his or her initiatives to control these risks are grounded in the organization's operating strategy. Doing so will lead not only to measures with a greater likelihood of avoiding and reducing loss, but also to more effective communication of risk control's importance to physicians, nurses, and other healthcare providers within the organization.

A healthcare organization's operating strategy has several dimensions:

- The degree of organizational centralization or decentralization, either functionally or by clinical unit or service
- The degree of operational flexibility, i.e., how swiftly the delivery of services can

be modified or moved into a setting more convenient to the patient
- The ratio of skilled to unskilled workers in the labor force, as well as the concentration of union versus non-union workers

To illustrate the effect of a hospital's operating strategy on its risk-assessment and risk-control strategies, consider the example of an organization that has two deeply ingrained operational strategies:

1. It uses the technique of stockless inventory, or just-in-time delivery of supplies for surgical services.
2. It has recently instituted a comprehensive patient safety program focused on creating a culture that supports the caregivers in their goal to provide safe care to patients.

Risk-assessment and risk-control efforts for this organization would need to recognize that stockless inventory and the culture of safety principles create strong webs of interdependency within the organization as well as between the organization and its suppliers. Furthermore, a risk assessment rooted in its mission and competitive strategy would pay close attention to the potential interruption of service, losses, or injuries stemming from lack of proper equipment or supplies during unplanned or emergency situations. It also would focus on exposures arising from poor quality—in both the service and product areas—that affect the ability to ensure safe, high-quality care and timely service. These potential risks would be weighed against the benefits of instituting a stockless inventory system within the organization.

Similarly, risk-control initiatives grounded in the hospital's operating strategy would center risk-avoidance and risk-reduction techniques on supplier partners. It might take the form of assisting in the risk management efforts of these suppliers, or it could involve seeking multiple suppliers of critical products or supplies. Because of the rigorous requirements placed on suppliers by stockless production and patient safety, the pool of qualifying vendors could be limited, making it especially difficult to find suitable alternates.

Financial Strategy and Risk Finance

The third element of any risk management strategy is risk finance. To be truly effective, the financing of a hospital's risks should be tailored to its financial strategy, which in turn influences its ability to survive in the future.

A healthcare organization's financial strategy is embodied in its policies and decisions with respect to such things as:

- Profit goals. Although most healthcare organizations are "not for profit," it is essential that they maintain fiscal viability to survive. Some organizations stress the need to show a year-end "profit" to continue to be able to provide community education, indigent care, and other special or new services. Financial strength is critical to ensure that payroll is met and that suppliers and vendors are compensated for the services and products they provide. In the hospital setting, patient mix, payer mix, and appropriate use of tests and procedures influence an organization's earning potential.
- Capital structure. All organizations establish target ratios for maximum total indebtedness to total capital.
- Tax policy. Some hospitals seek to maximize current deductions, whereas others (those experiencing operating losses, for example) do not. Also, some organizations are more willing than others to assume audit risk, or the risk that aggressive deductions will invite Internal Revenue Service scrutiny.
- Investment strategy. Each organization has a distinct risk personality when it comes to the kinds of businesses, assets (e.g., medical technology), and securities in which it is willing to invest.

Furthermore, each of the decisions healthcare organizations make regarding profit goals, capital structure, tax policy, and investment strategy helps to determine its overall cost of capital, which is a key yardstick for senior managers when considering the merits of alternative financing decisions.

In designing a risk finance program for an organization, some tentative conclusions can be made. Firstly, any surprises in the form of large unforeseen losses that might constrain or cripple the organization's ability to grow would invite senior management's wrath, suggesting the need to transfer significant amounts of risk. Secondly, increases in total indebtedness, in the form of large self-insured reserves, might conflict with the company's capital-structure targets. Thirdly, current deductions for insurance premiums would assist in the sheltering of income. Lastly, investments in any risk financing vehicle (e.g., in the form of funds dedicated to a captive insurer or other alternative risk finance program) would be weighed vis-à-vis other investments the organization could make. Any scenarios that did not measure up to its cost of capital or other appropriate cost-of-funds benchmark would likely be rejected.

Although there are many risk financing schemes that could support the conclusions drawn from this simple example, to fit snugly with the organization's financial strategy, at a minimum its risk finance program would have to transfer significant amounts of risk. Furthermore, although it may be simple, the example reinforces the need to match risk finance with financial strategy, and it highlights the framework's usefulness in engineering a risk finance program and communicating its importance to senior management.

In addition to the framework for linking risk management strategy and operational strategy, another way for risk management to gain currency among senior managers is to ensure that its elements—assessment, control, and finance—incorporate the key

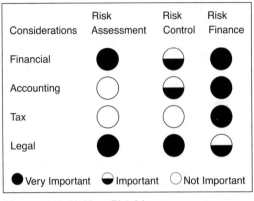

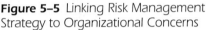

Figure 5–5 Linking Risk Management Strategy to Organizational Concerns

financial, accounting, tax, and legal considerations used by the organization when making any strategic or tactical decisions (Figure 5–5).

MAJOR CONSIDERATIONS

Financial Considerations

As has been discussed already, financial considerations are very important when assessing an organization's risks. Identifying and quantifying the potential losses of earnings and resources arising from operational exposures is the first step to building an effective risk management program. They are important, too, when designing and implementing risk-control measures. An effective way to measure the success, prospectively or retrospectively, of an investment in risk control is to quantify its cost and its benefit.

Accounting Considerations

Accounting considerations generally are not important when assessing risk. They are more important when making risk-control decisions, inasmuch as the controls imposed by the organization's inside and outside auditors contribute to controlling its fidelity, fiduciary, and directors' and officers' risks.

In contrast to risk assessment and control, however, accounting considerations are very

important to risk financing decisions. To be consistent with financial strategy, any proposed risk finance program should recognize and incorporate the organization's tax and financial accounting policies. A basic example of the importance of accounting considerations is that of the organization weighing the benefits of a loss-portfolio transfer. If the cash required to transfer the presently self-insured liabilities to an insurer is less than the book value of those liabilities on its balance sheet, the organization can recognize an accounting gain, and thus boost profits. If, however, the book value of the liabilities is less than the cost of risk transfer, the transaction will have an adverse effect on earnings.

Tax Considerations

Tax considerations are not important to risk assessment and generally are not important to risk-control decisions. An exception to this might be if an investment in risk control were to provide an investment tax credit. In this case, a risk-control decision should incorporate its relevant tax consequences. Tax considerations are very important to risk finance decisions, as is illustrated in the section on financial strategy and risk finance.

Legal Considerations

Legal considerations are very important in assessing an organization's risks. Key questions include: What is the legal climate in the jurisdictions where the hospital operates? What types of tort reform are available in those jurisdictions? What legal liabilities could arise from the pursuit of new or additional services or marketing strategies, now and in the future (e.g., satellite facilities, telemedicine services, state-to-state transfer programs)? Legal considerations are also important when making risk-control decisions, especially with respect to the protection of workers, customers, and the environment. Workers' compensation risk control is governed by Occupational Safety and Health Administration regulations. Federal and state medical-product safety laws help guide liability risk control, and federal Environmental Protection Agency requirements and state laws drive environmental risk control.

Legal considerations must be taken into account when making risk financing choices. The central question to answer is: What are the state and local legal requirements, restrictions, and opportunities with respect to any proposed risk financing program?

Healthcare risk managers, like everyone in today's leaner organizations, must do more with less. Furthermore, with flattened and more decentralized organizational structures, they must influence through persuasion rather than fiat; therefore, the advantage goes to the risk manager who can craft a potent risk management strategy and communicate its vitality to senior management. In the end, effective risk management requires top-management commitment and is the result of a sound risk management strategy that is grounded in the realities, mission, and culture of the healthcare organization.

APPENDIX 5–A: SAMPLE JOB DESCRIPTIONS

Exhibit 5–A–1 Sample Job Description for Director of Risk Management

Qualifications

1. Minimum of a bachelor's degree in business or health-related field

2. Master's degree preferred in business, hospital administration, or other health-related field

3. Excellent oral and written communication skills essential

4. Insurance and claims-management experience a plus

Reporting Relationship

1. Reports directly to the chief executive officer or her/his designee

2. Reports to legal counsel on matters involving hospital professional liability

Responsibilities

1. Management of insurance program for all hospital coverage:

   - Responsibility of program components, including professional liability, general liability, workers' compensation, motor-vehicle liability, property, directors and officers, fiduciary liability (ERISA), electronic data-processing coverage
   - Identification and evaluation of markets and options
   - Allocation of risk through the purchase of commercial insurance, deductibles, self-insured funds; evaluation of financial feasibility
   - Allocation of premium among insured entities
   - Oversight of reserves in relation to limits

2. Loss control and claims management:

   - Monitor incidents and claims-reporting systems
   - Coordinate with carrier the investigation and defense of all claims and suits
   - Cooperate with medical peer-review and institutional committees on issues related to standards of care
   - Develop programs and systems necessary for self-insurance
   - Provide guidance as required to security and environmental safety personnel

3. Coordination with hospital quality management and patient safety programs:

   - Develop a system to share hospital-wide quality-management and patient safety data with appropriate departments and administrative personnel
   - Develop a system for tracking and trending of generic screening monitors to assist in the identification of potentially high-risk behavior leading to patient, staff, and visitor injuries
   - Develop appropriate operational linkages to correct actual and potential problems that have been identified

(continues)

Exhibit 5–A–1 (Continued)

4. Resource for education on risk management:

- Develop a formal program for ongoing education for all hospital staff
- Respond to crisis situations that have risk management implications and assist staff with problem solving

5. Administrative duties and responsibilities:

- Supervise all professional and support staff in the risk management department
- Monitor department budget and assets of self-insurance funds
- Represent department on appropriate hospital committees as assigned

---

Exhibit 5–A–2 Sample Job Description for Patient Safety Manager

Qualifications

1. Minimum of a master's degree with focus on organizational development, patient safety, or human-factors engineering. Training in Six Sigma or Lean a plus.

2. Healthcare and patient safety experience preferred

3. Knowledge of other high-hazard industries that have incorporated high-reliability concepts to create a culture of safety

4. Excellent interpersonal skills

5. Good oral and written communication skills

6. Ability to make independent judgments and pay close attention to detail

7. Ability to analyze large data sets and design a process to identify cause and solution (may require the ability to perform analytic root-cause analysis, failure mode, and effects analysis, or to institute detailed analysis to determine the origin of errors)

Reporting Relationship

1. Reports directly to the chief medical officer

2. Reports indirectly to senior administrative staff and chief risk officer

Responsibilities

The person would be responsible for all aspects of the hospital patient safety program, including the following:

1. Review and analyze all near-miss and sentinel events to identify system factors contributing to error. Discuss incidents with individuals involved and challenge them to explain how the process of care needs to be redesigned to prevent recurrence. Maintain statistical tabulations and summaries of patient-safety-related occurrences and make appropriate reports to various agencies (or Patient Safety Organizations) as required by law or determined by the organization.

2. Develop a process to share lessons learned across the entire organization so that problems resolved in one area of the organization do not reappear elsewhere.

3. Serve as coach or primary data resource for individual units seeking to engage in focused patient safety projects. Encourage collaboration with other areas as appropriate.

4. Conduct routine tours of the entire hospital to foster transparency and to hear from staff what their greatest concerns are about the environment in which they work. Use this process to develop a list of priorities for staff education and resource allocation.

5. Chair and document the proceedings of the hospital patient safety committee and disaster-planning committee.

6. Develop, implement, and maintain educational patient safety programs for all hospital personnel.

7. Perform other duties as related to the risk management and patient safety programs as assigned.

8. Prepare formal reports for senior management and hospital board as required.

Exhibit 5–A–3 Sample Job Description for Workers' Compensation Specialist

Qualifications

1. Bachelor of Arts or Sciences, or the equivalent in experience
2. Prior workers' compensation claims experience
3. Excellent oral and written communication skills
4. Excellent judgment
5. Ability to work independently

Reporting Relationship

1. Reports directly to the director of risk management
2. Reports indirectly to patient safety officer

Responsibilities

The responsibilities involve identifying systemic issues that give rise to an unsafe environment for staff, processing workers' compensation claims, and maintaining insurance requirements mandated by state law and internal hospital guidelines. Specific duties include the following:

1. Coordinate and process work-related incident reports, claims, and related expenses. Maintain an aggregate database so trends can be identified and resolved.
2. Establish and maintain employee claim files and files related to occupational safety and health administration requirements.
3. Design reports using the risk management information system for analyses, trend tracking, and interdepartmental communications.
4. Assist in the coordination of workers' compensation insurance.
5. Serve on committees associated with workers' and patient safety.
6. Implement new workers' compensation programs as necessary.
7. Act as liaison with health, safety, and security personnel, and with the human resources department.

Exhibit 5–A–4 Sample Job Description for Claims Manager

Qualifications

1. Bachelor's degree in health care, business, or law
2. Minimum of 5 years of professional liability-claims experience
3. Database-management experience desirable
4. Excellent interpersonal skills
5. Good oral and written communication skills
6. Ability to communicate effectively with physicians, nurses, and other healthcare professionals
7. Excellent negotiating skills
8. Working knowledge of insurance coverage a plus

Reporting Relationship

1. Reports directly to the director of risk management
2. Reports indirectly to hospital legal counsel

Responsibilities

The person assumes responsibility for all aspects of claim and lawsuit management, including the following:

1. Evaluating the litigation potential of all incidents and adverse outcomes occurring within the hospital
2. Conducting a thorough investigation to determine elements of disclosure and whether an early offer of settlement is appropriate
3. Establishing claim files and estimate reserves
4. Coordinating the preparation of staff who may be called as witnesses at trials or depositions; identifying those who may need emotional support in light of being involved in the event
5. Acting as a representative of the hospital at selected legal proceedings
6. Assuming responsibility for settlement negotiations under the direction of the director of risk

(*continues*)

Exhibit 5–A–4 (Continued)

management with settlement authority up to $50,000

7. Identifying problem areas related to particular claims that may indicate staff educational needs

8. Preparing and reviewing all disbursements for approval from the various self-insurance funds

9. Managing the preparation of a database to include all claims information

10. Designing claims reports for use by hospital department heads, administration, and appropriate committees

---

Exhibit 5–A–5 Sample Job Description for Quality Manager

Qualifications

1. Minimum of a bachelor's degree in nursing (master's preferred)

2. Clinical expertise in critical care, obstetrics, or emergency department a plus

3. Minimum of 5 years of clinical or teaching experience

4. Performance-improvement or quality-assurance experience desirable; must be able to analyze large data sets and understand processes for statistical analysis

5. Excellent interpersonal skills

6. Good oral and written communication skills

Reporting Relationship

1. Reports directly to the chief medical officer and/or chief nursing officer

2. Direct working relationship with the director of risk management and patient safety officer

Responsibilities

This position focuses on the identification, evaluation, and modification of high-risk clinical activities occurring within the hospital that may give rise to

patient injury or suit. The following duties are required to accomplish these goals:

1. Implementing an early-warning system to identify areas of potential clinical exposure

2. Reviewing all quality-assurance or performance-improvement data with quality-assurance personnel to identify significant risk trends

3. Coordinating of communications among various departments and committees to enhance problem resolution, facilitate corrective action, and prevent recurrences

4. Processing reports of incidents, claims, suits, and complaints for review by medical staff and quality-assurance committees; referring specific behavioral issues to appropriate peer-review committees to ensure that staff are accountable for actions, as appropriate

5. Working closely with individual clinical departments and assisting in the development of appropriate department-specific clinical monitors

6. Assessing the educational needs of the hospital staff and participating in risk management education programs

7. Serving as a resource to staff and department heads

Reference

1. Porter, M. (1980). *Competitive strategy: Techniques for analyzing industries and competitors*. New York: Free Press.

PATIENT SAFETY: THE PAST DECADE

Lisa Saar, JD, MSN

INTRODUCTION

The Institute of Medicine's (IOM) 1999 report, "To Err Is Human: Building a Safer Health System," identified as many as 98,000 deaths attributable to medical errors.[1] That report opened with an account of two horrific headline cases of patients who died because of medical error. It is now more than 10 years later and the number of deaths related to medical errors remains a significant healthcare concern. News headlines across the nation continue to report horrific patient deaths due to medical error, and in turn, continue to lead to litigation. Health care has never been more expensive. Medical-malpractice litigation continues to be a major contributing factor to the expense of healthcare. According to Statehealthfacts.org, in 2007, there were 11,478 paid malpractice claims in the United States.[2] Improving patient safety has never been more impera-

tive, yet the risk manager's role in this process remains unclear.

Ten years ago, the IOM report made a number of recommendations for improving patient safety laid out in a four-tiered approach.[3] This chapter summarizes some of the most prominent changes in the field of patient safety 10 years after release of the IOM report. Presentation of these changes, many of which align closely with the traditional role of the healthcare risk manager and some of which create some tension in light of concerns related to our current legal system, uses the IOM report's recommendations under the four-tiered approach as a guide. The four tiers are as follows: (1) leadership and knowledge in the causes of medical error; (2) identifying and learning from errors; (3) setting performance standards and expectations for safety; and (4) implementing safety systems in healthcare organizations.

THE INSTITUTE OF MEDICINE'S FOUR-TIERED APPROACH

Leadership and Knowledge

Under the IOM's first tier, establishing a national focus to create leadership to enhance a knowledge base about safety, the IOM recommended that Congress create a Center for Patient Safety within the Agency for Healthcare Research and Quality (AHRQ).[4] In 2001, the AHRQ renamed the Center for Quality Measurement and Improvement (CQMI) as the Center for Quality Improvement and Patient Safety (CQuIPS).[5] Under the direction of the AHRQ, the CQuIPS was established to improve the quality of life and safety of all Americans. The goal of the CQuIPS is to conduct and disseminate patient safety research through collaboration with healthcare systems to implement evidence-based practices.[6] An important CQuIPS initiative in the past decade, the development of the Patient Safety Organizations rule, is discussed below (with the final PSO regulation discussed in Chapter 8).

Yearly, since 2003, the AHRQ has published the "National Healthcare Quality Report" and the "National Healthcare Disparities Report." These reports measure, among other things, trends in patient safety and present, in chart format, data on quality and access to care.[7] In 2005, the AHRQ and Department of Defense Health Affairs jointly sponsored a compendium of 140 articles, publishing "Advances in Patient Safety: From Research to Implementation," describing what federally funded programs have accomplished in understanding medical errors and implementing programs to improve patient safety since the IOM report.[8] In 2008, another AHRQ study, "Advances in Patient Safety: New Directions and Alternative Approaches," was released. This four-volume set of 115 articles put together by patient safety researchers and others includes, among other topics, articles on reporting systems, risk assessment, safety culture, med-

ical simulation, and medication safety.[9] Risk managers who are unfamiliar with these reports should review them and share with staff the lessons learned.

Although leadership and knowledge is important, it is not enough. It has taken a decade to compile volumes of articles and reports on the nation's status regarding patient safety. We need to take a critical look at the reports and literature and move forward, taking action to apply their recommendations in order to improve patient safety in all venues where patients receive care.

Identifying and Learning from Errors

The second tier, identifying and learning from errors, recommends a nationwide mandatory reporting system and encourages voluntary reporting of medical errors. The report recommends that the nationwide mandatory reporting system provide standardized information by state governments about adverse events resulting in death or serious harm.[10] Many states have already instituted mandatory reporting programs and are sharing what is being learned both within their state and to healthcare organizations throughout the country. Most are also contemplating how they become part of the national database established through AHRQ.

Patient Safety and Quality Improvement Act of 2005

The federal government, in response to IOM recommendations and the profound number of medical errors estimated in "To Err Is Human," enacted the Patient Safety and Quality Improvement Act of 2005 (PSQIA). The duties of this act are as follows:[11]

1. Provide for the certification and recertification of Patient Safety Organizations
2. Collect and disseminate information related to patient safety
3. Establish a patient safety database

4. Facilitate the development of consensus among healthcare providers, patients, and other interested parties concerning patient safety and recommendations to improve patient safety

5. Provide technical assistance to states that have (or are developing) medical-error reporting systems, assist states in developing standardized methods for data collection, and collect data from state reporting systems for inclusion in the patient safety database.

The ultimate goal of this act was to improve the nation's overall patient safety by encouraging confidential, voluntary reporting of events that adversely affect patients. Policymakers thought that if they promoted the systematic collection of medical-error data, under a theory that improved patient safety, information based on the data, with a subsequent awareness of those errors, would lead to prevention of errors and minimize their recurrence.[12] The AHRQ published the Patient and Safety Quality Improvement final rule on November 21, 2008 (73 FR 70732), and it became effective on January 19, 2009 (42 CFR Part 3).[13]

The PSQIA authorizes creation of Patient Safety Organizations (PSOs) and specifies each PSO's role and requirements in the collection, compilation, analysis, and maintenance of confidential medical-error information, voluntarily reported by healthcare providers. The United States Department of Health and Human Services, specifically AHRQ, currently lists 70 PSOs. Additionally, many states have enacted specific statutes specifying adverse-event reporting and monitoring, investigation, and inspection requirements in response to patient safety problems within the individual state. Chapter 8 describes in detail the specific provisions of the final regulations and provides some guidance about both the creation of a PSO and participation in one. It is essential that risk managers be aware of the type of data that is protected under these regulations and the specific limitations that relate to information gathered in anticipation of litigation.

National Quality Forum

The National Quality Forum (NQF), established in 1999 to improve the quality of American health care by setting national standards, is a non-profit organization based in Washington, D.C. Members of the NQF include hospitals, physicians, businesses and policymakers, and national, health, government, and consumer organizations committed to specific, measurable actions and goals for performance measurement and public reporting regarding patient safety. The NQF was spurred to action by the IOM report and in 2002 published a report, "Safe Practices for Better Healthcare," with an update in 2006 and again in 2009.[14] The report identifies safe practices that should be universally used by healthcare organizations and providers to reduce the risk of harm to patients. As of the 2009 report, there are 30 identified safe practices ranging from creating and sustaining a culture of safety to medication reconciliation and specific evidence-based practice protocols.

In addition to these reports, the NQF also completed other projects in pursuit of improved patient safety. One such project, "Serious Reportable Events in Healthcare: 2005–2006 Update," provides a list of 27 adverse events that were deemed "never events."[15] A never event, according to the NQF, is an error in medical care that is clearly preventable, and if allowed to occur, it indicates a problem in patient safety within a healthcare facility. The Centers for Medicare and Medicaid Services (CMS) announced in 2008 denial of payment for selected never events and hospital-acquired conditions.[16] These events are discussed in further detail in Chapter 7.

Another patient safety project produced an NQF-endorsed standardized taxonomy for patient safety. One of the largest problems in working with the plethora of data regarding patient safety is the multitude of meanings placed on various terms such as adverse event, medical error, etc. Standardizing the terms across reporting systems will assist in making the data more meaningful and support patient safety data-management innovation.[17]

Setting Performance Standards and Expectations for Patient Safety

The third tier, setting performance standards and expectations for patient safety, includes a recommendation for professional societies that make a clear commitment to improving patient safety.[18] Additionally, the IOM report recommended that the Food and Drug Administration (FDA) increase attention to the safe use of drugs and devices.[19] Professional groups that were already working on improving patient safety include the National Patient Safety Foundation (NPSF) and the Anesthesia Patient Safety Foundation. A leading professional society, the American Medical Association (AMA), is a strong supporter of improving patient safety through the AMA's Quality of Care Program. This program includes initiatives that the AMA has undertaken for America's patients under the categories of safety, advocacy, measurement, and education.[20] The AMA founded, and is a sponsor of, the NPSF, a group dedicated to improving patient safety through research, communication, and development of solutions to identified problems. The AMA also aggressively lobbied in support of federal legislation that would create voluntary confidential error-reporting systems, specifically, the Patient Safety Quality Improvement Act of 2005.

The American Nurses Association (ANA) is committed to patient safety. In the past decade, the ANA launched a campaign to assist in achieving safe-nurse-staffing legislation. Since 2004, the ANA has been relentless in support of legislation establishing safe nurse–patient ratio requirements. Although previous submissions failed, H.R. 2273 Nurse Staffing Standards for Patient Safety and Quality Care Act 2009 was introduced in May 2009 for initial processing in the legislative chain.[21]

The FDA, in response to the IOM report, formed a Drug Safety Board in 2005. This board consists of FDA staff and representatives from the National Institutes of Health and the Veterans Administration. The board advises the director of the Center for Drug Evaluation and Research, FDA, on drug-safety issues and works with the agency in communicating safety information to health professionals and patients. The Drug Safety Board and the FDA Web page, "Postmarket Drug Safety Information for Patients and Providers," is an effort to meet the intention of the IOM recommendation for improved transparency and communication.[22]

Creating Safety Systems Inside Healthcare Organizations

The fourth and final tier—and ultimate target of all the IOM's recommendations—is creating safety systems inside healthcare organizations. The nation's predominant standard-setting and accrediting body in health care, The Joint Commission, established the National Patient Safety Goal program in 2002 with the first set of goals taking effect in January 2003.[22] The Joint Commission and the Patient Safety Advisory group developed the national patient safety goals (NPSGs). Depending on the type of facility, there are approximately 13 goals with multiple elements of performance. The goals were developed based on an analysis of sentinel events and common issues in health care that give rise to errors. According to the Joint Commission, there will be no new goals for 2010, presumably because current goals are not being met.[23]

The Joint Commission is committed to improving safety in health care, with over half of its standards directly related to safety. Through the NPSGs, a universal protocol for preventing wrong site, person, or surgical procedure became effective in 2003. The universal protocol was updated in 2008 and took effect in January 2009.[23]

The AHRQ created a tool to assist hospitals in evaluating how well they establish a culture of patient safety within their institution. Hospital staff provides their opinions about various patient safety issues as well as medical-error and adverse-event reporting. The purpose of the report is to (1) allow hospitals to compare themselves with each other, (2) facilitate internal learning in patient safety improvements, (3) assist hospitals in identifying strengths and areas for improvement, and (4) show trends in patient safety over time.[24] The first report was released in 2007 and included data from 383 hospitals across the nation. The second report was released in 2008 and included data from 519 hospitals. The tool is still gaining momentum, because the 2009 report included data from 622 hospitals. The report allows hospitals to compare how well they are doing in establishing a culture of patient safety in their facility as compared with similar facilities across the United States.[24]

CONCLUSION

This chapter summarizes just a few of the most prominent patient safety initiatives since the publication of the IOM report 10 years ago. It is clear that the IOM report spurred the nation to action with the publishing of numerous reports and publications that discuss the problems identified. Patient safety and medical errors continue to be national problems with slow progress in correcting deficiencies. Continued efforts by the nation's leaders, businesses, policymakers, and national, health, government, and consumer organizations are required to improve patient safety. Standardizing collected data and effective use of technology are necessary to realize progress. It will be interesting to see what the next decade of patient safety efforts brings, and how the risk manager's role evolves in light of these challenges.

References

1. Kohn, L.T., Corrigan, J.M., & Donaldson, M.S. (Eds.). (2000). *To err is human: Building a safer health system*. Institute of Medicine (IOM) Committee on Quality of Health Care in America. Washington, DC: National Academies Press, p. vii.
2. Kaiser Family Foundation. State health facts. http://www.stateghealthfacts.org. Accessed June 1, 2009.
3. Kohn, L.T., Corrigan, J.M., & Donaldson, M.S. (Eds.). (2000). *To err is human: Building a safer health system*. Institute of Medicine (IOM) Committee on Quality of Health Care in America. Washington, DC: National Academies Press, p. 6.
4. Ibid, p. 7.
5. *Organizations, functions, and authority delegations*. Center for Quality Improvement and Patient Safety, Federal Register, January 24, 2001 (Vol. 66, No. 16).
6. Agency for Healthcare Research and Quality. (n.d.). *Center for Quality Improvement and Patient Safety: Mission statement*. http://www.ahrq.gov/About/cquips/cquipsmiss.html/. Accessed June 1, 2009.
7. Agency for Healthcare Research and Quality. (2008). 2008 National Healthcare Quality and Disparities Reports. http://www.ahrq.gov/qual/qrdr08.html/. Accessed June 1, 2009.
8. Agency for Healthcare Research and Quality. (2005, February). *Advances in patient safety: From research to implementation* (Vol. 1–4). AHRQ Publication Nos. 050021 (1–4). http://www.ahrq.gov/qual/advances/.
9. Agency for Healthcare Research and Quality. (2008, July). *Advances in patient safety: New directions and alternative approaches* (Vol. 1–4). AHRQ Publication Nos. 08-0034 (1–4). http://www.ahrq.gov/qual/advances2/.

10. Kohn, L.T., Corrigan, J.M., & Donaldson, M.S. (Eds.). (2000). *To err is human: Building a safer health system*. Institute of Medicine (IOM) Committee on Quality of Health Care in America. Washington, DC: National Academies Press, p. 9.
11. Agency for Healthcare Research and Quality. (2005). *The Patient Safety and Quality Improvement Act of 2005*. Overview 2008. http://www.ahrq.gov/qual/psoact.htm/. Accessed June 1, 2009.
12. Barringer, P.J., & Kachalia, A.B. (2008). Error reporting and injury compensation: Advancing patient safety through a state patient safety organization. *Wyoming Law Review, 8*, 349–371.
13. Agency for Healthcare Research and Quality. (2005). *Patient safety organizations (PSOs): Fast facts*. http://www.pso.ahrq.gov/psos/fastfacts.html/. Accessed June 1, 2009.
14. National Quality Forum. (n.d.). *About NQF*. http://www.qualityforum.org/about/. Accessed June 1, 2009.
15. National Quality Forum. (n.d.). *Serious reportable events in healthcare: 2005–2006 update*. http://www.qualityforum.org/projects/hacs_and_sres.aspx/. Accessed June 1, 2009.
16. Centers for Medicare and Medicaid Services. (n.d.). *Medicare and Medicaid move aggressively to encourage greater patient safety in hospitals and reduce never events*. http://www.cms.hhs.gov/apps/media/press/factsheet.asp?Counter = 3219/. Accessed June 1, 2009.
17. National Quality Forum. (n.d.). http://www.qualityforum.org/. Accessed June 1, 2009.
18. Kohn, L.T., Corrigan, J.M., & Donaldson, M.S. (Eds.). (2000). *To err is human: Building a safer health system*. Institute of Medicine (IOM) Committee on Quality of Health Care in America. Washington, DC: National Academies Press, p. 12.
19. Ibid, p. 13.
20. American Medical Association. *Patient safety: Quality of care program*. (n.d.). http://www.ama-assn.org/ama/pub/physician-resources/clinical-practice-improvement/patient-safety/quality-care-program.shtml/. Accessed June 1, 2009.
21. Govtrack.us. (2009). *Nurse staffing standards for Patient Safety and Quality Care Act of 2009*. http://www.govtrack.us/congress/bill.xpd?bill = h111-2273/. Accessed June 1, 2009.
22. United States Food and Drug Administration. (2007). *Postmarket drug safety information for patients and providers*. http://www.fda.gov/Cder/drugSafety.html/. Accessed June 1, 2009.
23. The Joint Commission. (2009). *Facts about the national patient safety goals*. http://www.jointcommission.org/PatientSafety/NationalPatientSafetyGoals/npsg_facts.htm/. Accessed June 1, 2009.
24. Sorra, J., Famolaro, T., & Dyer, N., et al. (2009). *Hospital survey on patient safety culture: 2009 comparative database report*. Agency for Healthcare Research and Quality. AHRQ publication no. 09-0030. http://www.ahrq.gov/qual/hospsurvey091.pdf/. Accessed June 1, 2009.

7

USING "NEVER EVENTS" TO REDUCE RISK AND ADVANCE PATIENT SAFETY

Terence McMahon, MBA

INTRODUCTION

For risk managers the use of financial incentives plays a major role in getting providers and administrators to create and measure the economic impact of patient safety. The "never-event" program, which influences reimbursement under the Centers for Medicare and Medicaid Services (CMS) and other payment-driven programs, has been created to motivate hospitals to reduce or eliminate preventable harm to patients. The various stakeholders, i.e., patients, providers, payers, professional organizations, and employers, are in agreement that there is a set of "never events," or preventable mistakes, that should not occur while the patient is under the care of a provider and therefore are not subject to reimbursement. Congress gave CMS the flexibility to make additions or deletions to this list as medical evidence justified. There is an expanding list of never events that includes hospital-acquired conditions (HACs) or complications where reim-bursement incentives are treated differently based on the contractual arrangement between the payer and provider.

CMS OVERVIEW

One of the nation's largest healthcare consumer stakeholders is the federal government, with an annual budget for 2010 of over $511,033 billion (http://www.cms.hhs.gov/PerformanceBudget/Downloads/CMSFY11CJ.pdf, accessed March 24, 2010). The Health and Human Services agency's Center for Medicare and Medicaid Services is charged by Congress to administer and oversee the programs. Growing healthcare costs, which are an increasingly significant percentage of the gross national product, have been recognized as a national crisis. The publication of "To Err Is Human: Building a Safer Health System" (Kohn, Corrigan, & Donaldson, 2000) brought to light the negative impact, on quality of patient care and overall costs, of the health-care practices that were not recognized as contributing to accepted patient safety levels. The economic impact and reporting of high-risk injury by patients who were hospitalized forced the healthcare industry to halt rising costs while finding protocols to provide quality health care at lower cost.

In 2007 the Bush Administration announced the first eight conditions considered reasonably preventable by hospitals, and for which Medicare would stop reimbursing, beginning in October 2008. According to a spokesman for CMS, the intent is to become an active purchaser, not a passive payer, of health care (Zhang, 2007). The federal government expects to hold healthcare providers more accountable for quality while containing the rising costs of Medicare.

Since October 2006 hospitals have been required to report certain quality data or face a penalty. Numerous studies have captured the sizeable dollars spent on patient care for preventable events, illnesses, or complications. In 2006 it was estimated by a Health Affairs study that five adverse events accounted for $300 million in extra payments. The Agency for Healthcare Research and Quality found that adverse events during surgery cost employers $1.5 billion a year in 2001 and 2002, with 4,140 of 161,004 adult major surgeries having at least one preventable adverse event (Brown, 2008). According to a CMS press release, hospital payments are, on average, increased from a low of $700 per case for decubitus ulcers to $9,000 for postoperative sepsis (CMS, 2006). The data collected from mandatory reporting of events supports the use of incentives in reimbursement.

CMS "Never Event"

The Deficit Reduction Act of 2005 (Appendix 7–A) mandated a CMS policy eliminating reimbursement to hospitals for 10 events (Appendix 7–B) on the National Quality Forum's (NQF) "never-events" list:

1. Surgery on the wrong body
2. Objects left in the body during surgery

3. Mismatched blood transfusion
4. Cause serious injury or death
5. Air embolism
6. Injuries from patient falls
7. Pressure ulcers
8. Urinary-tract infections
9. Vascular-catheter-associated infections
10. Mediastinitis, an infection following heart surgery (Zhang, 2007)

The CMS adheres to the NQF definition that never events are (1) errors in medical care that are clearly identifiable and preventable, (2) serious in their consequences for patients, and (3) indicate a real problem in the safety and credibility of a healthcare facility (CMS, 2006). To be included, the event has to be unambiguous or clearly identifiable and measurable, and thus feasible to include in a reporting system. The event is usually preventable, which recognizes that some events are not always avoidable. The effect is serious in that it results in death or loss of a body part, disability, or more than transient loss of a body function. Finally, the event's impact is either adverse and/or indicative of a problem in a healthcare facility's safety systems and/or important for public credibility or public accountability (CMS, 2006).

CMS Reimbursement

Enforcement of the 2005 Act was in several steps spanning several years. In October 2007 Inpatient Prospective Payment System (IPPS) hospitals were mandated to report, under the present-on-admission (POA) coding, whether the diagnosis was made in a timely manner; if it was not, the assumption is that the illness was acquired during the hospital stay. The number of quality measures started at 10 in 2004 and grew to 43 measures in 2009 for the 3,500 IPPS hospitals paid under the system. Under the hospital reporting rules, entitlement to the full market-basket update reimbursement was tied to reporting of CMS quality measures. Not participating or not being successful in reporting hospital reimbursement is equal to the hospital market basket less two percentage points. Today hospital participation is at 99%, with those participating receiving 97% of the full annual payment update.

The following year, October 2008, CMS stopped payment for cases assigned the higher diagnosis-related group (DRG) when the condition was acquired during hospitalization. Hospitals are now penalized such that CMS does not reimburse them and the patient is not liable. The importance of accurate identification and coding at admission has to be stressed to physicians and nurses for proper billing and reimbursement to occur. Compliance with procedures for admission should be reviewed periodically with needed operational improvements made, if necessary.

CMS specified that the POA indicator must follow two general requirements. Firstly, POA is defined as present at the time the order for inpatient admission occurs; therefore, conditions that develop during an outpatient encounter, including emergency department, observation, or outpatient surgery, are considered POA. Secondly, the POA indicator is assigned to the principal diagnosis, secondary diagnoses, and external causes of injury codes.

Claims will not be denied when submitted using an HAC-related DRG, rather than the original non-HAC DRG, if a lower reimbursement is processed. The identification of the "never claim" begins with the submission of DRG used during the pre-authorization for the inpatient stay. The final DRG for reimbursement has to be the same as the admitting DRG or a DRG resulting in a lower reimbursement. The hospital will be paid for the initial-diagnosis DRG even if a DRG for an HAC event is submitted.

CMS partnered with the Agency for Healthcare Research and Quality (AHRQ) in developing a standardized hospital survey of inpatients. The national implementation in early 2006 provides public reporting of comparable data across hospitals and assists the hospitals with a set of survey measures to support quality improvement. The survey results of 927 hospitals are available to the public on the Web (http://www.hospital compare.hhs.gov/Hospital/Search/Welcome .asp?version=default&browser=IE%7C8%7C Windows+Vista&language=English&default status=0&MBPProviderID=&Target Page=&ComingFromMBP=&Cookies EnabledStatus=&TID=&StateAbbr=&ZIP& State=&pagelist=Home). For example, in the 2007 survey 54% of respondents said "always" to the two questions asked about how often hospital-staff-provided explanations regarding the purpose of any new medicines given and their possible side effects (CMS, 2007).

Non-CMS Quality Initiatives

The two incentives for the never-event program that the various stakeholders in health care agree on is the need for improvement in quality of care and that hospitals should not be rewarded through reimbursement of never events. Patients want the best care available, healthcare professionals want patient care to be exemplary, employers and insurers want quality care at affordable costs, and the governments, both federal and state, are responsible for regulating the institutions to further achievement of these goals. A key element of care is building trust, which is the result of a reduction in never events and, through evidence-based medicine, means identifying additional areas as opportunities for improvement. In addition to reimbursement, Medicare has programs, such as the one cosponsored with Premier, the hospital purchasing-alliance project, for 250 hospitals, aimed at better compliance to prevent blood clots, deep-vein thrombosis, and pulmonary embolism following knee or hip surgery (Landro, 2009 April). Increased quality of patient care through these types of programs will also contribute to cost control of the country's healthcare expenditures.

NATIONAL QUALITY FORUM

In a report issued in 1998, the President's Advisory Commission on Consumer Protection and Quality in the Health Care Industry proposed the creation of the NQF as part of an integrated national quality-improvement agenda. Leaders from consumer, purchaser, provider, health plan, and health service research organizations met as the Quality Forum Planning Committee convened throughout 1998 and early 1999 to define the mission, structure, and financing of the NQF. The NQF was incorporated as a new organization in May 1999 (NQF, 2009). CMS used the NQF original never-events list as a source for the original reportable and non-reimburseable list.

The NQF believes that reporting is a key element and resource for hospitals to learn from other hospitals' experiences. The NQF identifies these lessons learned and in a 2006 report listed 30 safe practices to be adopted to reduce the risk of harm to patients, stating, "These practices range from creating and sustaining a culture of safety to information management and continuity of care to matching healthcare needs with service capability. The eventual goal . . . would be to improve the things that help and prevent the things that harm" (NQF, 2009).

According to the NQF, medical errors kill 98,000 Americans each year. In their words, that is the equivalent of a 270-passenger jumbo jet crashing every day—more deaths than breast cancer, AIDS, or car accidents cause. There is also the economic toll that preventable medical errors cost, estimated to be from $17 to $29 billion annually. The NQF believes that these consequences disproportionately impact minorities and low-income patients (NQF, 2009).

The NQF also believes that while progress has been made in improving safety, the gains have to be more prevalent. Hospital goals of zero preventable errors with zero harm to patients means a culture of safety willing to learn from past mistakes.

The future of reimbursement is beyond the immediate known harm and costs of never events. The NQF is currently working on national standards for hospital care related to outcomes and efficiency to be used for both public accountability and quality improvement. The project will focus on safety, effectiveness, efficiency, timeliness, equity, and patient-centered care. Hospitals play a central role in coordinating care between ambulatory care, home care, and skilled-nursing facilities. The focus will be on readmissions of Medicare patients through the transition points and tracking care in the healthcare home. This project, funded by the CMS, will have an expansive view of potential measures of hospital outcomes including, for example, quality of the hospital transition, improvement in health-related quality of life and functional status, palliative-care symptom control, surgical outcomes, and efficiency (NQF, 2009). Definitely once standards are attached to reporting and meeting these targets, more incentives through reimbursement will follow.

LEAPFROG GROUP

The Leapfrog Group was founded in November 2000 by the Business Roundtable and is supported by its members, the Robert Wood Johnson Foundation, the Commonwealth Fund, the AHRQ, and other sources. Each year the Leapfrog Group survey solicits data from American hospitals concentrating on safety practices, efficiency, quality, and patient outcomes. Leapfrog, which represents approximately 37 million people in both the private and public sectors, accounts for "tens of billions of dollars in annual healthcare expenditures" (Paoletti, 2009). Participation in the survey is voluntary. The importance of the survey is the competitive nature that hospitals have in comparing themselves. Public reporting of the data from groups such as Leapfrog and CMS motivates hospital administrators who are "paying greater attention broadly to providing high-quality care" (Paoletti, 2009).

According to Leapfrog, use of their standards for ICU staff, medication-ordering systems, and use of higher-performing hospitals for high-risk procedures would save 57,000 lives, avoid 3 million adverse drug events, and save up to $12 billion in healthcare costs per year (Paoletti, 2009). Leapfrog members represent the consumer's point of view in contracting benefits design, employee education, and pay-for-performance programs. Hospitals will see the impact of Leapfrog in their private payer's more aggressive contract negotiations, not unlike the CMS direct approach.

In computerized prescriber order-entry (CPOE) the Leapfrog estimates the number of adverse drug events (ADE) could be reduced up to 88% or 3 million medication errors a year. The CPOE system compares the physician-entered order with the system's database of laboratory and prescription data. Potential errors or problems are indicated upon physician entry, preventing the ADE. For a risk manager the opportunity costs by reducing ADE goes beyond the $2,000 average additional hospital costs with associated reduced events leading to lawsuits.

Hospitals performing or considering high-risk procedures should be aware of their peers' performance in evaluating hospitals' entry into, or continuation of, these procedures. The Leapfrog standards go beyond the CMS never-events list in the standard of patient care for high-risk procedures. They recommend that certain high-risk procedures be performed at hospitals with a higher volume, as these hospitals tend to have better outcomes. Low-volume hospitals should weigh the expected outcomes when deciding if the procedure(s) should be done. For the low-volume hospital, referring patients for a better outcome is an option to be weighed against the risk of HAC.

The 2008 survey results on hospital-acquired infections reported that 65% of the hospitals did not have all of Leapfrog's recommended policies in place. Their data estimates that 2 million people contract an infection and 90,000 die each year during care (Paoletti, 2009). Survey results for HACs found that 30% of hospitals had fewer than 0.25 hospital-acquired pressure ulcers per 1,000 patient inpatient days and 25% of hospitals have fewer than 0.07 hospital-acquired injuries per inpatient days. There was a wide dispersion of reported results between hospitals. Compared with hospitals that meet the standards for hospital-acquired pressure ulcers, 6% reported rates at least 10 times higher, and for hospital-acquired injuries 10% had at least 10 times as many events (Paoletti, 2009). The reporting of data on the Web has to be considered whether or not the patient will become an informed consumer making choices based on such information, which would give the best hospitals a competitive advantage.

In Leapfrog's never-events policy four steps are suggested when an event occurs: "apologize to the patient and/or the patient's family, conduct a root cause analysis of the event, report the event to a patient safety organization and waive incremental costs associated with the events." These recommended steps are not new but should be standard protocol in hospitals from a risk manager's perspective because they place the hospital in the best possible position to manage the event.

PRIVATE INSURANCE

Some private insurers are following CMS's quality push when contracting with providers not to pay for never events and not permitting patients to be billed for the charges. The insurers will ban reimbursement for the gravest mistakes. Most insurers agree that over time they will adopt stronger policies, such as that of Medicare, which includes the less clear-cut problems (Fuhrmans, 2008).

The insurers model their programs after the NQF 28 never-event list. Aetna, the nation's third largest insurer, is including the NQF 28 when their contracts come up for renewal with their hospitals. WellPoint, a parent for many Blue Cross Blue Shield plans and the largest insurer, is using four errors in Virginia with plans to include hospitals in New England, New York, and Georgia. United Health Group and also Cigna are expected to follow suit. Most insurers agree that the savings from banning reimbursement for the initial never events will not significantly reduce healthcare costs. The intent is to improve quality by preventing these events from occurring (Fuhrmans, 2008).

The greater opportunity for significant gains in patient safety and reduced costs are in the more common errors. Medicare has taken the lead in including infections in their never-events list. Insurers will include a never-events claim payment ban partly in answer to employers' expectations for payers to initiate quality improvements through networks and hospital contracts. Employers looking to improve quality and patient safety with an affordable cost do not want to pay the costs of medical errors and never events but expect payers to stimulate improvements through network relationships, contracting and payment and want to know what actions health plans are taking.

Insurers following the lead of organizations such as NQF, Leapfrog, and the CDC now compile statistics of patient quality results from various sources. Although they are in agreement with CMS that reducing patient harm is possible, the insurers have taken different approaches toward that end.

Comparison of hospital-acquired complications or infection rates shows that the best can achieve almost zero rates in some categories. The future focus will be prevention with the continued use of adverse payment mechanisms for never events and for HAC when lower HAC rates are found to be achievable. However, non-payment for insurers has legal implications when working within the current contracts. Where Medicare issues rules, private insurers renegotiate contracts to accomplish the same result. In comparison, Medicare's use of the DRG payment is suited for reporting the uneventful stay and

HAC/never-event stay. Current private payments based on per diem has one bill with mixed costs and is hard to differentiate between normal and the never-events/HAC charges. Estimating the potential impact of payment incentives is hard to determine for both the hospital and the payer.

Providers

For providers, reducing the occurrence of never events to zero is achievable. The costs are estimated at $91 million per year or $23,772 per hospital or $4,114 per patient for HAC (Wilson, 2008). The surveys and reporting show that hospitals that exhibit good quality of care produce results that patients expect and healthcare professionals want to provide. It takes hospital administration and physician staff to challenge the status quo and rely on evidence-based methods to accomplish the change. The alternative is lawsuit awards in the millions for infections acquired in hospitals, for example, St. Anthony's Medical Center in St. Louis with a jury award of $2.5 million and Tenet Healthcare settlement of 106 lawsuits for $31 million (McCaughey, 2008); thus, the potential final cost to a hospital is substantially more than the lost reimbursement.

According to Ray Zielke, an American Society for Quality Health Care market manager, this approach to better quality when compared with employing the "carrot or the stick" is the stick: "When Medicare provides 46 or 47% of your revenue, and hospitals run on a 4 or 5% margin, that can be big, big money" (Krzykowski, 2008).

The publishing of outcomes brings quality of care to the attention of the hospital's board of trustees. Some hospitals have taken unique approaches to reduce events related to physicians. At the Nebraska Medical Center, a three-tier credentialing process separates physicians into groups that are clean with no errors, a second group of physicians with one problem found to be acceptable, and a final group having multiple behavioral or malpractice issues. This grouping focuses attention where it belongs. Nebraska Medical Center also introduced a "crew resource-management program" that is used in the aviation industry, where a dynamic similar to that between surgeons and operating-room nurses exists (Pellet, 2007).

Hospitals that have, since 2005, been preparing by implementing patient safety programs set with higher standards believe that costs of the never-events policy should be minimal. The quality improvements range from the simple checklists intended to halt wrong-sided surgeries to enabling technology with surgical sponges containing radio trans-mitters (RFI tags) detectable with wands passed over the patient (Krzykowski, 2008). Still, the Leapfrog report found that 87% of hospitals are not following recommended guidelines, causing 2 million hospital-acquired infections and 90,000 deaths accounting for the majority of preventable adverse events (Sloane, 2007). Most of the steps necessary to prevent infections are simple but require train-ing and a corporate culture that instills compli-ance. "As a small but growing band of institutions has found, it can be the start of something bigger, the realization of patient-centered care" (Sloane, 2007).

Patients

For the patient, receiving the best quality of care is the ultimate goal. Health care is no longer just considered the community hospi-tal; it is categorized as an industry. Consider patients having greater access to hospital peer reporting, for comparison, when ser-vices are non-emergency. Considering patients as a consumer group, society now encourages the use of various resources, such as the Internet, for purchasing data. Hospital decision makers will need to know how they rank in these comparisons and what the expected impacts are. In addition, providers have to keep their patients' loyalty while knowing that insurers find difficulty in restricting provider entry into their networks when their employers seek a full-access provider network.

CONCLUSION

Since the original publication of "To Err Is Human," the healthcare industry has been self-regulated in terms of improving quality of care to reduce harm to patients. Public availability of various sources of information provides patients with the consumer data needed to decide which hospitals to choose for their care. Given this knowledge, patients can make an informed decision based on medical evidence. The uncertain factor is the personal nature of the patient–physician rela-tionship, which relies on the trust placed in the physician by the patient. This particular relationship dynamic usually overrides any rational decision to choose the highest-quality hospital. Another consideration is the nature of the patient's needs when time or the patient's financial situation does not per-mit an informed consumer decision.

Medicare is leading the way with stringent rules on never events. Many people would agree that some are truly events that should never occur; others claim that hospital-acquired complications are part of the hospi-tal setting. Peer comparison shows that steady improvement can result in minimal or zero adverse-event occurrences in hospitals with a culture of safety. One stakeholder, The Joint Commission on Accreditation of Health-care Organizations (TJC, 2008), is well posi-tioned to take the lead in setting appropriate risk-adjusted standards. Their role as the major hospital accreditator could be instru-mental in using evidence-based medicine to decide if hospitals meet the test. They state the following (TJC 2008):

> Over the next year, the current National Patient Safety Goals will undergo an extensive review process; as a result, there will be no new NPSGs developed for 2010. The Joint Commission and the

Patient Safety Advisory Group . . . have heard from the field and determined that now is the time to look at current NPSGs and review the process for development of NPSGs. Some of The Joint Commission's most visible and effective requirements, the NPSGs, highlight serious patient safety issues that need to be addressed by healthcare organizations. Compliance with the NPSGs is a critical and demanding part of the accreditation process. NPSGs have evolved over time, becoming more specific and detailed in some cases, and therefore require more time and resources to implement. The field is struggling to meet some of the current NPSGs.

The admission that healthcare professionals are struggling to meet patient safety goals is confirmation that hospitals will continue to be subject to pressure from CMS and other payers.

References

Brown, S.B. (2008). Never events in surgery prove costly. *Hospitals & Health Networks, 82*(10), 72.

Centers for Medicare and Medicaid Services (CMS). (2006, May 18). *Eliminating serious, preventable, and costly medical errors: Never events* (press release). Retrieved April 13, 2009, from http://www.cms.hhs.gov/.

Centers for Medicare and Medicaid Services (CMS). (2007). *2007 CAHPS hospital survey chartbook*. Retrieved May 5, 2009, from http://www.ahrq.gov/.

Centers for Medicare and Medicaid Services. (n.d.). *Downloads*. Retrieved from http://www.cms.hhs.gov/HospitalAcqCond/Downloads/HAC_HOP-HAC_LS_Slides.zip/.

Fuhrmans, V. (2008, January 15). Insurers stop paying for care linked to errors. *The Wall Street Journal* (eastern edition), p. D.1. Retrieved April 5, 2009, from ABI/INFORM global database (document ID: 1412798451).

Haynes, A.B., Weiser, T.G., Berry, W.R., Lipsitz, S.R., Breizat, A.H.S., Dellinger, E.P., et al. (2009). *A surgical safety checklist to reduce morbidity in a global population*. Retrieved April 28, 2009, from http://www.nejm.org/.

Illinois General Assembly. (2005). *Illinois compiled statutes*. Retrieved May 5, 2009, from http://www.ilga.gov/legislation/ilcs/ilcs.asp/.

Kohn, L.T., Corrigan, J.M., & Donaldson, M.S. (Eds.). (2000). To err is human: Building a safer health system. Institute of Medicine (IOM) Committee on Quality of Health Care in America. Washington, DC: National Academies Press.

Krzykowski, B. (2008). Hospitals prep for policy change. *Quality Progress, 41*(4), 14.

Landro, L. (2009, February 4). The informed patient: Lax needle use in clinics raises alarm—recent hepatitis outbreaks from reuse of syringes spur efforts to improve practices. *The Wall Street Journal* (eastern edition), p. D.1. Retrieved April 5, 2009, from ABI/INFORM global database (document ID: 1637889531).

Landro, L. (2009, April 1). The informed patient: In the hospital, facing a scourge of killer clots—Medicare move spurs efforts to improve screening for risk of pulmonary embolism. *The Wall Street Journal* (eastern edition), p. D.1. Retrieved April 5, 2009, from ABI/INFORM global database (document ID: 1670679991).

McCaughey, B. (2008, August 14). Hospital infections: preventable and unacceptable. *The Wall Street Journal* (eastern edition), p. A.11. Retrieved April 5, 2009, from ABI/INFORM global database (document ID: 1531362451).

National Quality Forum (NQF). (2009). Safe Practices for Better Healthcare. Retrieved April 26, 2009, from http://www.ahrq.gov/qual/nqfpract.pdf.

Paoletti, C. (2009). Leapfrog Hospital survey results 2008. Retrieved April 30, 2009, from http://www.leapfroggroup.org/.

Pellet, J. (2007). A prescription for health care. *Chief Executive, 230*, 52–57.

Sloane, T. (2007). The start of something big. *Modern Healthcare, 37*(51), 22.

TJC. (2008). The Joint Commission. *National patient safety goals.* Retrieved May 5, 2009, from http://www.jointcommission.org/.

Wilson, L. (2008). The cost of errors: You break it, you pay for it. *Modern Healthcare,* 8–9.

Zhang, J. (2007, August 20). Medicare to stop paying for some hospital errors. *The Wall Street Journal* (eastern edition), p. B.2. Retrieved April 5, 2009, from ABI/INFORM global database (document ID: 1568438951).

APPENDIX 7–A: DEFICIT REDUCTION ACT SEC. 5001. HOSPITAL QUALITY IMPROVEMENT

(c) QUALITY ADJUSTMENT IN DRG PAYMENTS FOR CERTAIN HOSPITAL ACQUIRED INFECTIONS

(1) IN GENERAL- Section 1886(d)(4) of the Social Security Act (42 U.S.C. 1395ww(d)(4)) is amended by adding at the end the following new subparagraph:

(D)(i) For discharges occurring on or after October 1, 2008, the diagnosis-related group to be assigned under this paragraph for a discharge described in clause (ii) shall be a diagnosis-related group that does not result in higher payment based on the presence of a secondary diagnosis code described in clause (iv).

(ii) A discharge described in this clause is a discharge which meets the following requirements:

(I) The discharge includes a condition identified by a diagnosis code selected under clause (iv) as a secondary diagnosis.

(II) But for clause (i), the discharge would have been classified to a diagnosis-related group that results in a higher payment based on the presence of a secondary diagnosis code selected under clause (iv).

(III) At the time of admission, no code selected under clause (iv) was present.

(iii) As part of the information required to be reported by a hospital with respect to a discharge of an individual in order for payment to be made under this subsection, for discharges occurring on or after October 1, 2007, the information shall include the secondary diagnosis of the individual at admission.

(iv) By not later than October 1, 2007, the Secretary shall select diagnosis codes associated with at least two conditions, each of which codes meets all of the following requirements (as determined by the Secretary):

(I) Cases described by such code have a high cost or high volume, or both, under this title.

(II) The code results in the assignment of a case to a diagnosis-related group that has a higher payment when the code is present as a secondary diagnosis.

(III) The code describes such conditions that could reasonably have been prevented through the application of evidence-based guidelines.

The Secretary may from time to time revise (through addition or deletion of codes) the diagnosis codes selected under this clause so long as there are diagnosis codes associated with at least two conditions selected for discharges occurring during any fiscal year.

(v) In selecting and revising diagnosis codes under clause (iv), the Secretary shall consult with the Centers for Disease Control and Prevention and other appropriate entities.

(vi) Any change resulting from the application of this subparagraph shall not be taken into account in adjusting the weighting factors under subparagraph (C)(i) or in applying budget neutrality under subparagraph (C)(iii).

(2) NO JUDICIAL REVIEW- Section 1886(d)(7)(B) of such Act (42 U.S.C. 1395 ww(d)(7)(B)) is amended by inserting before the period the following, including the selection and revision of codes under paragraph (4)(D).

APPENDIX 7–B: "NEVER-EVENT" LIST

Hospital-Acquired Conditions

Medicare has selected conditions that are reasonably preventable—and either costly or common—by following evidence-based guidelines. These conditions include:

- A foreign object (such as a sponge or needle) inadvertently left in a patient after surgery
- An air embolism (an air bubble that enters the bloodstream and can obstruct the flow of blood to the brain and vital organs)
- Transfusion with the wrong type of blood
- Severe pressure ulcers, i.e., deterioration of the skin due to the patient staying in one position too long, that have progressed to the point that tissue under the skin is affected (stage III), or that have become so deep that there is damage to the muscle and bone, and sometimes tendons and joints (stage IV)

Injuries from falls and trauma include:

- Fracture
- Joint dislocation
- Head injury
- Crushing injury
- Burn
- Electric shock
- Catheter-associated urinary-tract infection
- Vascular catheter-associated infection
- Manifestations of poor control of blood-sugar levels
- Surgical-site infection following coronary artery bypass graft
- Surgical-site infection following certain orthopedic procedures
- Surgical-site infection following bariatric surgery for obesity
- Deep-vein thrombosis (a blood clot in a major vein) and pulmonary embolism (blockage in the lungs) following certain orthopedic procedures
- Insemination of wrong donor sperm

APPENDIX 7–C: LEAPFROG PATIENT SAFETY INITIATIVES

- Prevent Medication Errors (formerly Computer Physician Order Entry)
  - Does the hospital use an electronic prescribing system with the ability to intercept errors at the time medications are ordered?
- Appropriate ICU Staffing (formerly ICU Physician Staffing)
  - Are the hospital ICUs staffed with intensivists—doctors and other caregivers with special training in critical care?
- High Risk Treatments (formerly Evidence-Based Hospital Referral)
  - Does the hospital have lots of experience and the best results for specific procedures, surgeries, or conditions?
- Steps to Avoid Harm (Formerly National Quality Forum-Endorsed Safe Practices)
  - Has the hospital put in place procedures to reduce 13 preventable medical mistakes?

- Managing Serious Errors (formerly Adherence to Never-Events Policy)
  - Has the hospital agreed to do the following if a never event occurs?
    1) Apologize to the patient and/or family
    2) Report the event to a specified agency within 10 days
    3) Perform a root cause analysis
    4) Waive costs directly related to the adverse event
- Transparency Indicator
  - Does the hospital make its quality and safety record public?
- Reduce Pressure Ulcers
  - Does the hospital have a low rate of pressure ulcers?
- Reduce In-Hospital Injuries
  - Does the hospital have a low rate of patients injured during their hospital stay? Possible injuries include falls, fractures, and burns.

Source: www.leapfroggroup.org

8

THE PATIENT SAFETY AND QUALITY IMPROVEMENT ACT: TENSION BETWEEN IMPROVING QUALITY OF CARE AND ACKNOWLEDGING RESPONSIBILITY FOR ERROR

Michelle M. Garvey, MEd, BA

INTRODUCTION

The Patient Safety and Quality Improvement Act emerged in July 2005 to provide the framework for a broader, more uniform system for medical-error prevention and reporting nationwide.[1] The Act appeared after individual states responded to the 1999 Institute of Medicine report, "To Err Is Human: Building a Safer Health System," by passing legislation aimed at improving medical-error reporting.[1] The state error-reporting statutes provided some evidentiary privilege for information reported to state agencies, but state agencies were often required to reveal that events or incidents had been reported or to notify involved patients and patients' families of events or incidents.[1] As a result, hospital legal counsel often advised against voluntary disclosure of information about medical errors to patients or their families, fearing that such information would be discoverable by plaintiffs' attorneys. In addition, organizations often failed to disclose what

was learned to their own staff and limited any meaningful dialogue about error and near-miss events or the sharing of information with staff following adverse events out of fear of loss of protection. This practice impeded the ability to learn from errors and to design appropriate strategies to prevent their recurrence. The Patient Safety and Quality Improvement Act responded by providing blanket confidentiality and privilege protections for such information if the information was developed for reporting to Patient Safety Organizations (PSOs), organizations that work with healthcare providers to identify, analyze, and reduce the risks and hazards associated with patient care.[2] Risk managers must clearly understand the benefits and limitations of this legislation in order to know what information can receive the benefit of protection against discovery under this Act.

Although the Act was signed into law on July 29, 2005, it remains unclear how far it goes to actually shield providers from liability by providing confidentiality and privilege protections to information defined as patient safety work product. This chapter provides a brief overview of the federal confidentiality and privilege protections for patient safety work product and argues that the Patient Safety and Quality Improvement Act should be read narrowly to limit the scope of information that is privileged and protected under the Act.

OBJECTIVES OF THE PATIENT SAFETY AND QUALITY IMPROVEMENT ACT OF 2005

According to the Agency for Healthcare Research and Quality (AHRQ), the Patient Safety and Quality Improvement Act of 2005 was created with three distinct goals: (1) to encourage the development of PSOs, (2) to foster a culture of safety by establishing federal confidentiality and privilege protections for reported patient safety information, and (3) to identify and publicize solutions for the risks and hazards associated with patient care.[2] The PSOs are certified public and private organizations that engage in patient safety activities, such as collecting and analyzing patient safety work product and utilizing data from patient safety work product to minimize patient risk.[3] Hospital systems, medical societies, group practices, registries, and large for-profit entities may become PSOs.[4] Although PSOs are not federally funded, AHRQ certifies and lists PSOs, and the Office for Civil Rights (OCR) investigates and enforces confidentiality provisions.[5]

The Act encourages provider organizations and other public and private entities to partner with PSOs by providing privilege and confidentiality protections for patient safety work product that is developed for reporting to PSOs. Thus, by becoming PSOs or partnering with PSOs, healthcare-provider organizations obtain privilege protections for reported information about patient safety events. By providing a secure environment for

reporting, PSOs receive, analyze, process, and publicize data to identify and reduce the risks and hazards associated with patient care. By the end of 2009, 69 PSOs were listed with AHRQ.[4]

DEFINITION OF PATIENT SAFETY WORK PRODUCT

In order to receive privilege and confidentiality protections under the Act, information must be classified as patient safety work product. Patient safety work product is defined as any data, reports, records, memoranda, analyses (such as root-cause analyses), or written or oral statements that (1) are assembled or developed by a provider for the purpose of reporting to a patient safety organization and are reported to a patient safety organization, or (2) are developed by a patient safety organization for the conduct of patient safety activities and that could result in improved patient safety, healthcare quality, or healthcare outcomes; or that identify or constitute the deliberations or analysis of, or identify the fact of reporting pursuant to, a patient safety evaluation system.[6]

The Act is clear that patient safety work product does not include medical records or billing and discharge information, or information that is collected, maintained, or developed separately from a patient safety evaluation system:[7]

> Information described [as patient safety work product] does not include a patient's medical record, billing and discharge information, or any other original patient or provider record. Information described [as patient safety work product] does not include information that is collected, maintained, or developed separately, or exists separately, from a patient safety evaluation system. Such separate information or a copy thereof reported to a patient safety

organization shall not by reason of its reporting be considered patient safety work product.[6]

The only provider-supplied information classified as patient safety work product under the Act, therefore, is patient safety information assembled or developed for the purpose of reporting to a PSO and subsequently reported to a PSO. The Patient Safety and Quality Improvement Final Rule clarifies that patient safety work product includes information not yet reported to a PSO, if that information is documented within a provider's patient safety evaluation system and is later reported to a PSO.[8] Additionally, retrospective analyses could constitute patient safety work product if the initial unanalyzed information was itself patient safety work product.[9]

Medical records, billing information, and other original provider records are not patient safety work product, because they are not specifically developed for the purpose of reporting to a PSO. According to this provision, information about patient safety collected by healthcare organizations for other purposes, such as defense of liability claims, medical-staff peer review, and quality improvement, is not patient safety work product (B. Youngberg, interview with D. Cousins and L. Patton, Center for Quality Improvement and Patient Safety, AHRQ). Because such information might be important to the analysis of a patient safety event, information contained in these records may be incorporated into patient safety work product, but the original record must be maintained separately.[10] Furthermore, copies of patient safety event information are not classified as patient safety work product if later reported to a PSO (B. Youngberg, interview with D. Cousins and L. Patton, Center for Quality Improvement and Patient Safety, AHRQ); thus, information that is not initially patient safety work product cannot later become patient safety work product by virtue of reporting to a PSO.

FEDERAL PRIVILEGE AND CONFIDENTIALITY PROTECTIONS FOR PATIENT SAFETY WORK PRODUCT

The Patient Safety and Quality Improvement Act of 2005 states:

> Patient safety work product alone is privileged and shall not be: (1) subject to a Federal, State, or local civil, criminal, or administrative subpoena or order, including in a Federal, State, or local civil or administrative disciplinary proceeding against a provider; (2) subject to discovery in connection with a Federal, State, or local civil, criminal, or administrative proceeding, including in a Federal, State, or local civil or administrative disciplinary proceeding against a provider; (3) admitted as evidence in any Federal, State, or local governmental civil proceeding, criminal proceeding, administrative rulemaking proceeding, or administrative adjudicatory proceeding, including any proceeding against a provider; or (4) admitted in a professional disciplinary proceeding of a professional disciplinary body established or specifically authorized under State law.[11]

Similarly, patient safety work product is confidential under the Act:

> Notwithstanding any other provision of federal, state, or local law, and subject to [limited exceptions] patient safety work product shall be confidential and shall not be disclosed.[12]

In order to obtain the above mentioned privilege and confidentiality protections, information must be specifically identified as patient safety work product, assembled or developed for reporting to a PSO and subsequently reported to a PSO. The limited definition of patient safety work product is critical in this context, because it prevents providers from protecting information from discovery or disclosure by sending the information or a copy of the information to a PSO.[13] Information that is not initially patient safety work product cannot become patient safety work product and gain privilege protections simply by virtue of reporting.

The Final Rule defines "disclosure" for the purpose of applying and enforcing the privilege and confidentiality provisions. According to the Rule, disclosure is "the release of, transfer of, provision of, access to, or divulging in any other manner of, patient safety work product, by an entity or natural person holding the patient safety work product to another *legally separate* entity or natural person, other than a workforce member of, or a physician holding privileges with, the entity holding the patient safety work product" (emphasis added).[14]

The sharing of patient safety work product from a component PSO to the entity of which it is a part, however, does constitute a disclosure, even though such a disclosure is internal to the entity and would be permitted according to the definition above.[14] The Final Rule emphasizes that the sharing of patient safety work product between a healthcare provider with privilege protections and the entity with which it holds the privileges does not constitute a disclosure.[14] The Act contains this provision because providers' participation with PSOs is voluntary and because the Act was created to promote the reporting and analysis of patient safety events.[14]

The Act provides for civil monetary penalties of up to $10,000 assessed against any person who knowingly or recklessly divulges patient safety work product in violation of privilege and confidentiality protections.[15] Equitable relief and compensatory damages are to be awarded to individuals adversely affected because of their good-faith reporting.[16] These sanctions encourage the reporting of patient safety events and protect

providers' interests by discouraging improper disclosure of patient safety work product.

EXCEPTIONS TO FEDERAL PRIVILEGE AND CONFIDENTIALITY PROTECTIONS

Exceptions to privilege and confidentiality protections may arise in criminal proceedings or civil actions due to violations of reporters' rights and with the authorization of identified providers:

> [Privilege and confidentiality protections] shall no longer apply to . . . one or more of the following disclosures: (a) disclosure of relevant patient safety work product for use in a criminal proceeding, but only after a court makes an in camera determination that such patient safety work product contains evidence of a criminal act and that such patient safety work product is material to the proceeding and not reasonably available from any other source; (b) disclosure of patient safety work product to the extent required to [obtain equitable relief for an adverse employment action based on good faith reporting of patient safety information to a PSO]; (c) disclosure of identifiable patient safety work product if authorized by each provider identified in such work product.[17]

Confidentiality protections do not apply to disclosures of patient safety work product for conducting patient safety activities or to disclosures to entities carrying out research authorized by the Secretary of the Department of Health and Human Services.[17] In addition, providers may voluntarily disclose patient safety work product to an accrediting body, and the Secretary may disclose patient safety work product as necessary for business operations and furthering the goals of the Act.[17]

In general, disclosure is not treated as a waiver of privilege or confidentiality protections; however, if patient safety work product is disclosed in a criminal proceeding or if the work product is non-identifiable, confidentiality protections no longer apply:[18]

> Patient safety work product that is disclosed . . . shall continue to be privileged and confidential . . . and such disclosure shall be treated as a waiver of privilege or confidentiality, and the privileged and confidential nature of such work product shall also apply to such work product in the possession or control of a person to whom such work product was disclosed. [However], if patient safety work product is disclosed in a criminal proceeding, the confidentiality protections . . . shall no longer apply . . . and if patient safety work product is disclosed [and is nonidentifiable], the privilege and confidentiality protections . . . shall no longer apply. . . .[19]

The Act provides limited exceptions to privilege and confidentiality protections, because these protections motivate providers to create or partner with PSOs to develop cultures of safety within healthcare organizations.

ADDITIONAL INCENTIVES FOR PROVIDERS

In addition to providing privilege and confidentiality protections, the Act prohibits accrediting bodies from taking action against providers because of providers' relationships with PSOs:

> An accrediting body shall not take an accrediting action against a provider based on the good faith participation of the provider in the collection, development, reporting, or maintenance of patient safety

work product . . . an accrediting body may not require a provider to reveal its communications with any patient safety organization . . .[20]

Accrediting bodies cannot identify providers who work with PSOs and subsequently pursue investigation of patient safety events involving those providers. Moreover, the Act encourages providers to work with, and report to, multiple PSOs in order to facilitate protection for providers and analysis of patient safety data.[21]

ARGUMENT FOR A NARROW READING OF THE ACT

The Supreme Court has cautioned that privilege and confidentiality protections be strictly construed, especially when Congress has considered competing concerns and has chosen not to extend such protections.[22] Here, the Act is clear about what can and cannot be privileged and confidential patient safety work product, and the Final Rule further clarifies the terms and provisions of the Act (B. Youngberg, interview with D. Cousins and L. Patton, Center for Quality Improvement and Patient Safety, AHRQ). It cautions against over-inclusiveness, stating:

> The fact that information is collected, developed, or analyzed under the protections of the Patient Safety Act does not shield a provider from needing to undertake similar activities, if applicable, outside of the ambit of the statute, so that the provider can meet its obligations with non-patient safety work product.[23]

Because the original records underlying patient safety work product are not actually patient safety work product, providers gain no privilege protections for such records and must submit them to fulfill state and other reporting requirements for patient safety events.[24] The Act cannot relieve a provider of responsibility to provide data to external authorities seeking information about how it has instituted corrective action following a reported threat to the quality or safety of patient care.[24] The provider must respond with information that is not patient safety work product; thus, the Act assumes that required patient safety information is available in an original record or another source maintained by the provider or provider organization.

IMPLICATIONS FOR PROVIDER LIABILITY

Although the Patient Safety and Quality Improvement Act was enacted in 2005, the Act has not been widely invoked in judicial proceedings throughout the past 4 years. Only one major case and a limited number of court documents have cited the Act, but none has prevented disclosure of patient safety information based on the privilege and confidentiality protections available for patient safety work product. This section and the sections that follow discuss that case and argue that the Act cannot be used to shield providers from liability for patient safety events.

In *Schlegel v. Kaiser Foundation Health Plan*, the plaintiff, a kidney-transplant patient, motioned to compel production of documents relating to the overall operation of Kaiser's transplant program, including documents relating to any investigation and audits of the transplant center by Kaiser, California's Department of Managed Health Care (DMHC), the Department of Health and Human Services Centers for Medicare and Medicaid Services (CMS), and the United Network for Organ Sharing (UNOS).[25] The defendants objected to the production of these documents, asserting that they were protected by the peer-review privilege and the "self-critical" analysis privilege.[25] Specifically, defendants asserted that state law peer-review privileges should apply and that Congress created a broad peer-review privilege

when it enacted the Patient Safety and Quality Improvement Act.[25]

The court granted the motion to compel based in part on the unique and narrow privilege created by the Act.[26] The court held that there was no indication that investigations conducted by defendants were prepared for, and reported to, a PSO and determined that none of the involved entities were PSOs.[26] Additionally, there was no evidence that the "mission and primary activity" of any of the relevant entities concerned the goal of patient safety as defined by the Act.[26] Because the documents requested were not patient safety work product according to the definition provided by the Act, they were not privileged and confidential and therefore were not protected from discovery.

The district court construed the definition of patient safety work product narrowly and emphasized that patient safety work product must be developed for reporting to a PSO. The court determined that the Act "carves out a narrow peer review privilege for work product prepared by a patient safety organization or prepared for, and reported to, a patient safety organization."[26] Although *Schlegel* is the only recorded case to interpret the Act, future courts will be challenged to apply the Act to situations where patient safety information appears more like patient safety work product than that at issue in *Schlegel*; however, if courts properly apply the limited definition of patient safety work product as stated in the Act, they will not extend privilege and confidentiality protections to shield providers from liability for adverse patient safety events. Applying the Act to several scenarios that might arise in litigation illustrates the narrow scope of the privilege and confidentiality protections.

COPIES OF PATIENT SAFETY WORK PRODUCT

Because the word "copy" is used in two senses in the Act and does not adhere to its plain-language meaning, courts will likely be challenged to determine whether or not copies of patient safety work product and copies of non-patient safety work product are privileged. The Act is clear that copies of patient safety records do not become patient safety work product if not originally developed for the purpose of reporting to a PSO; however, providers might choose to provide copies of these records to a PSO in order to support the PSO's analysis of a medical error. For example, a provider might develop a root-cause analysis for a PSO and might also provide the PSO with a copy of a patient's medical record to facilitate the PSO's investigation. In this case, because it was developed for the purpose of reporting to a PSO, the root-cause analysis would fall under the definition of patient safety work product and would gain privilege protections. The original medical record would not fall under the definition and would not gain privilege protections, but a copy of the record would be protected in the hands of the PSO. Although a plaintiff's attorney could discover information about the medical error in the provider's original medical record, the attorney could not gain access to the medical record through the PSO. (All of the foregoing information was obtained by M.M. Garvey in a telephone interview with D. Cousins and L. Patton, Center for Quality Improvement and Patient Safety, AHRQ.)

Courts challenged to determine whether or not copies of records are discoverable should determine why the records were created and where the records are available. Copies of patient safety work product remaining in the hands of a provider are protected if not used for any other purpose. Copies of non-patient safety work product, such as original provider records, are not protected in the hands of a provider but are protected in the hands of a PSO.

PATIENT SAFETY WORK PRODUCT USED FOR OTHER PURPOSES

A related issue is whether patient safety work product is protected if it is first developed for reporting to a PSO, is reported to a PSO, and is subsequently used for other purposes. To address this question, the Final Rule reviews how information becomes patient safety work product. Information becomes patient safety work product when reported to a PSO or when collected within a patient safety evaluation system for the purpose of reporting to a PSO.[27] If such information is initially developed for reporting to a PSO but is later reported to fulfill state reporting obligations, the information is removed from the patient safety evaluation system and is no longer privileged patient safety work product.[27] Similarly, patient safety information cannot remain privileged and protected after reporting to a PSO if the information is needed to fulfill state reporting requirements.[27] The limited definition of patient safety work product further narrows the scope of information that is privileged and confidential. Patient safety information that is used in medical records, billing and discharge information, and other provider records is not protected as patient safety work product.[28] Furthermore, provider-driven analyses may not be protected if it is incumbent upon a hospital to inspect records for state reporting (B. Youngberg, interview with D. Cousins and L. Patton, Center for Quality Improvement and Patient Safety, AHRQ).

PEER-REVIEW CONCERNS

Although the definition of patient safety work product is limited in the Act and Final Rule, the definition has yet to be tested and applied; thus, it remains unclear whether information generated from peer-review activities falls within the parameters of patient safety work product. Peer-review committees generally consist of hospital-staff physicians who evaluate the performance of other physicians who treat patients at the hospital. Since the advent of peer-review committees in the early 1900s, providers have feared civil liability and loss of esteem among colleagues as a result of the peer-review process.[29] Today, if findings of peer-review committees were privileged and protected as patient safety work product under the Patient Safety and Quality Improvement Act, providers would be more willing to participate in peer review, a valuable process for improving quality of care and patient outcomes.

Even if the Act is interpreted narrowly, it is likely that courts would protect information developed in the peer-review process, if that information were developed for the purpose of reporting to a PSO. Although the words "peer review" do not appear in the statute, the Act's legislative history contains frequent references to expanding peer-review protections so that healthcare providers can report medical errors without fear of being sued.[30] If provider organizations established relationships with PSOs and participated in the peer-review process in order to collect information about patient safety events for reporting to PSOs, that information would be patient safety work product and would gain privilege and confidentiality protections under the law. Such protections would encourage providers to engage in peer-review activities without fear of being sued or losing prestige. Although the Act has yet to be applied to information produced in the peer-review process, it is likely that a court would view such information as patient safety work product if it were developed for, and reported to, a PSO.

CONCLUSION

Although the privilege and confidentiality protections in the Patient Safety and Quality Improvement Act have not been widely tested, the protections will not fully shield a provider from all liability due to medical errors. The narrow application of the privilege and confidentiality protections prevents the disclosure of patient safety work product, but plaintiffs and plaintiffs' attorneys would likely discover information about medical error in medical records, billing and discharge information, and other original provider records not protected under the Act. In addition, once litigation ensues it is likely that specific questions posed in written interrogatories or in depositions will be posed to defendants and witnesses in order to elicit the information needed to prove a deviation from the acceptable standard of care; however, the Act encourages providers to participate in patient safety activities by fully protecting information that is collected and ultimately reported.

As outlined herein, the primary purpose of the Patient Safety and Quality Improvement Act is to improve the quality of patient care and patient outcomes by encouraging providers to report patient safety events to PSOs. Although providers are not totally shielded from liability under the Act, the Act does protect them from liability based on reporting to PSOs; thus, the Act benefits providers by promoting the reporting and analysis of medical errors for future error prevention, not by shielding providers from liability. Providers who hope to learn from medical errors and to develop a culture of safety in their organizations can report patient safety information without fear that the information will later be used against them in a court of law.

References

1. Key, C.M. (2005). A review of the Patient Safety and Quality Improvement Act of 2005. *Health Law, 18*, 1–20.
2. Agency for Healthcare Research and Quality. (2008). *The Patient Safety and Quality Improvement Act of 2005.* Retrieved May 10, 2010, from http://www.ahrq.gov/qual/psoact.htm.
3. 42 U.S.C.A. §299b-21(4) (2005).
4. Ivill, D.S., & Hooper Kearbey, A. (2009). The rise of patient safety organizations: Reporting and sharing without fear of liability. *Medical Malpractice Law & Strategy, 23*(3).
5. Patient Safety and Quality Improvement Final Rule, 73 Fed. Reg. 70,732 (November 21,

2008) (to be codified at 42 C.F.R. pt. 3). Retrieved April 7, 2010 from http://www.pso.ahrq.gov/regulations/regulations.htm/.

6. 42 U.S.C.A. §299b-21(7).
7. Patient Safety and Quality Improvement, 73 Fed. Reg. at 70,738.
8. Patient Safety and Quality Improvement, 73 Fed. Reg. at 70,732.
9. Ibid, at 70,744.
10. Patient Safety and Quality Improvement, 73 Fed. Reg. at 70,743.
11. 42 U.S.C.A. §299b-22(a).
12. Ibid, §299b-22(b).
13. Gosfield, A.G. (Ed.). (2009). *Health Law Handbook, §12,* 57.
14. Patient Safety and Quality Improvement, 73 Fed. Reg. at 70,736.
15. 42 U.S.C.A. §299b-22(f)(1).
16. Ibid, §299b-22(f)(4).
17. Ibid, §299b-22(b)(2).
18. Ibid, §299b-21(3).
19. Ibid, §299b-22(d)(1).
20. Ibid, §299b-22(d)(4B).
21. Patient Safety and Quality Improvement, 73 Fed. Reg. at 70,779.
22. Leaman, K. (2007). *Let's give them something to talk about: How the PSQIA may provide federal privilege and confidentiality protections to the medical peer review process.* (Comment). *Michigan State Law Review, 11*(178), 186.
23. Patient Safety and Quality Improvement, 73 Fed. Reg. at 70,732.
24. Ibid, at 70,740.
25. Schlegel v. Kaiser Foundation Health Plan, No. CIV 07-0520 MCE KJM, 2008 WL 4570619, at *2 (E.D. Cal. October 14, 2008).
26. Ibid, at 3.
27. Patient Safety and Quality Improvement, 73 Fed. Reg. at 70,742.
28. 42 U.S.C.A. §299b-21(7)(B)(i).
29. Leaman, K. (2007). *Let's give them something to talk about: How the PSQIA may provide federal privilege and confidentiality protections to the medical peer review process.* (Comment). *Michigan State Law Review, 11*(178), 178.
30. Ibid, pp. 186–187.

9

THE ROLE OF GOVERNANCE IN HOSPITAL RISK MANAGEMENT AND PATIENT SAFETY

Patricia Meersman, MBA, MJ, BA

Leaders are responsible for every-thing in the organization, especially everything that goes wrong.

—Paul O'Neill, Former Secretary of the Treasury and Chairman and CEO of Alcoa

INTRODUCTION

There is no doubt that national reports and media coverage about the quality of inpatient hospital care in the United States have captured the attention of consumers, purchasers, and government agencies.[1] In response, health plans, employers, Internet-based information companies, and government agencies are publicly disseminating an unprecedented amount of information about the quality of hospital care, ranging from patient satisfaction and process quality to clinical outcomes.[2] The emerging picture of potential harm to patients has prompted local communities and government regulators to increase pressure on hospitals to improve quality and patient safety. As evidenced by a recent survey of senior hospital executives, the message is getting through and has focused the attention of hospital leadership on quality and safety issues.[3]

Once limited to case-by-case responses and reactions to individual incidents, patient-safety-improvement activities now permeate healthcare organizations. In particularly complex organizations like hospitals, quality-performance improvement and risk management activity is ideally based on a culture of safety and scientific systems of measuring and reporting data.[4] Systematic change in organizational culture, no matter how urgently needed, is unlikely to happen unless the organization makes that change a top priority. Since setting organizational priorities is a governance function, the task of firmly engaging a hospital in an ongoing culture of patient safety falls squarely on the governing board. Boards adopting an arms-length oversight approach to patient safety, risk management, and quality improvement cannot meet this responsibility; instead, boards must actively participate in leading the establishment and support of strategies for systemic change. By law and regulation, the ultimate responsibility for hospital performance, including the quality and safety of patient care, resides with the governing board. This responsibility is also reflected in accreditation requirements, as reflected in standards set by The Joint Commission.[5]

As Don Berwick, president of the Institute for Healthcare Improvement (IHI) puts it, "The buck stops in the board room."[6]

Nevertheless, hospital governing board members have been reluctant to probe too deeply into the quality and safety of the care delivered in their hospitals. Board members may feel more comfortable in the traditional role of dealing with a hospital's financial issues because they have experience dealing with financial issues in their business and personal lives. It is much less common for board members to believe that they bring similarly informed experience to addressing the complexities of clinical quality improvement and patient safety. Even those boards that view their primary duty as protecting the financial health of the hospital are increasingly aware that patient safety and quality have an impact on the financial health of the organization. Any board that keeps a watchful eye on trends in patient revenue streams can see the direct cost of non-compliance with quality reporting and performance requirements imposed by both government and private payers. When major lenders in the capital markets make it perfectly clear that they take a hospital's leadership on clinical quality and safety outcomes into serious consideration when determining bond rating, a fiscally responsible board cannot ignore the impact of their own decisions on securing the long-term financial health of the hospital.[7]

Hospital boards will have to overcome their inclination to view quality and patient safety as a clinical matter best left to clinicians and find a way to bring the same level of discipline and rigor to quality oversight that they bring to financial oversight. Although it may be disconcerting at first, board members may very well find that more substantive engagement in quality improvement and patient safety fits naturally into the commitment they made to the organization when they accepted a position on the hospital board. This chapter describes the traditional role of governing boards in hospital quality and patient safety to set the context for understanding the board's responsibility for addressing emerging expectations for systematic quality improvement, risk reduction, and patient safety. Afterward, some specific ideas about board actions and best practices, as taken from the current research and findings in the growing body of literature about hospital governance and quality improvement, patient safety, and risk reduction, are presented.

CORPORATE RESPONSIBILITY, HOSPITAL QUALITY, AND PATIENT SAFETY

Hospitals are incorporated under state law as either for-profit or non-profit corporations governed by a board of directors, trustees, or commissioners. Whether the board consists of paid directors in a for-profit entity, voluntary trustees in a community hospital, or elected commissioners in a public facility, board members have the ultimate responsibility for the operation of the organization, including oversight of mission, strategy, executive leadership, quality, and safety. Boards are responsible for performing these activities within all applicable licensure standards, relevant law, and all governmental regulations. The following section is a brief overview of hospital duties and responsibilities as a corporate entity related to the organization's accountability for the quality of patient care, including corporate liability, shifting hospital standards of care, transparency and accountability, and the emerging concept of "quality fraud."

Corporate Liability

Ensuring safe care to patients is now viewed to be the very core of a hospital's responsibility to the general public and its patients, but there was no institutional liability for medical negligence until the decision of the 1965 case, *Darling v. Charleston Community Memorial Hospital*,[8] resulted in courts recognizing a new doctrine of hospital corporate liability. The Darling case concerned a teenage boy who was taken to Charleston Community Memorial Hospital for treatment of a fractured leg. His leg was placed in a cast, but then he suffered from gangrene and had to have his leg amputated below the knee. The boy's father sued both the physician and the hospital. The hospital countered that it did not practice medicine and thus could not be found negligent; however, the plaintiff claimed—and the court agreed—that the hospital was negligent for two reasons: it failed to properly review the work of an independent doctor, and its nurses failed to administer necessary care.

The court held that the hospital bylaws, licensing regulations, and standards for hospital accreditation were sufficient evidence to establish a standard of care for the hospital; therefore, the jury was able to conclude from the evidence that the hospital had breached its duty to act as a reasonably careful hospital because it had not provided adequately trained medical and nursing staff and had not established policies and procedures for monitoring the quality of medicine practiced within its walls. The Darling case established that the primary duty of the hospital is to provide the proper standard of care owed to patients—that is, while a patient is in the hospital, the organization owes a duty

directly to the patient to ensure the individual's safety and well-being.[9] Corporate negligence occurs when a hospital fails to perform those duties. Examples of hospital-specific duties include the maintenance of safe facilities and equipment, the selection and retention of competent providers, the supervision of all persons who practice medicine within hospital walls, and the formulation, adoption, and enforcement of rules and policies that ensure quality care.[9]

Shifting Standards of Care

In the Darling case, the court based its determination of the applicable standard of hospital care on Charleston's own bylaws, the licensing regulations in the state of Illinois, and The Joint Commission standards for hospital accreditation. The standard of care is an essential element in medical liability cases, since this is the standard against which the actions of a provider are judged as either appropriate or negligent. As more and more hospitals participate in national quality reporting and improvement programs, legal interpretations of what constitutes the hospital standard of care may shift. Over 4,000 hospitals are reporting quality data on process and outcome measures for the CMS program, Reporting Hospital Quality Data for Annual Payment Update.[10] While the federal government currently imposes no penalty for substandard performance on these measures (although there is a penalty for not reporting), it is conceivable that courts may accept the argument that these measures are established national standards of care.

What may be even more compelling to the courts are broad-based voluntary efforts by hospitals themselves to adopt common practices. For example, the 100,000 Lives Campaign was a nationwide initiative launched by the IHI to reduce hospital morbidity and mortality through evidence-based best practices.[11] As IHI summarizes the success of this campaign, "The 3,100 hospitals that participated in this initiative achieved a remarkable goal. Through their work on the Campaign's interventions, combined with other national and local improvement efforts, these facilities saved an estimated 122,000 lives in 18 months. Along the way, *nothing less than new standards of care began to emerge.*"[12]

Transparency and Accountability

In the early 2000s, the unscrupulous business practices of Enron, WorldCom, and Global Crossing cast a very harsh light on the consequence of irresponsible corporate oversight.[13] Given the magnitude of the harm caused by the failures of these organizations and their boards of directors, it is only natural that questions came up about the basic value and impact of corporate governance for any organization. The federal government responded by raising the bar on corporate transparency and accountability by enacting the Sarbanes–Oxley Act of 2002.[14]

The Sarbanes–Oxley provisions specifically target improved accountability and transparency from publicly traded companies, but that is not to say that non-profit corporations have escaped scrutiny on the issues of transparency and accountability. Most hospitals incorporated as non-profit organizations also apply for federal tax-exempt status as charitable organizations. As a tax-exempt charitable organization, a hospital places itself under the jurisdiction of the Internal Revenue Service (IRS), which requires a hospital to have well-crafted governance and management policies and procedures to earn its federal tax exemption.[3] The IRS has significantly ramped up its commitment to make non-profit governance a "pillar" of its compliance activity for the tax-exempt non-profit sector.[15] This is just one reflection of the heightened legislative and regulatory focus on the governance practices of all American businesses, including non-profit healthcare organizations.

Quality Fraud

If a hospital is not delivering high-quality care, it may be at risk for what commentators have recently called "quality fraud."[16] The Secretary of the Department of Health and Human Services can terminate a hospital's participation in the Medicare program for failing to meet the conditions of participation, which include quality requirements. For example, a hospital can be excluded from Medicare for providing excessive unnecessary items or services to patients or for failing to meet professionally recognized standards of care. Although terminations of hospital participation in the Medicare program have been rare to date, the threat of being excluded or suspended from Medicare is taken quite seriously due to the potentially devastating financial consequences for a hospital. Moreover, there are indications of increased government interest in pursuing cases of quality fraud.[16] Additional liability may arise under federal false-claims statutes that penalize any claim based on false information that is submitted to the federal government for reimbursement (i.e., under the Medicare and Medicaid programs). A pattern of quality or patient safety failures may be construed as false claims if it can be shown that the hospital knew, or should have known, about the problems but continued billing for substandard care without taking steps to correct the problem. Fraud may also be alleged based on hospital practices, including submitting false reports about quality or the failure to make required reports, ignoring practices or providers delivering profitable services of poor quality, and patients harmed by, or given false information about, the quality of their care.[17]

BOARD RESPONSIBILITIES AND HOSPITAL QUALITY

The job of meeting the duties and obligations of a corporation such as that described previously falls on governing boards composed of individuals from inside and outside the organization. In hospitals, "inside" board members include individuals on the hospital management team, physicians practicing at the hospital, and anyone receiving income from the institution. "Outside" board members, typically required to be the majority, could be community and religious leaders, volunteers (including individuals who receive care at the institution), governmental officials, local business people, or political figures from the area served. Hospital boards vary in size, composition, and how members are appointed, but a commonality is that most have a majority of members who are not healthcare professionals.

Individual board members are fiduciaries of the organization, which means that they must act in the best interest of the corporation (and not in their own best interest, if conflicts of interest arise) and ensure that the corporation's resources are used in a reasonable and legal manner. Day-to-day operational responsibilities are delegated to management, but it is the responsibility of the board to make sure that sound management practices are in place. It has been argued that the long-established legal duties of hospital fiduciaries demonstrate the higher standards of accountability and transparency that existed in the non-profit sector well before the scandals of Enron and others prompted similar standards in the for-profit sector.[18] Two of the duties of a fiduciary—the duty of care and the duty of obedience—are particularly relevant to the board's responsibilities in the overseeing of quality and patient safety.[19]

Duty of Care

In essence, duty of care requires the board to make responsible and informed decisions on behalf of the organization. To do so, the board must take time to learn about issues and understand facts before making decisions. Since much of this information is presented to the board by management, there is an additional obligation to make inquiries if there is any question of the validity or completeness of the information presented. Board members are not required to become experts on every issue put before them. In determining whether the duty of care is met, courts tend to apply the "business judgment rule" and do not second-guess board members in cases of good-faith decisions made by disinterested, reasonably informed directors who believe the decision to be in the best interests of the corporation. In short, the board is expected to act in good faith and follow rational decision-making processes.[20] With regard to quality and patient safety, duty-of-care principles apply to both specific decisions, such as physician-credentialing decisions, and to more global activities of the board, such as leadership in improving quality of care and patient safety.[21] Adherence to compliance programs also implicates the duty of care.[21] As quality, risk reduction, and patient safety are increasingly linked to hospital payment through pay-for-performance programs regulated by state and federal law, an effective compliance program to detect and deter legal violations will have to encompass quality issues. Executive staff are obligated to brief the board about new payment developments and related legal issues, and it is the obligation of the board to ensure that the organization's compliance program is in place to monitor emerging legal risks.

Hospital boards also have a duty to keep informed about national trends and evidence-based best practices for healthcare quality improvements and how other hospitals are responding to the increasingly public focus on quality. The Office of the Inspector General, which has authority to exclude hospitals from participation in the Medicare and Medicaid programs for substandard care, has stated that hospitals should "continually measure their performance against comprehensive standards."[22] As discussed in the comments about shifting standards of care, performance review may not be limited solely to standards established by federal agencies and accreditation organizations.

Duty of Obedience to Corporate Purpose and Mission

The fundamental nature of the duty of obedience is the obligation to further the purposes of the organization as set forth in its articles of incorporation or bylaws.[23] In turn, board members must comply with applicable laws, rules, and regulations, and honor the terms and conditions of the organization's mission, bylaws, policies, and procedures. The majority of hospitals in the United States are incorporated as non-profit organizations for a purpose recognized under state non-profit corporation laws. In addition, hospitals that apply for tax-exempt status do so as having the charitable purpose of health promotion. The articles of incorporation of a non-profit healthcare provider often describe its principal purpose in terms such as "the promotion of health through the provision of inpatient and outpatient hospital and healthcare services to residents in the community." Given the purpose and mission of hospitals, it is reasonable to suggest that the concept of delivering high-quality, safe patient care is inseparable from the mission of the organization.

BOARD LEADERSHIP IN HOSPITAL QUALITY AND PATIENT SAFETY

The previous discussion of the legal aspects of certain duties of a hospital board does not fully capture the meaning of the fiduciary responsibility of a hospital board. Fundamentally, the board is responsible to the community for all activities of the organization, including the ethical obligation to do everything possible to keep patients safe and offer the highest-quality care. This confers on the board the responsibility to oversee the hospital's quality of care by setting quality-

improvement plans and goals, monitoring progress toward those goals, and accepting the ultimate accountability for making sure that those goals are realized. The board does this by exercising its right and authority to ask for details about adverse incidents or data that suggest less-than-optimal performance, to ask for evidence of effective measurement and improvement, and to require that effective mechanisms be in place to measure, maintain, and improve quality and safety. The board does not have to master the details of clinical medicine or make clinical decisions to fulfill their responsibilities toward quality patient care. What they do have to do is make sure that appropriate staff at the hospital are accountable for the clinical details, and that these staff are doing their jobs effectively. The board can only reach the conclusion that the organization's actions are effective if, upon hearing about a problem, they are provided evidence that a solution has been implemented that has corrected the problem. The following sections describe some of the specific actions taken by the board, including leadership activity, credentialing, and best practices in board operations.

Leadership Activities

Built on the leadership concepts of "will, ideas, and execution," the IHI developed a list of five core leadership activities that focus the organization on improving quality and patient safety.[24] These activities are listed below as subsequently adapted by IHI in its advice to governing boards:[25]

- *Establish the mission, vision, and strategy.* Set direction and monitor performance, i.e., integrate strategy and quality, monitor the culture of quality and safety, and establish aims for safety and quality improvement.
- *Build the foundation for an effective leadership system.* Establish an interdisciplinary Board Quality Committee. Bring

knowledgeable quality leaders onto the board. Set and achieve educational standards for the board members. At board and committee meetings, with physician and nursing leaders, as well as with administration, build a culture of real (not pro forma) conversations about improving care. Allocate adequate resources to ongoing training of employees and medical staff about quality improvement.

- *Build will.* Establish a policy of full transparency about data on quality and safety. Insist on the review of both data and stories from patients and families. Help patients and families tell their stories directly to staff, senior leaders, and the board. Establish policies and practices with respect to errors and injuries that emphasize thorough communication, respectful practice, disclosure, apology, support, and resolution. Understand both the current performance of your organization and the performance levels of the best organizations in the world. Show that you own the problem and are driving the agenda by placing quality first on the board agenda and devoting 25% or more of the board's agenda to it. Show courage and do not flinch.

- *Ensure access to ideas.* Boards should ask management four idea-generating questions when reviewing progress against quality and safety aims. Those questions are: (1) Who is the best in the world at this? (2) Have you talked to them to find out how they do it? (3) How many ideas have you tried out? (4) What ideas did our patients and families and frontline staff have for improvement?

- *Attend relentlessly to execution.* Establish executive accountability for achievement of aims. Establish an effective supervisory process: devote 25% of board meeting time to quality and safety; monitor your own system-level measures for improvement (rather than being comforted by benchmarks);

review data generated weekly, or, at a minimum, monthly; ask hard questions. (Are we on track to achieve the aim? If not, why not? What is the improvement strategy? What are key steps planned toward full-scale execution?)

Physician Credentialing

One of the most essential roles of the board in safeguarding the quality of patient care is approving only the recommendations for physician appointments and clinical privileges that are based on a reliable and well-documented credentialing process. Credentialing has grown into a complex and detailed activity that must also meet accreditation standards. The board sets clear policies and procedures to guide all credentialing activities, including the collection and verification of all required information about an applicant. That information must be evaluated thoughtfully, exercising all due diligence in acting to grant, deny, or restrict medical-staff membership and the specific privileges being sought.

Board Best Practices

There is extensive discussion in the healthcare-governance literature about what board actions specifically constitute board "engagement" in quality improvement and patient safety, and what are the most effective and significant actions hospital board members should be taking. The search for specific board practices that make a significant contribution to successful quality improvement in a hospital is necessarily a work in progress as boards test various approaches. One of the advantages of the recent explosion in the public reporting of quality data is that earlier research about board practices based on qualitative observations, case studies, and self-reported survey data is beginning to be augmented with statistical analyses of the relationship between board practices and quality outcomes. This development of evidence-based best practices of hospital governing boards patterns the development of evidence-based best practices in clinical quality improvement. Some preliminary findings are described below.

Hospital Leadership Summit: Moving from Good to Great[26]

In 2006 CMS and the Oklahoma Foundation for Medical Quality sponsored a summit on the impact of hospital leadership on quality improvement. During the summit, results were presented on the first phase of an extensive national study of healthcare system and hospital governing-board practices related to the overseeing of quality (The Governance Institute and the Solucient Center for Healthcare Improvement). One of the purposes of the study was to determine whether specific practices contribute to better hospital quality performance and better organization-wide performance. The board practices found to be correlated to high-quality performance are summarized below.

1. Board practices of hospitals that perform very well on a composite measure based on quality outcomes, patient safety, efficiency, financial stability, and customer response:
   - CEO-performance evaluation is tied to both clinical-improvement goals and patient safety goals.
   - The board sets the agenda for discussions that concern quality.
   - Patient satisfaction scores are reviewed at least annually.
2. Board practices of hospitals that perform very well on a composite measure based on mortality, complications, patient safety, and length of stay:
   - CEO-performance evaluation is tied to patient safety goals.
   - The more time spent on quality during board meetings, the higher the composite score.

- The board quality committee chair or chief of staff presents quality reports to the entire board.
3. Board practices of hospitals that perform very well on both composite measures:
   - Board participates in medical-staff appointments, reappointments, and clinical privilege setting specifically by developing and/or approving explicit criteria.
   - Medical staff are involved in setting agenda for board discussion of quality.

Quality

In 2006 Lockee, Kroom, Zablocki, and Bader[27] found direct correlations between the following practices and high performance in hospitals:

- The CEO is held accountable for quality and safety goals.
- The board participates in developing criteria to guide medical staff credentialing and privileging.
- The board quality committee annually reviews patient-satisfaction scores.
- The board sets the board agenda for quality.
- The medical staff are involved in setting the board agenda for discussions about quality.

Executive Quality Improvement Survey

The Executive Quality Improvement Survey[28] identified the following characteristics of board engagement in quality improvement and patient safety as most likely to strengthen quality-improvement activities in top-performing hospitals:

- The board spends more than 25% of its time on quality issues.

- The board receives a formal quality-performance-measurement report.
- There is a high level of interaction between the board and the medical staff on quality strategy.
- The senior executives' compensation is based in part on quality performance.
- The CEO is identified as the person with the greatest impact on quality, especially when so identified by the executive in charge of quality.

THE RISK MANAGER'S ROLE IN EDUCATING THE BOARD

What is provided to the board to foster their education related to quality and safety concerns is undoubtedly fueled by the organization's position as it relates to the concept of transparency. Ideally, a board should be provided with any and all information that suggests problems with the structure and process of care and with the culture that is in place to support both patients and providers. In the past, although presenting this type of information to a board might have seemed very threatening to the leadership of an organization, many organizations now recognize that this level of detail is necessary to prevent a board member from being blindsided when a story about an adverse event is covered by the press, and to ensure that board members can focus and fund priorities. The need to provide this type of information, however, must be balanced in order not to overwhelm the board with pages of needless details that lack focus with regard to the true root cause of a problem and the solution being employed to address it. In addition, the risk management report shared with the board should keep important issues in the forefront until they have been resolved, so that the board can be assured not only that action is being taken, but that it is the appropriate action to successfully resolve those issues.

SUMMARY AND CONCLUSION

Hospital boards have long had the duty of overseeing the delivery of patient care in their organizations, and are ultimately responsible for the quality and safety of that care. The traditional reluctance of boards, particularly the outside directors, to fully exercise their authority for quality supervision is breaking down in the face of growing awareness that the success of quality-improvement and patient safety activities involves more than medical decision making. As quality issues become more tightly intertwined with the financial health of hospitals, board members may find it easier to take a more active leadership role on the hospital's quality agenda and firmly establish quality improvement as a top priority for the organization. The adoption of national quality-reporting and quality-improvement programs, and the development of evidence-based best practices for the board, are raising the quality bar for both hospitals and their governing boards. Not only do these initiatives reveal what can be accomplished, they are beginning to demonstrate how. Boards have the authority, responsibility, and skill to insist on the implementation of effective and accountable quality-improvement and patient safety systems and processes. It is hoped that advances in the field, and that a transparent sharing of relevant and necessary information, will give them the tools and confidence to do so.

References

1. Institute of Medicine. (n.d.). *Crossing the quality chasm: The IOM hospital quality initiative.* http://www.iom.edu/?id=35957/. Accessed December 9, 2008.
2. Shearer, A., & Cronin, C. (2005). *The state-of-the-art of online hospital public reporting: A review of fifty-one websites.* Easton, MD: Delmarva Foundation.
3. Laschober, M., Maxfield, M., Felt-Lisk, S., & Miranda, D.J. (2007). Hospital response to public reporting of quality indicators. *Health Care Financing Review 28*, 61.
4. Institute of Medicine. Committee on Quality of Health Care in America. (2001). *Crossing the quality chasm: A new health system for the 21st century.* Washington, DC: National Academies Press.
5. The Joint Commission. (1995). *The 1995 accreditation manual for hospitals.* Oakbrook Terrace, IL: The Joint Commission.
6. The Joint Commission. (December 2006). An interview with Donald Berwick. *Journal on Quality and Patient Safety 32(12)* , 666.
7. Levy, J. (2008). *Moody's special opinion.* http://runningahospital.blogspot.com/2008/02/quality-and-bond-ratings.html. Accessed December 9, 2008.
8. Darling v. Memorial Community Hospital, 211 N.E.2d 253 (Ill. 1965).
9. Thompson v. Nason Hospital, 591 A.2d 703, 707 (Pa. 1991).
10. Hospital Quality Alliance. (n.d.). *Resources for the national public–private collaboration committed to making hospital quality performance information accessible to the public, including the CMS* Hospital Compare *initiative.* http://www.hospitalqualityalliance.org/. Accessed December 1, 2008.
11. Institute for Healthcare Improvement. (n.d.). *Overview of the 100,000 Lives Campaign.* http://www.ihi.org/IHI/Programs/Campaign/100kCampaignOverviewArchive.htm/. Accessed December 9, 2008.
12. Institute for Healthcare Improvement. (n.d.). *5 Million Lives Campaign.* http://www.ihi.org/IHI/Programs/Campaign/Campaign.htm?TabId=1/. Accessed December 9, 2008.
13. Eichenwald, K. (2005) *Conspiracy of fools: A true story.* Portland, OR: Broadway Books.
14. Public Company Accounting Reform and Investor Protection Act §§302, 401, 404, 409, 802, 906, 15USC §7201, et. Seq. (2006).
15. Internal Revenue Service (n.d.). *Governance of charitable organizations and related topics.* http://www.irs.gov/charities/article/0,,id=178221,00.html/. Accessed December 1, 2008.
16. Gosfield, A.G., & Reinertsen, J.L. (2008). Avoiding quality fraud. *Trustee 61(8)*, 12, 14–15, 1.
17. Callender, A.N., Hastings, D.A., Hemsley, M.C., Morris, L., & Peregrine, M.W. (2007). *Corporate responsibility and health care quality: A resource for health care.* http://www.oig.hhs.gov/fraud/docs/complianceguidance/CorporateResponsibilityFinal%2094-07.pdf/. Accessed December 1, 2008.
18. Entin, F.J., Anderson, J.A., & O'Brien, K.S. (2006). *The board's fiduciary role: Legal responsibilities of health care governing boards.* Chicago: Center for Healthcare Governance.
19. Gosfield, A.G., & Reinertsen, J.L. (2008). Avoiding quality fraud. *Trustee 61(8)*, 12, 14–15, 1.
20. Revised Model Nonprofit Corporation Act §8.30 (1987). http://www.muridae.com/nporegulation/documents/model_npo_corp_act.html. Accessed April 8, 2010.
21. *In re* Caremark International Inc. Derivative litigation, 698 A.2d 959 (Del. Ch. 1996).
22. Office of the Inspector General. (2005, January 21). *Supplemental compliance program guidance for hospitals.* Washington, DC: Federal Register.
23. Kurtz, D.L. (1988). Board liability: Guide for nonprofit directors, 84, citing *Commonwealth of Pennsylvania v. The Barnes Foundation*, 398 Pa. 458, 159 A.2d 500, 505 (1960). *In re* Manhattan Eye, Ear & Throat Hospital, 715 N.Y.S.2d 575 (1999).
24. Provost, L., Miller, D., & Reinertsen, J. (2006). *A framework for leadership of improvement* (IHI). http://www.ihi.org/. Accessed December 9, 2008.
25. Institute for Healthcare Improvement. (2008). *5 Million Lives Campaign. Getting started kit: Governance leadership "Boards on Board" how-to guide.* http://www.ihi.org/. Accessed December 9, 2008.

26. Centers for Medicare and Medicaid Services. (2006). CMS leadership summit. *Moving hospitals from good to great. Summary of meeting proceedings.* http://www.safetyleaders.org/CMS/summitproceedingsV1%20_2_.pdf. Accessed April 8, 2010.

27. Lockee, C., Kroom, K., Zablocki E., & Bader, B. (2006). Quality. The Governance Institute, Baltimore, MD.

28. Vaughn, T., Koepke, M., Kroch, E., Lehrman, W., Sinha, S., & Levey, S. (March 2006). Engagement of leadership in quality improvement initiatives: Executive Quality Improvement Survey results. *Journal of Patient Safety 2(1)*, 2–9.

10

THE CULTURE OF MEDICINE, LEGAL OPPORTUNISM, AND PATIENT SAFETY

Drew McCormick, MA, BA

INTRODUCTION

In its often-cited report, "To Err Is Human: Building a Safer Health System," the Institute of Medicine (IOM) gives a staggering statistic: between 44,000 and 98,000 persons die from medical errors in hospitals in the United States every year.[1] This report catalyzed a media frenzy, placing the issue of medical error at the forefront of the nation's health-care consciousness. Subsequently, many research studies have been devoted to examining numerous subjects, including what contributes to medical error, how to analyze adverse events, and what the most effective techniques are for systemic risk prevention.[2] A significant proportion of studies and writings on the topic have lambasted the medical community for its errant behaviors.[3]

This chapter analyzes the practices of both the culture of medicine and the legal system in creating an environment of risk. The first part contains an analysis of how the predis-positions of physicians intersect with cultur-ally ingrained behaviors and have con-tributed to the staggering rate of adverse incidents cited by the IOM. The second part examines the complicity of the legal system, demonstrating how it has helped to foster a culture of risk by disincentivizing open dis-closure about risks and adverse events while incentivizing "defensive medicine," which may more often cause iatrogenic illnesses than improve care. The third section begins by providing an overview of previous medical-liability reform movements. This section explores the particular reform demands of the present environment and discusses the uniqueness of the current tort-reform crisis. Finally, the section identifies the tension between medical liability and patient safety by examining the benefits and detriments of several proffered reforms, pointing to reform efforts that will place patient safety at the forefront of medicine well into the future.

THE CULTURE OF MEDICINE

Traditionally, the individual-focused model of medicine has credited any and all diagnostic and treatment results to the skill of the provider; thus, errors and their consequences are also ascribed to a moral failure on the part of the provider.[4] This individualistic model of error is reflected in, and reinforced by, the system of medical-malpractice liability. This conception of medical outcomes serves to pressure physicians not only to avoid making errors, but to avoid admitting to making errors.[5]

In one 2006 survey published in the *Archives of Internal Medicine,* although 98% of physicians endorsed the need to disclose serious errors to patients, only 42% would actually use the word "error," and only 33% would explicitly apologize for their mistake.[6] This resistance to disclosure has many causes, including fear of blame, loss of trust, and loss of professional status, among others.[7] In a 1997 paper published in the *Journal of Clinical Ethics,* Daniel Finkelstein and his colleagues claimed that physicians responded to adverse events caused by error most commonly by withholding information, lying, or eluding discussion about the incident.[8]

The widespread tendency of physicians to avoid disclosing the commission of errors is not merely the result of commonly felt pressures. It is also entrenched in the culture of medicine to the extent that physicians are taught to strive for the unrealistic ideal of an error-free practice.[9] Because physicians deal with error, risk, and fatality on a daily basis, they have developed a language and culture that normalizes their mistakes.[10] Perhaps as a coping mechanism, physicians have donned a "mask of infallibility."[11] Society is complicit in this behavior, with people preferring to place their care in the hands of error-free, infallible caricatures of physician-heroes, rather than in those of fellow human beings capable of error.[10]

There are two interesting aspects of physician behavior that contribute to their shared culture. Firstly, there are the common personality traits and early life experiences among those who choose to enter the medical profession.[8] One example is the inordinately high percentage of physicians raised in households in which at least one parent is a physician.[12] Generally, many students who enter medical school have high-achieving parents. The need to obtain attention from distracted parents with busy professional lives may play a role in driving both independence and the need for validation through professional achievement that are common characteristics of physicians.

The second aspect pertains to learned and shared behaviors, which are acquired during the socialization process of young physicians as they rise through medical school and into residency. In *The Scalpel's Edge: The Culture of Surgeons,* Pearl Katz depicts in great detail her insightful observations of a group of surgeons in a university hospital. Katz documents culturally endowed behaviors and postures, such as a propensity toward action, a heroic self-image, and a tendency to alienate and patronize patients as a result.[13]

As noted by John Banja, many of the error-related behaviors physicians exhibit have developed out of psychological necessity in a system that attributes both success and failure to the skill and competency of the individual.[14] For instance, Banja describes the process of "rationalization," through which physicians use euphemistic language, distort the consequences of their actions, displace responsibility, and make advantageous comparisons, as a means to affirm their self-image as good people. He argues that these behaviors are triggered by a professional's narcissistically based need to maintain his or her self-esteem.

It is not surprising, given the intersection of the demand for perfection[15] and the attribution of blame on an individualistic basis, that physicians have erected psychological defense mechanisms to preserve the esteem necessary to make the life-and-death decisions that they must make on a daily basis;[16] however, the fact remains that dishonesty, patronization, arrogance, and other self-defense-oriented behaviors are damaging to the physician–patient relationship and can be harmful to patients by inhibiting communication and preventing appropriate error analysis.[17] Moreover, as discussed in the next sections, withheld information, perceived dishonesty,[18] and poor communication are commonly cited reasons that claimants pursue litigation after an adverse event.

THE COMPLICITY OF LAW IN CREATING ERROR

The tendency to point the finger at the medical community for creating an environment of error seems at times to be the province of the legal profession. Much of the analysis that has occurred subsequent to the IOM report has been in the form of blandishments directed at medical professionals. Such overzealous legal critics have failed to recognize the significant role of the legal system in creating the culture of risk.[19]

Medical malpractice, a professional-liability subset of negligence law, has been criticized since the early 1970s on the grounds of inefficiency and poor distribution.[20] Even worse, litigation is a primary impetus within the culture of "blame and shame," which many advocates perceive as ineffective and counterproductive to shifting the medical paradigm toward greater patient safety.[21] Experts have long contended that medical-malpractice litigation is an inefficient way to deter medical error,[22] although the purported purpose of the legal system is to provide incentives for safe healthcare delivery by utilizing tort law.[23] These trends in litigation are largely a function of the behavior of the plaintiff's lawyers, who act as the system's gatekeepers because claims rarely move forward without the stewardship of counsel.[24]

Recognition of medical malpractice is the longest-standing social-incentive structure that attempts to promote safety in healthcare delivery and represents an ethos of individual responsibility;[25] however, recent criticisms by physicians allege that not only does this system fail to promote safety, it may

even prevent them from reporting errors and making health care safer.[26] In addition, there is convincing evidence to suggest that medical malpractice actually influences physician behavior in negative ways.[27] Ironically, it has encouraged physicians to practice defensive medicine to reduce the risk of liability, even by ordering tests and procedures that are of "marginal or no medical benefit."[28]

The problem with a climate of individual responsibility, cultivated by the current medical liability system, is that it tends to ignore systematic causes of adverse events in medical institutions.[29] This tendency is fatally nearsighted. Admonishments of individual healthcare practitioners are doled out where system-wide analysis of the multiple causes of an error should be occurring.[30] Moreover, the individual model of responsibility, reinforced by the legal system, no longer appropriately fits the healthcare environment. The individual-practitioner model of yesteryear[31] has been substantially supplanted by complex healthcare delivery systems with cross-disciplinary treatment across multiple providers.[32]

As a result of the law's failure to evolve in parallel with medicine, the current legal system represents a significant impediment to ensuring and promoting patient safety.[33] For instance, the culture of blame and shame inhibits discussions about error, thus precluding the discovery of relevant information and lessons that could be gleaned from more transparent error analysis.[33]

If the avoidance of blame and professional castigation is not sufficient, the oppressiveness of medical-malpractice insurance costs and pressures, such as cooperation clauses,[34] as well as the professional and personal tribulations presented by litigation, provides incentive for physicians to withhold information that might be valuable for addressing error.[11] Not only do physicians feel pressure to hide error because of the harm that legal reprisal might inflict on their career, they may be pressured by their institution or malpractice insurer to deny wrongdoing.[35] In addition, rising insurance costs caused by medical malpractice litigation are forcing physicians in high-risk specialties to leave their practices or move to more hospitable jurisdictions, thus imperiling patients.[36]

Adding insult to injury (quite literally), what little information about error the adversarial legal system may produce during litigation[11] is often inaccurate because of crafty manipulation by a legal advocate in the context of a trial.[37] Lastly, but certainly equally important, is that the perpetually looming fear of devastating legal consequences of error is a dominant force in depriving patients of the open, honest communication about error. This is particularly unfortunate when considering the essential importance of a provider–patient relationship, which is grounded in trust and the fact that monetary compensation is limited in its ability to redress the "internal" hurt experienced by victims of medical malpractice.

One additional noteworthy problem with the way that the legal system interacts with medicine is that it predominantly fails to make most patients "whole again" because it only provides compensation to a small number of patients who are victims of medical error.[38] While the many barriers to the legal system deter meritorious claims by victims of error,[39] the abuses of the system by opportunistic plaintiffs' lawyers have increased the tension between the medical and legal communities.[40] Moreover, physicians are negatively impacted by the staggering cost of malpractice insurance as a result of excessive litigation.[11] This observation serves to suggest that a shift toward non-punitive models of identifying, evaluating, and preventing medical error will not be adverse to the rights of plaintiffs.

RESHAPING THE HEALTHCARE PARADIGM: INCENTIVIZING ERROR REPORTING AND IMPROVING PATIENT SAFETY

This chapter has analyzed thus far the multiple layers of the modern medical context that shape the culture of risk. Now, it will explore the history of malpractice reform movements and then posit several considerations for restructuring the medical-care paradigm around a core of patient safety.

Although it is a modern-day Titan, medical malpractice had humble beginnings. Until the 1950s, suing a physician was an onerous undertaking. But when the judiciary began dismantling barriers to bring claims to the American Bar Association, such as rolling back charitable immunity for hospitals and moving toward nationalized standards of care, medical malpractice began to flourish. Moreover, the expansion of plaintiff-favoring doctrines, such as *res ipsa loquitur,* and the separate tort of negligent failure to provide informed consent, led to steady growth in litigation.[24]

Because of the aforementioned surges in litigation, many states began to experience malpractice crises, causing insurance claims, and correspondingly premiums, to soar. Consequently, many major insurers left the market, leaving physicians without coverage. As a result, the legislatures of several states created quasi-public bodies, called joint underwriting associations, to serve as insurers of last resort and fill gaps in the underwriting market, abating the crisis by the late 1970s.[24]

This trend seemed to repeat itself in the mid-1980s when premium costs spiked, prompting another round of tort reform, this time focusing on caps on non-economic and punitive damages.[41] Industrial self-insurance and "bedpan mutuals" became the dominant players in malpractice indemnity, holding steady through the 1990s with no sizable growth in malpractice litigation. While 70% of claims close with no payment, there were increases in average settlement amounts.[42]

THE CURRENT CRISIS: THE TENSION BETWEEN MEDICAL LIABILITY AND PATIENT SAFETY

Increases in the frequency of claims, the downturn in the economy, and dramatic increases in plaintiff payouts in the past

10 years have all contributed to the present tort crisis. The predominant problem is the decreasing availability of insurance coverage as insurers leave the market in response to deteriorating loss ratios and the decreasing affordability of policies offered by the remaining insurers.[27]

Although there are many evident similarities between the previous crises and the present one, there are also important differences; one is that the healthcare industry today has a diminished capacity to absorb sudden increases in insurance premiums. A second reason that the present crisis is unique is that it is arising amidst the patient safety movement, which has goals and initiatives seemingly at odds with the malpractice system.[27] The threat of litigation in the "punitive, individualistic, adversarial approach of tort law" is diametrically opposed to the increased transparent, system-oriented, cooperative, and non-punitive strategies of the patient safety movement. For this same reason, the tort-liability system undermines efforts to improve patient quality, a point that is the foundation for the subsequent discussion that compares and contrasts alternative compensation systems.[27]

Safety analysts point to the necessity of greater transparency and the need for systematic error analysis as one of the most important facets of patient-safety-centered medicine.[29] In order to learn from errors, we must first identify them, which necessitates a healthcare environment conducive to openness about mistakes.[17] In part, particular characteristics of medical culture, such as the tendency for physicians to divert blame, impede the open sharing of error; however, the threat of litigation has also been quite effective in dissuading physicians from openly disclosing and discussing error. In contrast to the faulty-systems model of error espoused by the patient safety movement, the tort-liability system targets individual physicians and ascribes blame on the basis of failure to meet the duty of care (negligence).[17]

Recent works on patient safety stress that error underreporting is a hindrance to collecting and analyzing data in order to develop systematic strategies. These works emphasize that patient safety must go beyond addressing deterrence of error and extend to creating reporting incentives.[29] Moreover, systems analysis has been underrepresented in remediation efforts since the IOM report.[43] In order to properly address the present error-prone environment of medicine, public policy should establish incentives to collect, analyze, and share error, as advocated in the IOM report.[5]

In addition to facilitating the study and prevention of error in the medical system, the legal system must be changed so that it adequately addresses the needs of injured patients and their families.[37] A study performed during the 1980s at Harvard Medical School, by a research team that reviewed medical records from over 30,000 hospital discharges, found a troubling disparity: only 2% of negligent injuries resulted in claims, and only 17% of claims appeared to involve a negligent injury.[42] Other studies, including those conducted in Utah and Colorado in the late 1990s, indicated similar injury rates and nearly identical disparity between injury and litigation. The overall impression of medical malpractice based on professional liability seems to paint a picture of an "incredibly inefficient" and "profoundly inaccurate mechanism for distributing compensation."[42]

LIABILITY SYSTEM REFORMS: COMPARED AND CONTRASTED

As discussed previously, our present medical-liability system fails to adequately compensate injured patients, impedes the development of a patient safety culture of sharing and preventing error, and has been largely responsible for constructing yet another crisis demanding system reform. The current system also demonstrates another inefficiency: nearly 60 cents of every dollar spent is absorbed by administrative costs, predominantly legal fees.[27]

It is clear that change is needed; the twofold question then becomes: What are the deficiencies in the current medical culture that we want to ameliorate (or, couched in positive terms, what positive elements do we want to engender), and what augmentations will we make to reach our goal?[44] The leading recommendations include tort reform, alternative dispute resolution, dispensing with negligence as the basis of fault, and locating liability at the institutional level (called enterprise liability). We examine each in turn, with the goal of identifying systems that will maximize patient safety, particularly by facilitating error disclosure and open physician–patient communication, as well as systems that will provide fair compensation for injured patients.

Conventional tort reform, which can come in many forms, has been a hotly debated issue as a part of the broader debate over healthcare reform.[45] Some approaches to tort reform include caps on non-economic damages, sanctions for frivolous filings, screening panels, and limits on contingency fees. Although intended to limit litigation (thus facilitating error disclosure), economic arguments against tort reform suggest that it will make medical-malpractice cases more expensive, riskier, and less rewarding for claimants while making them less frequent and less expensive for physicians.[46]

It has been argued that the nexus between tort reform efforts and error disclosure is more tenuous than might be hoped given the drawbacks, because the primary effect of tort reform is to reduce malpractice costs rather than incentivize improvement in care.[47] For the same reason (reducing the costs of litigation), tort reform may remove some of the fear surrounding litigation, thus promoting candor in error disclosure.[46] In addition, some studies indicate that reforms, such as damage caps, can reduce liability-insurance premiums;[48] however, as some scholars have pointed out, it is unrealistic to expect that decreasing the number of lawsuits or the amount of damages will achieve the goals of promoting patient safety and making injury compensation fair.[49]

Properly ensuring that patients are justly compensated for their injuries might involve a shift away from litigation and toward an administrative system that will support a no-fault model for injury that would provide timely compensation.[37] One alternative is early-offer programs, in which the patients and healthcare organizations have incentives to negotiate a private settlement immediately after an adverse event occurs. Subsequent chapters in this book not only describe these types of programs but also provide evidence of their success. This way, routine malpractice claims could be settled through structured mediation, administrative hearings, or medical courts.[50] In addition to enabling a more equitable distribution of plaintiff awards, these types of systems would have the benefit of accelerating the speed at which injured patients receive their settlements, which is currently on average nearly 5 years.[51]

Enterprise liability and no-fault compensation were two suggestions of the IOM's 2001 report, "Crossing the Quality Chasm," under the theory that these alternative systems will drastically change the legal environment, making it more conducive to uncovering and resolving quality problems.[11] No-fault compensation would emulate the model of workers' compensation and remove negligence as the basis of eligibility for compensation, replacing it with a standard of determining whether or not an event was avoidable.[50]

Proponents of this model suggest that the costs of increased payouts, resulting from the more permissive standard of avoidance increasing the pool of injuries eligible for compensation, would be offset by savings in other areas, such as administrative and legal expenses. They also tout the closer fit between the standard of avoidance and the system focus of the patient safety movement, as well as the likelihood of fairer compensation for injuries associated with this model.[50]

Enterprise liability shifts the locus of legal responsibility from the individual physician to the healthcare institution. This would ameliorate the stultifying medical-malpractice insurance premiums currently inflicted upon physicians. Moreover, such a model might engage more collaborative efforts in patient safety. It is argued that this organizational approach to compensation and deterrence would also underscore the value of systemic approaches to quality improvement.[52]

All in all, research overwhelmingly supports the contention that limits on malpractice suits would have a significant impact on what physicians will admit. Consequently, a further advantage of non-traditional, more patient-safety-focused forms of recourse after adverse incidents are that they provide a forum to receive an apology as well as a fuller explanation of the event, as well as an opportunity for the healthcare institution to analyze (and theoretically prevent in the future) the error.[53] Research supports the legal pragmatism and system-wide benefits of this type of full and prompt disclosure of error.

Organizations that have begun programs that encourage transparency over more traditional adversarial posturing have reported significant benefits. For instance, of 37 cases at the University of Illinois where the hospital acknowledged a preventable error and apologized, only one patient filed suit.[22] Similarly, at the University of Michigan Health System, existing claims and lawsuits dropped from 262 in August of 2001 to 83 in August 2007, and legal costs for the institution fell by an astounding two thirds. The foregoing studies demonstrate that not only does greater physician candor positively impact error analysis and prevention, it also can decrease the appeal to legal redress for harm due to error, and correspondingly, decrease the costs associated with defending lawsuits.[22]

The importance of restoring trust in the era of medical error is a notion that has been largely lost amidst the milieu of other post-IOM movements, namely, system-analysis approaches to risk assessment.[2] Not only is the restoration of provider–patient trust through communication about error necessary to prevent feelings of isolation in patients, it has more basic practical implications as well. For instance, withholding information from patients can lead to lawsuits if patients feel that a mistake has not been taken seriously. In addition, it can provide valuable insight into eliminating errors by providing a diverse perspective on the series of events that led to a medical error.[2] In the post-report era of medicine, patients are increasingly aware of error, which strips medicine of its previous ability to sweep it under the carpet.[54]

REMEDIATING THE CULTURE OF RISK: RECTIFYING THE CULTURE OF MEDICINE

As demonstrated in the preceding section, the current mechanisms of legal liability have significantly impacted the healthcare system, disincentivizing error transparency and communication, and significantly influencing the behavior of physicians;[55] however, shifting the fulcrum of the healthcare system toward patient safety will require efforts beyond liability reform, as discussed previously. As the problems identified in "The Complicity of Law in Creating Error" indicated, fundamental changes in the culture of medicine must also be effectuated in order to facilitate a paradigm shift toward a system of medicine that focuses on patient safety and quality of care.

Firstly, the ethics of the provider–patient relationship should reflect mutual respect, trust, and responsibility, rather than the unidirectional, authoritarian model of physician dominance embraced in centuries past.[53] While alternative liability systems may facilitate this type of physician–patient dynamic, certain changes in the posture of physicians will also be instrumental in reshaping clinical interactions. Patients have a right to know their past and present medical status, placing an ethical duty on physicians to ensure that patients understand adverse events and the effect they have had on the patient's condition.[56]

One study that examined the sociological[57] reasons that patients seek legal redress for injury will be helpful in articulating the disparity between the general collective perceptions of physicians versus those of patients. Marginalization, the tendency for physicians to push their patients' social concerns related to treatment to the periphery, was a central theme among patients interviewed in the study. Some examples include not listening to, or discounting, patients' perspectives, patronizing patients, ignoring patients' personal concerns, and avoiding patients or withholding information after an adverse event.

As outlined in "The Complicity of Law in Creating Error," physician behaviors of this kind are responsible for harming patients as well as frequently correlated with a decision to seek legal action against a physician, as noted previously. In order to truly effectuate a shift toward patient-centered, safety-focused care, the medical community will have to address the dominant, defensive, patient-alienating posture that many physicians have adopted to cope with the extreme consequences of their human errors.[58] Physi-

cians must learn how to have open, candid conversations with patients and their families when errors occur.[59]

CONCLUSION

This chapter has examined the combined roles of the culture of medicine and the medical-liability system in creating an environment of risk for patients. Most importantly, it has illuminated the need for reform in our current liability system in order to ensure compensation to harmed patients, repair the damage to the physician–patient dynamic, and enable open disclosure regarding error to enhance efforts to maximize patient safety. Changes within the culture of medicine that will be necessary to effectively leverage the shift of medicine toward patient safety have also been highlighted.

Just as the post-IOM-report climate of risk assessment has shifted toward system-level analysis of error and the avoidance of finger pointing at individual players, so must we make the shift toward holistic, systemic analysis of the factors that created the current environment where patient safety has been stifled and unnecessary risk has flourished.[60]

References

1. Kohn, L., Corrigan, J., & Donaldson, M. (Eds.). (2000). *To err is human: Building a safer health care system*. Committee on Quality of Health Care in America, Institute of Medicine. Washington, DC: National Academy Press.
2. Delbanco, T., & Bell, S.K. (2007). Guilty, afraid and alone: Struggling with medical error. *New England Journal of Medicine, 357,* 1682.
3. Editorial. (2002, December 18). Errors that kill medical patients. *New York Times.* http://www.nytimes.com/2002/12/18/opinion/errors-that-kill-medical-patients.html?scp=1&sq=Errors%20That%20Kill%20Medical%20Patients&st=cse/. Accessed September 27, 2009.
4. Sharpe, V.A. (2000). Behind closed doors: Accountability and responsibility in patient care. *Journal of Medicine and Philosophy, 25*(28), 47.
5. Liang, B.A. (2004). A policy of system safety: Shifting the medical and legal paradigms to effectively address error in medicine. *Harvard Health Policy Review, 5,* 9.
6. Editorial. (2006, September 9). When doctors hide medical errors. *New York Times,* A 14.
7. Quick, O. (2006). Outing medical errors: Questions of trust and responsibility. *Medical Law Review, 14,* 27.

8. Banja, J. (2005). *Medical error and medical narcissism* (p. 26). Sudbury, MA: Jones and Bartlett Publishers.

9. Hilfaker, D. (1984). Facing our mistakes. *New England Journal of Medicine, 310,* 118.

10. Quick, O. (2006). Outing medical errors: Questions of trust and responsibility. *Medical Law Review, 14,* 28.

11. Hyman, D.A., & Silver, C. (2005, spring). Speak not of error. *Regulation, 52,* 52.

12. Banja, J. (2005). *Medical error and medical narcissism* (p. 61). Sudbury, MA: Jones and Bartlett Publishers.

13. Katz, P. (1999). *The scalpel's edge: The culture of surgeons* (pp. ix–xi). Boston: Allyn and Bacon.

14. Banja, J. (2005). *Medical error and medical narcissism* (p. 34). Sudbury, MA: Jones and Bartlett Publishers.

15. Merry, A., & McCall Smith, A. (2002). Errors, medicine, and the law. *Medical Law Review,* 230, 232.

16. Banja, J. (2005). *Medical error and medical narcissism* (pp. 63–68). Sudbury, MA: Jones and Bartlett Publishers.

17. Studdert, D., Mello, M., & Brennan, T.A. (2004). Medical malpractice. *New England Journal of Medicine, 350,* 283, 287.

18. Fielding, S.L. (1995). Changing medical malpractice and medical malpractice claims. *Social Problems, 42,* 38, 43.

19. Merry, A., & McCall Smith, A. (2002). Errors, medicine, and the law. *Medical Law Review,* 230, 31–32.

20. Grepperud, S. (2005). Medical errors: Getting the incentives right. *International Journal of Health Care Finance & Economics, 5,* 307, 308.

21. Mello, M.M., Studdert D.M., & Brennan T.A. (2003). The new medical malpractice crisis. *New England Journal of Medicine, 348,* 2281–2284.

22. Editorial. (2008, May 22). Doctors who say they're sorry. *New York Times,* A30.

23. Liang, B.A. (2004). A policy of system safety: Shifting the medical and legal paradigms to effectively address error in medicine. *Harvard Health Policy Review, 5,* 8.

24. Studdert, D., Mello, M., & Brennan, T.A. (2004). Medical malpractice. *New England Journal of Medicine, 350,* 284.

25. Mello, M.M., Studdert, D., & Brennan, T.A. (2003). The new medical malpractice crisis. *New England Journal of Medicine, 348,* 2281–2284.

26. Liang, B.A., & Ren, L. (2004). Medical liability insurance and damage caps: Getting beyond band aids to substantive systems treatment to improve quality and safety in healthcare. *American Journal of Law & Medicine, 30,* 501–505.

27. Studdert, D., Mello, M., & Brennan, T.A. (2004). Medical malpractice. *New England Journal of Medicine, 350,* 286.

28. Kessler, D., & McClellan, M. (1996). Do doctors practice defensive medicine? *The Quarterly Journal of Economics, 111,* 353, 390.

29. Grepperud, S. (2005). Medical errors: Getting the incentives right. *International Journal of Health Care Finance & Economics, 5,* 320.

30. Institute of Medicine. (2000). *To err is human.* http://www.nap.edu/catalog.php?record_id=9728/. Accessed October 3, 2009.

31. Bodenheimer, T. (2008). Coordinating care: A perilous journey through the health care system. *New England Journal of Medicine, 358,* 1060, 1064.

32. Haggerty, J.L., Reid, R.J., Freeman, G.K., Starfield, B.H. Adair, C.E., & McKendry, R. (2003). Continuity of care: A multidisciplinary review. *British Medical Journal, 327,* 1219.

33. A policy of system safety: Shifting the medical and legal paradigms to effectively address error in medicine. *Harvard Health Policy Review, 5,* 10.

34. Banja, J.D. (2005, February). *Does medical error disclosure violate the medical malpractice insurance cooperation clause?* Advances in patient safety: From research to implementation. http://www.ncbi.nlm.nih.gov/books/bv.fcgi?rid=aps.section.5340/. Accessed October 8, 2009.

35. Delbanco, T., & Bell, S.K. (2007). Guilty, afraid and alone: Struggling with medical error. *New England Journal of Medicine, 357,* 1683.

36. Liang, B.A., & Ren, L. (2004). Medical liability insurance and damage caps: Getting beyond band aids to substantive systems treatment to improve quality and safety in healthcare. *American Journal of Law & Medicine, 30,* 502.

37. Liang, B.A. (2004). A policy of system safety: Shifting the medical and legal paradigms to effectively address error in medicine. *Harvard Health Policy Review, 5,* 10.

38. Weiler, P.C. (1991). *Medical malpractice on trial.* Boston: Harvard University Press.
39. Hyman, D.A., & Silver, C. (2005). Speak not of error. *Regulation, 52,* 54.
40. Dodds, P. (1993, May 16). Quantity of lawyers; quality of justice. *New York Times.* http://www.nytimes.com/1993/05/16/nyregion/1-quantity-of-lawyers-quality-of-justice-059493.html?scp=2&sq=quantity%20of%20lawyers%20quality%20of%20justice&st=cse. Retrieved April 20, 2010.
41. Kinney, E. (1995). Malpractice reform in the 1990s: Past disappointments, future success? *Journal of Health Politics and Political Law 20,* 135.
42. Studdert, D., Mello, M., & Brennan, T.A. (2004). Medical malpractice. *New England Journal of Medicine, 350,* 285.
43. Liang, B.A. (2004). A policy of system safety: Shifting the medical and legal paradigms to effectively address error in medicine. *Harvard Health Policy Review, 5,* 7.
44. Gostin, L.O., & Jacobson, P.D. (2005). *Law and the health system.* Foundation Press, 500.
45. Hiltzik, M. (2009, October 1). Tort reform is the health care debate's frivolous sideshow. *Los Angeles Times.* http://www.latimes.com/business/la-fi-hiltzik1-2009oct01,0,7502095.column/. Accessed October 3, 2009.
46. Hyman, D.A., & Silver, C. (2005). Speak not of error. *Regulation, 52,* 56.
47. Todres, J. (2006). Toward healing and restoration for all: Reframing medical malpractice reform. *Connecticut Law Review, 667,* 669–673.
48. Nelson L.J. III, et al. (1997) Damage caps in medical malpractice liability. *The Millbank Quarterly, 85*(2), 259.
49. Hyman, D.A., & Silver, C. (2005). Speak not of error. *Regulation, 52,* 288.
50. Studdert, D., Mello M., & Brennan, T.A. (2004). Medical malpractice. *New England Journal of Medicine, 350,* 289.
51. Emanuel, E.J. (2008). Health care, guaranteed. *Public Affairs,* 23.
52. Studdert, D., Mello M., & Brennan, T.A. (2004). Medical malpractice. *New England Journal of Medicine, 350,* 290.
53. Liang, B.A. (2004). A policy of system safety: Shifting the medical and legal paradigms to effectively address error in medicine. *Harvard Health Policy Review, 5,* 11.
54. Quick, O. (2006). Outing medical errors: Questions of trust and responsibility. *Medical Law Review, 14,* 34.
55. Liang, B.A., & Ren, L. (2004). Medical liability insurance and damage caps: Getting beyond band aids to substantive systems treatment to improve quality and safety in healthcare. *American Journal of Law & Medicine, 30,* 531–533.
56. Banja, J. (2005). *Medical error and medical narcissism* (p. 22). Sudbury, MA: Jones and Bartlett Publishers.
57. Fielding, S.L. (1995). Changing medical malpractice and medical malpractice claims. *Social Problems, 42,* 45.
58. Banja, J. (2005). *Medical error and medical narcissism* (p. 20). Sudbury, MA: Jones and Bartlett Publishers.
59. Banja, J.D. *Discussing unanticipated outcomes and disclosing medical errors.* http://www.gha.org/phaold/video/index.asp/. Accessed October 8, 2009.
60. Gilmour, J.M. (2006, May). *Patient safety, medical error and tort law: An international comparison.* The Health Research Policy Program. Ottawa, Ontario: Health Canada. http://www.hc-sc.gc.ca/sr-sr/pubs/hpr-rpms/2006-gilmour-eng.php. Retrieved April 20, 2010.

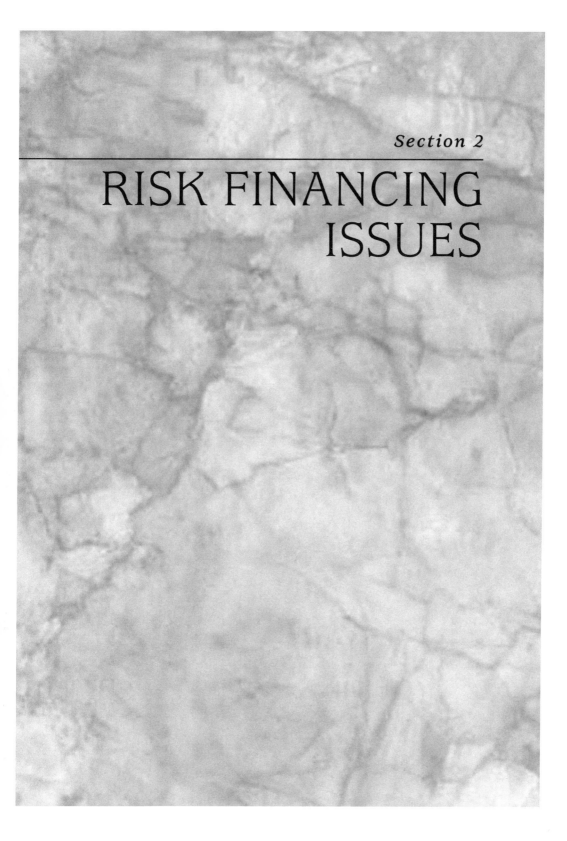

RISK FINANCING
ISSUES

11

ENTERPRISE RISK MANAGEMENT: THE IMPACT ON HEALTHCARE ORGANIZATIONS

Roberta Carroll, MBA, ARM, CPCU

INTRODUCTION

Enterprise risk management (ERM) is a topic of much discussion recently, but it is not often described in terms that are understandable for people who work in health care. Enterprise risk management needs to be defined, clearly understood, and personalized by each organization to fit their unique culture and environmental climate. There is no single right model that fits all. Enterprise risk management is "not a stop on the road, but a journey." With that adage in mind, let us start the journey.

ENTERPRISE RISK MANAGEMENT DEFINED

The first step in developing and implementing an ERM program is to define what it means to the organization. Enterprise risk management can be described in several ways: firstly, it is a business decision-making *process* used to identify and manage the risks across the continuum of an organization's structure and function; secondly, it is a *discipline* that engages professionals; and thirdly, it is a *practice* that embraces organizational risk identification, analysis, mitigation, monitoring, and evaluation. Several common definitions of ERM include the following:

> Enterprise risk management is a comprehensive process which evaluates all risk exposures confronting an organization from the top down. It is a discipline broad in scope reflecting an organizational-wide, ongoing commitment. To be most effective, it should be part of strategic planning for the organization and a *proactive* as well as *reactive* process.

> Enterprise risk management is a process, effected by an entity's board of directors, management and other personnel, applied in

strategy setting and across the enterprise, designed to identify potential events that may affect the entity, and manage risks to be within its risk appetite, to provide reasonable assurance regarding the achievement of entity objectives.[1]

The ERM process is a broad-based discipline requiring the active involvement of all in healthcare and has risk identification and analysis, risk prioritization, and the implementation and monitoring of risk mitigation initiatives at its core.

Enterprise risk management is an enterprise-wide process designed to identify potential events that may affect the entity, determine the enterprise's appetite for risk, and manage the event risk according to enterprise objectives.[2]

Enterprise risk management can best be described as an ongoing business decision-making process instituted and supported by the healthcare organization's board of directors, executive administration and medical staff leadership. ERM recognizes the synergistic effect of risk across the continuum of care, and has as its goals to assist the organization, reduce uncertainty and process variability, promote patient safety, and maximize the return on investment (ROI) through asset preservation and the recognition of actionable risk opportunities.[3]

When examining these definitions of ERM, it becomes clear that the language is similar in most examples and includes terms and concepts such as comprehensive, broad-based, ongoing, process driven, top-down, committed involvement, and risk identification.

Enterprise risk management utilizes a series of ongoing interrelated activities designed to identify, assess, manage, and monitor events and risks that an organization faces. Risks identified may or may not be insurable and may be handled by different departments, units, or divisions within the organization. Once all risks are identified, evaluated, and measured, the organization can develop prioritized, organization-wide solutions and strategies for dealing with those risks. Peter Bernstein, a noted historian and author, remarked that "risk management is about making choices, not preventing losses."[4] With the acceptance of identifiable and manageable risks, organizations may grow and often realize a competitive advantage. Today's emphasis on prevention and control, as opposed to avoidance, places importance on controlling, mitigating, and monitoring risks on an ongoing basis; therefore, the choices we make regarding risks and the management of risks in an ERM program are inherently different than those we make in conventional risk management programs.

The ERM process allows an organization to step back from the minutia of risk and take a more global or strategic perspective. This new top-down, bottom-up process should result in a more efficient treatment of risk, a better understanding of future risk, use of common risk taxonomy, and a strategic risk framework. Regardless of how the organization defines ERM, the goal is to help the organization better understand its risks so that exposure and loss can be reduced and overall corporate stewardship, reputation, and shareholder value improved.

This chapter discusses the need that is prompting healthcare organizations to develop ERM programs, the differences from a conventional risk management program, actionable steps for program development, necessary resources and benefits, and impediments of program implementation. The chapter offers a basic overview of ERM and concentrates on activities for the novice to "get started."

A DISCUSSION ABOUT RISK

Risk is uncertainty, which has both upside and downside potential. It can erode, create, or enhance value. If you have ever placed a bet on a sporting event, gambled at cards, placed money in the stock market, or been on a junket to Las Vegas, you will understand the concept of risk as uncertainty. There are two types of risk: speculative risk and pure risk. Speculative risk offers both the potential for loss as well as gain. Speculative risk is at the heart of ERM and a concept that supports competitive advantage and opportunity. Pure risk creates only the potential for loss. Not all pure risks will necessarily result in a loss, but there will never be the opportunity for gain. Pure risk maintains the status quo at best, and in the worst-case scenario, it creates a loss.

One of the great disservices done to the development of the risk management profession has been the division of risk into pure and speculative subsets with risk management relegated to the management of pure risk only as reported by James Davis in 1998.[5] Holistic risk management (now called ERM) was promoted as the solution to combine those subsets and look at a portfolio of risk for the total organizational. Risks do not exist in isolation; they have a synergistic effect. Having no boundaries, their impact can affect the total organization.

RISK CORRELATION

It is helpful when discussing risk to understand the concept of risk correlation. Risk correlation is the relationship that risks have together. It is just this concept that is missing in conventional risk management programs. Risk in conventional risk management programs focuses on one risk at a time, or one category of risk at a time, and fail to take into account how risks relate to each other.

Risk can be negatively or positively correlated. In risks that are positively correlated, as the probability or impact of one risk increases, so does that of an associated risk. When risks are negatively correlated, the probability or impact of one risk increasing triggers a corresponding decrease in another risk.

Types of Risks

Inherent risk, control risk, and residual risk are important concepts to understand when discussing ERM programs. Inherent risks are those risks that are associated with the activity. Appropriate risk control mitigation (including prevention, reduction, separation, and duplication) can have a positive effect on risk minimization. Control risks are those risks such that errors in systems, processes, or activities will not be prevented, detected, or corrected before an error occurs. The lessons learned from "good catches" will help alleviate control risks, as will the performance of Failure Mode and Effects Analysis on risky processes and activities. Residual risks are those risks that remain even after controls are put into place to mitigate inherent risks. It is important to accept that residual risk exists, and that striving for "no risks" is not achievable. An organization's unwillingness to take risk is a risk itself.

Risk Appetite

The term risk appetite refers to the degree to which an organization's management is willing to accept the uncertainty of loss for a given risk when it has the option to pay a fixed sum to transfer that risk to an insurer (Figure 11–1). The organization's board and senior leadership have to determine the acceptable level of residual risk that they are comfortable assuming against the cost of implementing additional controls.

Risk Domains

Many ERM programs refer to categories or areas of risks called "domains." These

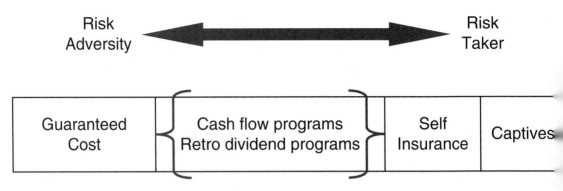

FIGURE 11–1 Organizational Risk Appetite

domains are simply one way of grouping similar risks (including opportunities) and are used as a tool to guide the risk management professional in identifying organizational risks. Most conventional risk management programs focus on clinical-care variability, which fails to account for the synergistic effect of other risks. Risk domains can help in this regard by acting as a prompt to remind the risk management professional to consider other categories of risk beyond the conventional clinical risks with which they are most familiar. Risk domains can also represent areas of interest to the board and senior leadership as having high potential for opportunity or loss. Most domains are the direct responsibility of one or more of the organization's senior leaders. For example, with most organizations the finance domain is under the purview of the chief financial officer and responsibility for the human capital domain resides with the organization's chief human resources officer; both are senior-level executives in most organizations. Responsibility for the operations domain may be separated into functional roles such as the chief medical officer, chief nursing officer, chief administrative officer, or chief operating officer, depending on organizational structure and setting. Risk domains can be expanded or consolidated as appropriate for the organization; however, the most common domains are listed next with a brief description of each.

Operational Risks

The business of health care is the delivery of care that is safe, timely, effective, efficient, and patient centered within diverse populations; therefore, operational risks relate to those risks that result from inadequate or failed internal processes, people, or systems that affect business operations.

Financial Risks

These risks affect the profitability, cash position, access to capital or external financial ratings through business relationships, or the timing and recognition of revenue and expenses.

Strategic Risks

Strategic risks are those risks associated with brand and reputation, business strategy, and failure to adapt to a changing healthcare environment, changing customer priorities, and competition.

Human Capital Risks

Human capital risks refer to the organization's most valuable asset: its workforce. This is an explosive area of exposure in today's tight labor and economic markets. Included are risks associated with employee selection, retention, turnover, absenteeism, productivity, and compensation. The focus of human capital risks has expanded and may include risks associated with the recruitment, retention, and termination of members of the medical staff.

Legal and Regulatory Risks

Legal and regulatory risks include those that arise out of licensure, accreditation, statutes, standards, and regulations, Centers for Medicare and Medicaid Services (CMS) Conditions of Participation (CoPs), product liability, management liability, as well as issues related to intellectual property. Legal and regulatory risks are continuously changing as new laws and requirements are passed.

Technology Risks

Those risks associated with the use of machines, hardware, equipment, devices, and tools, but can also include techniques, systems, and methods of organization, are technology risks. Health care has seen an explosion in the use of technology for clinical diagnosis and treatment, training and education, information storage and retrieval, asset preservation, and so forth.

Hazard Risks

Physical loss of an asset or a reduction in its value created by natural hazards or business interruptions are considered hazard risks. Traditionally, these risks are insurable risks.

THE ENVIRONMENT PROMOTING ERM

A confluence of factors has created an environment ripe for the development of health-care ERM programs. This section highlights just a few of those factors as they impact the availability, or lack thereof, of resources necessary for implementation of efficient and effective programs. These resources include time, money, and people.

Committee of Sponsoring Organizations of the Treadway Commission

The Committee of Sponsoring Organizations of the Treadway Commission (COSO) has

published two documents that are valuable background material when developing an ERM program. One document is an older, but robust, report entitled "Internal Control: Integrated Framework," developed by COSO in 1992 to assess and enhance internal control systems for businesses. This framework has long served as a blueprint for establishing internal controls that promote efficiency, minimize risks, help ensure the reliability of financial statements, and comply with laws and regulations. It has been embraced by many organizations for its comprehensiveness, effectiveness, and universal principles in support of strong internal control.

A preliminary draft of "Enterprise Risk Management: Integrated Framework," including an ERM definition as described previously, was published in July 2003 with the final draft released in 2004. This framework was published in response to growing support for standardizing ERM procedures by developing a conceptually sound framework that provides integrated principles, common terminology, and practical implementation guidance. Regardless of the applicability of the COSO framework in health care (some people feel it is too complex and cumbersome), it supports ERM principles, promotes the concept and principles on a broad basis, and enlists support at the board and senior leadership level: "Although the traditional audience for COSO has been internal auditors and members of the accounting community, the audience for the framework also includes CEOs, CFOs, strategists, board members, and operation leaders. There is also a high degree of relevance for risk managers, many of whom may still be struggling to understand their role in the ERM process."[6] This is particularly true in healthcare organizations.

Sarbanes–Oxley Act of 2002

The Sarbanes–Oxley Act of 2002 (SOX) requires management of public companies, both large and small, to annually assess and report on the effectiveness of internal control over financial reporting. Many not-for-profit organizations have voluntarily complied with the requirement under SOX in promotion of sound business practices and to promote transparency. Once again the emphasis is on internal controls.

Standard & Poor's

In November 2007 Standard & Poor's proposed the introduction of ERM analysis into the corporate credit-ratings process for non-financial companies. They started with incorporating ERM discussions with rated companies and then began to include commentary in their reports in the fourth quarter of 2008. Their reviews focus predominantly on two widely accepted aspects of ERM: risk management culture and strategic risk management. They will defer formal scoring of companies' ERM capabilities (e.g., "strong," "adequate," "weak") until they have conducted a sufficient number of reviews to permit reliable benchmarking and published evaluation criteria. Credit ratings and rating outlooks would be affected in the meantime only if they observe extraordinary conditions that change our existing perception of a company's business profile. An ERM quality score would be assigned and factored into each firm's credit rating. This coincides with increased interest and initiatives by many organizations in risk management practices that:

- Increase risk-adjusted returns
- Improve strategic judgment
- Avoid extraordinary losses due to lawsuits, fines, operational failures, or negligence

Healthcare organizations require access to capital in order to fund projects such as new construction or facility rehabilitation, the purchase of new or updated obsolete technology for information management, clinical-decision support or clinical diagnostics, and the development of advanced patient-care programs. This creates a need to maintain an appropriate credit rating for continued access to the markets. Other rating agencies, such as Moody's and Fitch, are also focusing on ERM in the non-financial sector.

Economic Downturn

Due to the pervasiveness of the credit-market crisis, hospitals and health systems that typically have had broad access to capital are now finding it difficult to finance capital expenditures, according to a survey by the Healthcare Financial Management Association published in 2009. Almost 30% of institutions with typically broad access to capital experienced a substantial increase in the cost of debt, 18% reported difficulty securing letters of credit, and 24% had to withdraw or delay the issuance of bonds. More than half of all organizations report declining inpatient volumes, and increased patient bad debt and charity care are negatively impacting the financial performance of the vast majority of hospitals, according to the survey.[7]

Detailed results from another survey conducted by the American Hospital Association (AHA)[8] continues to highlight the constraints that healthcare organizations are experiencing due to the economic downturn, as follows:

- Borrowing has been constrained.
- Charitable donations are down.
- Capital decisions have been affected as uncertainty mounts, operating performance declines, and the value of reserves fails due to stock market and other investment woes.
- Half of the organizations that responded have put capital projects on hold (82% facility projects, 65% clinical technology, and 62% information technology).
- The ability to meet community needs and goals, such as improved quality, efficiency, and coordination of care, has been affected.

According to a study[9] published in *Health Affairs*, 19.2% of all non-elderly Americans will be uninsured in 2010. This 2% increase from 2007 is due to increases in both the population and the percentage of uninsureds, and brings the number of uninsured to a high of 52 million non-elderly Americans. This increase further stresses an already overburdened healthcare system in an area of vulnerability: the emergency department, the gateway for many hospital admissions.

Connecting the dots between these issues (regulatory, environmental, and economic) strengthens the impetus for the development of ERM programs. Healthcare organizations, more now than ever, need to be fiscally prudent as well as efficient and effective in how care is delivered. Waste of precious resources cannot be tolerated.

WHAT IS DIFFERENT ABOUT ERM PROGRAMS?

The differences between a conventional risk management program and an ERM program are vast (see Table 11–1). The ERM programs promote early identification and can give an organization a competitive advantage. It is no longer good enough to perform as expected for the national average on quality outcomes and patient satisfaction; organizations need to exceed the results of their competitor(s) down the road in order to maintain and grow market share.

Table 11–1 Risk Management Transition to Enterprise Risk Management

Risk Management	Enterprise Risk Management
Pure risk	Speculative risk
Individual error	System/process error
Disciplinary/punitive	Learning/caring/non-punitive
Closed	Transparent/open
Obstructing	Enabling
Tactical	Strategic
Department/unit/division	Organization-wide
Separate	Holistic
Reactive	Proactive
Focused	Comprehensive
Risk silos	Risk integrated
Avoidance	Prevention/mitigation
Transactional	Consultative
Independent	Interdependent
Loss	Opportunity

ACTIONABLE STEPS IN PROGRAM DEVELOPMENT

The following steps are necessary in developing an ERM program:

- Obtain board- and senior-leadership support.
- Integrate ERM with strategic planning.
- Develop a well-articulated vision and plan.
- Maintain a positive culture and environment.
- Implement cross-functional teams.
- Develop and implement a communication plan.
- Offer education on risk.
- Determine availability of internal and external resources.
- Identify performance metrics.

Obtain Board and Senior Leadership Support

The implementation of an ERM program requires high-level commitment throughout an organization, including those in the executive or "C-Suite"* and the board. Without this support, ERM programs are in jeopardy of failure. An ERM is not the "flavor of the month," changing on a whim and at a moment's notice. It is more akin to a favorite meal—always savored, enjoyed often, remembered long, and repeated frequently.

Integrate with Strategic Planning

Every adverse event has repercussions that affect the entire organization. The cost of a bad outcome (e.g., quality failure) is not lim-

---

* "C-Suite" refers to the senior leadership team and generally includes the following positions: chief executive officer, chief medical officer, chief financial officer, chief nursing officer, chief risk officer, chief operating officer, chief administrative officer, chief human resources officer, chief information officer, and so forth.

ited to the check written for a legal settlement. Staff morale drops, absences increase, mandatory reporting increases, care costs go up, and the organization's reputation may suffer. Effective ERM programs are integrated with the strategic-planning process, budgeting cycle, outcomes measurement, and performance reviews.

Develop a Well-Articulated Vision and Plan

A defined vision and plan can start with something as simple as a values doctrine (Exhibit 11–1). Having a well-articulated vision and plan promotes the communication plan, is the foundation of all educational initiatives, and should be revised as needed.

Maintain a Positive Culture and Environment

Healthcare organizations struggle to change the work environment to one that is non-punitive and non-disciplinary. Terms that are often used to reflect this new environment and culture are transparent, fair, trusted, open, and learning. The ERM programs can flourish in the new environment, but they will quickly fade under the previous culture of individual blame and shame.

High-reliability organizations (HROs) are inherently related to high-performing organizations. In health care, reliability is defined as the "measurable ability of health-related process, procedure, or service to perform its intended functions in the required time under commonly occurring conditions."[10] "HROs have a (1) preoccupation with avoiding failure, (2) reluctance to simplify interpretations, (3) sensitivity to operations, (4) commitment to resilience, and (5) deference to expertise."[11] The HROs are well positioned to implement ERM because they already support a healthy work environment and culture that is open to new ideas, promotes best practice, and is collaborative and communicative. The characteristics of high reliability and specific strategies for managing the most common operational failures of them are addressed in detail in the final section of this book.

Implement Cross-Functional Teams

The ERM programs cannot be developed, implemented, monitored, or evaluated without the collaborative effort of cross-functional teams within the organizations. The collective power and support of cross-functional teams allow for innovation, as well as rapid support for, and assistance in, the deployment of strategies and solutions, which facilitates employee communication and builds employee empowerment.

Develop and Implement a Communication Plan

The development of a communication plan is an important function in the early stages of ERM development. How will the organization describe its ERM activities to outside stakeholders when questioned? How will the organization communicate the ERM program to all employees? And then keep them up to date with new developments? Newsletters, E-mails, town-hall meetings, Webinars? How can the organization use education as a communication tool? How will the organization engage all employees, answer questions that arise, and respond to comments?

Most organizations still focus primarily on senior leadership when implementing ERM, and have not taken the next step to reach out to employees who, in many cases, are at the "sharp end" of the process, which is, after all, where many of the risks occur. Until the employees are truly engaged in the risk management process, the full value and impact of ERM will not be realized. Enterprise risk management is a top-down and bottom-up program that requires the active support of all healthcare employees.

Exhibit 11–1 *Sample Values Doctrine for Enterprise Risk Management*

- Quality care is at the center of all that we do and is the core to our business objectives.

- Creating a culture that supports a safe environment for all is paramount to the organization's mission and objectives. This includes not only our patients/residents and their families and caregivers, but also our employees, board members, medical staff, volunteers, and contractors.

- We promote an enterprise-wide early-warning system and framework for the comprehensive identification and resolution of all organizational risks.

- We reward the reporting of risk (potential and real), adverse events, and near misses/good catches.

- We adhere to an early-intervention program that supports patient safety, prompt investigations of adverse events, open and honest communication, transparency, disclosure, apology, and fair compensation (when appropriate) to injured patients/residents.

- Employee empowerment and service recovery are principles with which all employees are trained and encouraged to practice.

- In promotion of our organization as a learning environment, we will share with all stakeholders the lessons learned from patient safety and other risk-related issues.

- To safeguard the delivery of patient-centered care, we will strive for patient/family/caregiver participation in strategy setting and membership on functional teams designed to identify and mitigate the potential for loss.

This values doctrine is endorsed by the organization's board of directors, executive leadership, and medical staff, and is supported by all employees and volunteers.

Offer Education on Risk

Education is a key part of ERM development and implementation at all levels of the organization. Employees throughout the organization need to have a general understanding of risk, how the organization views ERM through definitions, a common taxonomy, an articulated values doctrine, defined goals and benefits, and understanding and support for the resources necessary to carry out the program. Education should be ongoing and track the process as it evolves over time. Initially, education may start with the board and senior leadership. As committees and teams are developed, education will be pushed further down in the organization, where eventually all employees will understand the basic concepts. In this manner, employees understand individual and organizational expectations and become risk managers within their areas of responsibility.

Determine Availability of Internal and External Resources

Most organizations will have a wealth of talent within their ranks that can support the ERM program. How to identify this talent so that it can be tapped when necessary is the challenge. Knowing what expertise or services may be required from outside sources should be identified early in the process so that resource costs can be included in the budget cycle. Most organizations outsource the complex financial modeling used to quantify the fiscal impact on an organization, whereas others are not comfortable in identifying risk and request outside assistance. Outside consultants are often contracted to supplement internal efforts particularly with education for the board, senior leadership, and medical staff.

Chapter 12 addresses more specifically the best way to utilize the talents of external service providers to optimize the value and quality of an ERM program.

Identify Performance Metrics

A common problem with most ERM programs is the failure to determine how success will be measured as you develop the program. Developing performance metrics starts with an understanding of the program's goals and objectives, as well as the organization's strategic plan. Is the organization trying to decrease its cost of risk? How will improvement be measured? How do you measure what you have prevented? (This is an old question with a new twist.) The steering committee should determine performance metrics specific to their ERM program.

GETTING STARTED

The following steps are a broad-based concept to review as the organization moves forward with developing and implementing an ERM program:

1. *Identify and engage an executive-level champion.* The concept of ERM program development can be suggested by a variety of professionals, including the CEO, CFO, general counsel, and the risk management professional. Quite possibly a board member may promote ERM by querying senior leadership because of something they may have read or heard. Regardless of who suggests the program, development and implementation of an ERM program will need a champion. If the organization has a professional that fits the criteria for a chief risk officer (CRO), this person is in the best position to champion that charge. For all individual projects that are identified to reduce or mitigate risk, an individual champion should be tasked with project responsibility, follow-through, as well as monitoring and evaluating success. This champion may be a member of the leadership team with current responsibilities closest to the risk.

2. *Select a steering committee and working task force.* A steering committee composed of four to six members who represent senior leadership should be tasked with the responsibility for:

- Defining ERM for the organization
- Setting realistic goals, objectives, and expectations
- Determining the organization's risk tendency
- Establishing an ERM framework (Figure 11–2)
- Determining risk-quantification tools to prioritize identified risk, and defining a range for frequency, severity, time to impact, and risk mitigants
- Establishing performance metrics
- Approving the membership of the working task force

Depending on the reporting level of the risk management professional within the organizational structure and skill set, he or she may sit on the steering committee. The steering committee will also develop a timeline for program development taking into account the strategic-planning cycle, budgeting process, timing of board meetings, medical-staff meeting and key departmental meetings, and risk financing program renewals. The steering committee will generally meet quarterly to review and approve projects, approve resource allocation, and receive status reports on existing projects (see Exhibit 11–2).

A working task force, representative of the major risk domains (finance, legal, regulatory, technology, operations [nursing and medical staff], and human resources), along with the risk management professional, will meet monthly but may meet more often in the early stages of program development. The working task force will manage the risk-identification process, develop and implement identification tools, review the results, and develop a risk list. From this risk list they will prioritize/rank the identified risk and determine the top 5 to 10 risks the organization should address in individual project teams. This risk list and recommended risk prioritization will be reviewed and approved by the steering committee before individual teams and project champions are chosen. The

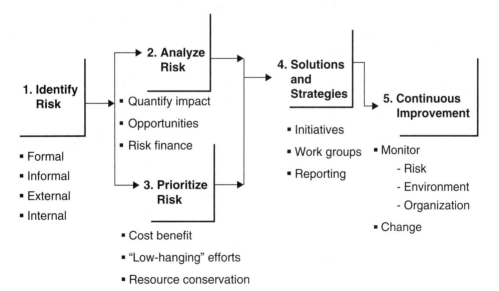

FIGURE 11–2 ERM Framework

working task force also plays a significant and ongoing role in employee education.

3. *Review strategic plan for organization.* Far too often the process of developing an ERM program is begun without many of the key players being aware of the organization's strategic direction. The strategic plan should be reviewed with the steering committee and the working task force to ensure that the goals and objectives are clearly stated, that the ERM program supports the existing plan, and that conflicts do not arise. Initiating an ERM program may necessitate a revision or updating of the strategic plan for the organization. This is a perfect opportunity to ensure that both are in sync. The ERM should be built into future revisions of the plan. It is also helpful for both teams, the steering committee, and the working task force to review and understand the approval process for resource deployment and the system by which new policies, procedures, protocols, and best practices are developed and implemented.

4. *Identify and review current risk-identification tools.* The working task force should review all existing methods to identify risk. These methods may be internal or external to the organization, and may be formal or informal (see "Risk Identification"). The working task force will also be charged with the development of any new tools such as surveys, questionnaires, and interview guides.

5. *Compile and share resource lists and reference materials, and identify subject-matter experts.* There is a wealth of information available about ERM. The working task force may be responsible for compiling the reference materials in an online library for easy reference.

RISK IDENTIFICATION

Developing a process to identify organizational risks will assist management in determining what risks can impact strategy and the achievement of organizational goals. Some of the same methodologies used to identify risks in conventional risk management programs can be deployed in an ERM program and include both formal and informal methods. The incident report, the cornerstone of most conventional risk management programs, is one such formal method. Although the incident report is not an often-used reporting format for significant risks, it offers information on a variety of risks in a consolidated manner. It can be particularly useful in identifying "good catches." The use of the Institute for Healthcare Improvement's (IHI) Global Trigger Tool is another formal method of risk identification through occurrence screening.[12] Regardless of the method used, no single procedure will uncover all risks to the organization. Risks can be internal within an organization or external to it. They can be identified retrospectively, concurrently, pre-interventionally, or prospectively.

Two other methods successfully used in ERM programs to identify risk are risk surveys and risk interviews (Exhibit 11–3). The development of risk surveys requires thoughtful consideration as to the types of questions you want the respondent to answer and to whom the survey will be sent. General demographic information should be solicited to allow for comparison. For example, answers from a manager of a non-clinical unit, such as the admitting office, will differ from a manager of a high-risk clinical area such as the operating room. Identifying reporting level within the organization and length of service are also important to ensure an accurate understanding of the results. Surveys will offer a mix of direct questions (yes/no, multiple-choice answers) as well as

Exhibit 11–2 Sample Board-Status Report

Project Name (brief narrative description of initiative):			
#_____			
Project Leader:	Name	Position/Title	Department
Initiative Champions (board member, senior leadership, physician)	Name	Position/Title	Department
Initiative Team Members	Name 1. 2. 3.	Position/Title	Department
Resource Deployment (to date: amount, number, items)	Financial	Human Resources	Technology
	$	$	$
	Item	Number (FTE)	Item
Identified Constraints	1. 2. 3. 4.		
Review Dates:	1.	2.	3.
	4.	5.	6.
Project Status			
Action Items Identified	1.	2.	3.

open-ended questions. Open-ended questions are asked so that the tool is not limiting or perceived as guiding the respondent's answers.

One-on-one and small group interviews are an effective way to solicit risk informa-tion from a wide variety of staff/personnel. Interviewing for risk has the added benefit of being able to follow up immediately on sig-nificant risks, alters subsequent questioning based on real-time answers, and adds the personal touch a personal interview can

Exhibit 11–3 Risk-Identification Interview Tool

Interviewer:

Interviewee:

Department:

Date:

Risk Identification:

1. How do you define risk?

2. How do you identify risk in your area? (Early-warning system)

3. What do you feel are the top five real or perceived risks in your department, division, or organization?

4. What is the impact of identified risks in your area? (Inadequate staffing, inefficient use of resources, diminished capital, etc.)

5. How often do they occur?

Risk Ownership:

6. How do you (or will you) engage employees in risk initiatives?

7. How will each division/unit/team contribute to meeting the goals of the ERM strategy?

8. How will teams/individuals be held accountable for success?

Risk Prioritization:

9. What method(s) do you use to prioritize risk? (For example, costs, benefit, resource consumption, easy to implement)

10. How are the identified risks ranked? (For example, frequency, impact, severity)

11. Are the identified risks material? (Important)

12. What are the consequences if these risks are not addressed?

Risk Treatment:

13. How are the identified risks currently managed?

14. Is the approach effective?

15. Given limited resources, what criteria are used to choose initiatives to implement?

16. Do you feel resources are being wasted or used inefficiently? If so, where and how?

Risk Solutions:

17. What action plans should be in place? How are responsible parties assigned for follow-through?

18. How are risks monitored?

19. How is success measured?

offer. It is important to keep in mind that interviewing for risk takes time—more time than conducting a survey. With both methods, the results need to be consolidated and compared. Some organizations may choose to survey management staff and then conduct interviews to dig deeper into risk identified in the survey. The results of the surveys and interviews will identify organizational, departmental, unit, and divisional risks depending on the respondents chosen. When preparing a survey or interview tool, care should be taken to include all areas/domains of risk. Open-ended questions should also be asked during the interview to solicit additional comments not covered by survey questions. Other questions might include (1) "What other aspects of your position keep you awake at night?" (2) "Would you go to your emergency department if you were ill? If not, why?" (3) "Given unlimited resources, what would you implement that could impact patient safety?" (4) "What would you change first?" and (5) "Where are you wasting resources and, if possible, where can you redeploy them?"

Additional instructions may also ask the respondents to identify current risk mitigation initiatives and who has assigned responsibility. Asking respondents to identify the significance of risks (frequency/severity) will also be helpful in knowing how they prioritize and view risks within their area of responsibility. Always encourage the participants to call back with questions, additional comments, or if they have forgotten to mention an important item. During the risk-identification phase you want to ensure that every possible effort has been taken to identify all risks to the organization.

The identification of all organizational risks is a critical phase in ERM and one from which all other activities stem. It is important to be thorough. From the prepared surveys, personal interviews, and other formal and informal methods to identify risks, a preliminary risk list is developed. At this stage, the risk list has not been analyzed or quantified.

Keep in mind that this list may be quite long initially, and until some filters are incorporated in the assessment phase, it may appear cumbersome. Initially, the working task force can combine similar risks as well as identify, track, and eliminate duplication, and look for quick fixes or "low-hanging fruit"—risks that have an obvious and easy fix. Risks on the list should be categorized by domain and numbered for easy reference.

RISK ASSESSMENT

Once all organizational risks have been identified and placed on the risk list by domain, the next phase is to:

- Understand and attempt to quantify the potential magnitude or materiality of each identified risk
- Consider the positive and negative consequences of events that underlie identified risks across an organization
- Incorporate at least two dimensions of risk: likelihood and severity
- Evaluate risk-control mitigation strategies for each risk and determine how they influence the likelihood and impact of the risk occurring
- Recognize that there may be a range of possible results associated with an event

The outcome of this phase will be an inventory of risks ranked and prioritized.

Risk Scoring and Risk Prioritization

Given limited resources, particularly with the economic downturn of 2008–2009, organizations need some methodology by which identified risks can be separated into those that require attention and those that do not. For those risks determined to be of some significance to the organization and therefore require attention, how are they analyzed to see which ones are addressed first? Most ERM programs use a scoring or ranking system to prioritize identified risks. A simple, commonly used risk-ranking system is created by adding the probability rating (frequency that an event will occur) to its time-to-impact rating (the period of time to respond or how long the impact will be felt) and then multiplying this total by the severity (financial consequences of loss) to identify key risks that require immediate attention:

Frequency + Time to Impact
× Severity = Risk Score

Using this risk-ranking system requires the organization to define the range of options for each point. The frequency (likelihood of an incident occurring) generally has a range from 1 to 5, with 1 equal to occurrence only in rare circumstances, whereas 5 equals occurrence in most circumstances. Under the time-to-impact scoring, a range of 1–3 is used, with 3 meaning that you have no warning and the results are felt for a long time. For example, an earthquake might be categorized as a 3 on the range of time to impact. The severity range (financial impact or consequences) can be equated with the financial consequences or relate to a patient/resident harm index. This range is most often considered on a scale of 1–5, with 5 being the most costly or catastrophic in terms of injury. A death due to medical error would be a 5 on the severity scale and would most likely be a 5 on the financial severity scale as well.

Just as the organization needs to define ERM within its environment and culture, it also needs to define the descriptors within each of the ranges. Those descriptors need to be meaningful to them. For example, on the severity scale, some organizations may consider a $50,000 loss to be major (a 4 on the range of values), whereas other organizations may find this to be a minor loss (a 1 on the range of values).

Another key factor used to determine the priority of risks to address is the evaluation of the use of internal control or mitigants. With no risk mitigants to manage known risk, risks take on a higher significance (priority) than if you have appropriate controls in place that are working to minimize the potential frequency and severity; thus, while

the actual risk may not increase, the priority for action may elevate this risk before other risks with a higher score but with effective internal controls in place. Some ERM programs measure current controls that reduce the likelihood of the event occurring (frequency) and measure the effect of the controls that reduce the impact of the event if it occurs (severity).[13]

For risk prioritized as a high priority for intervention, additional detailed modeling may be necessary. This modeling may require company-specific data combined with external data to create detailed risk models. Through the use of sophisticated financial-modeling tools, including dynamic financial analysis and other catastrophic risk simulation used to determine the potential impact of risk events on critical financial measures, such as cash flow, financial ratings, and earnings per share, senior leadership and the board can review various scenarios and their impact on the organization. Although they are valid and important, these detailed financial-modeling tools are not discussed further because they are beyond the scope of this chapter.

Risk Mapping

A picture is worth a thousand words." Risk maps are tools that help "message" risks to the organization. They are easy to read, colorful, and quick to prepare with software programs or developed on one's personal desktop. They graphically depict an organization's risk by displaying the relationship between frequency and severity. This relationship often takes the form of a two-dimensional grid with frequency (or likelihood of occurrence) on one axis and severity (degree of financial impact or harm) on the other axis (Figure 11–3). Risk maps prioritize risks and are useful for:

- Data collection
- Risk-mitigation strategies (Risks that fall in the high-frequency/high-severity quadrant are given priority risk management attention.)

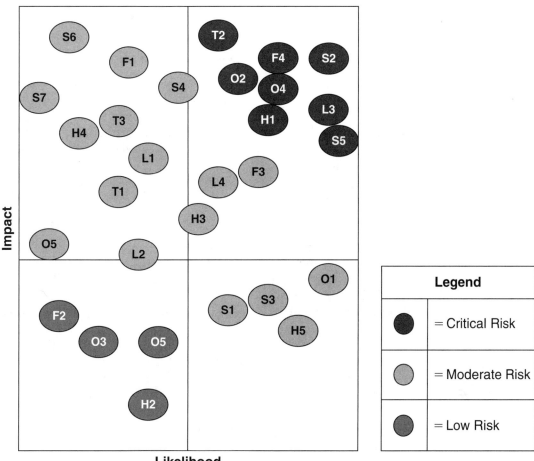

Figure 11–3 Risk Map and List

RISK LIST

Financial Risks
F1 – Loss of payor/
      reimbursement cuts
F2 – Increased expenses
F3 – Rating Agency Perception

Legal/Regulatory Risks
L1 – Corporate compliance
      program
L2 – Local legal environment
L3 – Billing fraud
L4 – Electronic physician
      consultation
L5 – HIPAA compliance
L6 – Monitoring of legislative
      market
L7 – Potential for Stark violations

Technology Risks
T1 – Separate medical records
T2 – Lack of redundancy in IT
T3 – Loss of connectivity
T4 – Unauthorized access

Operational Risks
O1 – Lack of emphasis on patient-
      centered care
O2 – Pandemic outbreak
O3 – Lack of information sharing
      between partners
O4 – Lack of communication
      between executives and
      physicians/staff
O5 – Inaccurate provider list
O6 – Lack of comprehensive risk
      management program
O7 – Ineffective communication
O8 – Inadequate policies,
      procedures, and protocols
O9 – Clinical errors in Interventional
      Radiology
O10 – Lack of standardization
O11 – Space constraints
O12 – Inefficient operating rooms

Human Capital Risks
H1 – Aging physicians
H2 – Staff turnover
H3 – Physician fatigue
H4 – Continuity of leadership
H5 – Physician behavior
H6 – Leadership and management
      skills
H7 – Physician recruitment
H8 – Physician retention

Strategic Risks
S1 – Clinical quality scores
S2 – Negatively publicized event
S3 – Monitoring of local market
S4 – Key partner dependencies
S5 – Loss of market share
S6 – Lack of strategic identity
S7 – Decreasing demand for in-patient
      services
S8 – Inability to capture profit
S9 – Loss of key clinicians
S10 – Integration with partners
S11 – Internal controls development

- Capital allocation
- Helping to exploit a competitive edge
- Board and senior leadership presentations to support short commentary

The development of risk maps requires a team effort. They improve knowledge of exposures and facilitate risk-control techniques.

BENEFITS OF AN ERM PROGRAM

Enterprise risk management may be seen as a route to helping organizations demonstrate compliance with governance and reporting requirements, yet it is also increasingly perceived as affecting the organization's culture. Other benefits identified from a recent Aon study include improvement of operational efficiencies, reduction in cost of risk, improvement in organizational efficiency, securing of growth opportunities, and enhancement of behaviors and commitment.[14]

IMPEDIMENTS TO IMPLEMENTATION

Length of Time to Complete

The development and implementation of an ERM program is not for the "faint hearted" or the "quick fixer." Implementation of ERM into strategic planning and firmly embedded in the culture of the organization is a daunting task for many risk management professionals, because it can take from 2 to 5 years on average for full implementation. "ERM is not strictly a serial process, where one component builds upon the next. Rather, it is a multidirectional, interactive process where any component can and does influence the other."[15]

Failure to Adequately Define ERM

The ERM needs to make sense for the organization, with a definition that is understandable, easy to communicate, and consistent with the strategy. The ERM process and plan also need a communication plan to enlist the support of everyone within the organization.

Lack of Access to Key Resources

Implementing an ERM program requires a multidisciplinary approach and the active involvement and support of a wide variety of professionals, both internal and external. The inability to access needed assistance from key resources can be a limitation. This inability to access key resources may be due to time constraints on the resource, not knowing of a qualified resource, unbudgeted resource costs, and having no particular individual designated as the responsible "go-to" person for approval.

Lack of Education

Education is an important factor to consider when developing an ERM program. Education starts with the board and senior leadership and eventually trickles down through the organization to all employees. Education can help sell the message to the employees and staff, and it can embed ERM in the fabric of the organization.

No Champion or Defined Responsibility

A risk management steering committee and task force will be assigned to do much of the initial preparatory work; however, on an ongoing basis, champions need to be identified for each project developed. Without this accountability and responsibility, most projects falter due to a lack of leadership and direction. The same is true for the overall ERM program. Eventually, the responsibility and oversight for the day-to-day activities need to be assigned to an individual or unit within the organization at a high enough level to keep the program moving forward. This is generally the CRO or the Enterprise Risk Management Department.

THE NEW RISK MANAGEMENT PROFESSIONAL: CHIEF RISK OFFICER

Because the journey to full implementation of an organization-wide ERM program has changed the focus of previous risk programs to now include both pure risk and speculative risk, the necessary skills for the risk management professional have changed as well. It is assumed that the technical skills associated with risk financing, insurance concepts and principles, claims management (including incident investigation and litigation support), risk management information systems (RIMS), and risk control are proven skills. "The likelihood of finding an individual with the background and time to get to grips with every sub-discipline of risk management from credit risk and market to network and operational risk, is unrealistically ambitious."[16] Therefore, the risk management professional, regardless of his or her experience, background, and educational credentials, will need to collaborate with others in the organization, or in parallel, for support and guidance. The seasoned professional will know when and where to obtain assistance. Helpful business skills include finance, legal, human resources, security, patient and environmental safety, marketing, operations, compliance, technology, and clinical.

Necessary Skills

The risk management professional, in this new environment, takes on greater visibility within the organization and draws upon competency skills, such as those described in a recent RIMS ERM publication,[17] that had not been previously valued to the same extent. This includes two sets of competency skills: (1) interpersonal, including leadership, motivator, negotiations, consensus builder, and team builder; and (2) personal, including motivated, innovative, experienced, articulate, and consultative.

A new title, chief risk officer (CRO), has emerged in recognition of the complexity of responsibilities. It is a position on the senior leadership team. The CRO, in this new environment, becomes a facilitator, orchestrator, ringleader, teacher, presenter, educator, strategist, problem solver, decision maker, and collaborator. Although many risk managers responsible for conventional risk management programs possess many of these personal and interpersonal skills, these skills have not been celebrated, embraced, or sought after as they are today.

Health care has been slow in adopting ERM, and therefore it is no surprise that there are not many CROs available to organizations that want to implement a program. The people who are functioning in the role of CRO will readily admit that their responsibilities are far different from those that they had with a conventional risk management program. A concern for organizations as they move forward with development of ERM programs is their ability to attract and retain talent. Talented people with an appropriate mix of skill sets are critical to developing a sustainable and successful ERM program. Recruitment, professional development, succession planning, and competency training are key strategies to ensure that the organization will have the people that it needs to advance and fully realize the potential of their ERM program.

CONCLUSION

Enterprise risk management in health care is more important than ever. The risks that threaten healthcare organizations are constantly changing and becoming more complex. It has been said often that nothing in risk management ever goes away—we just keep adding to the list of tasks and responsibilities; thus, the development of an ERM program is truly a journey, and the road may be a bit rocky for a while until there are enough other successful programs that can point the way for other organizations with the same goal.

References

1. COSO. (2004). Enterprise risk management: Integrated framework. http://www.coso.org/documents/COSO_ERM_Executive Summary.pdf. Accessed April 21, 2010.
2. Carroll R.L., & Nakamura, P.A. (2008). *Key elements, stakeholders and responsibilities in an ERM plan.* Presentation ASHRMs annual meeting and education conference, 2008, Boston, Massachusetts.
3. Carroll, R.L. (2009). Enterprise risk management: What's it all about. *ERM Handbook.* Washington, DC: American Health Lawyers Association, Chapter 1.
4. Bernstein, P. (2008, November 20). The remarkable story of risk. *International Herald Tribune.*
5. Davis, J.V. (Winter 1998). The trend to holistic risk management. *The John Liner Review, 11(4)*, 39.
6. Kaufman, C. (2004). *An urgent call to action: COSO, ERM and the role of the risk manager.* Chicago: Aon Enterprise Risk Management Consulting.
7. American Hospital Association. (2009, January 26). *News now.* http://www.hfma.org/financialhealth/swf/sldDeck.pdf/. Accessed November 9, 2009.
8. American Hospital Association. (November 2008). *The capital crisis: Survey of impact on hospitals.* http://www.aha.org/aha/content/2008/pdf/081119econcrisisreport.pdf/. Accessed November 9, 2009.
9. Gilmer, T.P., & Kronick, R.G. (2009). Hard times and health insurance: How many Americans will be uninsured by 2010? *Health Affairs, 28*(4), w573–w577.
10. Hughes, R.G. (Ed.). (2008). Nurses at the "sharp end" of patient care. *Patient safety and quality: An evidence-based handbook for nurses.* AHRQ publication no. 08-0043. Rockville, MD: Agency for Healthcare Research and Quality.
11. Ibid, p. 7.
12. Institute for Healthcare Improvement. (2009). *Global trigger tools for measuring adverse outcomes.* http://www.ihi.org/IHI/Topics/PatientSafety/SafetyGeneral/Tools/IHIGlobalTriggerTool forMeasuringAEs.htm/. Accessed May 30, 2009.
13. The University of New England Armidale. (n.d.). *Risk identification and assessment worksheet.* http://www.une.edu.au/risk-management/riskworksheet.pdf/ . Accessed May 30, 2009.
14. Aon Global Survey Results. (2007). Enterprise risk management: The full picture. http://www.aon.com/netherlands/risk services/pdf/ERM.Survey.Report_Final_2010 .pdf. Accessed April 12, 2010.
15. Moody, M.J. (2007). Enterprise risk management's future is brighter. *CPCU Risk Management Quarterly, 23*(4), 10–12.
16. The Economist Intelligence Unit. (2005). The evolving role of the CRO: A report from the Economist Intelligence Unit Sponsored by ACE, Cisco Systems, Deutsche Bank and IBM. http://www.aceeuropeangroup.com/NR/rdonlyres/F206B4A7-C9F9-4223-82BA -BBA03268014C/0/EVOLVING_CRO_REPORT. pdf. Accessed April 12, 2010.
17. Coffin, B. (Ed.). The 2008 financial crisis: A wakeup call for enterprise risk management. RIMS executive report, *The risk perspective,* January 2009.

DEVELOPING A REQUEST FOR PROPOSAL AND WORKING WITH INSURANCE PROVIDERS

Michael Sheppard, MBA

INTRODUCTION

One of the issues that keeps risk managers awake at night is how they will continue to manage the costs associated with a changing insurance marketplace, the continued escalation of malpractice verdicts and settlements, and an unstable economy. Each factor is dramatically changing the way healthcare risk managers or chief risk officers (CRO) structure risk financing programs, and each directly affects the costs associated with providing medical professional-liability (MPL) insurance coverage. The amount of self-funding required in the current market is forcing many organizations to, in effect, operate their own insurance companies. Commercial coverage at any level may not be available for certain classes of risk or for organizations in specific areas where the tort system is out of control. Commercial coverage, even if it is available, may be unaffordable, particularly in light of the other financial pressures faced by individual providers and healthcare organizations.

DEVELOPING A PLAN TO MANAGE MEDICAL PROFESSIONAL-LIABILITY RISK

The basic goal behind the financing of MPL risk is to ensure that an organization can meet all of the financial obligations that arise from that risk. Chapter 11 sets out the strategy for conceptualizing organizational risk and should be completed before the activities described in the present chapter occur. This will increase the likelihood that the program created by the risk manager or CRO and external insurance providers meets the strategic objectives of the organization. The most common methods used to ensure that all claims can be paid when they arise include purchasing commercial insurance that transfers the risk to a third party, self-insuring all the risk, and a combination of commercial insurance and self-insurance. In today's economy, most healthcare organizations use the combination of self-insurance and commercial insurance.

Analyzing the appropriateness of a combined insurance structure and implementing it is complex. It requires a professional risk manager or chief risk officer and assistance from professionals outside the organization. The primary professionals that an organization should use in formulating the risk financing plan are:

- *Insurance brokers or consultants.* These professionals are most critical in the development of a risk financing plan and represent a significant professional relationship for the organization. They provide information regarding the insurance marketplace, new products, and concepts in self-insurance, and, most importantly, they serve as the intermediary to the commercial-insurance marketplace. Many insurance brokerage firms can also provide related services such as loss control, claims management, and actuarial services.
- *Attorneys.* A healthcare organization will need to engage attorneys who specialize in administrative matters and have knowledge of the state laws that govern how organizations can create self-insured or partially insured programs.
- *Actuaries.* These professionals will help predict an organization's risk based on the exposure information collected. Actuaries then create models that will assist the organization in making decisions about risk retention. Most large actuarial firms have comprehensive databases for MPL risks that help them analyze and predict an organization's expected level of loss. Since today's commercial-insurance marketplace requires some form of self-insurance, a healthcare organization may be required by auditors or insurance underwriters to have actuarial assistance in establishing and funding its program.
- *Investment brokers or money managers.* These professionals help the organization obtain the maximum return on investment.

Selecting and Managing the Insurance Broker

Since the insurance broker is so critical to the development and implementation of the risk financing plan, selecting a broker should be undertaken in a highly structured manner. Most organizations have an established competitive bidding process for outside service procurement, and the selection of an insurance broker for MPL risk should follow the established process. This process usually entails a request for qualifications (RFQ), a request for proposal (RFP), and an interview; however, the scope of each varies from one organization to another. Within the organizational bidding process, the following basic materials should be developed to describe the program and to target the needs of the program with an appropriate insurance broker:

1. An introduction of the healthcare organization that includes:
   - The background of the organization, including its history, operation, and place in the community.
   - A description of the risk management function of the organization, including mission and strategy statements.
   - An outline of the current risk financing program, with information about the level of insurance and self-insurance. It is often helpful to caution competing brokers not to contact any insurers, particularly the organization's current insurer, during the broker-selection process.
   - The term of the proposed agreement and a request that the broker submit the bid to comply with the length of the agreement.
2. A full explanation of the scope of services required from the broker.
   - Identify and explain in detail the MPL risk exposure in the organization.
   - Specifically identify and explain each of the services that will be required of the broker in the program. If the orga-

nization is focusing solely on risk financing, state in detail the expectations of the broker in the program design, insurance negotiation, and program administration. If the organization requires services beyond risk financing, such as an actuarial analysis or claims management, identify the scope and expectations for each of those services.

3. A detailed summary of the selection criteria that the organization will use.

- A formal explanation of the bidding process and the timeline should be presented.
- The response format and specific rules should be explained clearly. Always request references and a detailed cost breakdown for each service the broker is to provide.
- List the specific criteria on which the bidders will be rated; these can include cost, quality of the account team, and perceived quality of the proposed services.

The broker-selection process in most organizations is normally via a committee of the stakeholders. Establishing a rating system that is fair to the competing candidates is very important. Exhibit 12–1 is a sample broker-selection scorecard that can be used to assist committee members in rating the broker candidates.

Broker compensation is widely discussed and debated. Since the insurance brokerage is a significant professional relationship for the organization, the level of compensation is often quite large. There are two basic methods for compensating a broker: commission or fee.

In the commission strategy, the insurer pays the broker for the placement of an insurance policy. The commission is based on a fixed percentage of the premium and is part of the total premium charged to the buyer. The normal range for these commissions is 5–12.5% of the premium. This strategy carries the stigma that a broker has an incentive to seek higher premiums when, in fact, the broker's duty is to get the buyer the best deal at the lowest rate. Commission remuneration usually only applies to insurance placement, and brokers require separate fees for other services they may provide. Although this method of payment is the easiest to carry out, it can result in the perception that "it's not the client compensating the broker, but rather the insurer." It is important to remember that whatever amount of commission determined to be acceptable is added to the premium and this should be communicated to the insurer by the buyer.

The fee-for-service approach is the preferred strategy in today's market. It is a predictable cost and can be more easily justified in terms of services provided. This strategy allows the buyer to identify and control the costs of both the placement of insurance and other ancillary services the broker may provide.

When the selection process is complete, be certain to document all the services required in a formal agreement with the broker. This will avoid any disputes over scope of services or remuneration at a later date. Brokers often have global capabilities for placements offshore, and such placements require additional fees. Make certain to include any fees associated with offshore placements in the initial agreement to avoid having to pay additional fees if international insurance markets are used.

Once the brokerage agreement is executed, the organization must take responsibility for the proper management of the broker within its risk financing program. Make certain that the broker is fully aware that the organization controls the process. Always reinforce the "client-in-control" concept to avoid situations in which the broker is asserting too much influence on the program. Develop expected performance standards with the broker to include such areas as responsiveness and work product. It is a good idea to schedule either face-to-face or telephone meetings at least monthly with the

Exhibit 12–1 Broker-Selection Scorecard

Maximum Points	Trait	Broker 1	Broker 2
	Insurance-company relationships		
3	Relationship with current carrier		
3	Relationship with property insurer		
3	Relationship with Directors and Officers (D&O) insurer		
6	Other		
	International insurance-placement capability		
3	Explained international abilities		
	Claims expertise		
3	Demonstrates success		
	Delivery of complete and correct policies		
3	Explained effective process		
	Resources to help complete insurance applications		
3	Offers helpful resources		
Supplementary services			
	Actuarial service for liability exposures		
3	Can provide		
	Review of actuarial reports		
3	Has capability in-house		
	Medical risk management consulting services		
1	Has capability in-house		
	Property-loss-prevention consulting services		
3	Has capability in-house		
	Captive formation and management		
3	Has capability in-house		
	Risk management information-system consulting		
1	Has capability in-house		

(continues)

account executive to discuss the program. Finally, it is highly recommended that the organization formally document in writing (letter, E-mail) to the broker all critical deci-sions and instructions regarding insurance placement to avoid misunderstandings.

Many larger brokers have additional com-pensation schemes with carriers whereby

Exhibit 12–1 (Continued)

Maximum Points	Trait	Broker 1	Broker 2
	Business-operations qualifications:		
	Qualifications of the employees assigned to account		
	Account executive		
3	General insurance experience		
3	Experience with healthcare organizations		
3	Appropriate rank within firm		
	Lead assistant		
3	General insurance experience		
3	Experience with healthcare organizations		
3	Appropriate rank within firm		
	Other support staff		
5	Overall qualifications		
	Firm qualifications		
1	Financial strength adequate (Y or N)		
1	Public/private (circle)		
1	MBE/WBE firm (minority/woman business enterprise)		
1	MBE/WBE participation		
1	MBE/WBE functions described		
1	Local entity		
1	Local area staffing		
	Expertise with comparable healthcare clients		
5	Experience with similar entities		
	Health care (Y or N)		
	Education (Y or N)		
	Certificate of professional-liability insurance (Y or N)		
	Total		

they receive financial incentives for placing large volumes of business. In the interest of full disclosure, it is important to discern whether such deals exist with your broker to ensure that they do not influence your broker's recommendations for coverage or insurance carrier.

Evaluating Risk-Financing Options

For self-insurance (either total or partial), the organization places a predetermined sum of money into a fund, which it controls, to pay for future losses. Obviously, the more accurately an organization can quantify the potential risks, the more likely that funds set aside will be adequate to pay for these risks. The advantage of this system is that, if the risks prove less costly than anticipated, dollars can be returned to the general operating budget of the organization.

The potential disadvantage of this type of risk financing program is that it requires a sound risk management and loss-control program and a commitment from administration to hire appropriate staff and to provide appropriate support to ensure that the program functions well. In addition, there is always the possibility that the amount of money set aside is less than the ultimate cost. In that case, the organization will have to fund the additional cost.

Most organizations structure their risk financing programs to include both purchased commercial insurance and self-insurance. In these types of programs, a layer of risk commonly known as the self-insured retention (SIR) is financed by the organization, and commercial insurance is purchased to finance the risks above the level of the SIR.

Choosing the Appropriate Level of Risk Retention

The appropriate level of self-insurance is determined by the organization's financial ability to bear loss, its philosophy concerning risk assumption, and a comparison of the predictable against the catastrophic loss probabilities. Risk-retention capacity is determined by examining the organization's measures of liquidity, profitability, and balance-sheet strength.

One of the initial steps in evaluating how much risk to self-insure is to compare the organization's information to that of similar organizations. The best benchmarks for MPL retentions are found through information compiled by industry associations and brokers or consulting firms. It is recommended that an organization compare its proposed level of self-insurance with those of organizations of similar structure and organizations in the same geographic location.

Another key litmus test to determine whether the organization is taking the appropriate level of risk retention is to review the cost of its current commercial-insurance coverage. If the premiums equal or exceed 20% of the policy limits, a change in the level of self-insurance may be warranted. High premium-to-limit ratios are a red flag indicating an opportunity to consider retaining more risk.

The decision process regarding self-insurance requires the organization to retain the services of an actuary. The actuary should perform a number of simulations and tests to assist the organization in determining the appropriate level of risk retention. Using loss-probability distributions, computer simulations, and other techniques, the actuary can forecast losses and the potential variability for a range of self-insured levels.

Loss-Analysis Modeling

Using sophisticated financial models, statistical and actuarial analyses are used to determine the organization's expected losses. These models take into account several variables, including actual incurred losses (frequency and severity), loss development (incurred but not reported and reserve growth in open cases), exposure changes (payroll, sales, etc.), and inflation trends. Figure 12-1 shows a sample loss projection.

The loss-analysis model enables the organization to:

- Project expected losses

- Identify frequency and average severity trends in claims

- Determine reserve liabilities and letter-of-credit requirements

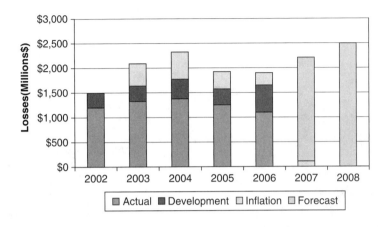

Figure 12–1 Sample Loss Projection

- Negotiate risk financing programs with insurers
- Select an appropriate risk financing vehicle

Variability Analysis

Once the expected losses are determined, the organization can then examine the risk of higher-than-expected losses at various levels of self-insurance. By calculating frequency and severity probability distributions based on the organization's actual loss experience, the actuary can show the variability of expected losses. Figure 12–2 illustrates variability of losses at various confidence levels.

Risk-Retention Analysis

Retention-capacity analysis provides support for deciding the organization's maximum risk-retention level. The optimal balance between risk retention and risk transfer can be achieved by combining traditional actuarial analysis with investment-decision principles and insurance-market pricing. The results of this analysis illustrate the most cost-effective retention level that optimizes the trade-off between premium savings and the increased risk associated with higher

retention levels. Figure 12–3 illustrates this analysis at various levels of risk retention at the 95th-percentile confidence level.

Once the organization has determined (with the assistance of its actuary and insurance broker) the basic parameters of the level of self-insurance, the most cost-effective type of retention must be determined. The retention type is often dictated by the commercial insurance market that assumes the risk beyond self-insurance. Within the boundaries set by the commercial market, several strategies can be used (see Figures 12–4 and 12–5). The most common types of retention strategies used today are:

1. *Each occurrence.* This type of retention applies once for each occurrence, and there is no maximum. This type of retention is being dictated by many MPL insurers in venues or jurisdictions that the insurer believes are particularly volatile. The each-occurrence retention does not protect the organization against a higher-than-expected number of claims in a particular year.
2. *Each occurrence/aggregate retention.* This type of retention disappears after a

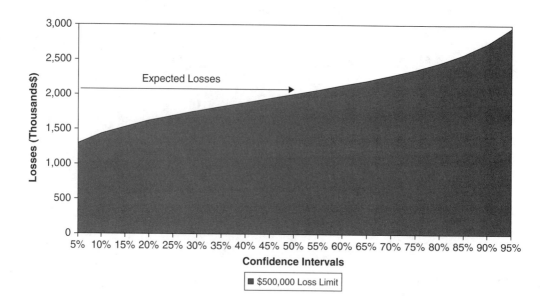

Figure 12–2 Sample Risk Variability Analysis

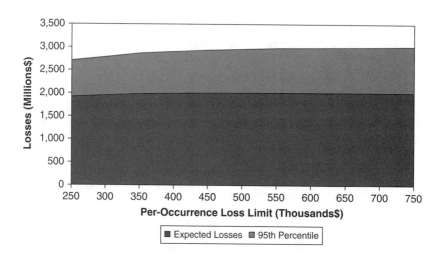

Figure 12–3 Sample Retention Level Analysis

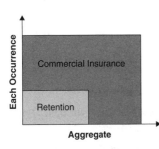

Figure 12–4 Sample of Program Structures

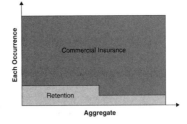

Figure 12–5 Sample of Program Structures

certain threshold of losses is reached. This level of self-insurance is still offered in the MPL market, but the retention level is usually dictated by the commercial insurer. The aggregate stop point is often a key point of negotiation when transferring risk to the commercial market. The aggregate feature protects the organization from both higher frequency and greater severity of claims than expected in a single year.

3. *Aggregate retention with maintenance deductible.* This type of retention does not completely disappear when a certain threshold is met; instead, when the threshold is met, the level of the retention drops and then continues on a per-occurrence basis. Commercial insurers like this form of aggregate protection because the insured continues to participate in the payment of losses during the policy year.

Mechanisms for Self-Funding

Several forms and variations of mechanisms are available to structure risk retention within an organization. The most basic types are simple trust and captive insurance company.

Simple Trust

The most common vehicle for the funding of a self-insured obligation is the simple trust.

Under a trust agreement, a specified level of funds is set aside to pay for losses as they occur. In most cases, annual or periodic contributions to the trust are made based on an actuarial determination of the expected value of actual losses, losses incurred but not reported (IBNR), and future losses. In most situations, persons who determine whether the amount of funding necessary to ensure that the trust will indeed cover losses first analyze the time required for cases that arise in their jurisdiction to actually come to trial or to be resolved otherwise. This allows for a discounting of the ultimate value of the final resolution of a claim due to the amount of investment return that will be gained before resolution of the claim.

Setting up a simple trust for financing MPL losses requires less administrative overhead than many of the other models. In most cases, using a simple trust eliminates the need to budget for premium taxes, brokerage fees, acquisition costs, or sophisticated management fees. Also, the establishment of a simple trust does not require state approval, which must be obtained when establishing other types of insuring vehicles, although there may be exceptions in states whose legislatures have established patient compensation funds or that have specific professional-liability-insurance requirements.

Organizations that set up a simple trust will want to determine the impact that this type of self-insurance program may have on bond-indenture requirements and the need to produce certificates of insurance for any capital-funding programs. Generally, these issues can be clarified in the trust documents.

Captive Insurance Company

A more sophisticated form of self-insurance involves setting up a captive insurance company. By definition, a captive insurance program is a limited-purpose licensed insurance company whose primary business is insuring the risks of its owners. Captives can be set up "onshore" (within the contiguous United States) or "offshore" (outside the contiguous United States) and can be either for-profit or not-for-profit companies. The selection of domicile and captive type determines the laws governing its operation and may also dictate funding requirements, capitalization, and tax status.

Setting up a captive insurance company necessitates a high level of staff sophistication. It also requires administrative commitment that this will be a long-term initiative that may, for the first few years, cost more than a basic program.

Organizations elect to form a captive for many reasons. Some are appropriate; others are not. One appropriate reason is the desire to encourage cooperation among the persons and entities insured to enable them to develop and implement a joint program based on sound risk management, quality improvement, and loss-control initiatives. The common financial interest shared by all participants in the captive helps ensure that such principles are taken seriously.

A captive should not be considered a short-term solution to ride out the high cost of malpractice premiums or as a way to save money paid in insurance taxes or fees. It is also inappropriate to think of a captive as a shelter for money not subject to taxation that will never be called up to pay for losses. This is unlikely to materialize and should not be presented as a reason for establishing this type of self-insurance program.

Taking the Plan to Market

Figure 12–6 provides a summary of the primary steps in the insurance-marketing process. To be successful in today's marketplace, the organization must actively pursue these steps.

Step 1: Review the Existing Risk Financing Plan

Before beginning the marketing process, an organization should discuss with its broker the objectives and strategies for transferring risk to the commercial-insurance marketplace. This discussion should address:

- The existing MPL program placement, including program structure and coverage terms
- The plan for risk retention
- The organization's current exposures, including any operational changes or mergers and acquisitions
- The clinical risk management program and objectives
- The claims management practices
- The organization's current loss history
- The organization's financial considerations

An organization should be thorough in conveying thoughts and directives to the broker during this initial discussion. Both parties should come away with a firm knowledge of the current risk financing plan and the expectations for the commercial-insurance placement process.

Step 2: Identify and Analyze Potential Insurers

The insurers chosen as candidates to underwrite the risk transfer program must meet all of the organization's objectives. The broker and the organization should discuss in detail all potential carriers before selecting the final candidates that will receive submission. This collaborative review should include a written comparative summary of each carrier's underwriting position, capacity, financial strength and size, policy maintenance and service capabilities, longevity and experience

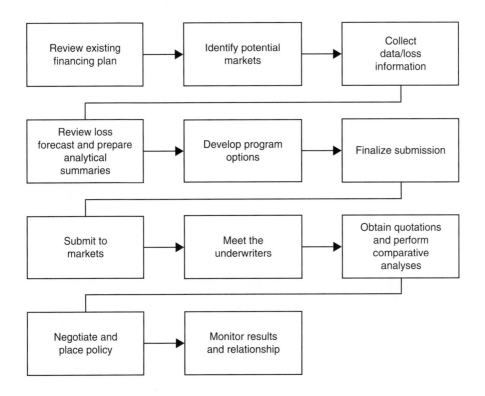

Figure 12–6 *Primary Steps in the Insurance Marketing Process*

in the marketplace, and other factors that affect the selection. More specifically, the review process should include the following items:

1. Financial strength of the insurer, including any recent changes
   - Review published accounts, such as balance sheet and operating results.
   - Review public financial reports filed with regulatory agencies.
   - Review information available from insurer financial rating services.
2. Financial solvency analysis (conducted if there is any question about financial strength)
   - The ratio of net premium written to policyholders' surplus
   - Any significant changes in gross or net written premiums

   - The amount and quality of reinsurance recoverables
   - Underwriting earnings compared with investment income
   - Cash flow from operations and liquidity
   - Historical loss data
3. Determination of state licensing, country of origin, or domicile
4. Identification of parent company and any intercompany relationships
5. Identification of the quality-of-reinsurance arrangements
6. Examination of the insurer's management competence
   - Identify key underwriting management changes.
   - Identify changes in underwriting philosophy.

7. Analysis of any other types of risks underwritten and their impact on company performance
   - Are rating and underwriting changes in these areas relevant?
   - Are these risks still relevant given changes in the insurance structure?
8. Present or past government supervision and regulation
9. Existence of any agency agreements (pools and underwriting agents) and the impact they have on company performance
10. Perceived place in the market structure and performance position
    - Risk management services
    - Maintenance of past commitments

Two rating agencies are the recognized leaders in rating the financial stability of insurance carriers: A.M. Best and Standard & Poor's.

A. M. Best's Rating System

A. M. Best's ratings provide an overall opinion of an insurer's ability to meet its obligations to policyholders. The rating is derived by evaluating a company's financial strength, operating performance, and market profile. The ratings (see Table 12–1) are divided into two broad categories: secure (high ratings: A++ to B+) and vulnerable (low ratings: B to S).

The higher an insurer's rating, the greater its ability to withstand adverse changes in underwriting and economic conditions over longer periods.

Best assigns "S" ratings to companies that have experienced sudden and significant events that affect their financial position or operating performance, and to companies whose rating cannot be evaluated due to a lack of timely or adequate information.

A. M. Best assigns each insurer a financial-size category (FSC). The FSC is designed to provide a convenient indicator of the size of an insurer in terms of its statutory surplus and related accounts (see Table 12–2).

Standard & Poor's Rating System

A Standard & Poor's Insurer Financial Strength Rating is a current opinion of the financial security of an insurance company regarding its ability to pay claims (see Table 12–3).

Step 3: Collect Data and Loss Information

It is neither feasible nor realistic to complete multiple applications for submission, but in today's marketplace it is not uncommon for insurers to request that their own applications be completed before binding coverage; therefore, it is a good idea to begin the submission process using an application that is initially acceptable by the majority of insur-

Table 12–1 A. M. Best's Ratings

Secure Ratings		Vulnerable Ratings	
A++, A+	Superior	B and B–	Fair
A and A–	Excellent	C++, C+	Marginal
B++, B+	Very good	C, C–	Weak
		D	Poor
		E	Under regulatory supervision
		F	In liquidation
		S	Rating suspended (replaces the former category of NA-11)

Table 12–2 A. M. Best's Financial-Size Categories

Financial-Size Category (Class)	Adjusted Dollar Amount of Policyholder Surplus
I	< 1,000
II	1–2,000
III	2–5,000
IV	5–10,000
V	10–25,000
VI	25–50,000
VII	50–100,000
VIII	100–250,000
IX	250–500,000
X	500–750,000
XI	750,000 to 1 million
XII	1 to 1.25 million
XIII	1.25 to 1.5 million
XIV	1.5 to 2 million
XV	> 2 million

ers. The broker should be able to identify one easily, and the organization can fulfill a specific insurer's requirements once a determination has been made to place insurance with them.

The data-collection process begins by assembling general information about the organization. This information includes:

- The history of the organization, along with any promotional materials deemed necessary. Specific information regarding key personnel may be included. Remember, the organization is trying to sell itself to the underwriter and therefore should always attempt to present itself in the most favorable light.
- A description of operations and services, including geographic scope.
- An organizational chart.

- The latest audited financials for all entities to be insured.
- Current financial information that may be relevant.
- The most recent internal-audit risk report.
- The most recent Joint Commission report.
- Information regarding key personnel, if deemed significant to the underwriting process by your insurance broker.

Exposure information, usually 10 years' worth, needs to be assembled in a concise format that will enable an underwriter to fully review and rate the risk. The following information is required:

- Total number of hospital beds, licensed and occupied, for acute care, cribs and bassinets, psychiatric care, and extended care.
- Total number of outpatient visits, by department.
- Physician roster by specialty and employment status (employed, staff/attending, contracted, resident). The roster should also reflect the date of employment for each physician listed. If some or all of the physicians purchase insurance separately, list the limits of coverage that they carry and identify their current insurance carrier.

Loss information, customarily 10 years' worth, should be assembled in electronic format, and a disk containing the data should be attached to your submission. The most commonly accepted software is Microsoft Excel (Microsoft, Redmond, Wash.). The electronic loss data disk enables an underwriter or actuary to easily sort your information into a format that can be easily analyzed. Always remember that the market is flooded with submissions, and the underwriters do not have time to input loss information from paper copies. Risk submissions with paper loss information are often not even quoted because of the underwriter's time limitations.

Table 12–3 Standard & Poor's Ratings

Secure		Vulnerable	
AAA	Extremely strong financial security	BB	Marginal financial security: positive attributes exist, but adverse business conditions could lead to insufficient ability to meet financial commitments.
AA	Very strong financial security	B	Weak financial security: adverse business conditions will likely impair insurer's ability to meet financial commitments.
A	Strong financial security	CCC	Very weak financial security: insurer is dependent on favorable business conditions to meet financial commitments.
BBB	Good financial security	CC	Extremely weak: insurer is not likely to meet some of its financial commitments.
		R	Regulatory action: insurer is under supervision.
		NR	Not rated.

The loss data should be presented on a per-claim basis and sorted by loss date. Amounts paid and reserved by all excess carriers must be included, on a per-claim basis. Do not submit only the self-insured portions of your losses; all losses should be reported from the ground up. The mandatory fields for your loss information spreadsheet are:

- Loss date (date of incident or occurrence)
- Claim date (date claim made)
- Report date (date reported to insurance carrier)
- Loss description (in detail if claim reserved and/or paid in excess of $100,000)
- Expenses paid
- Expense reserve
- Indemnity paid
- Indemnity reserved
- Total incurred (expenses paid + expense reserves + indemnity paid + indemnity reserved)

Finally, to help the underwriter understand the organization better, include the following items in the submission:

- A copy of the organization's claims-handling procedures. It is also helpful

to make a formal statement of the organization's philosophy regarding claims. A detailed list of the malpractice defense attorneys used by the organization should be compiled and made part of the claims-handling procedures.

- A detailed description of the risk management department that includes an organizational chart, biographies of key personnel, and an outline of the educational program.
- A detailed description of quality improvement and patient safety initiatives.
- A copy of the risk management plan, with an emphasis on the clinical risk management operations.

If the organization is self-insured for any portion of malpractice risk, include a copy of the current trust fund agreement. If the organization is self-insured through a captive, include a copy of the captive policy and an explanation of the captive structure. In addition, include a copy of the most current actuarial study for the self-insured trust fund or captive.

Step 4: Review Loss Forecast and Prepare Analytical Summaries

Whether the organization is currently self-insured or is considering the move to self-insurance, the risk manager and the insurance broker must thoroughly understand the organization's loss forecast and be prepared to present analytical summaries to support negotiations with the underwriters.

In addition to the retention-analysis tools described previously, a loss-stratification diagram should be developed. Although it is quite simple, it can be an extremely effective visual tool in negotiating with underwriters.

Step 5: Develop Program Options

After determining the parameters of risk retention, the organization needs to focus on the structural options available for the risk transfer portion of the program. Often the organization can gain access to preferred insurance markets through participation in group purchasing organizations or associations. Some insurance markets offer preferred pricing and other features to group purchasing participants based on the economies of scale the group brings to the market. Group purchasing organizations also often offer alternative risk financing programs that make use of risk sharing among the participants. These programs often take the form of captives or shared excess-liability layers. The organization should discuss and explore in detail with the broker the potential financial advantages of participation in a group program.

As an individual buyer, or as part of a group, numerous structural options are available for risk transfer. The following options should be reviewed in an effort to minimize the cost of commercial insurance and address issues that might be specific or unique to the organization:

- Purchasing excess limits on a multiyear finite-layer basis
- Using inner aggregate structures

- Employing a commutation or profit-sharing feature
- Using loss-sensitive buffer layers
- Using quota-share layers both between carriers and between the insured and the carrier
- Using stretched or multiyear excess layers
- Purchasing lower limits but with an aggregate limit reinstatement at a predetermined cost
- Changing the treatment of defense costs within or outside the limit of excess coverage or within or outside the retention level
- Purchasing tail of prior policies as an option, particularly if the organization is moving off a multiyear pricing arrangement

Figure 12–7 illustrates examples of creative options that address organizations' specific needs or issues.

Step 6: Finalize the Submission

The submission is the "anchor" in the marketing process and program implementation and must be skillfully drafted. It will become the record from which to negotiate with the underwriters.

Every effort should be made to produce the entire submission in electronic format. This will provide the underwriters with easy access to information and may make the difference in whether they decide to even review the submission.

A typical submission table of contents is as follows:

1. Executive summary, i.e., a statement of what the organization is looking for in the marketplace and the type of partnership with the commercial-insurance market it wishes to establish. If the submission is part of a group-sponsored program, identify that program and the organization's relationship to it.
2. History and general description of operations (step 3)

Option I

Issues

- Limited capacity from individual insurers
- Fluctuation of market from year to year
- Unavailability of aggregate protection from most insurers
- Escalating insurance costs

Creative Solutions

- Three year stretched policy limit
- Variable per-occurrence retention
- Predetermined reinstatement feature
- Premium payable over three years

Benefits

- Eliminates fluctuation of market
- Stabilizes self-insured retention over three years
- Availability of reinstatement of limits allowing for
- varying SIR's based on exposure for a known cost

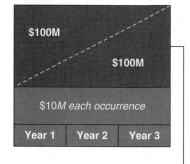

Includes a predetermined reinstatement feature as an option

Option II

Creative Solutions

- Aggregate protection to the trust offered through second layer excess
- Quota share layer on lead umbrella
- Three year stretched policy limit
- Commutation features may also be available

Benefits

- Aggregate protection through second layer excess allows greater selection of lead umbrella carriers
- Quota share lead umbrella creates market leverage while also increasing the amount of available markets for lead umbrella
- Stretched three-year limit for excess capacity stabilizes cost over three-year period. Use of layer is typically remote
- Commutation allows an insured to increase the SIR over time as warranted

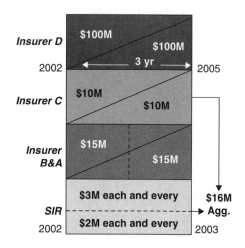

Figure 12–7 Options for Addressing Needs/Issues

Option III

Creative Solutions
- 1st two claims are subject to $5M peroccurrence retention
- 3rd claim and others subject to a $2M per-occurrence retention

Benefits
- Smoothes the effect on assuming a much larger per-occurrence self-insured retention than anticipated

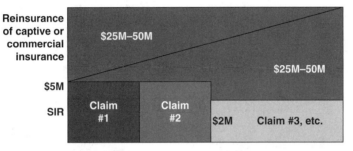

Figure 12–7 (Continued)

3. Description of current insurance-program structure (step 3)
4. Description of proposed program-structure options (step 5)
5. Coverage specifications, i.e., named insured, claims made versus occurrence, anticipated coverage, terms and conditions (a sample is provided in Appendix 12–A)
6. Exposure data (step 3, including completed application)
7. Loss information (step 3)
8. Appendixes, which should include:
   - Latest audited financial report for the organization(s).
   - Current financial information that might be relevant.
   - Most recent internal audit risk report.
   - Most recent Joint Commission report.
   - Claims philosophy and claim-handling procedures.
   - Clinical risk management plan highlighting most recent risk management focus. It is also helpful to include samples of materials devel-

oped to educate staff relating to loss-prevention activities.
   - Copy of current trust agreement for self-insurance or the policy, if self-insured through a captive.
   - Current actuarial study for self-insured structure.

Step 7: Submit to Insurers

As a general rule, the marketplace should receive the submission no earlier or later than 90 days before your renewal. This will allow them ample time, typically 30 days, to review the submission and decide if they will be able to provide a quotation. The broker should use this time to set up face-to-face meetings with interested underwriters.

Step 8: Meet the Underwriters

Meeting with the underwriters of interested and viable insurers is a critical component in the marketing process. This meeting is the organization's opportunity to tell its story and to probe the capability and willingness of the underwriter to become the risk transfer partner. Because these meetings are of critical importance, every effort should be made to include the organization's CEO, CFO, risk manager, and, if appropriate, a member of the medical staff, particularly if the hospital employs physicians or residents. If possible, these meetings should take place at the underwriter's office; however, if the underwriter suggests that the meeting take place at the healthcare facility, take advantage of this opportunity to provide the underwriter with a well-planned tour.

Step 9: Obtain Quotations and Perform Comparative Analyses

If the insurers received the submission by 90 days before renewal, and meetings with interested insurers have taken place, the organization should begin to receive formal proposals about 60 days before the renewal date. In addition to pricing indications, the responses will include proposed coverage terms and conditions, possibly a request for additional information, and perhaps a statement that certain criteria must be met before binding coverage.

Develop a scorecard for performing a comparative analysis of competing quotations. Develop weighted criteria based on the organization's goals and objectives. Possible criteria include:

1. Company financials and general information
   - A. M. Best's rating
   - Standard & Poor's rating
   - Years in business
   - Total premium written
   - Percentage of premium written related to hospital professional liability
   - Combined loss ratio
   - Location of underwriting office
   - Experience within your geographic region
   - Experience with similar risks
   - Admitted or surplus lines paper

2. Limits and structure
   - Attachment points per occurrence and aggregate
   - Limits offered
   - Maintenance deductible
   - Defense costs within or outside self-insured retention
   - Defense costs within or outside limits
   - Reinstatement features, if any
   - Tail options
3. Coverage specifications
   - Type of coverage offered
     - Excess hospital professional liability
     - Umbrella liability
     - Claims made (retroactive date)
     - Occurrence
   - Terms and conditions
4. Coverage enhancements, if any
5. Proposed premiums and payment plans
   - Annual or multiyear premium
   - Applicable taxes
   - Tail pricing
   - Payment terms
6. Risk management
   - Location of service office
   - Educational programs or print material
   - Assessments
   - Other services
7. Claims management
   - Location of service office
   - Timing of audits
   - Claim representative's experience
   - Philosophy

Step 10: Negotiate and Place Policy

After conducting a complete comparative analysis, the organization can begin negotiations with the insurers of choice. The art of negotiation in today's marketplace is difficult at best. A few thoughts that might assist in reaching a reasonable outcome are as follows:

- If the organization has a good and fair relationship with its existing carrier, that insurer will most likely be the easiest partner with which to negotiate. The underwriter knows the organization, having already provided coverage with terms and conditions and at a premium the organization was willing to accept.

- Always try to leverage the insurance broker's relationships with carriers of interest to the organization. Even though in today's marketplace most underwriters evaluate a risk based on its own merits, the insurance broker might have a working relationship, usually based on volume, with those carriers with which the organization is negotiating.

- Understand the losses and use the actuarial analysis to your advantage. It is all about the numbers in today's marketplace. The art of underwriting has taken a back seat to actuarial underwriting. A thorough knowledge of the organization's loss picture and analyses will position it better to justify negotiating points with an underwriter who is focused primarily on the numbers.

- Emphasize the organization's risk management and claims-handling abilities. Insurers today are placing more emphasis on these activities than ever before. The ability to portray these activities with demonstrated positive results will give the organization leverage in negotiations, especially with markets that are concerned about the level of self-insurance.

In the end, selecting the final carrier will hinge on comparative analysis, a bit of subjective expertise, and any price negotiation the organization and its broker are able to accomplish. Once the organization is comfortable with the final terms of the proposal,

bind the coverage in writing through the broker. Be certain to specify the proper terms and conditions of the deal along with the price agreed upon. Make a written record of the organization's understanding of the deal to protect against changes or alterations.

The implementation of the program will vary depending on whether there is a change in insurance carriers, change in the structure of the current program (occurrence to claims made), buying out the tail from the expiring carrier, raising self-insured retentions, or purchasing lower excess limits.

If the organization is not buying out the tail from the expiring carrier, changing insurers will require it to report all known incidents/claims to the current carrier before expiration. Raising self-insured retentions or purchasing lower excess limits may require additional funding.

Step 11: Monitor Results and Relationship

It is important to monitor the performance of the insurer throughout the term of the policy instead of waiting until the next renewal cycle comes around. Table 12–4 provides guidelines that can be used to monitor the insurer's service. This is not an all-inclusive model, and it can be amended to meet different needs.

The insurance carrier is the organization's risk transfer partner. A successful partnership depends on clear communication, whether it be scheduled or ad hoc. Quarterly claim meetings should be scheduled to keep the underwriters up to date about the organization's loss activities. Ad hoc meetings should be held as needed to discuss risk management, underwriting, and service issues.

Table 12–4 Insurance-Carrier Service Requirements

Service	Standard
Notice of any significant program change	Minimum 90-day notice before renewal
Request information needed for renewal	Minimum 90 days before renewal
Oral proposals (new and renewal)	Within 45 days after receipt of underwriting information, except on new business (60 days)
Complete written confirmation of proposal including premium, fees, taxes, commission rates, and sample side-agreement wording	Within 2 days after oral proposal
Policy number assigned	At the time of binding coverage before effective date/time
Written confirmation of binding	Within 24 hours after receipt of order to bind
Invoice	Within 24 hours after receipt of order to bind, except for installments (then within 3 days)
Identification cards, posting notices, legal filings	Immediately after receipt of order to bind
Side legal agreements (Letter of Credit [LOC], indemnity agreements, etc.)	Within 30 days after inception of coverage
Return premiums (policy release)	Within 30 days of receipt of letter from Insured
Initial loss-control service plan in place	Within 30 days after inception of coverage
Claim instructions delivered to you	Within 10 days after receipt of order to bind
Receipt of policy	(1) Within 45 days after effective date or date upon which insurer has all information necessary for completion of policy, and (2) 100% accurate
Policy endorsements	(1) Within 30 days after request for endorsement, and (2) 100% accurate
Audits and adjustments	Receipt by us within 3 months after expiration of policy, except retroactive adjustments at 8 months
Loss payments	Paid to Insured in accordance with policy terms
Claims services (including loss runs; form and timing)	Delivered in accordance with claims-service instructions
Loss-control services (form and timing)	Delivered in accordance with loss-control service plan
Security calculations for primary casualty programs	Within 20 months after inception and every 12 months thereafter
Return of phone calls	Within 24 hours at most
Document transmission to our office	Include a contact name (first and last name) on every piece of correspondence

APPENDIX 12–A: ANTICIPATED COVERAGES, TERMS, AND CONDITIONS

Broad Form Named Insured

"Broad Form Named Insured" should include, without limitation, ABC Hospital, and its subsidiaries and affiliates; any/all past, present, and newly created subsidiaries, affiliated institutions, organizations or companies, predecessors, successors, or other business which any of the Named Insureds own, operate, control, or manage; employees, directors, officers, stockholders, or partners of the Named Insured; any partner, executive officer, administrator, member of an Insured, stockholder, or member of the board of directors, trustees, or governors of the Insured; any intern or fellow while acting within the scope of their duties; any employed physician or physician the Insured has agreed to provide coverage for, including locum tenens; any student, volunteer, or temporary or leased employee of the Insured; any member of a professional board or committee of the Insured; any real estate manager acting for the Insured; and any person or entity to which the Named Insured is contractually obligated to provide insurance. Coverage should be extended to provide 90 days' automatic coverage for newly acquired or formed entities.

Provide Coverage for Joint Ventures Where Specified

Coverage should be provided on an "indemnify" basis. The non-concurrence endorsement is as follows:

Whereas, the underlying policy(ies) listed in the Schedule of Underlying Insurance including renewals or replacements thereof, are non-concurrent with the policy period hereunder, and

Whereas, the Insured has no knowledge of accidents or occurrences having taken place during the period(s) of the underlying policy(ies) listed in the Schedule of Underlying Insurance to the inception of this excess policy;

Now therefore, in consideration of the premium charged, in the event of reduction or exhaustion of the aggregate limit(s) of the underlying policy(ies) listed in the Schedule of Underlying Insurance by reason of losses in respect of occurrences or accidents before the inception of this excess policy, it is agreed that such insurance as is afforded by this policy shall, subject to the terms and conditions of the underlying insurance:

1. In the event of reduction, apply in excess of the reduced underlying limits.
2. In the event of exhaustion, continue in force as underlying insurance.

Anything in this endorsement to the contrary notwithstanding, this policy applies only to occurrences happening during the policy period.

Knowledge of Occurrence or Claim

Knowledge of an occurrence or claim by your agent, servant, or employee shall not constitute knowledge by you unless the designated person (i.e., Risk Manager) has received such notice.

Designated person TBD

Notice of Occurrence

The company shall not deny coverage as the result of an unintentional failure by you to give notice as respects any occurrence, provided notice is given as soon as practicable after becoming aware that this policy may apply to such occurrence.

Notice of Cancellation

In the event reinsurance is canceled at the request of the reinsurer company, 120 days' notice will be provided to the reinsured, except in the event of nonpayment of premium, in which case notice will be 10 days.

Intentional Injury

Amend intentional injury to include bodily injury and property damage and delete the word "reasonable."

Notice of Material Change

In the event the policy is materially changed at the request of the company, 120 days' notice will be provided, except in the event of nonpayment of premium, in which case notice will be 10 days.

Non-Owned Watercraft

Coverage for watercraft to 125 feet in length.

Fellow Employee

Delete any fellow-employee exclusion as concerns employees.

Broad-Form Property Damage

Delete any exclusion relating to property damage to the insured's products, completed operations, or work performed by others on the insured's behalf, or relating to property in the insured's care, custody, or control, and replace with the following:

Coverage is not provided for the insured liability for damage:

(I) To property owned or occupied by or rented to the insured, or except with respect to the use of elevators, to property held by the insured for sale or entrusted to the insured for storage or safekeeping;

(II) Except with respect to liability under a written sidetrack agreement or the use of elevators
   a. To property while on premises owned by or rented to the insured for the purpose of having operations performed on such property by or on behalf of the insured,
   b. To tools or equipment while being used by the insured in performing his operations,
   c. To property in the custody of the insured which is to be installed, erected, or used in construction by the insured,
   d. To that particular part of any property, not on premises owned by or rented to the insured,
      i. Upon which operations are being performed by or on behalf of the insured at the time of the property damage arising out of such operations,
      ii. Out of which any property damage arises, or
      iii. The restoration, repair, or replacement of which has been made or is nec-

essary by reason of faulty workmanship thereon by or on behalf of the insured.

With respect to the completed operations hazard, to property damage to work performed by the named insured arising out of the work or any portion thereof, or out of materials part of equipment furnished in connection therewith.

Coverage for integrated batch.

Pre- and post-judgment interest included.

Defense expenses outside the limit as an option.

Coverage for sexual and physical abuse.

Amend nuclear exclusion to provide coverage for medical incidents.

Evaluate "terrorism" exclusive language to ensure that it *does not* include waivers for acts of professional negligence that may be against victims of terrorism.

Amend loading and/or unloading exclusion to provide coverage for patient loading and/or unloading.

Amend any "insured vs insured" exclusion to provide coverage for credentialing and peer review activities and for employees getting professional care in an insured institution.

Coverage for punitive damages where legally permitted to insure.

Provide separation of insureds (severability of interests clause).

Provide a waiver of subrogation: "In the event of any payment under this policy, the company waives its rights of recovery against any entity when any insured has agreed in writing, before the date of loss, to obtain a waiver of subrogation from the insured's insurer in favor of such entity."

Notice of Non-Renewal

Insurer must provide 120 days' notice.

Unintentional Failure to Disclose

Unintentional failure of the Named Insured to disclose all hazards existing at the inception of this policy shall not be a basis for denial of any coverage afforded by this policy.

Covered Persons

The following persons are covered under the protected persons on the policy:

- *Administrators.* The following are insured while acting solely within the course and scope of their administrative duties for you: your chief executive officer; your superintendent; your administrator; your department heads; and medical directors.
- *Committee or board members.* Members of your boards or committees are insureds for claims that result directly from their duties as members. Those who carry out the orders of such committees or boards are insureds while in the course of executing the orders. Those who provide information to such boards or committees to help them evaluate applicants for staff membership or privileges, or to conduct corrective or disciplinary action, are also insureds.
- *Medical staff.* Members of your medical staff are insureds. But each is an insured only while acting within the course and scope of his or her duties to supervise, teach, or proctor others at your request or as an obligation of medical staff membership.
- *Employees.* Your employees (including temporary employees), students, and authorized volunteers are insureds while acting within the course and scope of their duties.
- Any physician, intern, resident or fellow for whom a "Named Insured" has elected to provide coverage but solely while acting within the scope of their

duties for the "Named Insured." Coverage applies excess of any valid and collectible insurance.

Good Samaritan Endorsement

Present and former employees are protected persons while rendering emergency first aid outside the scope of their duties as employees as long as the aid is rendered without the receipt or expectation of remuneration.

Tail Options

Tail options include:

- Predetermined cost
- Unlimited reporting
- Refreshed limits

13

THE IMPORTANCE OF DEVELOPING A MEDICAL LIABILITY COST-ALLOCATION SYSTEM

Barbara J. Youngberg, JD, MSW, BSN, FASHRM

INTRODUCTION

The effective financial management of any organization requires that costs be identified and attributed to their sources. Most healthcare organizations seek to allocate their risk management costs to individual departments or organizational units and to develop systems or structures with incentives for achieving specific risk management or patient safety objectives. Similarly, many entities, such as pools or trusts, seek to allocate the group's risk management costs to all entities within the group. The system used to allocate these costs is commonly known as a cost-allocation system. A properly designed risk management cost-allocation system encourages proactive loss or risk control, early claims reporting, heightened systematic mindfulness, transparency, and good claims management.

A risk manager's starting point when designing an allocation system for a medical liability program is to set realistic objectives that the organization can meet. This poses a particular challenge for large or complex organizations or other large healthcare systems that have residency or teaching components and operate many ancillary businesses to manage patient care across the continuum, because of the interrelationships among the faculty, residents, fellows, hospital staff, and various business entities. The key objectives of an organization's medical liability cost-allocation system are to promote participation in risk management and patient safety programs and balance risk bearing and risk sharing across all aspects of the healthcare business operation.

PROMOTING PARTICIPATION IN RISK MANAGEMENT PROGRAMS

The primary purpose of a cost-allocation system is usually to encourage participation in risk management and patient saftey programs, to reduce overall costs and the frequency and severity of losses, and to share proportionately in the cost of the program. The easiest way to

159

achieve this is by allocating the costs to the parties (e.g., hospital, physician business entities of the healthcare enterprise) that generate them, which can be done through a number of approaches. Among the results of implementing a cost-allocation system are the focus of attention on a health system's clinical encounters, the inherent risk associated with the service being provided, the actual adverse loss experience of the entity, the ability to reward favorable loss experience, and the development of proactive risk-control strategies. Furthermore, a cost-allocation system provides information that can help a complex health system decide how to best utilize risk management activities and how to adjust or improve risk management programs to better meet the needs of the organization, network partners, faculty, and residents.

BALANCING RISK BEARING AND RISK SHARING

An effective cost-allocation system strikes the right balance between risk bearing and risk sharing for the organization. A system that is entirely risk bearing allocates all medical liability costs directly to their sources. This type of system, however, does not take into account that some losses are matters of chance and may unfairly penalize the hospital's business department for an unusual catastrophic loss. In addition, such a system provides little support for new business ventures that are established by the organization but have yet to develop any loss history. Charging such losses only to the department that generates them creates an imbalance in the financial results of that department from one period to the next. Small departments, in particular, may be unduly penalized for a single expensive catastrophic loss, and new or innovative businesses may have too little business experience to calculate their ultimate loss potential. This underscores the need for a risk-sharing allocation system to preserve their financial integrity along with that of the organization to which they belong.

A risk-sharing system allocates all medical liability costs in proportion to each department's exposure. It facilitates accurate budgeting and does not subject individual departments to large payment fluctuations from period to period. This system does not, however, provide an incentive for participation in risk management programs, because individual loss experience is not recognized.

The proper allocation system for most organizations lies somewhere between these two extremes. Success in balancing risk sharing and risk bearing is dependent on the goals for cost allocation, and the management philosophy, of an organization or complex health system. The most important factor is that all individuals and entities that create the risk must be encouraged to participate in risk management costs and activities, a requirement that tilts the scale toward a risk-bearing system.

Other Goals

Other goals of a healthcare system's medical liability cost-allocation system include recognizing and rewarding behavior that reduces risk and promotes patient and provider safety, and identifying and assessing those departments that fail to comply with the organization's risk management program and whose behavior creates liability for the organization.

Attributes of a Sound Cost-Allocation System

A comprehensive cost-allocation system usually identifies an organization's loss-frequency and loss-severity problems. The information can be used by management to analyze and determine the effectiveness of a healthcare system's current risk management activities and to highlight new areas that might benefit from a risk-control program.

An effective cost-allocation system is not subject to manipulation, a fact that presents a particular challenge in a complex health-care system or academic environment, where political or financial pressures within the organization may attempt to influence the amounts allocated to specific groups. For instance, prestigious practice plans or highly coveted services, or niche programs with strong financial returns, may attempt to use the revenue they generate as a bargaining chip to negotiate their allocated amounts downward in exchange for their continued loyalty to the organization. The health system or hospital administration, on the other hand, might feel that it has firm control of the faculty physicians or business entities and attempt to pass back to them the full cost of losses that the organization incurs. In other situations, the faculty or physicians may actually control the organization and attempt to allocate the bulk of the costs back to the hospital; therefore, the risk manager must take care to craft a fair system that is sensitive to the organization's political structure or to the business goals of a complex health system while maintaining a non-manipulative, easily explainable, consistently applicable cost-allocation structure.

Finally, a sound cost-allocation system is simple to administer and easy to understand. With today's technology, very complicated cost-allocation systems can be administered relatively easily; however, if the system is so complex that it cannot be easily understood, its influence in motivating staff to participate in a risk-control program may be greatly diminished.

APPROACHES TO A RISK MANAGEMENT PROGRAM

One of two broad approaches to establishing a risk management program for cost allocation is generally followed; the first involves evaluating losses prospectively, and the second involves a retrospective review. A complex health system must determine which approach will best serve its risk financing and risk management programs.

The Prospective Approach

With a prospective approach, costs are allocated before the beginning of the funding year in which they are expected to be incurred and are not changed for that period. This is similar to the experience-rating approach used by the insurance industry. The funding costs are allocated primarily on the basis of potential loss exposure and secondarily on the basis of historical loss experience. The chief disadvantage of the prospective approach is that actual expenditures may be much different from those allocated, and any corrections will not be linked with the period to which they are charged. Furthermore, because the average experiential period for a prospective system is 2–5 years, it is difficult to immediately measure the effectiveness of risk management activities.

The Retrospective Approach

A retrospective system estimates and allocates costs at the beginning of the funding year in which they are expected to be incurred; however, they may be reallocated several times during or after the end of the year. Therefore, final allocated costs are not determined until well after the end of the year in which they were incurred. This approach is similar to the retrospective rating system used by the insurance industry. Actual loss experience is the primary basis for allocation, and potential loss exposure is the secondary basis. The average experiential period for a retrospective system is 1–3 years, thus making it easier to measure the impact of risk management activities.

DETERMINING THE COSTS TO BE ALLOCATED

After an organization defines its goals for cost allocation and determines the approach that best serves the risk financing program, it must decide what costs to allocate. The first decision it must make is whether the health system will allocate for costs paid during the year, for occurrences reported during the year, or for occurrences incurred during the year.

The most common decision is to base contributions to the risk financing program on incurred losses. Because any one of the three methods can have a significant impact on an organization's financial statement, it is critical to enlist the support of finance and accounting personnel when making any decisions about the funding or cost strategies.

After the funding decision has been made, the organization must decide whether to fund the liability program for expected costs only or expected costs plus a margin. This margin is often referred to as a risk margin and is similar to the surplus held by an insurance company. It represents money not expected to be spent but which should be available in case actual costs exceed projections. The risk margin also has the potential to affect the financial statement, further underscoring the need for consulting the appropriate financial personnel to ensure that the organization's objectives are met.

Often organizations dedicate the income anticipated from investments to cover their risk margin; however, some organizations fund their programs without using investment income for their margins. Investment income can be recognized only when it is earned and reported appropriately on the financial statements.

IDENTIFYING SPECIFIC COSTS

The next step in implementing a risk financing program for medical liability is to decide what specific costs to allocate. The three dominant cost categories are:

- The cost of excess insurance premiums
- The cost of funding retained losses (self-insured retentions) and associated expenses
- The cost of administrative overhead for operating the insurance program(s),

including risk management program support, actuarial, brokerage services, and loss-control expense

The cost-gathering process for each cost category should be very specific. Historical data are most helpful in developing the projected cost of the medical liability program and can be used to develop benchmarks for each category. The cost of insurance should include any brokerage or consulting fees that were incurred in placing the coverage with an insurer. It is recommended that these costs be attributed to specific services provided by the broker and negotiated up front, as opposed to being set as a percentage of the policy premium.

AREAS OF EXPENDITURES COVERED

The cost of funding a self-insured retention (SIR) usually covers several areas of expenditure. The healthcare organization should pay attention to capturing all charges pertaining to actuarially determined funding requirements for indemnity losses within the SIR, costs carried over from previous years, allocated loss-adjustment expenses, unallocated loss adjustment expenses, and administrative overhead.

Actuarially Determined Funding Requirements for Indemnity Losses Within the SIR

This area usually represents the largest component of the funding amount and is based on an independent actuarial study of prior years' loss development and the organization's specific risk tolerance (confidence level).

If additional funding of the SIR is required (e.g., due to costs carried over from previous years), these costs usually are the result of unexpected settlement amounts or potential impairment of the annual aggregate retention level.

Allocated Loss-Adjustment Expenses

Allocated loss-adjustment expenses (ALAE) are charges associated with the settlement or conclusion of individual claims. The largest outlay is usually for outside legal fees incurred in the defense of litigated claims. Other costs typically allocated to claims are independent adjuster fees, expert-witness fees, and court costs.

Unallocated Loss-Adjustment Expenses

Unallocated loss-adjustment expenses (ULAE) are expenditures associated with the settlement of claims that are not incurred on any individual claims. An example is fees paid to a third-party claim administrator. Some organizations choose to treat ULAE as an overhead cost.

Administrative Overhead

Administrative overhead may cover a myriad of costs, depending on the individual organization's philosophy and cost-accounting structure. Administrative charges usually allocated in a medical liability program include consultant costs such as those for actuaries and auditors, corporate attorney fees associated with the insurance program (these may be significant if the SIR is a trust or a captive), salaries paid to risk management and claims staff to administer the program, and costs of office space, equipment, and supplies.

COMMON METHODS OF ALLOCATION

Costs may be allocated on the basis of loss exposure or loss experience. An exposure-based system allocates costs solely on exposure, with no regard to loss experience or the political climate of the organization. Exposure rates generally are based on industry-wide data. An experience-based system allocates costs based solely on pro rata shar-

ing of historical losses. The most advantageous basis for a medical liability program is a blending of the two methods.

The Exposure-Based System

To allocate costs based on exposure, an organization must determine what exposure base would accurately reflect losses and other costs being allocated. All cost-allocation systems must weigh experience against expected costs. This is accomplished by weighting costs based on experience with costs based on exposure and producing a credibility factor.

Physician Allocation

For physicians and practice plans, the organization should compile a numerical listing of all physicians by department or specialty. The listing should contain an appropriate classification and rate for each listed specialty or department. This listing is calculated in full-time equivalents (FTEs) based on the number of hours spent in clinical practice. This is important because many academic physicians spend time in non-clinical teaching activities. Such non-clinical teaching activities rarely pose a threat to loss experience, so discounting them in the allocation process should not create an imbalance. An organization should not view research and teaching activities as being risk free, however, as many high-exposure lawsuits have resulted from failures in these areas; thus, some attribution to program costs is appropriate. In addition, an argument can be made that faculty members who spend most of their days in a lab and spend little time with patients might be higher risks when they actually do see patients. This argument again supports the need to allocate funds for these risks.

One of the most commonly used classification and rating systems is that of the Insurance Services Office (ISO). The ISO is considered to be the major rate-making organization for property and casualty insurance.

It produces rates for all classifications of an organization's medical liability program. The organizations that do not have access to ISO classifications and rates can obtain them from their insurance broker, actuary, or excess carrier. It is also appropriate to substitute other classifications and rates produced by an organization that best meet an organization's needs. Most medical liability insurers produce hospital and physician rates that are classified by specialty and are geographically adjusted. Geographical adjustment is usually helpful when an organization is operating in a market noted for either extremely high or extremely low verdicts. It is very important to make certain that each rate applied is for a specified level of coverage, such as $1–3 million, and that the level remains constant throughout the weighting process.

When the physician listing is completed, an organization will note that specialties that have a high degree of risk of harm, such as neurosurgery or obstetrics, will have the highest premium rates. This information generates a weighted premium by which to allocate physician costs based solely on their exposures.

Resident and Fellow Allocation

Residents and fellows in a healthcare organization present a unique allocation challenge. If possible, they should be noted in the physician FTE listing, or a separate listing should be created and rated for them. For weighting purposes, the organization must decide whether it wants to consider them as part of the faculty practice plan or the hospital. The most common decision is to include the residents and fellows as part of the hospital allocation and weight them as a set percentage of the physician rate, usually 0.5 for residents and 0.75 for fellows.

Hospital Allocation

For hospital exposures, an organization must determine the average bed occupancy and the number of outpatient visits per year. The ISO and various insurers produce rates for both categories that, when combined, result in the weighted premium for the hospital exposure. Again, it is important to ensure that the rates are applied at a consistent level, such as $1–3 million. In addition, other business entities owned by the organization, such as a blood bank or a durable medical equipment (DME) program, present risk to the organization but may be more difficult to gauge in terms of their exposure.

Arriving at the Final Allocation

The final steps of allocating costs entail applying the costs or funding amounts to the weights and allocating them accordingly. The easiest method for a teaching hospital or healthcare organization is to reach a mutually agreeable split of the costs of the funding amount before the final allocation. For example, if the funding level is set at $8 million, the parties may agree that a 60% physician and 40% hospital split is politically desirable; therefore, the total allocated to the hospital would be $3.2 million and the amount designated for the physicians would be $4.8 million. These costs would then receive an additional allocation to account for the various entities comprising each group.

A fairer or truer method might be to attain a properly weighted credibility factor for the hospital, business entities, and physician split. The facility premium is derived from the bed and outpatient premiums along with the premiums for fellows and residents. The physician premium is the total of the rated physician FTEs. The appropriate percentages are then apportioned. In the $8-million-example, 0.499 ($3,992,000) would be allocated to the hospital and 0.501 ($4,008,000) would be allocated to the physicians.

Finally, the healthcare organization can allocate to the individual departments the appropriate amounts based on the exposure factors derived. The hospital can use the same exposure factors derived for the residents and fellows, and can allocate among the various departments if so desired.

Frequency of Claims

The frequency of claims helps to determine whether more or fewer occurrences are causing losses. It is a good measure for gauging the impact of risk management programs, but it does not truly demonstrate the cost impact of claims. Claims frequency also lack a certain fairness because some departments may incur a large number of smaller claims. If loss experience is measured by frequency of claims, such a department could actually be penalized for having lower costs than other departments.

The Experience-Based System

Loss experience is often used to measure the success of a risk management program. The usual measuring points are loss frequency (the number of claims that occurred) and aggregate loss severity (the amount of the total claims cost). To allocate based on loss experience, an organization must decide what type of measuring point will be used.

Aggregate Loss Severity

The preferred choice for measuring loss in an experience-based system is severity—usually in an aggregate format. Under this method, losses are recorded with a set ceiling for individual claims, usually $50,000. For example, a department may have incurred three losses in the past year with values of $2,500, $22,000, and $135,000. The aggregate charge to that department would be $74,500. The ceiling amount is flexible but should be set at an amount that reasonably reflects the overall loss picture of the organization and penalizes for unfavorable loss experience.

Loss-development factors must be applied to each year's aggregate historical losses to compensate for the possibility of both late-reported claims and a future increase in the incurred amount for reported claims. They are a key element in the forecasting process because an estimate must be made of the

amount that will eventually be paid for each historical-loss year. Loss-development factors are applied to historical incurred losses for each year to estimate ultimate losses—the amount that is eventually paid after all the claims for a particular year are closed. Loss-development factors are available from a number of insurance industry sources; however, it is recommended that, whenever possible, a healthcare organization use factors calculated based on its own loss data.

Calculating Allocations for a Severity-Based Experience System

The most important criterion of a severity measure is that the claims data be accurate, especially when attributing reserves and payments. The appropriation of charged fault must be made fairly and accurately. The integrity and success of an experience-based allocation system depends on such fairness and accuracy. A healthcare organization must ensure that claim charges allocated to any individual department, business unit, or physician are equitable.

Allocating by Department

The final step involves allocating the designated portions by department or business unit.

Problems Associated with an Experience-Based System

Two key problems arise when a healthcare organization uses an experience-based system. The first problem concerns timing, as the allocations made based on the previous year's loss experience seldom give a truly accurate prediction of the costs for the year being funded. The second problem is that some departments receive no allocation amounts because they are loss free; yet, by the nature of their profession, they have loss exposures. This hurts the timeliness of risk management activities and may lead to lax performance in the premium-free years for certain departments; thus, it appears that a blended approach might be a more comprehensive method.

A Blended Approach

A blended approach takes into account both the exposure and experience models and can be weighted in a manner that best fits the organization's needs and political philosophy. Using the previous examples, a blended approach can be illustrated. The starting point is to determine the weight factors to use. In this first example, the weights will be a 50/50 split between exposure and severity of loss experience.

The next step is to gather the information related to actual and potential losses and exposures and make the appropriate calculations to determine the proper split between the faculty allocation and the hospital allocation.

The formula uses 0.5 as a multiplier because this example demonstrates a 50/50 split for exposure and experience. The multipliers or weights can be changed to reflect the organization's own philosophy. For example, an organization without sound loss information may decide on a 75% weight for exposure and a 25% weight for severity experience. Using this split, the allocation would be 0.25 as a multiplier.

The use of a blended formula can be taken one step further with the addition of claim frequency as a factor. Factoring in the number of claims made makes it possible to use the healthcare organization's total loss picture in the allocation process. Again, weights can be set in a manner that best suits the organization's philosophy.

The final step in applying the blended approach is to allocate the costs to the individual departments.

OTHER ALLOCATION METHODS

Other exposure-based methods are available to healthcare organizations in allocating costs for medical liability risk management programs. One such method can utilize physician billing information that can be detailed utilizing common procedural terminology (CPT) codes down to the level of a specific encounter or intervention. CPT codes are numbers assigned to every task and service a medical practitioner may provide to a patient including medical, surgical, and diagnostic services. They are used by insurers to determine the amount of reimbursement that a practitioner will receive by an insurer. Since everyone uses the same codes to mean the same thing, they ensure uniformity.

Using MGMA Data to Allocate Medical Group Costs

Another exposure-based allocation system for organizations that share risk financing program exposure with faculty practice groups can be developed in which the division of the allocated amount between the hospital and the medical group is predetermined. This methodology allocates costs within the medical group.

This system uses annual charges by department along with data from the MGMA's Physician Compensation and Production Survey. Gross fiscal-year charges are identified for each department. The MGMA median gross charges per physician are identified and divided into the fiscal charges per department. This produces the number of FTEs it would take to staff each department based on the gross charges. This number is then used to generate a premium amount by applying a geographically adjusted classification and rating system. The ISO ratings are then applied to each practice group. The specific rates are multiplied by the staffing FTE number for each department, producing a premium amount. This amount is then weighted for each department and multiplied by the group allocation amount that produces departmental allocations.

Because the basic objective of an allocation system is to promote participation in risk management activities, this system might benefit from the integration of loss severity and loss frequency data. This would produce a fairer methodology and promote risk management activities based on the loss portion of the allocation.

ALLOCATING OUTSIDE THE SYSTEM

Designing an appropriate allocation system presents many additional challenges. These challenges increase in complexity as complex healthcare organizations, through managed care contracts, assume responsibilities for exposures outside the home facility. These exposures include situations where care is either provided in facilities outside the primary setting (under contract), additional services such as home or hospice care are provided to patients outside the primary facility, or situations in which residents rotate through network facilities or in which non-faculty or non-employed physicians supervise residents.

The first step in managing risk in such situations is to determine which party is responsible for funding the insurance under the contract. If it is the healthcare organization, a decision must be made to allocate these contracted exposures to the organizational entity, the physician practice group, the clinical faculty, or a combination of all entities. The existing methodology for allocating can easily be adjusted to fit the contracted exposure. Initially, however, legal counsel should review all contracts in an attempt to determine who is assuming liability under the contract. For instance, if non-faculty physicians supervise residents outside the primary organization and that organization has responsibility for funding the insurance for that exposure, the hospital can assign a weight similar to the fellow/resident allocation already described. The weighted premium can then be charged to either the hospital- or the faculty-allocated amount.

Determining the appropriate allocation for new business ventures may become challenging and contentious given the lack of data that would be available for a new business venture. When this is the case, risk managers can seek assistance and data from external actuarial firms or from their insurance partners' underwriters to determine appropriate benchmarks for contributions to the organization's risk financing program.

14

MANAGING THE RISKS OF WORKERS' COMPENSATION

Mark G. Schneider, MBA

INTRODUCTION

Workers' compensation represents a growing area of responsibility for risk managers. The management of workplace injuries is synergistic with the principles of patient safety, which focus on maintaining a safe workplace with the necessary systems in place to ensure that employees can provide the safest care possible. What was once just another employee benefit is now more fully understood by upper management for its litigation potential and its ultimate financial impact. Many organizations now look to the discipline of risk management to oversee claims handling and to manage the costs associated with workers' compensation claims.

What is workers' compensation? It is a program created by state or federal law requiring employer-paid benefits for employee injury or illness that occurred in the course and scope of employment. Benefits include lost wages, healthcare costs, and awards for loss-of-earning capacity.

BRIEF HISTORY[1]

Workers' compensation laws were part of a significant evolution in the relationship of employers to their employees at the beginning of the twentieth century. The rise in industrial accidents drew attention to the inadequacies of common law rights available to an injured employee against his or her employer. Common law defenses, such as contributory negligence, assumption of risk, and negligent acts of fellow servants, were seen by the public as unfairly limiting an employee's recovery. Employers' liability laws, which modified common law defenses, were passed in a number of states between 1900 and 1910. The first state workers' compensation programs were enacted in 1911, and most states quickly adopted this format.

The principle embodied in the legislation is that employers should bear the costs of industrial accidents, without any regard to fault. Losses are included in the cost of production, and employees can consider this an employment benefit. In exchange for granting this benefit, employers are, for the most part, exempted from liability claims arising from these accidents.

Most statutes are designed to accomplish the following objectives:

- Provide prompt income and medical benefits to work-accident victims
- Provide a single remedy for the victim's cause of action
- Establish the mechanism for adjudicating disputes regarding benefits
- Encourage employer interest in safety
- Promote statewide analysis of accident causes

These precepts are consistent from state to state; however, the schedules for payments of lost wages and for medical expense vary considerably. Different minimum and maximum compensable wage levels are set by each state. Many states have established medical-fee schedules, and some now mandate managed-care programs.

HOW DOES WORKERS' COMPENSATION WORK?

The following example illustrates the benefits to be paid: an employee sustains a severe injury while performing his assigned duties. He obtains treatment from a physician, who performs surgery and keeps him home for a number of weeks. Although the employee returns to work performing the same job, the physician reports that the injury will result in a permanent limitation.

Under a typical workers' compensation statute, the employee would expect to receive temporary disability payments during the period he could not work, which are roughly equivalent to his take-home pay. He would expect that all reasonable hospital and physician charges would be paid. He would also expect to receive a settlement (usually calculated as a percentage of the loss of use of a part of the body) to compensate him for

future limitations caused by this accident. If he were represented by an attorney, that attorney would typically receive his fee as a percentage of the permanency settlement. Employers may challenge any of the following matters:

- Compensability of the injury
- Extent of time off work
- Reasonableness of medical expenses
- Extent of permanent injury

WORKERS' COMPENSATION AS AN INSURANCE PRODUCT

Coverage for workers' compensation was developed as a line of business by property and casualty insurers. Underwriting and claims handling became highly specialized, and single-line workers' compensation insurers formed to compete for this business with multiline insurers. Many large corporations decided to self-insure the predictable levels of workers' compensation losses, using third-party administrators to provide claims-handling services.

At the present time, there is a sophisticated array of insurance and related services available to assist an employer with its workers' compensation exposure. These services include:

- Primary workers' compensation insurance
- Excess workers' compensation insurance
- Unbundled claims and loss-prevention services from insurers
- Third-party claims administrators
- Loss-prevention consultants
- Case-management coordinators and claims administrators
- Medical-utilization-review analysts
- Workers' compensation managed-care providers
- Transitional duty consultants
- Disability-management coordinators and claims administrators
- Vocational-rehabilitation specialists

WHAT DEPARTMENT ADMINISTERS WORKERS' COMPENSATION FOR THE EMPLOYER?

Confusion arises because workers' compensation might be considered a benefit or a liability. Arguing in favor of its role as an employee benefit is its statutory grant of payments, with established schedules of payment; however, workers' compensation could also be viewed as a contingent liability, because the employer is not obligated to make any payment unless certain conditions occur, and even those conditions are subject to challenge. Because there is no predominating view and workers' compensation has characteristics of both a benefit and a liability, there has been no universal agreement as to the most effective organizational locus. Human resources, risk management, and finance, respectively, are the most frequently cited departments. Most often, the administering department actually oversees a third-party claims administrator or the claims handling performed by a primary insurer. The risk manager can add value to the administration of workers' compensation, regardless of its organizational structure, particularly in the following areas:

- Risk financing
- Claims administration
- Loss prevention
- Loss mitigation

Risk Financing

The same decision process used to decide whether to self-insure professional liability can be applied to workers' compensation. The first step is to determine the magnitude of the annual losses and then to see what portion of these losses is predictable. This expected layer of losses would become the self-insured retention. Excess insurance would be purchased to safeguard against losses that exceed the retention. If there are legal reasons why an organi-

zation cannot qualify as a self-insurer in a particular state, or if the organization has multistate exposure and does not want to qualify as a self-insurer in all locations, an alternative approach would be to engage a fronting insurer and reinsure the fronted exposure through a captive. During periods of intense competition for workers' compensation premiums, many insurers offer two notable incentives to insureds to forego self-insurance: scheduled premium credits and gainsharing. Subject to state insurance-department oversight, insurers are able to offer substantial discounts off the standard premiums for attractive accounts. Gainsharing has become a popular adjunct to benchmarking, in which the insurer will receive a negotiated premium surcharge for targeted favorable outcomes and will remit premium if it fails to achieve specified outcomes.

Claims Administration

Handling workers' compensation claims bears some resemblance to handling professional-liability or general-liability claims, except fewer issues are subject to dispute and the payments are controlled by statutory schedules. The extensive medical knowledge gained from professional-liability claims becomes very beneficial in workers' compensation, because most issues are resolved by medical opinion. The basic file-handling mechanics of proper reserving, monitoring progress, and periodic reporting are also valuable in overseeing workers' compensation claims. Figure 14–1 provides a sample flowchart for workers' compensation claims. This chart tracks the interaction of the employer or "manager," the claims administrator, and the medical provider. Figure 14–2 shows a similar process from the vantage point of the claims administrator.

If the organization is self-insured, one critical question to be addressed is whether claims should be self-administered or handled externally by a third-party administrator (or insurer

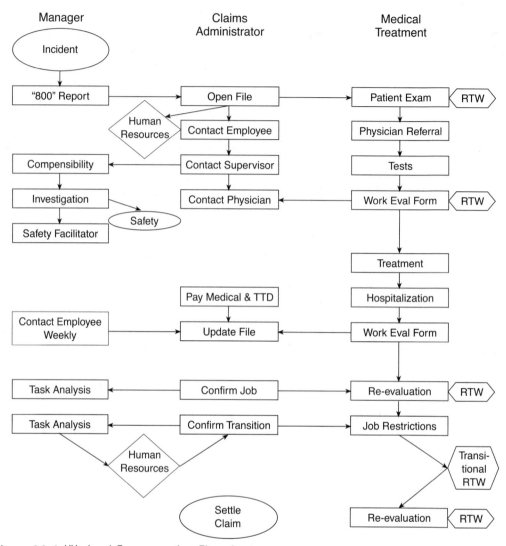

Figure 14–1 Workers' Compensation Flowchart

on an unbundled basis). The volume of case activity in workers' compensation is considerably greater than in professional liability, requiring efficient information processing, check writing, and accounting systems. Also, two different levels of specialty expertise are usually required: a claims-processor level for the majority of claims and a claims-manager level for a small volume of complicated cases; thus, a large volume of workers' compensation claims is necessary to permit the hiring of both levels into an internal-claims department.

When there is not an adequate volume of complex cases to warrant a full-time claims manager, some organizations assign that role to professional-liability staff as part of their duties. Other organizations in the same circumstance opt for third-party administrators.

If the organization elects to have a third-party administrator handle its claims, it can choose between third-party administrators and unbundled insurer claims services. Although the differences between them have rapidly narrowed, third-party administrators

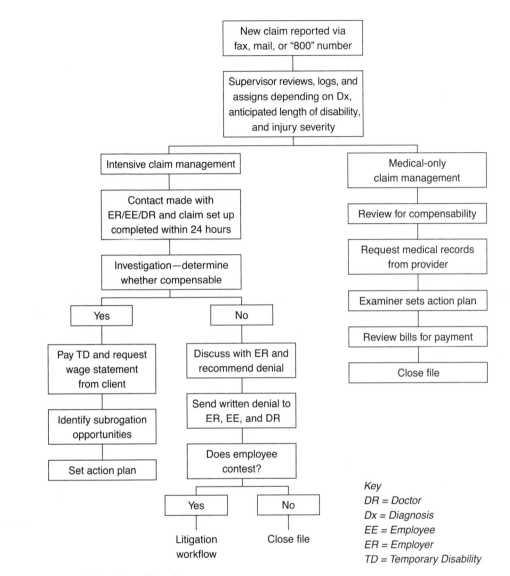

Figure 14–2 Claims Handling Process

are generally more flexible in designing their services around the requirements of the organization, whereas the insurers are generally large enough to offer a larger variety of services in an integrated system. Self-insurers typically use some combination of claims management, medical-case management, information-management systems, utilization review, bill review, vocational rehabilitation, insurance, banking, and legal services.

At the same time an organization is assessing third-party administrator services, it should also address internal issues that affect claims handling, including the following:

- Promptness of reporting. Can the lag time between accident and the date the claim is reported to the claims administrator be reduced to improve the claims administrator's ability to manage the claim?

- Workers' compensation communications coordinator. Is there a designated workers' compensation coordinator within the organization to enhance the flow of information and to increase the effectiveness of handling in the early phases of a claim?
- Directed medical treatment. Are injured workers immediately directed to physicians preferred by the employer? Does the emergency department refer the employees to these preferred physicians?

Loss Prevention

Reducing the accidents giving rise to workers' compensation claims can be incorporated easily into the risk manager's role. Given the volume of workers' compensation incidents, it is usually possible not only to analyze the loss history to pinpoint likely sources of problems, but also to demonstrate improvements using the loss data. Most workers' compensation information systems allow analysis of losses by using many variables. Even the simplest systems routinely analyze losses by department and by body part. Many systems also have standardized coding for causes and types of loss. Exhibit 14–1 is a sample quarterly report that focuses on the most prevalent types of incidents. Exhibit 14–2 is a sample investigation report used by supervisors to identify preventable incidents. It can also be used for trending.

Once the problems are identified, the more difficult task is to devise effective motivation for loss reduction. The most frequent methods adopted are the following:

- Recognition of better (or worse)-than-expected departmental results
- Tangible rewards to employees for improved performance
- System-wide cost allocations

A study by Towers Perrin Tillinghast[2] shows cost allocations to be the most prevalent method, customarily charging back to each department some share of the costs arising from that department's workers' compensation losses. The employers surveyed rated the cost-allocation method to be about 80% effective. Although used by less than 10% of the employers surveyed, gainsharing with employees and supervisors was considered particularly effective, rated as 100% effective in the case of employee gainsharing. Cash bonuses for reduced claims are similarly used by less than 10% of the employers but are also rated as highly effective.

Education, particularly at the department level, is necessary to train line supervisors in identifying and correcting accident-prone work routines. Routine reporting of loss summaries to departments maintains awareness of these issues and provides a feedback loop for noting improvements. Post-offer physical examinations are being used more frequently to determine if the prospective employee is able to perform the physical tasks of the job. There is uniform agreement that lifting injuries and repetitive-motion wrist injuries are the most significant problem areas for workers' compensation.

Loss Mitigation

How well the organization is positioned to manage the injured employee, from the standpoint of corporate operations, will have a large effect on the results of those handling workers' compensation claims. Prompt reporting of claims allows the claims administrator to manage the case at a critical stage, in terms of medical referral and employee confidence. Reporting lags permit increased lost time from work. Earlier rapport with the injured employee also reduces the likelihood that the claim will be litigated.

Clear communication of expectations between the injured employee and his or her supervisor also encourages earlier return to work and reduces the misunderstandings that sometimes prompt litigation. Exhibits 14–3 and 14–4 show examples of information sheets for supervisors and for employees. The employee's

Exhibit 14–1 Safety Analysis Report—By Injury Type (Period 7/1/96–7/1/97)

Category Frequency

Injury Type	Number of Claims	Percentage of Total Claims
1. Struck By	164	17.5%
2. Lifting	105	11.2%
3. Contact with Infectious Disease	78	8.3%

Category #1 **Struck By**

Location Frequency

Location	Number of Claims
Campus 1	158
Campus 2	6
Campus 3	0

Department	Number of Claims	Number of Medical-Only Cases	Number of Lost-Time Cases	Number of Lost-Time Days	Paid and Expected Costs
Department 32	6	25	1	97	$40,000.00
Department 28	20	17	3	72	$4,000.00
Department 10	14	13	1	10	$3,300.00
Other Departments	104	103	1	15	$25,000.00
Totals	164	158	6	194	$72,300.00

Category #2 **Lifting**

Location Frequency

Location	Number of Claims
Campus 1	104
Campus 2	0
Campus 3	1

Department	Number of Claims	Number of Medical-Only Cases	Number of Lost-Time Cases	Number of Lost-Time Days	Paid and Expected Costs
Department 10	18	12	6	109	$50,000.00
Department 28	16	10	6	250	$35,000.00
Department 31	11	10	1	32	$4,000.00
Other Departments	60	47	13	321	$90,000.00
Totals	105	79	26	712	$179,000.00

Category #3 **Contact with Infectious Disease**

Location Frequency

Location	Number of Claims
Campus 1	78
Campus 2	0
Campus 3	0

Department	Number of Claims	Number of Medical-Only Cases	Number of Lost-Time Cases	Number of Lost-Time Days	Paid and Expected Costs
Department 31	40	40	0	0	$1,500.00
Department 11	11	11	0	0	$500.00
Department 10	7	7	0	0	$250.00
Other Departments	20	20	0	0	$500.00
Totals	78	78	0	0	$2,750.00

Exhibit 14–2 Workers' Compensation Program

Supervisor's Investigation Report of Accident/Injury

Date: _____

Employee Name: _____ Occupation: _____

Employment Status: _____ New   _____ Part time   _____ Full time   _____ Contract

Date Injured: _____ Time Injured: _____ Department: _____

Location (Bldg., room, etc.): _____

Description of Injury: _____

_____

Part of body affected: _____

Supervisor:

How did this happen? Use extra sheet or sketch if needed.	
What task was involved?	
Was task performed per protocol and training? (personal protective equipment, etc.)	
Was there a defective or unsafe condition? (wet floor, improper lighting, broken equipment)	
What specifically did you do to prevent a similar injury? (If nothing, give reason.)	
Ask employee: What can be done to prevent this injury to others?	
	Supervisor's Signature: _____

DEPARTMENT HEAD/ADMINISTRATOR:

Please review, sign, and forward to Safety Department within 5 days.	Department Head/Administrator Signature: _____

SAFETY DEPARTMENT REVIEW:

_____

_____

_____

_____

Accident prevention is an important part of your job.

Exhibit 14–3 Workers' Compensation Program Supervisor's Information Sheet

Management Philosophy

Workers' compensation is a benefit required of every employer by state statute, in the event of injury or illness arising out of the scope of a person's employment. This program provides resources to the supervisor for loss prevention, management of workers' compensation claims, and returning the employee to work. When an injury or illness has been determined to be compensable, benefits will be paid based on the statute. The intent of this law is to provide employees with means to recover from injury or illness in an efficient and medically sound manner, so that they can return to the job.

It is the responsibility of every manager and employee to make certain that each task is performed in an approved and safe manner. This program is committed to providing a safe environment for all its employees, students, patients, and visitors. The supervisor is the primary link between the injured employee and the work environment.

Accountabilities

The supervisor of an employee who sustains a work-related injury is responsible for the following steps:

1. He or she must obtain immediate medical care for the injured employee.
   a. For non-ambulatory patients, the supervisor must call 911. The employee should be sent directly to an emergency department.
   b. The supervisor should send ambulatory patients to the assigned clinic during its hours of operation.

2. The supervisor must report the work-related injury immediately. Also, he or she must notify the human resources department.

3. The supervisor should investigate this incident and complete the incident-investigation report. If the injury involves serious trauma, chemical exposures, air-quality issues, repetitive trauma, or any other series of related incidents, the safety department should be contacted immediately; otherwise, the incident-investigation report should be completed and forwarded to the safety department within 5 days.

4. In analyzing the environmental factors that gave rise to this incident, the supervisor should perform an analysis of the tasks to determine if any changes to the work environment or employee training are necessary. The safety department can provide initial guidance in performing task analysis.

5. The supervisor should stay in weekly contact with an injured employee who remains off work. The employee is responsible for reviewing the work-evaluation form with the supervisor after each physician visit. At that time, the supervisor should determine if the employee can return to work or if transitional duty is available. The supervisor should notify human resources of any change in the employee's duty status.

6. When a physician releases the employee for full duty, that employee should contact the supervisor directly. On return to work, the employee will present the supervisor with a copy of the work-evaluation form. The supervisor should also notify human resources of the date of the employee's return to work.

7. If the work-evaluation form permits restricted work activities of the employee, the supervisor will need to conduct a task analysis to see if transitional duty can be offered within the department. If this does not appear to be feasible, the supervisor should check with human resources to see what other alternatives for transitional duty are available.

8. If a settlement for permanent partial disability is under consideration, the claims-administrator representative will review the employee's work status, and any restrictions, with the supervisor.

9. The supervisor's ongoing commitment to a safe environment should include the following steps:
   a. Periodic monitoring of the work area for indications of environmental and/or human factors that might cause problems.
   b. Evaluation of tasks in terms of the need for additional training, and evaluation of the use of related personal protective equipment.
   c. Redesign of task protocols that will reduce the potential for injury and improve employee efficiency.

Exhibit 14–4 Workers' Compensation Program Employee-Information Sheet

Benefits

Workers' compensation is a benefit required of every employer by state statute, in the event of an injury or illness arising from, and in the course and scope of, one's employment. This program has hired an independent company to act as the claims administrator, investigate, determine compensability, pay benefits, and monitor the progress of workers' compensation claims. When an injury or illness has been determined to be compensable, benefits will be paid based on the statute. The intent of this law is to provide an employee with the means to recover from an injury or illness in an efficient and medically sound manner. To that end, this program assists its employees in returning to work as quickly as possible.

Generally, reasonable medical expenses and temporary total disability after the prescribed waiting time will be paid on behalf of the employer. If a permanent disability results from the injury, employees may have the right to make a further claim.

Obligations

An employee who sustains a work-related injury or illness must take the following steps:

1. Report the injury or illness to the supervisor on the day it occurs. This information is required to report a workers' compensation claim.

2. Make sure a physician completes the work-evaluation form for each visit. After each visit, bring a copy to review with the supervisor, to determine return-to-work status. If needed, transitional duty may be available, either within the employee's department or facilitated elsewhere by human resources.

3. The employee is expected to maintain, at a minimum, weekly contact with his or her supervisor, regardless of return-to-work status.

4. The claims administrator gathers information and authorizes benefits on behalf of this program. The employee must cooperate with the representatives of the claims administrator.

5. Missed physician appointments must be cleared with the claims administrator in advance. Delays due to a missed appointment may not be compensated.

6. Medical bills for treatment of the work-related injury should be sent to the claims administrator.

7. The workers' compensation benefit checks for temporary total disability will be available in human resources on regular paydays. In general, the workers' compensation statute limits temporary total disability benefits to two thirds of the average weekly wage, after the waiting period.

8. Depending on the nature of the issue, the following resources are available to the employee, in addition to the supervisor:
   • Claims administrator
   • Human resources department
   • Safety department
   • Insurance department

---

information sheet (see Exhibit 14–4) is to be given to an employee at the time of injury, so he or she is aware of his or her benefits and responsibilities. The latest development is the establishment of transitional-duty programs, which enable an employee who is capable of performing some tasks to be returned promptly to the work force while he or she continues to recover fully. Case managers are instrumental in interpreting medical restrictions and explaining them to supervisors so that appropriate and productive transitional duty can be designed. An important consideration is to monitor progress toward full recovery after the

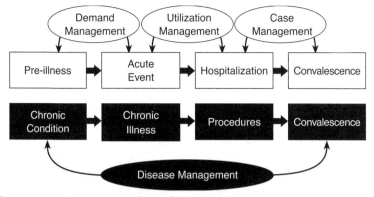

Figure 14–3 Strategies to Reduce the Cost of Medical Care
Courtesy of Tillinghast Towers Perrin.

employee is assigned transitional duty. This will limit the disruption of normal operations and prevent an employee's mistaking transitional duty for reasonable accommodation.

WORKERS' COMPENSATION: AMERICANS WITH DISABILITIES ACT AND FAMILY MEDICAL LEAVE ACT

Two federal laws that occasionally affect the management of workers' compensation claims are the Americans with Disabilities Act and the Family Medical Leave Act. An injured employee may claim that he or she is qualified to perform the essential functions of his or her job, even though the injury caused a permanent impairment of a major life function. That employee would request that the employer make a reasonable accommodation in the job; or an employee in a transitional duty may attempt to claim that the transitional duty is the de facto reasonable accommodation. Task-oriented job descriptions that clearly identify essential functions of the job are valuable in dealing with these requests. In transitional-duty cases, it is helpful to document expectations of the type and duration of the transitional job, as well as the reasons for its design.

If the workers' compensation injury can be considered a serious health condition, the Family Medical Leave Act can be granted, running concurrently with the workers' compensation absence.[3] The human resources policies should be reviewed to confirm that the Family Medical Leave Act and workers' compensation leaves can run concurrently. Proper notification must be given to the employee, telling him or her that the Family Medical Leave Act leave has been granted.

Financial Impact of Workers' Compensation

The actual expenses for workers' compensation typically fall between 1% and 2% of an organization's total payroll; however, indirect costs (e.g., hiring and training replacement personnel, replacing damaged equipment, rearranging departmental workloads) are estimated to be as much as four times that of direct workers' compensation expenses. With other types of disability expenses accounting for another 2–3% of total payroll, there is increasing interest in managing all forms of disability consistently. Proven return-to-work techniques in workers' compensation are being adapted to non-occupational disability management. This approach will also help to reduce the service gaps in "24-hour" coverage. Figure 14–3 is a Towers Perrin Tillinghast chart[4] that identifies the stages in which medical management can be applied for both occupational and non-occupational conditions.

Within the direct workers' compensation expenses, medical expense typically accounts for 45–50% of the cost. This explains the extent to which medical-utilization management has been applied to workers' compensation; however, lower cost is not the single criterion for effective medical utilization in workers' compensation. Prompt return to work, without relapses, is an additional critical outcome to be considered. As a result of these unique requirements, workers' compensation managed care tends to be more aggressive in its treatment modalities than a typical health-maintenance-organization model. A study by Intracorp in December 1995 demonstrated the advantages of managed care to be the following:[5]

- Costs dropped by 23% when managed-care techniques were applied within the first 3 months of the injury.
- Managed claims closed 27% sooner.

Ruth Estrich[6] has identified eight key managed-care components that she believes are necessary to run a successful managed-care program. These components include:

- Comprehensive loss prevention
- Provider network
- Occupationally oriented utilization management
- Nurse case management
- Vocational rehabilitation
- Managed prescription-drug program
- Comprehensive bill review
- Information

Successful managed care includes methods for quick transfer of medical information back to the employer. Many specialty medical providers use a single-page form to report work-status capability on the same day that treatment was rendered. Exhibits 14–5 and 14–6 show two examples of this type of form.

In addition to productivity issues, the employer has a direct financial interest in returning an employee to work. A large percentage of direct workers' compensation expense is payment for days lost from work. There is a strong correlation between the number of lost days and any eventual permanency settlement. A number of return-to-work strategies have been used successfully, including transitional-duty programs, volunteer organization assignments, case management, and employee incentives.

Workers' compensation becomes exceptionally important during corporate downsizing. There have been instances when employees have filed workers' compensation claims in an effort to extend payroll benefits or to improve a severance package. In these circumstances, claims-handling capability must be increased rapidly to adequately investigate and challenge these claims. Joseph P. Rainey[7] lists important steps to take, including the following:

- Put resources in place before the reduction is announced.
- Appoint a coordinator to work closely with the claims-service provider.
- Focus on returning restricted-duty employees to full duty.
- Preserve claim documentation.

Healthcare Organization as a User of Workers' Compensation Services

Any healthcare system is in an unusual position, because it provides workers' compensation medical services to many employers and uses workers' compensation services as a large employer in its own right. This dual role offers two important potential advantages in the management of workers' compensation: reduction of medical costs and ability to support a profit center.

When a healthcare system provides workers' compensation medical treatment to its own employees, it saves on expenses to the extent that it is not paying an external medical provider for the workers' compensation medical treatment. As a corollary, an internal "payment" of charges puts less pressure on the

Exhibit 14–5 Work Evaluation Form: Employee Workers' Compensation Claim

Section I: Employee Information TO BE COMPLETED BY EMPLOYEE

Last _____ First _____ MI _____

Social Security # _____

Address _____

City _____ State _____ ZIP _____ Home Phone _____

Date of Injury _____ Job Title _____ Department _____

Manager's Name _____ Ext. _____

Section II: TO BE COMPLETED BY PHYSICIAN

Attending physician: In an effort to ensure that employees return to work at the appropriate time from a claim for workers' compensation, please complete the following to determine if the employee is able to return to full duty or on a modified basis. An effort will be made to accommodate the limitations you have identified.

I saw this patient on _____(date)_____ and recommend:

Employee may:

❑ Return to work with no restrictions on _____(date)_____

❑ Return to work _____(date)_____ capable of performing

   (If frequency is limited, state duration in comments section)
   ❑ Stand/Walk   ❑ Sit
   ❑ Drive   ❑ Bend
   ❑ Lift   ❑ Weight (indicate #) _____

   Use of hand(s) for repetitive motion
   ❑ Single Grasping   ❑ One-Hand Work   ❑ Left   ❑ Right
   ❑ Pushing & Pulling   ❑ Data Entry   ❑ Writing

❑ Is unable to work at this time.

These restrictions are in effect until _____ or until patient is reevaluated on _____ or patient is referred to _____.

Comments: _____

Diagnosis/Condition (explanation): _____

Prognosis: _____

_____

Physician Signature: _____

Physician Phone Number: _____ Date Signed: _____

Print Name: _____ Address: _____

White—OHS   Yellow—Dept. Mgr.   Blue—Employee   Pink—HR   Green—Physician

Courtesy of Loyola University Medical Center.

Exhibit 14–6 Work Status Report

Occupational Health Network

A. TO BE COMPLETED AFTER EACH VISIT

Employee: _____ Today's Date: _____ Time In: _____ Time Out: _____

Social Security Number: _____ Job Title: _____ Date of Injury: _____

Employer: _____ Fax No.: _____ Work Schedule: _____

B. SELECT AS INDICATED BELOW

1. ❏ Unrestricted Duty _____/_____/_____ 2. ❏ Restricted Duty _____/_____/_____ (See Below)

3. ❏ Off Work _____/_____/_____

4. ❏ Referred to Specialist

5. ❏ Case Closed _____/_____/_____

C. RESTRICTED DUTY—THIS EMPLOYEE CAN:

N/A: Not Applicable; **FREQUENT**: 5–6 Hours per day; **OCCASIONAL:** 2–3 Hours per day; **RARE:** 1/2–1 Hour per day; **NONE:** 0 Hours per day.

Activity/Exposure		Freq.	Occas.	Rare	None
Lift/Carry	0–10 lbs				
Lift/Carry	10–20 lbs				
Lift/Carry	20–50 lbs				
Lift/Carry	50–100 lbs				
Perform a Sitting Job					
Climb Stairs					
Climb Ladders					
Kneel					
Stoop/Bend					
Work with _____ Foot Elevated					
Operate Foot Controls					
Operate Motor Vehicle					
Grip/Pinch/Twist with Right Hand					
Grip/Pinch/Twist with Left Hand					
Do _____ Hand Work Only					
Push/Pull up to _____ lbs					
Walking/Standing					

(continues)

Exhibit 14–6 (Continued)

INSTRUCTIONS:

❏ Change dressing daily   ❏ Keep dressing and wound clean and dry

❏ Medication may cause drowsiness   ❏ Must wear splint/sling

Can work eight (8) hour day   ❏ Yes   ❏ No   Can work twelve (12) hour day   ❏ Yes   ❏ No

If not eight (8) or twelve (12) hours per day, how many? _____

Expected time to achieve eight (8) hours. _____

GENERAL COMMENTS: _____

DIAGNOSIS: _____

Next Appointment _____/_____/_____ Completed by _____

(Physician's Printed Name)

_____

(Physician's Signature)

Work status communicated to _____ by _____ via   ❏ phone
                                                                      ❏ fax

Courtesy of West Suburban Medical Center.

system's cash flow, because it is an accounting entry rather than an actual payment.

Developing a center of excellence in occupational medicine could produce a win–win situation. There is a growing recognition of the need for physicians with concentrated experience in occupational medicine to anchor the burgeoning workers' compensation networks.[8] The budgeted workers' compensation medical expense can be considered by the occupational medicine department as a base of guaranteed income on which to build a strong treatment program with effective communication systems. As a user of these services, the organization will enjoy improved claims handling. This reliable base of revenue for medical services will allow the occupational-medicine department to expand its market to more area employers, with the healthcare organization itself demonstrating client satisfaction.

References

1. Aon Insurance Brokerage. (1996). Analysis of workers' compensation claims. Chicago: Aon Insurance Brokerage.
2. Towers Perrin Tillinghast. (1996, February). Reality testing.
3. Business Insurance. (1997, April 28). Leave Act shouldn't scare employers.
4. Towers Perrin Tillinghast. (1997). Emphasis.
5. Intracorp. (1996, March). Risk management.
6. Estrich, R. (1997, summer). Managed medical and managed disability. Liberty Directions.
7. Rainey, J.P. (1995, August 14). Preparing for downsizing costs. Business Insurance.
8. Business Insurance. (1996, February 12). Employers warned on Comp networks.

CLAIMS MANAGEMENT ISSUES: THE AFTERMATH OF ERROR

15

GUIDELINES FOR IN-HOUSE CLAIMS MANAGEMENT

Josephine Goode-Evans, MA, BSN
Barbara J. Youngberg, JD, MSW, BSN, FASHRM

INTRODUCTION

Early identification, investigation, and resolution of potentially compensable events are the major objectives of an effective claims-management program. Successful achievement of these objectives depends on strong commitment and support from all participants and an effective risk management program that maximizes the four basic components of identification, analysis, treatment, and evaluation. Because these components become the foundation of the claims-management process, the first step toward program development is an overall assessment. Subsequent chapters deal with an increasingly popular approach taken by healthcare organizations that seek to identify events that may be managed better outside the legal system because it has been determined that the provider or organization indeed caused or contributed to harming a patient. These programs foster candor with patients and their families, allow for early

offers of compensation, and seek to avoid engaging either the patient or the provider in contentious and protracted litigation. Of course, there will always be events where internal review suggests that the care provided met the standard and is defensible, or when the plaintiff's demands are disproportionate to the injury sustained. For these events, a rigorous process of claims management must be maintained, and that process is the basis for this chapter.

ASSESSING THE ENVIRONMENT

The risk or claims manager should first assess the environment in which the program is to be established. This assessment should include the following actions:

- Ensure top-level commitment and support of the system.
- Determine position of the organization regarding disclosure and early-offer programs.

- Review existing risk identification systems to ensure protection of information.
- Evaluate the scope of the proposed program as it relates to the requirements of insurance companies and other risk financing vehicles.
- Determine information-management-system needs.
- Survey existing resources and establish goals and objectives.

Top-Level Commitment

It is imperative that senior administration and the institution's, network's, or system's governing board understand the scope of responsibility and accountability necessary to develop and maintain an in-house claims-management system. The risk or claims manager, as applicable, should ensure that the people ultimately responsible for its success and support understand, at minimum, the following aspects of the proposed program:

- Structure of the program, including its relationships to other departments and external reporting requirements
- Procedures for obtaining and protecting required information
- Process for extracting learning from claims to advance patient safety goals
- Limitation of informational access (procedures and reasons). How does the organization protect information without jeopardizing a learning environment?
- Investigational policies and procedures
- Requirements of participants (insured or covered persons)
- Types of coverage, restrictions, and exclusions

This list is not meant to be all-inclusive but instead suggests basic guidelines for developing the governing board's education and interest to increase its support for the program.

Risk Identification Systems

Most institutions already have mechanisms in place to identify untoward patient occur-

rences ranging from basic incident reporting to elaborate networks that involve receipt of information from other in-house systems. The incident report remains one of the oldest methods of communicating information of adverse occurrences. Participants in the program should be encouraged to report information freely and objectively; they should be assured that reports are non-punitive. Depending on the program's structure and methods for protecting the confidentiality of the information, other methods, such as telephone reports and anonymous telephone lines, may be explored to supplement written reports.

Additionally, the risk or claims manager should educate non-clinical departments in the importance of providing information regarding potentially compensable events. Through this method, managers can extend beyond traditional sources to ensure prompt identification of these incidents. The following departments are often able to provide early-warning indicators:

- The medical-records department can advise the claims-management office of requests for records by plaintiffs' attorneys.
- The quality-management department can provide information from generic screening criteria and other medical-staff sources, as applicable.
- Billing offices can notify the claims office of serious medical-care complaints when following up on delinquent bills.
- Volunteer services and patient-relations departments can relay complaints about patient care. Volunteers are often the first to hear from disgruntled patients, because they are often viewed by the patients as neutral.

Prior to implementing any risk identification techniques, it is imperative to take measures to differentiate between patient safety information and information gained in anticipation of litigation. This could impact the manner in which information is shared and protected. (See Chapter 8 for a detailed discussion.) Legal counsel should be consulted to ensure that all program-identification methods, guidelines, structures, and documentation are appropriate and effective for the institution's particular circumstances and consistent with prevailing state and federal laws.

In self-insured programs, it is also helpful, if possible, to advise covered participants of their obligation to report adverse outcomes as a condition of their coverage.

Scope of the Program

The in-house program will be significantly affected by the organization's method of risk financing. For example, if the organization is self-insured, the risk or claims manager must ascertain whether excess or umbrella coverage will be purchased; if so, many of the program's reporting requirements, both internally and externally, will be affected by the excess policy. If the program will purchase first-dollar commercial insurance, the program requirements, structure, data collection, and other features will be defined by this primary policy. Consequently, a full review of the type of risk financing mechanisms should be conducted with an eye toward determining the scope of in-house responsibility that can and should be assumed in accordance with internal and external constraints.

Management Information System

Whether the institution will have first-dollar commercial insurance coverage (or self-insurance completely, in essence becoming a first-dollar insured) or use alternative risk-funding mechanisms will also affect the claims-management information system. If using commercial insurance coverage, the claims manager must ascertain the type of information the company requires and provides, and the regularity for reconciling these reports. At a minimum, it is recommended that the insurance company provide a loss experience and case-status update on a regular basis (see Exhibit 15–1). For those institu-

tions that use risk financing alternatives, detailed information regarding development of an in-house claims-management information system is discussed later. Having a comprehensive risk management information system that aggregates, tracks, and trends this information is becoming increasingly important and should be installed to ensure maximum efficiency and effectiveness of a claims management program.

GOALS AND OBJECTIVES

The success of the program is directly related to the manager's ability to formulate achievable, realistic, and measurable goals by using available resources. After the scope of the program is determined and it is clear where the in-house claims-program responsibilities begin and end, objectives should be established and clearly stated. The objectives must be consistent with the institution's goals and with the corporate culture. Planning at this stage should consider internal, external, and vertical communication; protocols; policies and procedures; and claims-management requirements.

PROGRAM DEVELOPMENT

When the manager has completed the overall assessment to determine the appropriate scope and structure of the program, a claims-management philosophy statement should be developed, setting forth the philosophy of claims handling for the institution. As previously mentioned, the statement must describe the organization's position relative to full disclosure, early-offer program, and full transparency. It might be helpful to share the organization's philosophy with attorneys in the community so that they know that the organization has a plan and a history of vigorously defending claims where expert review suggests an absence of negligence. The statement and subsequent policies should guide the staff in routine handling of claims and should also be in line with other relevant primary or excess coverage.

Exhibit 15–1 Sample Checklist for a Commercially Insured Institution

I. Read the complete insurance policy and pay particular attention to the following sections:

    A. Insuring agreements (defines the coverage granted by the policy)
    B. Exclusions (specific acts or events that the insurer eliminates from the coverage of the policy)
    C. Conditions (defines the rights, privileges, duties, and obligations of the insured and the insurer)
    D. Definitions (defines special meanings assigned to words or phrases in the contract)
    E. Declarations (contains fundamental information of the contract [e.g., name and address of insured, policy period, limits of liability])

II. Review specific reporting requirements of the policy, inclusive of:

    A. What constitutes a reportable claim
    B. Who is to report to the company
    C. How often and in what manner reports are made
    D. Who is to conduct an investigation in the event of a claim

III. Develop a system of classifications for incidents.

IV. Determine which incidents are to be reported to insurers and how often.

V. Request acknowledgment of receipt of incidents from insurer.

VI. Discuss with insurer reports to be received:

    A. Status report on open claims at least quarterly, inclusive of whether suit has been filed, attorney assignments, liability exposure, and other relevant factors
    B. Quarterly loss experience; details all reserved matters and should also include:
        1. Claimant name
        2. Claimant number
        3. Expense reserved
        4. Indemnity reserved
        5. Paid-to-date expense
        6. Date of loss
        7. Paid-to-date indemnity
        8. Total incurred
        9. Brief synopsis of claim

VII. Review loss experience quarterly to determine:

    A. Encroachment on aggregate policy limits
    B. Patterns of frequency and severity
    C. Areas for risk prevention and loss control
    D. Meaningful reports to governing board
    E. Departmental manager's involvement
    F. Time frames for action
    G. Performance criteria and monitors
    H. Control mechanisms

An efficient and effective risk identification mechanism is the foundation for development of the claims-management system. Guidelines must be developed to determine how the information is to be collected, trended, logged in, classified, and shared or transferred, as applicable, depending on the program's scope. Information received from all sources should be logged into the system (computerized or manual) upon receipt. The information log should include:

- Date of receipt
- Date of the incident
- Patient's name
- Patient's identification number
- Location of the incident

Within 24 hours of receipt, each incident should be reviewed and classified for further activity. A simple classification system establishing definitions for each classification in accordance with applicable primary or excess insurance definitions is needed. For example, the claims or risk manager may choose to use the following classifications and definitions:

- Incident: adverse occurrence having no loss potential; to be evaluated for loss prevention, education, statistical analysis, and trending purposes, as applicable
- Investigative incident: adverse occurrence appearing to have some potential loss exposure by description:
  - Will need further investigation to make risk-prevention or loss-control referrals, or liability determination; once this process is complete, a recommendation will be sought as to whether to engage the patient in settlement discussions or vigorously defend care should a claim arise.
  - If questionable exposure, will be suspended for further review, but if patient is questioning care, will describe the process for keeping the patient aware of the investigation

  - If no exposure, will be referred to the quality-assurance department, physician peer review, etc., or used to develop loss-prevention programs
  - If exposure exists, will reconcile with organizational philosophy to disclose and work toward settlement or establish file as potential claim
- Potential claim: adverse occurrence having definite loss potential and exposure; needs complete internal investigation; possible referral for educational purposes, statistical analysis, and loss prevention
- Claim: defined as a written demand for monetary reimbursement; could develop into formal legal action

These simple risk management definitions may be helpful in identifying and classifying information; however, for claims-management purposes, they should be refined further. Insurance companies and self-insured programs generally use three major definitions: incidents, claims, and suits. Consequently, the incident-classification system for claims-management purposes may merge incidents, investigative incidents, and potential claims into a category called incidents. When the manager receives a written demand for compensation, the incident then becomes a claim. If resolution is not achieved and formal legal action is pursued in the judicial system, the claim then becomes a suit.

ESTABLISHING THE CLAIMS FILE

A claims file should be established when it is determined that the possibility of financial loss, liability, or exposure exists. In the event that the institution is procuring coverage with a minimal deductible, this file may be established by the insurance company, and the claims manager's file may be only a monitoring file. The insurance company may require complete investigation by its own investigators but may rely on the claims manager for coordination of the insured's activities, such as locating all relevant records and scheduling staff interviews, and obtaining copies of relevant policies, procedures, and other data. It is important that the claims manager ensure that information in the files that are identified as potential lawsuits be protected from discoverability, whether they be monitoring files or complete in-house investigative files.

Usually the file jacket or folder contains basic identification information on the claim (e.g., claimant's name, claim number). Inside the file, a simple form can be developed manually or run from the computerized claims-management information system to provide pertinent information at a glance. The form should contain the following data:

- Date of incident
- Date of claim
- Allegation
- Claim number
- Date file opened
- Date file closed
- Current status
- Changes in reserves (indemnity and expense)
- Plaintiff's name
- Defendant's name
- Name of plaintiff's attorney
- Name of defense attorney
- Department
- Location
- Diary date
- Disposition of case

The body of the file should be organized and filed in chronological order. The following information should be included:

- Incident report or other source of information
- Date the incident occurred
- Date the incident was reported to the claims-management department
- Date reported to insurer (as applicable)
- Date reported to attorney (as applicable)
- How the information was reported

This information is useful in evaluating the effectiveness of the identification program at a later date. If a significant amount of time elapsed between the incident and when it was reported to the claims-management department, it may indicate a need to educate program participants in the necessity of early reporting and the advantages of prompt investigation and negotiation. The date that the incident is reported to the insurer must be noted for proof of compliance with the insurer's reporting requirements. If the information was reported by someone other than the individual involved, education may be necessary again.

Documentation of the investigation findings and any internal expert physician reviews or evaluations should be contained in the file. Many hospitals, particularly teaching programs, take advantage of the wide variety of faculty specialties and use this expertise to help screen incidents for deviations from standards of care and resultant exposures (see Exhibit 15–2). If a hospital uses this method, it is strongly suggested that education programs for all experts be conducted to discuss confidentiality and objective assessment.

A review of the medical record surrounding the events of the incident should be conducted in detail. The review should not only examine the clinical components of the record but also assess the following:

- Whether the incident is documented in the medical record
- Whether the information is recorded in an objective, factual manner
- Whether there are disparaging or other undesirable comments in the record regarding the patient or among services, consultants, and providers

A summary of the record highlights should be dictated and placed in the file for reference. All correspondence related in any manner to the incident should be included in chronological order in the file. Extremely

Exhibit 15–2 Guidelines for In-House Expert Evaluations

Request a review by the chief of department or designee where the incident occurred, including but not limited to:

1. Expert opinion of patient care, management, and treatment prior to incident or complication, surrounding the incident or complication, and following the incident and throughout discharge

2. Whether there is exposure or deviation from standard of care

3. Whether reasonable steps were taken to avoid incident or complication

4. Opinion of injury and prognosis; whether permanent or temporary

5. Whether complication or injury should have been anticipated

6. Whether policies, procedures, and protocols were observed

7. Whether informed consent was adequate

8. Whether laboratory tests, studies, and consultations were timely and appropriate

9. Whether initial history and physical examination were adequate to make diagnosis

10. Whether there are contradictions, inconsistencies, unnecessary time delays, and possible alterations

11. Whether the incident caused injury or an adverse outcome

---

sensitive information that causes concern to the risk or claims manager should be removed from the file and transferred immediately to the attorney if there is any question of protection of the information. Insureds should be strongly cautioned against keeping copies of sensitive information in their patient files. Plaintiffs' attorneys can legally obtain any information that is considered part of the routine hospital operation.

When it is determined that the file should be transferred to defense counsel for handling, a copy of the assignment letter should accompany copies of relevant information. All notices of claims, assignment of counsel, health-claim arbitration, and other relevant judicial proceedings should be maintained in the file. Copies of status reports from defense counsel and insurers should be reviewed, handled appropriately, and placed in the file, along with documentation of expense payments, medical bills, and other items.

The manager should request that the medical record, original X-ray films, pathology specimens, and other clinical evidence be sequestered in their respective departments. This ensures that the originals are available and have not been tampered with as legal proceedings progress. All equipment involved in an injury should be evaluated and sequestered (see Exhibit 15–3).

Sequestering can be as simplified as requiring that the items in question be placed in a locked area with limited, monitored access within the specific department. Requests for sequestering by the claims office can be refined to standard format, with copies of the requests placed in the file. Written notification should be requested from the departments if the information is not available, so the manager can begin an early and extensive search, if necessary. Lost or misplaced information may create difficulty in negotiating a claim.

At the conclusion of the initial investigation, a claim summary or brief of not more

Exhibit 15–3 Checklist for Equipment Incidents

1. Sequester the equipment involved in the incident under lock and key immediately.

2. Do not test or alter the equipment except under controlled circumstances.

3. Take pictures, if possible, under attorney supervision.

4. Obtain copies of maintenance contract and service records.

5. Review contracts for hold-harmless language from the manufacturer.

6. Determine responsibility for service and maintenance (internal and external).

7. Obtain independent testing, if necessary.

8. Obtain name of manufacturer, serial number, and purchase records.

9. Determine if alerts issued by manufacturer were known and observed.

10. Make determination in cooperation with the defense attorney as to whether equipment should be returned to service or repaired, or whether another action should be taken.

than three pages should be placed in the file. A checklist that details elements of the initial investigation should include:

- Claimant information: name, date of birth, gender, address, telephone number, marital status, occupation, employer, income, dependents, and other relevant social factors
- Insured defendant information: name, address, telephone number, medical staff or employment status, specialty, involvement in case, and insurance information (policy number, policy period, limits)
- Co-defendant information: name, address, telephone number, medical staff or employment status, specialty, involvement in case, and insurance information (insurance carrier, policy number, policy period, limits)
- Claimant's allegations of improper treatment
- Claimant's injuries: nature of injury, extent of injury (temporary or permanent, partial or total), additional treatment required as a result of the injury, medical examination results, and prognosis

- Medical-record review: medical-record number, dates of admission and discharge, admitting history, admitting and discharge diagnoses, chronology of treatment, review of physician and nursing notes, laboratory reports, consent forms, and other relevant documents
- Interviews of physicians, hospital staff, and other witnesses to the incident
- What information was disclosed to the patient concerning the event
- Copies of relevant hospital policies, procedures, and protocols
- Results of any expert review, peer review, or other administrative review of the incident
- Equipment incidents: name and address of equipment manufacturer, copies of purchase information and warranties, copies of equipment-maintenance contracts and equipment-maintenance reports, reports from clinical-engineering department subsequent to incident, reports of similar problems with type of equipment in question (from within the institution or from outside sources such as the Food and Drug Administration and the Emergency Care Research Institute)

- Evaluation of the damages claimed
- Evaluation of liability: applicable standard of care; responsibility of involved parties, including assessment of co-defendant's liability
- Settlement value and strategy

The summary saves lengthy reviews of the entire file by providing a brief synopsis of the following items:

- Pertinent points from the record of the clinical course
- Claimants
- Possible defendants
- Allegations
- Legal status
- Deviations from standard of care
- Plaintiff's counsel
- Defense counsel
- Witness testimony
- Demand
- Comments
- Future activity

The initial investigation should be completed within 30 days of notification of the incident and the file updated as additional information is received. Ongoing evaluation dates are necessary to ensure appropriate monitoring and evaluation. Monitoring of ongoing events (e.g., testimony of experts and witnesses) and regular updates of the patient's clinical status are necessary to keep abreast of significant factors that may influence liability and exposure. A status-report checklist should include:

- Current status of patient
- Autopsy report
- Medical-record deficiencies
- Follow-up activities conducted to date
- Documentation and status of all persons involved
- Medical bills or charges
- Patient profile including family history, employment status, insurance coverage, and dependents
- Patient and family response to incident

- Expert review
- Record review
- Sequestered medical records, X-ray, pathology specimens
- Source of incident

INVESTIGATIVE TECHNIQUES

Legal counsel should be consulted when the claim appears to be one that will proceed to litigation to ensure protection from discoverability of data and to review pertinent policies and the extent of the risk or claim manager's responsibility. It is necessary to decide, for example, whether the manager will take witness statements, discuss the case in detail with involved providers, make referrals, and gather specific information for in-house files. The attorney should aid in establishing these basic ground rules in accordance with legal and insurance restraints. The organization, in its intention to integrate robust patient safety practices with risk management, may need to differentiate between the investigation and analysis of near-miss events and those where a patient suffered harm and has threatened legal action.

If it is determined that the aforementioned activities are indeed within the scope of the claim manager's responsibility, he or she will discuss the facts of each incident with the physician and other involved staff members after a review of the medical record. Interviews should be concise, timely, and factual. For the sake of objectivity, it is important that the interviewer not lead the interviewee. All information should be verified and substantiated as far as possible without compromising the integrity of the investigation. Personnel with direct or indirect knowledge of the matter should be noted regardless of whether they are to be interviewed. Interview statements must become a part of the permanent claim file. It is recommended that the interviewer take detailed notes of a meeting rather than obtain a long written and signed statement. A summary of the meeting should be written and placed in the body of the claim file.

The investigation should identify all personnel involved in the care of the patient at the time of the occurrence. The current name, address, and telephone number of each person should be obtained. It is also useful to include his or her work status (e.g., full time, part time, contractual) and work location.

An objective report of the actual interview must be documented. The manager should determine how the patient and family were advised of the incident. It is important to record the patient's and family's reactions to the incident, their support system, interactions, and social factors, and their reactions to the staff before and after the incident. The staff should keep the manager aware of the patient's status, attitudes, and other significant information throughout the hospitalization. The manager should also determine the economic history of the patient, whether there are any dependents, the source of payment for clinical care, and whether there were any witnesses to the incident. Witnesses' names, addresses, and telephone numbers must be recorded (see Exhibit 15–4).

EVALUATION OF THE MEDICAL RECORD

The medical record should be reviewed, if possible, while the patient is still in the hospital. State statutes determine whether negotiations with the patient can take place during the hospitalization, but it is important to review the incident and effect risk-control and loss-prevention measures as quickly as possible.

If a formal complaint has been lodged, a meticulous review of all related medical records from the viewpoint of the allegations as presented in the complaint is necessary. If an early-warning identification system is in place, evaluation of the record may occur prior to presentation of any formal action. In these circumstances, the manager must assess the potential areas of liability and exposure. The record review should include any emergency and outpatient clinic records. It is helpful to find out exactly what is considered part of the patient's medical record (e.g., electrocardiogram tracings, fetal-monitoring strips), because hospitals are held increasingly accountable for the loss of this type of documentation.

Exhibit 15–4 Checklist for Conducting Staff Interviews

1. Obtain objective report of the incident.

2. Determine if, how, and by whom the patient was advised of the incident.

3. Determine patient's reaction to the incident.

4. Determine family's reaction to the incident.

5. Evaluate family's support system and interaction.

6. Evaluate social factors of patient.

7. Determine the patient's and family's interactions with, and attitudes toward, the staff before and after the incident.

8. Advise the staff to keep the manager informed of the patient's status and attitude as well as other significant factors throughout the hospitalization.

9. Ascertain the economic history of patient and any dependents, and the source of bill payment.

10. Determine if there were any witnesses to the incident; document names, addresses, and telephone numbers.

When reviewing the medical record, the entire record should be assessed, not just those facts surrounding the particular incident. There is always the possibility that the cause of an alleged claim is a result of a previously unidentified incident. Consequently, the review should be focused on all potential areas of liability, as well as those in the claim. The review should be accomplished by someone knowledgeable in acceptable standards of medical care appropriate to the case and should be supplemented by findings from interviews with providers directly involved in the patient's care.

Exhibits 15–5 and 15–6 provide general guidelines to follow when reviewing medical records.

BILL ABATEMENTS

Often the issue of medical-bill abatement surfaces in an adverse incident that involves a patient. Whether to abate a hospital bill is a matter of philosophy in many instances. Some hospital administrators feel that abatement of a bill acknowledges guilt, whereas others believe that it mitigates damages and establishes a sense of good will.

In hospitals where bill abatement is evaluated on a case-by-case basis, general guidelines and criteria should be established to ensure uniform evaluation. Among these criteria are the following:

- A review of the bill for adjustment
- A complete review of the medical record surrounding the alleged injury
- Independent evaluation of the treatment to determine specific deviations from the standard of care
- Consultation with, and recommendations of, the direct providers related to the alleged injury
- Objective assessment of the outcome of the incident or complication (e.g., prolonged hospital stay, damages, injury, additional procedures, additional incurred costs)
- Assessment of patient's and family's attitudes toward staff before the incident
- Assessment of patient's and family's attitudes toward the incident
- Availability of third-party coverage
- Liability and other negative exposures

The manager should consider whether abatement can make amends to the patient

Exhibit 15–5 Guidelines to Medical-Record Review

1. Always attempt to review the medical record while the patient is in the hospital.

2. Note documentation of the incident in the medical record.

3. Note any mention of an incident report being filed in the medical record.

4. Document any reference that the family and patient were advised of the incident, as well as any documented descriptive comments of the patient or family.

5. Check to see if an attorney has requested the record.

6. Observe whether there is any criticism of the treatment, management, or staff in the record.

7. Note any negative or unsubstantiated comments that have been written by the staff regarding the patient or family.

8. Note whether the record appears to follow a defined rationale or if it has loose ends.

9. Note legibility of documentation.

10. Note any area that could be construed as altered documentation.

Exhibit 15–6 Medical-Record Review Checklist

1. What was the date of admission (note prolonged stay)?
2. What was the reason for admission?
3. Is there any mention of previous incidents, complications, allergic reactions, and/or complaints regarding quality of care?
4. What was the admitting history?
5. Compare admitting diagnosis with treatment, appropriate tests, consultations, and other clinical actions.
6. If a change in diagnosis or condition warranted transfer to another area, was it accomplished in a timely manner?
7. When did the physician first see and examine the patient?
8. Is there appropriate correlation among physicians' orders, laboratory reports, nurses' notes, and progress notes?
9. Was original surgery or admission necessary?
10. Was the consent form signed by a physician?
11. What risks are specifically mentioned?
12. Does the consent form conform to performed surgery?
13. Were additional procedures done?
14. Do progress notes conform to the procedure and consent form?
15. What does the operative note state? Is it standard?
16. What were the dates when the operative notes were dictated and transcribed?
17. Is there a written progress note of the operation and does it describe the incident? If so, how?
18. Does the anesthesia note collaborate with the progress notes?
19. Does the anesthesia note indicate any difficulty in intubation, excessive anesthesia time, or other problems?
20. Were preoperative electrocardiogram and chest radiograph evaluations included in the anesthesia preoperative note?
21. How long was the patient in the recovery room?
22. Note nurses' notes on patient's arrival in unit, general status, and condition.
23. Are there long gaps in nursing observation notes?
24. Compare the time of surgery to the first indication of complication or incident discovery.
25. Was the patient appropriately monitored and observed by all involved staff?
26. Note any inconsistencies between the physician's and nurses' notes.
27. Note any delays in diagnosis, prescription for appropriate treatment, and implementation of treatment.
28. Were consultants used appropriately, and was there a timely referral?
29. Does the record reflect the patient's complaints or lack thereof at each visit?
30. Do the examination and disposition reflect attention to the complaint?
31. Is there follow-up documentation that test results were reviewed?

or family to the extent that it can stop costly litigation and promote an environment conducive to further negotiation. A signed release form from the patient should be considered, unless it would jeopardize an already fragile resolution.

EFFECTIVE COMMUNICATION

Communication is essential to effective claims control. In addition to notifying insurance carriers and defense counsel as applicable, claims management must keep appropriate senior administration aware of necessary information. As has already been noted, the claims manager must be aware of the policy of the organization relative to full disclosure and also have regular dialogue with the patient or the patient's designated representative. The manager should identify circumstances in which the administration and the organization's board requires notification of routine and unique claim matters.

Other issues should be brought immediately to the senior administrator's attention. Those issues include the following:

- Potential adverse publicity
- Cross claims and third-party actions
- Excessive difficulty with a particular program participant

- Possibility of a significant adverse verdict
- Notification of trial dates

SETTLEMENT NEGOTIATIONS

Many organizations with in-house programs choose to spread responsibility and authority for settlements between the claims manager and an advisory committee (often called a claims management or review committee). The committee reviews the outcomes of the claims-management process and provides ongoing internal review of active claims and settlements, whether handled by defense counsel or the claims manager.

The responsibilities of the committee may include the following:

- Provides expert evaluation in claims and suits as requested
- Aids in the development of claim management philosophy, policy, and procedure
- Reviews and approves claim strategies and settlements to the extent of approved reserves
- Evaluates the appropriateness of a structured settlement as a means for resolving a case involving serious injury (see Exhibit 15–7)

Exhibit 15–7 When to Use Structured Settlements

Using structured settlements for the payment of large or catastrophic claims can benefit both the plaintiff and the defendant. Some states now mandate the acceptance of structured settlements or periodic payments in cases where a large portion of the award relates to future medical costs. This form of award enables the hospital (or other defendant) to purchase an annuity or similar program that provides for future payouts at scheduled increments. Types of structured settlements include the following:

- Annuity contracts
- Trusts funded with U.S. Treasury bonds
- Funds for rehabilitation
- Lump-sum payments of cash to compensate for lost income, medical expenses, and attorney's fees (Generally these payments include past expenses and out-of-pocket losses.)
- Reversionary medical trust to pay for ongoing or future medical care
- Educational fund for the benefit of the victim's dependent children
- Term insurance to pay for funeral expenses

(continued)

Exhibit 15–7 (Continued)

Many cases are well suited for the use of structured settlements. The most common types include the following:

- Wrongful death, especially when there are surviving dependents
- Serious personal-injury cases in which substantial future medical expenses are anticipated, such as:
  - Irreversible brain damage
  - Quadriplegia or paraplegia
  - Injuries resulting in permanent disabilities that limit or prevent the injured from future gainful employment
  - Injuries in which it is anticipated that the injured party will require lifetime physical therapy
- All cases involving minors
- All cases involving incompetents
- All cases in which the injured party would be unable to pay for future education for himself or herself or for dependents' education
- Cases involving substantial judgments and large attorney's fees, especially if the fees represent one third or more of a judgment
- Cases in which an attempt is made to bridge the gap between high cash demands and realistic evaluations, especially in those where liability may be difficult to ascertain (including claims in which issues related to liability become overshadowed by the emotional impact of significant injury (e.g., a severely injured infant)

When the committee reviews a claim, it is often helpful to have the chief of service of the department in which it occurred at the meeting, in addition to the physicians assigned to the committee. The chief of service can assist in refining the clinical aspects of the claim, identify potential experts, and offer information about departmental claim activity that can be useful in quality and risk management assessments.

Whether claim reserving is conducted in-house or provided by an insurance company adjuster or a contractual service, it is necessary to determine whether the claims manager, the review committee, or both, have authority to approve payment of funds for settlement purposes. Many factors must be considered when claims are negotiated in-house. It is imperative that an objective and factual evaluation of the incident, damages, treatment, and prognosis be completed for each claim.

The risk or claims manager should specifically analyze the claims allegations and evaluate special damages (costs outside of clinical treatment, physical therapy, radiographs, and other hospital services). It is important to keep these damages under control. When possible, the institution's resources can be used for follow-up care.

The organization's liability through its employees and the exposure in relation to the verification and extent of injuries must be evaluated. It is necessary to verify coverage of the persons involved in the incident and identify any factors that may influence the plaintiff's posture. The manager should also consider other factors that may have a significant impact on the case, such as medical coverage and public attitudes.

State statutes should be reviewed to determine if any reform measures could affect the claim (e.g., a cap on non-economic damages).

It is important that the claims manager remain in control during discussions with the plaintiff's counsel. The manager should evaluate the plaintiff's position objectively, state his or her position, consider the attorney's response, and evaluate the demand. The manager should not feel pressured into any commitment before reevaluation and should be very careful not to educate the plaintiff's counsel.

When all aspects of the claim have been fully evaluated and the manager needs further guidance, defense counsel should be used whether or not it has been officially retained. Following this thorough investigative process, the claims risk manager and hospital administration may elect to notify the plaintiff and/or his or her attorney of their desire to settle or deny the claim. They may also elect to continue their investigation until further evidence of fault or injury can be established. Form letters can be developed to be used at this phase of the investigation process.

LITIGATION MANAGEMENT

Litigation management is an often-neglected area of claims administration. Specific guidelines for managing defense counsel should be established and discussed with counsel prior to retention. At minimum, the following seven factors should be considered in developing guidelines and objectives for sound litigation management:

1. Criteria used in the selection and assignment of counsel are:
   - History of prior success in the area of medical malpractice, especially in trials of complex injury cases. (Request a list of claims that were settled by the firm and those resolved via a defense verdict.)
   - Evidence of technical expertise of the firm's staff (e.g., a registered nurse/attorney or physician/attorney).
   - Evidence that senior partners with the most trial experience and expertise will be directly involved in handling appropriate cases. (Less-experienced, and hopefully, less-costly counsel should be available for routine motions and initial discovery.)
   - Evidence that the firm has access to quality medical experts and the respect of local physicians.

2. Preliminary evaluation from counsel, completed within 2 weeks from the date of case assignment, includes the following reports:
   - An analysis of each element of negligence
   - An identification of all potentially culpable defendants
   - An identification of the various potential defenses that might be successful
   - A list of the types of experts that would be most appropriate and the names of persons who could be engaged as experts
   - An analysis of the skill and expertise of opposing counsel, if that person has been identified
   - A timetable for the development of the case in anticipation of trial or settlement

3. Timetables for reporting actions. The risk or claims manager and defense counsel should share their timetables to allow them both to remain continually apprised of significant developments of the case. The manager should ask that defense counsel agree to abide by the timetables.

4. Motions that must be approved by the institution prior to the defense counsel's instigation include:
   - Any motion that might serve to affect the material elements of a case
   - Any motion that might serve to add additional parties to the litigation
   - Any motion that might seek to bring about an outcome not anticipated by the parties to the litigation

5. Copies of the following documents should be furnished to the risk or claims manager:
   - Original summons and complaints, and any amendments thereto
   - Summary of all expert depositions that are material to the successful defense of malpractice claims

- Any offers of settlement or dismissal, including offers to dismiss a single defendant when there are multiple parties involved in the litigation
- Evaluation of an injured plaintiff performed by a damage expert or by an economist
- Any other documents that the initial investigation and evaluation identify as being potentially material to the complete evaluation of the discovery process

6. Legal-fee and expense guidelines
7. Methods to evaluate the counsel's performance

CONCLUSION

Development of an effective claims-management system requires top-level commitment, establishment of clear goals and objectives, and an accurate assessment of resources, requirements, structure, corporate culture, and scope of responsibility. Managers should meet with legal counsel prior to development of the system so that it will be effective in maintaining confidentiality and protection from discoverability of collected data. Clear policies and procedures regarding the process must be developed and communicated to all participants. Full support of legal counsel, the administration, the professional staff, and the governing board is absolutely necessary. Their commitment serves as the foundation of the program.

16

Principles for Strategic Discovery

Stacey A. Cischke, JD
Stephen Pavkovic, JD, MPH, BSN

INTRODUCTION

Despite aggressive risk management techniques, including proactive disclosure policies and patient-focused care models, individual healthcare providers and institutions face a real threat of becoming defendants in malpractice lawsuits. While the majority of professional-negligence suits get resolved before jury disposition, few lawsuits get resolved without the initiation of court-mandated discovery.

Each professional-negligence complaint involves unique facts, parties, and venues. This chapter provides the healthcare risk manager with a survey of common professional-negligence discovery principles and recommends the steps risk managers can take to create coordinated, strategic discovery responses. Through a strategic approach to litigation discovery, risk managers can control unnecessary healthcare litigation losses and increase efficiency when answering inquires from legal, regulatory, or accreditation agencies.

LITIGATION FOUNDATIONS

In general, civil litigation results when a claimant ("plaintiff") files a civil claim ("lawsuit") against a defendant, stating that the defendant's actions, or omissions, caused the claimant's loss. A medical-malpractice lawsuit is a specific type of civil action in which the plaintiff seeks recovery for injuries that the plaintiff believes were caused by the defendant's failure to meet an established professional duty of care. Defendants in medical-malpractice lawsuits are usually individual physicians, hospitals, and physician or medical practice groups ("defendants"). In the two phases of discovery, written and oral, the plaintiff and defendants ("parties") collect and share information. Written discovery is the exchange of written questions ("interrogatories") and requests for the production of documents and tangible items. In the oral-discovery phase, the parties frequently identify and depose fact and expert opinion witnesses. In the absence of lawsuit dismissal or settlement, the facts collected during the discovery phase are presented to a judge or jury during a trial as the ultimate trier of fact.

State and federal courts follow specific procedural rules for all aspects of civil litigation, and the jurisdiction where a medical-negligence lawsuit is pending dictates how the pre-trial discovery process proceeds. The applicable civil-procedure rules dictate the type and format of produced documents, the timeliness of production, and the penalties for failing to produce those documents within a party's control. In some jurisdictions, professional negligence, including medical-malpractice claims, have specific interrogatories, production requests, and other rules that govern the use of healthcare information, treating-physician testimony, and the identification of medical experts. To increase accuracy and efficiency in future discovery responses, risk managers should be familiar with the rules that govern discovery and civil procedure in their particular jurisdiction.

LAWSUIT LOSSES

For healthcare defendants, lawsuits involve uncertain risks and the potential for significant loss. Lawsuit uncertainty arises from the inherent inability to predict either judicial rulings or jury decisions, and from the challenges of determining the actual dollar-exposure amounts. Direct economic losses can arise from defense costs including legal representation and expert fees, decreased personnel productivity, claim processing or administrative costs, and, ultimately, from claim disposition. Indirect litigation costs are always difficult to ascertain but can arise from opportunity and reputational losses related to lawsuit publicity and resolution. Risk managers should remain mindful that performing their daily investigations and discovery responses in an efficient, strategic manner could prevent avoidable losses from excessive fees and court sanction.

PROACTIVE RISK AND CLAIMS MANAGEMENT

Unlike defendants that rely solely on commercial insurance lines for professional-liability insurance coverage, healthcare defendants that retain "first-layer" coverage with a self-insurance retention (SIR) maintain more control over their pre-suit activities. For example, healthcare providers with an SIR can engage their risk managers to conduct a pre-suit investigation or retain experts without the need for external approval. This early proactive approach may provide insight into the appropriateness of patient disclosure, the identification of potential evidence, and cataloging concerns related to weaknesses of the anticipated defense. Pre-suit SIR-supported investigations may also identify unknown patient safety issues and lead to previously unidentified loss-prevention opportunities. Figure 16–1 illustrates the transition from the traditional discovery model to a discovery model that incorporates important information obtained through risk management and patient safety investigations.

LITIGATION POSTURE

Reliable and thorough pre-suit investigation provides valuable insight into a defendant's response if the investigated matter becomes a lawsuit. For those matters not investigated at the pre-suit stage, defendants' lawsuit response is determined by their litigation posture. Institutions and providers consider multiple factors to define their litigation posture. Although the majority of these factors involve the same enterprise-risk-management considerations as any business decision, the factors specific to healthcare defendants in professional-negligence litigation include:

- Governing board direction, if any
- A party's ability to control pre-suit activities via SIR

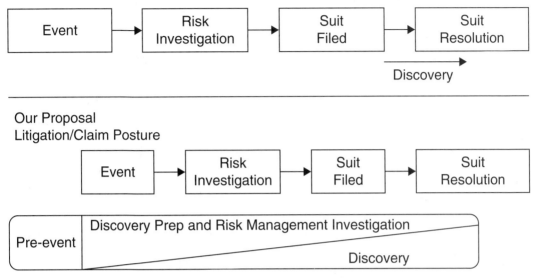

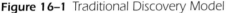

Figure 16–1 Traditional Discovery Model

- The insurance-market climate and the availability of commercial coverage ("soft" vs "hard" market)
- A defendant's litigation history and tolerance for publicity related to lawsuits
- Venue, including court and jurisdiction rules, recent jury decisions, and awards
- The requirement of physician (or other insured) consent to settle the case

LITIGATION RESPONSE

Once a lawsuit is filed, the healthcare defendant must consider the merits of the suit within the context of its litigation posture to determine a litigation response. At this early litigation stage, risk managers, the product of their investigations, and their organizational knowledge may play a critical role in defining a litigation response. Assigned defense counsel plays an additional critical role. Litigation counsel can provide valuable insight into how the known facts at the start of a lawsuit may play out during the life of the suit. Additional

factors that may direct a healthcare defendant's litigation response include:

- The quality of anticipated witnesses, anticipated discovery responses, and the product expert review
- The magnitude of injury
- The verdict potential
- The caliber of opposing counsel
- The likelihood of success on the merits
- Information learned through oral and written discovery
- In rare circumstances, the need to "send a message" to the plaintiff's bar and venue observers by trying a case with a high likelihood of success, even when the plaintiff's demand is reasonably exceeded by the anticipated costs of defense

Based upon these factors, some organizations have adopted absolute positions for all claims and others have adopted conditionally responsive ones.

The information provided through accurate and timely risk investigations and discovery responses can support a defendant's litigation posture and position. Poorly coordinated or inattentive discovery responses can result in serial discovery supplements and discrepancies between the written interrogatory responses and deposition testimony. When this occurs, a defendant's veracity may become an issue in the litigation and unnecessarily burden a defendant's standing before the court and jury. Inaccurate discovery responses can also lead to court-imposed discovery sanctions including monetary fines, exclusion of supportive evidence, and witness testimony.

SPOLIATION

Aside from a defendant's duty to produce evidence during the course of a lawsuit, the loss of medical information can lead to a *separate, independent action* against a healthcare provider, premised upon the theory of spoliation of evidence. A spoliation action seeks damages not for negligent medical care, but for a breach of the duty to preserve medical evidence. In the healthcare context, this type of action arises from the loss of key medical records or films, medical devices or instruments used during the care and treatment at issue, and even the loss of non-medical information such as phone records.

Risk managers can work to prevent spoliation actions with effective medical-information-maintenance policies and procedures. Consistent and established policies regarding the maintenance of health information, the preservation of medical devices, and communication protocols for preserving health information once there is reasonable belief that a lawsuit may be filed will assist in preventing a spoliation action. Some common potential-litigation warning signs include an executed patient authorization for release of medical records produced by an attorney, a request for films and billing records, and a patient and/or family that is very upset about an unexpected or dramatic outcome. To identify loss-control opportunities, these patient factors need to be considered within the context of an organization's litigation posture.

WRITTEN DISCOVERY

Written discovery is the first phase of the discovery process in a medical-negligence case. Written discovery usually involves two types of requests: an initial set of written interrogatories, and a request to produce documents and tangible items, such as records, films, and pathology slides. Many states have codified standard interrogatories and requests for production used in personal-injury and professional-negligence cases in their civil-practice code. The rationale behind the use of standardized interrogatories is that they make the written-discovery process more efficient, expeditious, and economical.[1] Form interrogatories and production requests help the courts manage the litigation of cases with issues that arise on a consistent basis. Standard interrogatories are not necessarily mandatory, and most jurisdictions allow parties to propound non-standard interrogatories with the court's permission. Risk manager knowledge of the applicable written-discovery interrogatories and the types of required information is the basis for a strategic discovery response.

STANDARD INTERROGATORIES AND REQUESTS TO PRODUCE

To respond consistently and efficiently to written discovery, a risk manager should anticipate the information typically requested in all medical-negligence cases and specific information related to the claim of professional or institutional negligence. The number and scope of standard interrogatories allowed varies from jurisdiction to jurisdiction. Nonetheless, common information requested of healthcare providers include:

- Medical-liability insurance coverage
- Prior litigation history
- Whether any peer-review or quality-improvement hearings were conducted

with respect to the care at issue in the lawsuit

- Information regarding the patient's medical history prior to the care at issue in the lawsuit
- Identification and disclosure of any hospital policies relevant to the care and treatment at issue
- Information regarding the identification and employment status of individuals involved in the relevant care and treatment of the patient or who have knowledge of the medical treatment at issue in the lawsuit
- Disclosure and production of all medical information that pertains to the patient, including records, letters/reports from healthcare providers, films, drawings, diagrams, photographs, and electronic data
- Witnesses who may be called to testify at trial
- Proof of The Joint Commission or other accreditation
- Medical-staff bylaws, policies, and procedures, or other documents that govern the scope of medical-staff practices

Most jurisdictions impose a continuing duty upon the parties to seasonally supplement their written-discovery responses with new or additional information identified during the course of discovery. The failure to fully and accurately respond to written discovery, or the failure to seasonably supplement prior discovery responses, can lead to sanctions, such as the exclusion of evidence, monetary sanctions, or in rare circumstances resolution by dismissal or summary judgment. Risk managers and litigation counsel need to coordinate efforts to timely complete any supplemental discovery requests and to evaluate the discoverability of any new or additional information identified during the pendency of the lawsuit.

MEDICAL RECORDS

In medical-malpractice cases, discoverability of medical records is determined by the record's relevance to the allegations. The medical records that pertain to the care and treatment at issue are always relevant, and records that document prior and subsequent care are likely to be considered relevant. Many state laws adopt a broad definition of "medical record" to include all communications in any form or medium, maintained for purposes of patient diagnosis or treatment, including medical records that are prepared by a healthcare provider or by other providers. Some state statutes specifically designate X-rays, laboratory tests, computed tomography imaging, magnetic resonance imaging, electroencephalograms, electrocardiograms, and other tests conducted within the hospital as part of a patient's "medical records."

To provide consistent and accurate responses to the patient and plaintiff's requests for medical records, risk managers participating in discovery need to work closely with medical-records personnel and know both their jurisdictional definition of a "medical record" and their own organization's definitions. Of particular concern in discovery is what are the elements that constitute the patient's "final" or "official" chart? When different versions of hospital documents are produced in discovery, or when medical records are not produced in an accurate, timely, and consistent manner, additional requests for discovery will likely follow. These additional requests may come in the form of a motion to compel with the potential for a contempt order and could include:

- An inspection of the original records by the plaintiff's attorney
- Production of the institutional record-keeping policies and procedures
- Production of electronically stored information (ESI) such as a medical-record electronic-audit trail, document-access information, etc.
- Testimony by a representative of the departments of risk management, medical records, and/or information technology

- Possible requests for access to hospital computers and databases for independent computer forensic-analysis mirror imaging or copying of a hard drive

RELEVANT MEDICAL INFORMATION THAT IS NOT THE MEDICAL RECORD

In addition to traditional medical records, other relevant medical information is commonly requested in the course of discovery. Examples include paper radiology or pathology requisitions, nursing-staff schedules, medical-staff privilege and credentialing files, change-of-shift reports, surgical-count sheets, and patient-satisfaction questionnaires.

Often, relevant medical information is automatically created and electronically stored without direct knowledge of care providers. For example, call-light utilization and response records, paging records, patient census and acuity records, electronic medical-record-access audits, draft-dictation reports, and electronic door access logs may be retained in some electronic form.

For the risk manager, this type of ESI can complicate the issue of identifying relevant and discoverable information. The ESI's litigation relevance is demonstrated when the retained information provides data that are not otherwise present in the patient's permanent medical records. Analysis of ESI may also provide insight into the thought processes that supported medical decisions. For example, ESI may indicate the order in which electronic medical records were accessed, the length of time that individual documents were opened for review, and the length of time between document review and report dictation.

The creation and storage of potentially relevant medical information, including ESI, may vary from department to department. Accurate and complete discovery responses require that the risk manager work closely with hospital personnel, survey the available

retained information, and understand the following:

- Where the organization may have potentially relevant medical information
- Where and how it is kept
- How long it is maintained
- Who is responsible for the maintenance of such information
- Any policies regarding the maintenance and/or destruction of these records

Once a survey of the available relevant medical information and ESI is completed, the risk manager will need to coordinate with defense counsel to create efficient, reliable discovery responses.

POLICIES AND PROCEDURES

Policies and procedures are frequently requested and produced during discovery. In fact, some states include the production of healthcare policies and procedures as part of the standard written medical-negligence discovery.[2] When analyzing a potential claim or even after litigation has already been initiated, it is important to anticipate and assess what policies, procedures, or protocols may be requested during discovery. Proactive risk manager identification and analysis of potentially relevant policies and procedures will help to further refine a defendant's litigation response.

Policies and procedures are often used in litigation to show whether the defendants followed expected protocols and may provide the basis for cross-examination of medical witnesses during trial. Early risk management evaluation as to whether any gross deviations from hospital policies or procedures, without reasonable medical justification for doing so, is a very important step in evaluating an institutional defendant's litigation response in a particular case. A gross or obvious deviation from policy/procedures on a key issue in a case may be very difficult to defend and may help identify that case as a candidate for early resolution in order to minimize public exposure and unnecessary litigation costs.

Policies and procedures are reviewed and modified at regular intervals. Risk management knowledge of an organization's process for policy review, assessment, and retention is key to preparing written-discovery responses and producing accurate documents. For discovery, it is important to produce only the applicable policies and procedures that were enacted at the time of the occurrence at issue. The plaintiff may frequently request past policies to lead to the discovery of other relevant information. Risk management should participate with clinical personnel to determine policy and procedure retention practices that comply with an organization's litigation posture.

QUALITY-IMPROVEMENT DOCUMENTS

The plaintiff may request the production of documents generated during quality-improvement activities. In many jurisdictions, these documents are privileged and not discoverable because of the larger public-policy objective that permits healthcare providers to improve the delivery of patient care without the threat that the product of a critical internal review will be used against the defendant in a civil suit. Risk managers should strategize with litigation counsel, in-house counsel, and other relevant quality directors on the best practices for structuring, documenting, and protecting a healthcare provider's quality-improvement activities. Specific issues to be considered for regular review include the organization, structure, and membership of various quality committees; how and by whom the quality process can be initiated; and who is responsible for managing the documentation of the quality processes. Risk managers should understand the particular privileges that may apply to protect a quality-improvement committee's work and the jurisdictional rules required to enable that protection. With this knowledge, risk managers can provide discovery responses that maintain the available privilege protections within their organization's litigation posture and response.

Some examples of materials that are protected from disclosure include:

- Medical journals used by a peer-review committee obtained as a result of assignments given during committee meetings and used by the committee in its deliberations[3]
- Recommendations and internal conclusions of committees that may or may not lead to ultimate decisions or actions taken by the committee or hospital[4]
- Letters of reference from doctors assessing physicians' professional competence generated at the request of the hospital credentialing committee for use in determining whether permanent privileges should be extended to a physician[5]
- Documents that consist of annual evaluations of physicians by the chairman of hospital's department, memorandum from the chairman to the credentialing committee, and a confidential physician-evaluation form[6]

Materials that are not protected from discovery in professional-malpractice lawsuits include:

- Hospital credentialing requirements as codified in its regulations and bylaws[7]
- Evidence of actual changes that were adopted because of the recommendations and internal conclusions of the committee[8]
- "Results" of a committee that take the form of ultimate decisions made or actions taken by the committee or hospital including revocation, modification or restriction of privileges, letters of resignation or withdrawal, and revision of rules, regulations, policies, and procedures[9]
- Applications for privileges and educational transcripts generated prior to the peer-review process[10]

E-DISCOVERY

The Federal Rules of Civil Procedure specifically address the scope of e-discovery in federal cases. Rule 26(b)(2)(B) of the Federal Rules of Civil Procedure governs the discovery of ESI providing that:

> A party need not provide discovery of ESI from sources that the party identifies as not reasonably accessible because of undue burden or cost. On motion to compel discovery or for a protective order, the party from whom discovery is sought must show that the information is not reasonably accessible because of undue burden or cost. If that showing is made, the court may nonetheless order discovery from such sources if the requesting party shows good cause. . . . The court may specify the conditions for the discovery.

The Seventh Circuit has formed an electronic discovery committee to address electronic discovery issues and establish agreed-upon principles for the discovery of ESI. The goal of the principles is to encourage the parties to participate in early and informal information exchange on commonly encountered issues.[11] These principles set the groundwork for litigants and thinking about e-discovery. Many state courts have adopted FRCP 26 (b)(2)(B) and incorporated the federal rule into their own discovery rules. Other states take a contrary approach to the federal rule and note that a party may be ordered to produce electronic information even when the party shows that the requested information is not reasonably accessible because of cost or undue burden.

In the absence of exceptional circumstances, courts generally are reluctant to impose sanctions for the failure to produce ESI lost as a result of the routine, good-faith operation of an electronic-information sys-tem. Risk managers seeking to claim that ESI was not retained due to the routine, good-faith systems maintenance, need to be prepared to provide evidence of their organization's information-destruction policy. Despite this good-faith defense, once a defendant has received notice of filed litigation, all risk managers should adopt a prudent approach to the routine destruction of potentially relevant information with, and coordinate all records activities with, defense counsel.

The Sedona Principles

The Sedona Conference is a charitable, research, and educational institute dedicated to the advancement of law and policy in the areas of antitrust law, complex litigation, and intellectual-property rights. As part of its attention to the area of complex litigation, the Sedona Conference has developed principles and best-practice recommendations for electronic-document retention and production. The Sedona Conference developed some basic principles that risk managers will find valuable in identifying and producing ESI in the course of, or in anticipation of, litigation.[12] The guidelines are as follows:

1. Where litigation is anticipated but no plaintiff has emerged or other considerations make it impossible to initiate a dialogue, the producing party should make preservation decisions by a process that conforms to that set forth in the Decision Tree.

2. As soon as feasible, preservation issues should be openly and cooperatively discussed in sufficient detail so that the parties can reach mutually satisfactory accommodation and also evaluate the need, if any, to seek court intervention or assistance.

3. In conjunction with the initial discussions or where appropriate in the response to discovery requests, the parties should clearly identify the inaccessi-

ble sources reasonably related to the discovery or claims that are not being searched or preserved.

4. A party should exercise caution when it decides, for business reasons, to move potentially discoverable information subject to preservation from accessible to less-accessible data stores.

5. It is acceptable practice, in the absence of an applicable preservation duty, for entities to manage their information in a way that minimizes accumulations of inaccessible data, provided that adequate provisions are made to accommodate preservation imperatives.

Additional ESI Considerations

With the explosion of ESI, some organizations are contracting with independent, third-party vendors to handle the storage and management of electronic medical data. Risk managers should consider including specific indemnification language in any written agreement with outside vendors, in the event that any ESI is destroyed in a manner that is inconsistent with the terms of the written agreement and/or provider's policies and procedures for ESI. The failure to appropriately retain and produce ESI may result in significant court-imposed sanctions, which can impact the outcome of a lawsuit.

Some of the possible sanctions that courts will consider are illustrated in the case of *Zubulake v. UBS Warburg LLC, et al.*:[13]

In a gender-discrimination suit against her former employer, plaintiff Zubulake sought discovery of e-mails relevant to her claim. After a lengthy course of litigation over ESI production, the defendant and defense counsel were sanctioned for failing to comply with discovery orders entered regarding numerous e-mails concerning the plaintiff. The

court found that a number of discovery breaches occurred, including: (1) the failure by counsel for UBS to communicate litigation-hold instructions to relevant UBS employees; (2) the failure by counsel for UBS to safeguard certain back-up tapes that might have contained some deleted e-mails; (3) the failure by UBS personnel to retain e-mails germane to plaintiff Zubulake's claims; and (4) the failure to disclose and produce specific e-mails regarding Zubulake for over 2 years.

The *Zubulake* court ordered that an *adverse inference instruction* would be given to the jury with respect to the deleted and lost e-mails. The court ordered that the jury would be instructed that they were permitted (but not required) to infer that UBS was in control of the lost e-mails, and that jury could also infer (or assume) that the lost e-mails were unfavorable to UBS. UBS was also ordered to pay any costs associated with any depositions or re-depositions required by the late production of certain e-mails.

The *Zubulake* decision illustrates how the failure to accurately and adequately produce ESI can lead to additional liability exposure and litigation expense. Favorable information may be barred as a consequence of a failure to comply, or as in *Zubulake,* an adverse inference instruction may be given to the jury, allowing the jury to infer that the organization did not produce ESI because it was unfavorable to the organization's defense in the case. To prevent court sanctions based on ESI discovery requests, risk managers need knowledge of their organization's ESI storage systems and management processes. Where appropriate, risk managers should promote best-practice models that comply with their organization's litigation posture.

Logistics of E-Discovery

More frequently, the plaintiff's discovery requests will specify that medical records and ESI be produced in electronic form only. This raises the issue of whether ESI can be produced without undue defendant expense or burden. Risk managers may have to assist litigation counsel in explaining to a court why certain ESI is unavailable in the requested format. For example, ESI may be created and stored on proprietary systems that run on critical vendor equipment and software.

The produced format of electronic-medical-records production may create another logistical issue. Although the data entered into an electronic medical record will remain constant, the formatting of the record may change significantly from the time of its entry by a clinician to its production in discovery. For example, when completing an electronic bedside-nursing assessment, multiple fields and drop-down options are available to the clinician; yet, when this same assessment is produced in discovery, only the selected fields may be printed. Additionally, information may appear on the printed version of the medical record that is automatically generated in an unfamiliar process for healthcare providers. For example, a lab report may contain various times to represent the actions, such as when the specimen was received, when the result was returned, and when the result was "reported" into the computer chart. These automatically generated data are not entered by the healthcare professional, and yet, the clinician may be expected to testify to the significance of the times in a deposition. Unfamiliarity with the electronic data contained in medical records can create issues with respect to a witness' ability to give a complete and accurate deposition, which could ultimately affect the witness' credibility before a jury.

ORAL DISCOVERY

Once written discovery is completed, the next phase of discovery is oral discovery, or depositions. As with other areas of discovery, statutes and jurisdiction rules control this process of which risk managers need to be aware. The number and scope of discovery depositions can vary widely depending on the presented lawsuit facts. While conducting investigations into matters that may become lawsuits, risk managers should begin determining the appropriate witnesses, their anticipated testimony, and the level of preparation that the witness would likely require to provide effective deposition testimony.

Risk managers also need to collaborate with defense counsel and, where possible, avoid unnecessary depositions to prevent unnecessary stress, expense, and lost productivity.

Deposition testimony permits the plaintiff's attorney(s) a chance to question the defense, and permits the defense counsel to evaluate the quality and presentation of the key persons in the case. The discovery deposition represents each witness's "statement" in the case, and to some extent, it sets the parameters for trial testimony. Deposition testimony can influence whether a case is defensible.

DISCOVERY CONSIDERATION FOR RISK MANAGERS

A planned, strategic approach to litigation discovery provides the risk manager with opportunities to control litigation losses and increase individual risk manger performance with improved efficiency and reliability.

Specific pre-suit risk management discovery considerations include:

- Defining an organization's litigation posture with objective enterprise risk management principles

- Conducting all risk investigations as if the product of such investigations will be used in future lawsuits, including the identification of potential witnesses and relevant medical information
- Knowing the applicable laws, regulations, and accreditation standards that relate to the creation, storage, and destruction of potentially relevant medical information, including medical records and ESI
- Knowing the applicable jurisdiction's statutory discovery rules, including the use of standard interrogatories, timelines for response, scope of discovery, and oral-discovery rules
- Preparing standard discovery responses for standard interrogatories to create reliable, accurate court filings
- Creating the documentation and processes required to support a claim to prevent the discoverability of documents through privilege
- Establishing close professional relationships with qualified external counsel for advice on pre-suit matters and potential discovery issues

After a suit is filed, specific risk management discovery considerations include:

- Establishing "litigation-hold" procedures to prevent the destruction of potentially relevant medical information, ESI, or evidence
- Engaging litigation defense counsel as soon as possible to aid in the early evaluation of potential exposure and creating a litigation position
- Notifying defense counsel of any discovery concerns, including missing or unavailable medical records, policies, ESI, or potential witnesses, that may require extensive deposition preparation
- Answering all written discovery promptly, accurately, and consistently
- Supplementing discovery responses when new information becomes available
- Conducting a critical internal review of specific department response to discovery requests, with a focus on improving future discovery responses

References

1. Moskowitz, S. (2007). Discovery in state civil procedure: The national perspective. *Western State University Law Review, 35,* 121.
2. See e.g. Ill. S. Ct. Rule 213 (f) (West 2009).
3. See *Anderson v. Rush-Copley Medical Center, Inc.*, 385 Ill.App.3d 167, 174–175 (1st Dist. 2008).
4. See *Ardisana v. Northwest Community Hospital, Inc.*, 342 Ill.App.3d 741, 747 (1st Dist. 2003).
5. See *Stricklin v. Becan*, 293 Ill.App.3d 886, 890 (4th Dist. 1997).
6. See *Toth v. Jensen*, 272 Ill.App.3d 382, 381 (1st Dist. 1995).
7. See *Frigo v. Silver Cross Hospital & Medical Center*, 377 Ill.App.3d 43 (1st Dist. 2007).
8. See *Anderson v. Rush-Copley Medical Center, Inc.*, 385 Ill.App.3d 167, 181 (1st Dist. 2008).
9. See *Ardisana v. Northwest Community Hospital, Inc.*, 342 Ill.App.3d 741, 747 (1st Dist. 2003).
10. See *Menoski v. Shih*, 242 Ill.App.3d 117, 120 (2nd Dist. 1993).
11. Seventh Circuit Electronic Discovery Pilot Program. Phase one: October 1, 2009 to May 1, 2010. *Statement of purpose and preparation of principles.* http://www.docstoc.com/docs/25685920/SEVENTH-CIRCUIT-ELECTRONIC-DISCOVERY-PILOT-PROGRAM/. Accessed April 21, 2010.
12. The Sedona Conference. (2008). http://www.thesedonaconference.org/dltForm?did=SedonaPrinciples200401.pdf. Accessed April 21, 2010.
13. See 229 F.R.D. 422 (S.D.N.Y 2004).

17

FULL DISCLOSURE AS A RISK MANAGEMENT IMPERATIVE

Nancy Hill-Davis, MJ, MA, BA, BSN

INTRODUCTION

With the 1999 release of "To Err Is Human: Building a Safer Health System," the Institute of Medicine (IOM) issued a wake-up call to healthcare organizations, providers, and patients alike, highlighting the startling prevalence of medical errors in the United States.[1] The IOM reported that as many as 98,000 deaths in hospitals each year were the result of preventable medical errors.[1] The IOM's report reverberated loudly throughout the medical community, in part because of the historical "culture of silence" in medicine under which physicians routinely failed to reveal medical errors to their peers, institutions, and, most notably, patients.[2] A 1999 New York Times article provided a chilling real-life illustration of this profound lack of transparency in medical culture.[3] Dr. Michael Leonard, an anesthesiologist and chief of surgery for Kaiser Permanente in Denver, was operating on a cancer patient when he administered the wrong medication. Dr. Leonard confused two medications because they were side by side and looked identical. Fortunately, the patient survived. Nevertheless, Dr. Leonard addressed the situation by disclosing the error to the surgeon, the scrub nurses, the patient's wife, and the hospital pharmacist responsible for drug labeling; however, when the surgeon spoke with his five partners, their reaction astonished him. Four of the five doctors said, "You know, I've done the same thing."[3] One of them said, "I did the same thing last week."[3] Dr. Leonard realized, "I am the chief of surgery. And nobody ever said to me, 'We have this problem.' A lot of it comes back to this culture of silence."[3]

A recent study on medical error found that while most physicians said they supported the concept of telling patients about errors, fewer than half had actually done so after a minor error, and only 5% of physicians had done so after a major event.[4] Physicians' historical reluctance to acknowledge medical errors to the public and to their peers has many bases.[5] Physicians have cited the anxiety of exposing individual fault, cost to their reputations, fear of loss of referrals, and fear of liability and exposure to malpractice litigations as just some of the reasons why they choose not to make disclosures when adverse events occur.[6] These fears of malpractice liability and confusion about causation and responsibility have long impeded comprehensive and bold initiatives designed to change the patient, family, and clinician experience with medical error.[7]

Lucian Leape cites two major reasons why healthcare providers historically have not revealed the occurrence of adverse events.[8] Firstly, many providers experience disappointment or shame in themselves for not being perfect. They experience a sense of failure that then triggers fear of theoretical consequences.[8] Secondly, revealing mistakes is simply difficult to do.[8] Few people have been trained to deliver bad news, particularly when they have at least some responsibility for causing it. Taking responsibility for one's actions when they result in injury is not easy. The healthcare provider, likewise, may be dealing with the emotional and psychological impact of the medical error.[8]

In spite of these obstacles, increasing interest has developed for changing the dynamics that surround medical error. This chapter undertakes analysis of the historical impediments to disclosure and recent ideas for responding to these impediments. Next, the chapter reviews the ethical, professional, and legal benefits and obligations of challenging the culture of silence and disclosing medical errors. The chapters which follow in this text provide a structure for successful, institution-wide disclosure programs and a summary of practical strategies for making the profound changes required to end the long-standing culture of silence that surrounds medical errors.

WHY DISCLOSE? WHY APOLOGIZE?

To truly bring an end to the culture of silence, two related but discrete concepts must be addressed: disclosure and apology. Disclo-sure refers to a process in medicine that involves reconstructing the events leading up to an adverse outcome and relating those events to the patient and family. It is often defined as, "as a prompt, truthful, and compassionate explanation of how the injury occurred, its short and long term effects, remedies available to the patient and steps developed following an analysis of the root cause of the error that will be taken to prevent its recurrence."[9] An apology is "a written or spoken expression of one's regret, remorse, or sorrow for having insulted, failed, injured, or wronged another," "an acknowledgement expressing regret or asking pardon for a fault or offense," or "an expression of regret" over a bad event.[10] There are several broad and compelling reasons why healthcare providers should both disclose medical errors and, in appropriate circumstances, apologize to their patients.[11]

It is ethical to disclose medical errors for the simple reason that patients have a right to know what happened to them.[11] There is no moral or legal right to withhold relevant information concerning the patient's care and treatment, and medical error constitutes information on the patient's care and treatment.[11] This information is a critical component of the continuum that makes up informed consent to treatment—a fundamental legal and moral concept in health care. Informed consent is the process by which a patient makes decisions about his or her health care based on full information regarding the risks and benefits of proposed treatment options.[12] Ongoing disclosure is part and parcel of updating the patient's understanding of risks and benefits and is paramount to continuing a trusting relationship between provider and patient.[12]

It is also therapeutic to disclose and apologize for causing preventable injury.[13] There is no question that serious injury can cause not only physical damage but also psychological trauma for both patient and provider.[13] The first step in dealing with the patient's and provider's emotional hurt is to explain what happened and take responsibility for it.[13] An apology starts to restore the emotional balance for both the patient and the healthcare providers involved in the medical error.[13] In disclosing medical errors, providers can faithfully discharge their ethical and fiduciary responsibilities to their patients. Providers also receive much-desired emotional relief from admitting the error to the patient and have the opportunity to obtain forgiveness. Additionally, the provider reaps an emotional and professional benefit from disclosures that lead to individual and institutional changes to facilitate patient safety.

As is discussed in more detail later, significant numbers of patients who have experienced a medical error state that they file lawsuits to get information about and understand their injury and the circumstances surrounding it. It has been established that disclosing error is less likely to lead to litigation than the "deny-and-defend" approach, or worse yet, the "silent treatment."[13] By disclosing and apologizing, the communication channels are open to discussion of appropriate compensation without resorting to filing a lawsuit. Furthermore, it has been demonstrated repeatedly that patients sue not merely because of the injury to their body, but also because of the insult to their dignity.[13] When patients are not treated with respect, when they are not told the truth, when the healthcare provider does not take responsibility for his or her actions, patients often feel that they have no alternative but to resort to litigation.[13] As Michael S. Woods states: "There is no evidence that reporting or disclosing medical errors actually leads to lawsuits."[14] On the contrary, research amply demonstrates that disclosing medical errors has the potential to result in a decrease in malpractice claims and lawsuits, as well as a decrease in malpractice liability and associated insurance premiums.[15]

The benefits of disclosure are also substantial for healthcare organizations. Disclosure of medical errors and the potential learning that results creates a critical opportunity to improve patient safety at an institutional level. Like providers, healthcare organizations may experience a decrease in malpractice claims, lawsuits, liability, and insurance premiums when they facilitate structured and systemic disclosure and apology programs. Furthermore, organizations may experience lower malpractice defense costs as a result of fewer claims and less-complicated settlements. Of considerable note is the increased patient and community confidence in the organization's integrity that can result from systemic disclosure initiatives.[15]

BARRIERS TO DISCLOSURE AND RESPONSES

Despite the numerous benefits outlined previously, there remain significant barriers to disclosure. The culture of silence is not easily dismantled. A recent study broke the culture of silence into four factors that impede willingness to disclose medical errors.[16] The first factor comprises attitudinal barriers, including perfectionism, a culture of blame and humiliation for error, professional arrogance, provider competitiveness, and doubt about the benefits of disclosure.[16] The second factor comprises concerns over lack of control on the provider's part once a disclosure is made. Providers also fear the lack of time to disclose errors, lack of confidentiality or immunity after disclosure, lack of institutional or collegial support after disclosure, and that error-reporting systems penalize those who are honest. Finally, providers feel helpless to address errors because they cannot control enough of the system of care to facilitate true preventative efforts.[16]

The third factor comprises uncertainties about how to disclose, disagreement about whether an error has in fact occurred, and most significantly, uncertainty about which errors should be disclosed.[16] In fact, defining which events to disclose is the topic of continued debate across and within organizations. Some organizations seek to disclose all unanticipated outcomes (including near misses) whether or not the patient was harmed or an error actually occurred, whereas others require disclosure of only medical errors that result in patient injury.[16] The fourth and final factor involves the professional and legal implications of disclosure. Providers fear legal and financial liability, professional discipline, loss of reputation, and loss of position. Providers also fear patients' and families' anger, anxiety, and loss of confidence. Professionally, providers fear looking foolish in front of colleagues, negative publicity, fallout on colleagues, and the sense of personal failure that threatens their self-identity as a healer.[16]

To eliminate disclosure barriers, institutions and individuals must address these four factors. The study by the National Patient Safety Foundation[16] concluded with the identification of a specific response to each barrier. These responses reinforce an existing value within the provider community, offering a counterbalance to the impulse toward silence in a vocabulary that providers can find accessible.[17] The first response builds on providers' existing sense of responsibility to patients, including the desire to communicate honestly with patients and to facilitate follow-up medical care for the harmed patient.[17] The second response reinforces providers' existing sense of responsibility to their profession, including the desire to share lessons learned from errors, to serve as a role model in disclosing errors or breaking bad news, and to change professional culture by accepting medicine's imperfections and lessening the focus on managing malpractice risks.[17] The third response focuses on providers' existing sense of personal accountability, integrity, and sense of fairness, altruism, and empathy. It also includes a willingness to accept one's fallibility and limitations, and to be vulnerable.[17] Finally, the fourth response reinforces providers' existing sense of responsibility to the community, including the desire to enhance the health of future patients, sustain patients' trust in the medical profession, foster physician–patient relationships that can absorb the shock of error, help patients be more realistic about medicine's imperfections, and help patients understand the complex causes of errors.[17] Encouraging providers to align their existing personal and professional values with the goal of enhanced communication with patients, even over something as difficult as error, may provide practical help to motivate providers to disclose errors when they do occur.

ETHICAL AND LEGAL BASES FOR IMPLEMENTING DISCLOSURE INITIATIVES

Healthcare providers owe a fundamental ethical duty to patients. Because patients must rely in significant part on providers' professional judgment for their health and safety, the provider–patient relationship is based on profound trust. Providers are therefore ethically bound to act in the patient's best interest and to justify that trust with honesty. Healthcare providers have a responsibility to disclose medical errors based on existing, but perhaps under-acknowledged, ethical, legal, and regulatory standards.

Ethical Codes

The majority of ethical codes that govern healthcare providers focus on the professional's responsibility to communicate openly and honestly with patients about their care and treatment, preserve patient dignity, and respect patient autonomy. The American Medical Association's *Code of Medical Ethics* states in part:

> It is a fundamental ethical requirement that a physician should at all times deal honestly and openly with patients. Patients have a right to know their past and present medical status and to be free of any mistaken beliefs concerning their conditions. Situations occasionally occur in which a patient suffers significant medical complications that may have resulted from the physician's mistake or judgment. In

these situations, the physician is ethically required to inform the patient of all the facts necessary to ensure understanding of what has occurred. Only through full disclosure is a patient able to make informed decisions regarding future medical care.[18]

Other professional organizations have adopted similar ethical requirements. For example, "the nurse owes the same duties to self as to others, including the responsibility to preserve integrity and safety";[19] "a pharmacist acts with honesty and integrity in professional relationships . . . [and] has a duty to tell the truth and to act with conviction of conscience";[20] the healthcare executive is expected to "work to ensure the existence of a process that will advise patients or others served of the rights, opportunities, responsibilities and risks regarding available healthcare services . . . and to provide a process that ensures the autonomy and self-determination of patients or others served";[21] and risk managers "will . . . communicate honestly and factually with patients and their families."[22] Embedded in each of these directives is a fundamental honesty with patients that arguably demands disclosure of medical error.

Accrediting Bodies

A clear disclosure requirement also exists for those organizations accredited by The Joint Commission. In 2001, The Joint Commission incorporated patient safety standards into its accreditation process for healthcare organizations, specifically requiring that "patients, and when appropriate their families, [be] informed about the outcomes of care, including unanticipated outcomes."[23] Additionally, The Joint Commission recognizes that adverse outcomes also have serious ramifications for the healthcare personnel involved. As a result, The Joint Commission Standard LD.5 requires that there be "defined mechanisms for support of staff who have been

involved in a sentinel event" as part of the organization's patient safety program.[23] Individual institutions have taken up The Joint Commission's mandates and created internal policies that encourage disclosure of medical errors. For example, the University of Michigan Health System adopted a policy that "[t]he responsible licensed independent practitioner or his or her designee clearly explains the outcome of any treatment or procedures to the patient[,] and when appropriate the family, whenever those outcomes differ significantly from the anticipated outcome."[24]

Case Law and Legislation

Another aspect of medical-error disclosure involves the concept of a provider's legal duty. The foundation of this duty arose in case law defining the physician–patient relationship.[25] Courts have generally held that physicians have a fiduciary duty to patients and must therefore disclose *all* relevant information regarding their care.[25] Some courts have ruled that the failure to disclose may be considered an act of fraud and fraudulent concealment.[25] These case holdings could logically be construed to suggest a legal duty to disclose medical errors to patients as well.

The second type of legal duty that pertains to disclosure are mandates in state law. Many states, including California, Florida, Nevada, New Jersey, Oregon, Pennsylvania, Vermont, and Washington, have enacted mandatory disclosure requirements. To illustrate, Nevada's law provides that:

1.   Each medical facility that is located within this state shall designate a representative for the notification of patients who have been involved in sentinel events at that medical facility.

2.   A representative designated pursuant to subsection 1 shall, not later than 7 days after discovering or becoming aware of

a sentinel event that occurred at the medical facility, provide notice of that fact to each patient who was involved in that sentinel event.

3. The provision of notice to a patient pursuant to subsection 2 must not, in any action or proceeding, be considered an acknowledgment or admission of liability.

4. A representative designated pursuant to subsection 1 may or may not be the same person who serves as the facility's patient safety officer."[26]

Underlying these laws is the belief that, for patients, disclosure can improve patient safety.[8] Being provided with complete information regarding their health can also facilitate patient autonomy and decision making. Equally importantly, open and honest disclosure can help to preserve and improve the integrity of the patient–provider relationship and help patients develop more realistic expectations about the limitations of medicine.[8] Furthermore, disclosure can prevent patients from blaming themselves for the results of the error and validate their suspicions of what is often obvious.[27]

Concomitant with laws mandating error disclosure, a variety of laws have also been proposed or enacted at the state and federal levels to address the issue of apologies. As discussed previously, apologies—either acknowledging responsibility or merely offering condolences at an unanticipated outcome—can be a critical part of the disclosure process. These laws offer some liability protection to the providers. Massachusetts was the first state to enact such a law in 1986. It reads:

Statements, writings or benevolent gestures expressing sympathy or a general sense of benevolence relating to the pain, suffering or death of

a person involved in an accident and made to such person or to the family of such person shall be inadmissible as evidence of an admission of liability in a civil action.[28]

Following Massachusetts' lead, more than 30 other states* enacted apology laws with a variety of components, some of which include immunity provisions. For example, the Illinois law states:

Any expression of grief, apology, or explanation provided by a health care provider, including, but not limited to, a statement that the health care provider is "sorry" for the outcome to a patient, the patient's family, or the patient's legal representative about an inadequate or unanticipated treatment or care outcome that is provided within 72 hours of when the provider knew or should have known of the potential cause of such outcome shall not be admissible as evidence in any action of any kind in any court or before any tribunal, board, agency, or person. The disclosure of any such information, whether proper, or improper, shall not waive or have any effect upon its confidentiality or inadmissibility.[29]

On the federal stage, in 2005 the National Medical Error Disclosure and Compensation (MEDiC) Act was proposed by Hillary Rodham Clinton and Barack Obama, both senators at the time.[30] As proposed, the MEDiC program would provide federal grant support

---

*Arizona, California, Colorado, Connecticut, Delaware, Florida, Georgia, Hawaii, Idaho, Illinois, Indiana, Louisiana, Maine, Maryland, Missouri, Montana, Nebraska, New Hampshire, North Carolina, North Dakota, Ohio, Oklahoma, Oregon, South Carolina, South Dakota, Tennessee, Texas, Utah, Vermont, Virginia, Washington, West Virginia, and Wyoming

and technical assistance to participant providers that disclose errors and offer fair compensation.[30] The bill provided that:

> Any medical error, patient safety event, or notice of legal action related to the medical liability of a health care provider, shall be reported to the patient safety officer. If it is determined that a patient was injured or harmed as a result of medical error or the standard of care not being followed, the Program participant would be required to disclose the matter to the patient, and offer to enter into negotiations for fair compensation to the patient. The terms of negotiation for compensation assure confidentiality, protection for any apology made by a health care provider to the patient within the negotiation period, a patient's right to seek legal counsel, and allow for the use of a neutral third party mediator to facilitate the negotiation. All negotiations must be completed within a six-month period, with the possibility for a one-time extension of three months. As part of the conditions of participation in the Program, medical liability insurance companies and health care providers would be required to apply a percentage of the savings they reap from lower administrative and legal costs to the reduction of premiums for physicians and toward initiatives to improve patient safety and reduce medical error.[31]

Although the bill did not pass, the possibility of future federal legislation on disclosure remains viable.

Disclosure Initiatives

In accordance with its mission to improve patient safety, the National Patient Safety Foundation issued "Talking to Patients about Health Care Injury: Statement of Principle," which reads in part:

> When a health care injury occurs, the patient and the family or representative are entitled to a prompt explanation of how the injury occurred and its short- and long-term effects. When an error contributed to the injury, the patient and the family or representative should receive a truthful and compassionate explanation about the error and the remedies available to the patient. They should be informed that the factors involved in the injury will be investigated so that steps can be taken to reduce the likelihood of similar injury to other patients.[9]

The Leapfrog Group also strives to encourage transparency and easy access to healthcare information through work with its employer members, as well as rewards programs for hospitals that have a proven record of high-quality care.[32] Through the 2007 Leapfrog Hospital Quality and Safety Survey, the Leapfrog Group encouraged hospitals to receive public recognition for agreeing to following "never-event" policy: ". . . apologizing to the patient, reporting the event to at least one reporting agency such as the The Joint Commission or a state reporting program, performing a root cause analysis, and waiving all costs directly related to the never event and refraining from seeking reimbursement from the patient or a third-party payor."[33]

DISCLOSURE AND APOLOGY AND MALPRACTICE CLAIMS

A recent study asked malpractice plaintiffs about any explanation that they had received following an adverse event, why they brought the claim, and what could have prevented them from filing a claim. The study found that nearly 40% of claimants who thought that something could have been done to prevent litigation indicated that litigation would not have been necessary if the medical provider had offered an explanation and apologized.[34] Another study interviewed family members who had filed claims against medical providers for perinatal injuries. The study found that 24% filed claims because "they realized that physicians had failed to be completely honest with them about what happened, allowed them to believe things that were not true, or intentionally misled them."[35] Several other studies have investigated the reasons that patients sue providers. Although medical malpractice claims are generally initiated because of an adverse event, many factors influence a patient's decision to sue. Patients report that miscommunication or a lack of communication adds insult to injury, so they pursue a malpractice case in order to get answers about what happened. For example, in one study 13% of respon-

dents believed that their physician would not listen, 32% felt that their physician would not talk openly, and 48% believed that their physician attempted to mislead them.[36] Furthermore, the same authors discovered that malpractice claims were causally linked to unsatisfactory communication and patient complaints.[37]

Chapter 18 provides specific details about organizations that have in fact implemented full disclosure and that have data that support the benefits of this approach.

Transparency and open communication between doctors, healthcare institutions, and patients is still a work in progress. Significant work remains to be done in the area of disclosure and apology. Rather than simply mandate disclosure policies and programs, institutions would do well to understand the rationale that underlies healthcare providers' fear of disclosure and help them come to an appreciation of the benefits of disclosure and apology.

References

1. Kohn, L., Corrigan, J., & Donaldson, M. (Eds.). (2000). *To err is human: Building a safer health care system*. Committee on Quality of Health Care in America, Institute of Medicine. Washington, DC: National Academy Press.
2. Woods, M.S. (2005). *Proceedings from the Quality Colloquium: What if we just said, "I'm sorry"?* Patient Safety & Quality Healthcare. http://www.psqh.com/novdec05/what-if.html. Accessed April 21, 2010.
3. Stolberg, S.G. (1999, December 5). Do no harm: Breaking down the culture of silence. New York Times, D1.
4. Osterweil, N. (Ed.). *To err is human, to disclose it to patients is optional*. MedPage, May 11, 2007.
5. Darr, K. (2001). Uncircling the wagon: Informing patients about unanticipated outcomes. *Hospital Topics, 79*(3), 33, 34.
6. Gallagher, T.H., Waterman, A.D., Ebers, A.G., Fraser, V.J., and Levinson, W. (2003). Patients' and physicians attitudes regarding disclosure of medical errors. *The Journal of the American Medical Association, 289*(8), 1001, 1003.
7. Full Disclosure Working Group. (2006). *When things go wrong: Responding to adverse events*. A consensus statement of the Harvard Hospitals. http://www.macoalition.org/documents/respondingToAdverseEvents.pdf. Accessed April 21, 2010.
8. Leape, L. (2005). Understanding the power of apology: How saying "I'm sorry" helps heal patients and caregivers. *Focus on Patient Safety, 8*(4), 1–3. http://npsf.org/paf/npsfp/fo/pdf/Focus2005Vol8No4.pdf/.
9. National Patient Safety Foundation. (2001). *Talking to patients about health care injury: Statement of principle*. http://www.npsf.org/rc/pdf/Statement_of_Principle.pdf. Accessed May 21, 2010.
10. The American Academy of Physician Assistants. (2007). *Acknowledging and apologizing for adverse outcomes manual*. http://www.aapa.org/images/stories/documents/about_aapa/policymanual/38-AcknowledgeAdverse Outcomes.pdf. Accessed April 21, 2010.

11. Leape, L. (2006). Full disclosure and apology: An idea whose time has come. *Physician Executive, 32*(2), 16–18.

12. Whitman, A.B. (2006). How do patients want physicians to handle mistakes? A survey of internal medicine patients in an academic setting. *Archives of Internal Medicine, 156* 2565–2569.

13. Leape, L. (2006). Full disclosure and apology: An idea whose time has come. *Physician Executive, 32*(2), 18.

14. Woods, M.S. (2007). *Healing words: The power of apology in medicine.* Oak Park, IL: Doctors in Touch.

15. Straumanis, J.P. (2007). Disclosure of medical error: Is it worth the risk? *Pediatric Critical Care Medicine, 8,* S42.

16. Kaldjian, L.C., Jones, E.W., Rosenthal, G.E., Tripp-Reimer, T., & Hillis, S.L. (2006). An empirically derived taxonomy of factors affecting physicians' willingness to disclose medical errors. *Journal of General Internal Medicine, 21,* 946.

17. Ibid, p. 945.

18. American Medical Association. (2006). Opinion E-8.12. Patient information. *Code of medical ethics.* Chicago: American Medical Association.

19. The American Nurses Association. (2001). *Code of ethics for nurses: Provisions.* Silver Springs, MD: Author.

20. American Pharmaceutical Association. (1994). http://www.pharmacist.com/Content/NavigationMenu2/LeadershipProfessionalism/ProfessionalDevelopment/CodeofEthicsforPharmacists/default.htm. Accessed April 20, 2010.

21. American College of Healthcare Executives. (2007). *Code of ethics.* http://www.ache.org/ABT_ACHE/code.cfm. Accessed April 20, 2010.

22. American Society for Healthcare Risk Management. (2007). *Code of professional conduct.* http://www.ashrm.org/ashrm/about/governance/files/codeconduct.pdf. Accessed April 20,2010.

23. The Joint Commission on Accreditation of Healthcare Organizations. (2002). *Revisions to Joint Commission standards in support of patient safety and medical/health care error reduction.* Oakbrook Terrace, IL: JCAHO.

24. University of Michigan Health System. (n.d.). *Disclosure: Accreditation standards.* http://www.med.umich.edu/patientsafetytoolkit/. Accessed April 20, 2010

25. Porto, G.G. (2001). Disclosure of medical error: Facts and fallacies. *Journal of Healthcare Risk Management, 21,* 72.

26. Nevada Revised Statute. (2008, December 5). *Section 439.855.* http://www.leg.state.nv.us/NRS/NRS-439.html#NRS439Sec855/. Accessed April 28, 2010.

27. Rosner, F., Berger, J.T., Kark, P., Potash, J., & Bennett, A. (2000). Disclosure and prevention of medical errors. *Archives of Internal Medicine, 160,* 2090.

28. The General Laws of Massachusetts. (2008, December, 3). *Chapter 233, §23D.* Accessed April 20, 2010.

29. Illinois Compiled Statutes. (2008, November 30). *735 ILCS 5/8-1901.* http://www.ilga.gov/legislation/ilcs/fulltext.asp?DocName = 073500050K8-1901/. Accessed April 20, 2010.

30. Clinton, H.R., & Obama, B. (2006). Making patient safety the centerpiece of medical liability reform. *The New England Journal of Medicine, 354,* 2206.

31. The National Medical Error Disclosure Act of 2005 (draft effective September 28, 2005). http://www.who.int/patientsafety/highlights/USbillonpatient_safety.pdf/. Accessed April 20, 2010.

32. The Leapfrog Group. (n.d.). *About us.* http://www.leapfroggroup.org/about_us/. April 20, 2010

33. The Leapfrog Group. (2007). *Leapfrog hospital quality and safety survey.* http://www.leapfroggroup.org/for_hospitals/. Accessed April 20, 2010

34. Vincent, C., et al. (1994). Why do people sue doctors? A study of patients and relatives taking legal action. *Lancet, 343,* 1609.

35. Hickson, G.B., Clayton, E.W., Githens, P.B., & Sloan, F.A. (1992). Factors that prompted families to file malpractice claims following perinatal injuries. *The Journal of the American Medical Association, 267,* 1359.

36. Hickson, G.B., Clayton, E.W., Githens, P.B., & Sloan, F.A. (1992). Factors that prompted families to file malpractice claims following perinatal injuries. *The Journal of the American Medical Association, 267,* 1360–1363.

37. Hickson, G.B., Federspiel, C.F., Pichert, J.W., Miller, C.S., Gauld-Jaeger, J., & Bost, P. (2002). Patient complaints and malpractice risk. *The Journal of the American Medical Association, 287,* 2951–2957.

The Development of Full-Disclosure Programs: Case Studies of Programs That Have Demonstrated Value

Katherine V. Schostok, JD, LLM

INTRODUCTION

It would be hard to imagine a practicing risk manager who would admit to believing that the traditional way in which claims were managed—where full transparency to patients was not fostered—was the preferred way to do business; however, many who have read the studies described in Chapter 17 believe in the underlying principles but either are unclear as to the consequences or unsure about how to implement a comprehensive operational strategy. This chapter describes in detail a number of organizations across the United States that are leaders in moving the concept of full transparency forward and have shared their process for doing so. It is hoped that this chapter will help move the concept of transparency from theory to practice. It is obvious from reading these case studies that although the concept makes perfect sense, the passion and commitment of a champion is necessary to bring

it to life. In many cases, the chief risk officer is that person.

THE DEVELOPMENT OF FULL DISCLOSURE PROGRAMS

Veterans Affairs Medical Center (Lexington, Kentucky)

The Veterans Affairs (VA) Medical Center in Lexington, Kentucky, developed one of the first disclosure programs in the United States. This hospital began using humanistic risk management approaches in 1987 after paying $1.5 million in judgments for two malpractice cases.[1] Steve Kraman, Chief of Staff at that time, created a risk management committee charged with developing procedures that would decrease medical-malpractice litigation against the hospital. The group reviewed the facility's litigation history and found that when the hospital failed to handle the patient's concerns, the potential for a lawsuit increased.[2]

The committee determined that the hospital had a duty to remain as a caregiver even after an adverse event occurred. In that capacity, the hospital should fully disclose information to the patient.

The VA Medical Center has had great success with this policy. During the period from 1990 through 1996, the Center had 88 malpractice claims and paid an average of only $190,113 per year in settlements. The average payment per claim was $15,622.[2] In 1995, the Department of Veterans Affairs followed this example and rewrote the risk management portion of its policy manual. The Department added a Patient Safety section that stated: "The medical center will inform the patient and/or family, as appropriate, of the event, assure them that medical measures have been implemented, and that additional steps are being taken to minimize the disability, death, inconvenience, or financial loss to the patient or family."[1] The manual also explained that this standard does not remove the patient's right to subsequently file suit, and the patient and family should be notified of this option.

In 1997, Kraman conducted a comparative analysis of the payments made by the VA Medical Center and those of similar institutions. Although the VA facility compensated more patients, the overall cost to the hospital was in the lower quartile of the centers reviewed.[3] The results of these programs vary depending on a number of factors, but Kraman's experience has been very positive. Patients appear to be satisfied at the end of discussions and appreciative of the information they received and the attention given to their concerns. When asked about the patient response to the program at the VA Medical Center, Kraman responded: "In almost every case, and we've done this, it must be 200 times, they're pleasant. . . . We end up, after a meeting, shaking hands, hugging. Most all of them behave in a very rational and decent way afterwards. They basically respond in kind. And even their attorneys respond in kind."[3]

University of Michigan Health System (Ann Arbor, Michigan)

Background of the Facility and History of the Program

The University of Michigan Health System (UMHS) is a renowned health system and medical school. The UMHS comprises a large number of hospitals, health centers, clinics, a medical school, and a faculty group practice. The hospitals and clinics alone have 913 licensed beds. Annually, the facilities provide for 43,173 admissions and over a million visits to its clinics.[4]

The UMHS and Richard Boothman, Chief Risk Officer at UMHS, designed a risk management program that was introduced in 2001. By 2004, UMHS's program was regarded as one of the most successful and innovative in the field.[5] Boothman was motivated by the statistics that disproved that a "deny-and-defend" approach to malpractice claims is effective for decreasing litigation and protecting heathcare systems. This strategy is also costly and time-consuming. Boothman and UMHS designed the program in response to a general failure of healthcare providers to assume accountability when appropriate, and an overall reluctance to open communication with patients and families.[6]

Malpractice laws in the state also support investigation of events and engaging patients in discussions. In Michigan, a plaintiff seeking to file a malpractice suit must provide written notice of the specific allegations to the defendants. By statute, this notice must include the factual basis for the claim, the standard of care, the alleged breach, the compliant conduct that should have occurred, the manner in which the breach proximately caused the harm, and the names of all providers involved.[6] Subsequently, the plaintiff cannot file suit for a 6-month period following this notification to allow for a proper investigation, potential discussions between parties, and reevaluation of the lawsuit.[7]

Guiding Principles

The UMHS adopted three guiding principles as the basis of its risk-management and full-disclosure program. The UMHS articulated its overarching goal as "Apologize and learn when we're wrong, explain and vigorously defend when we're right, and view court as a last resort."[8] The general principles developed are as follows:

1. We will compensate quickly and fairly when inappropriate medical care causes injury.

2. We will defend medically appropriate care vigorously.

3. Reduce patient injuries (and therefore claims) by learning from mistakes.[6]

In the policy statement UMHS published in 2001, the system declared the intention to remain open and honest with its patients in all communications and contact. This includes the full disclosure of information, even for unanticipated outcomes. The UMHS employs a reasonable test in reviewing events. Under this standard, UMHS holds that a "medical error occurs when a patient is injured as a result of medical care that is unreasonable under the circumstances."[7]

Description of Program Elements

In general, the process for responding to unanticipated outcomes is to gather all the facts of the situation, presume good intentions of those involved, be truthful and open in disclosure conversations, maintain patient privacy, focus decisions on the patient and the patient's interests, refrain from speculation, and plan follow-up communications.[9] The UMHS defines unanticipated outcomes as "[a] result that differs significantly from what was anticipated to be the result of a treatment or procedures."[9]

Reporting

The first step in the UMHS process is reporting the event to the risk management office.

This notification may occur through an incident report or phone call from the staff administrator or nurse on duty. The risk management office is charged with stabilizing the situation and beginning the investigation process.

Investigation

A full investigation requires interviewing those health professionals involved, notifying the necessary administrative staff, and determining whether the event qualifies as a sentinel event. This decision must be made within 5 business days after the event is first reported.[10] A sentinel event is defined by The Joint Commission as "an unexpected occurrence involving death or serious physical or psychological injury, or the risk thereof."[11] Under this definition, serious injury includes the loss of a limb or full function of a limb. The risk portion refers to a substantial possibility of a serious adverse outcome should the event reoccur. This label is not synonymous with medical error but instead triggers the need for an investigation and prompt reaction. If the event does potentially qualify, the chief of staff or designated executive makes a final determination of whether a report to The Joint Commission is necessary. If the event is reported, organizations accredited by The Joint Commission, such as UMHS, are required to perform a root-cause analysis, implement necessary changes to prevent recurrence, and monitor improvements to the facility. Some of these events are reviewable by The Joint Commission. If the event is not reported as a sentinel event, the risk management office continues the standard process for event response. This includes a complete investigation, meetings with the patient and family, and full-disclosure practices.

Initial Meeting

Once the situation is stabilized and the investigation stage has begun, the risk management team has an initial meeting with the patient and possibly the patient's family. In this meeting, the risk manager is to introduce all of the parties, explain the confidentiality of the communication, review and confirm the facts and chronology of events, and discuss any subsequent actions and potential system improvements. The conversation should be summarized at the end of the meeting and the risk manager should welcome comments or criticisms of the process at that juncture.[12] The risk manager should then continue investigation of the event and maintain communication with the patient. The priority throughout the process is the patient's needs. The UMHS will offer an apology for true mistakes. For any event, the patient is entitled to a comprehensive explanation. Follow-up discussions regarding the event and future care are also important elements to the process when an adverse event does occur.

Committee Review

The UMHS expanded a committee of six health professionals, originally formed to aid attorneys representing the health system, to 32 clinicians with various medical backgrounds. The committee members represent over 20 specialties. This group is charged with evaluating if (1) the care provided was reasonable and (2) the care negatively affected the treatment outcome.[13] The committee is also responsible for reviewing each case to determine if peer review, quality improvements, or additional education and training are appropriate.[13] The committee discussions and findings are not discoverable, as they fall under the Michigan legal protection of those materials created in anticipation of litigation and in the course of quality improvement and peer review. A UMHS attorney is present for all meetings to address any legal concerns that may arise and provide additional protections for the information discussed.

Disclosure

As articulated in the foundational principles, full disclosure to the patient is necessary to maintain an open and honest relationship between patient and provider. In recent years, UMHS has shifted its focus to perfecting the method of disclosure. Published guidelines and trained risk managers are available to aid clinicians in communicating empathy and remorse to patients, when necessary, and to effectively address patient concerns in emotionally charged situations. Counselors are also available to provide psychological support for the health professionals.

Who Is Responsible for Disclosure? The patient's attending physician is responsible for maintaining full disclosure with the patient. This process begins with informed consent before and throughout the treatment but is continued even after an unanticipated outcome is reported. The risk management team is available to guide the health professional through the disclosure process. The physician is required to document the discussions with the patient or family in the patient's record.

What Should Be Included in Disclosure Discussions? At a minimum, full disclosure includes the facts surrounding the unanticipated outcome, how the result occurred, any subsequent or consequential health concerns, respective treatment plans, and contact information for questions. To ensure protection of this information from discovery, details collected from peer review or regarding quality assurance cannot be shared with the patient or documented in the medical record. If any information is withheld from the patient, the health professional should note the reason for this decision in the medical record.

When Should Disclosure Discussions Occur? Disclosure should be made promptly after the unanticipated outcome is discovered. At the latest, full disclosure should be completed before the patient is discharged or at the end of the medical treatment. The UMHS allows for the use of professional judgment in determining the specific disclosure details and timeline.

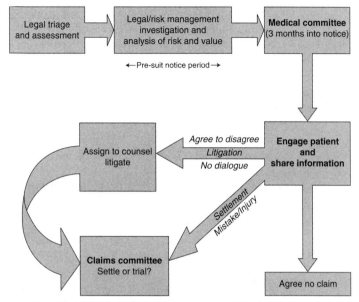

Figure 18–1 University of Michigan Claims Management Model
These diagrams were created by the University of Michigan Health System and are used with their permission.

How Should Disclosure Occur? The attending physician is responsible for ensuring that information be fully disclosed. The physician may consult the department chairpersons or the office of clinical affairs for assistance. The health professional should have access to all pertinent facts and answers to anticipated questions. The UMHS published "Guidelines for Disclosure" along with the 2001 policy statement. These guidelines stress that preparation is essential. The physician must expect questions and conduct necessary research before entering the meeting. The disclosure conversations should involve detailed recommendations about the outcome, future treatment, and follow-up communication. An important component is differentiating between reasonable and unreasonable care during the investigation and responding accordingly. If the care was unreasonable, accountability should be communicated. The appropriate response and level of disclosure depends on the severity and whether the care is determined to be unreasonable under the surrounding circumstances.

Figure 18–1 is a basic depiction of the claims management model, including the change in response once litigation is pursued, prepared by UMHS.[13] A detailed and comprehensive flowchart of the review and analysis of patient safety reports is given in Appendix 18–A.[6]

University of Illinois Medical Center at Chicago (Chicago, Illinois)

Background of the Facility and History of the Program

The University of Illinois Medical Center at Chicago (UIMCC) is a 450-bed state-of-the-art academic medical center in Chicago, Illinois.[10] The UIMCC provides highly specialized medical care for over 19,000 inpatients and 45,000 outpatients each year. The UIMCC began implementation of a patient safety incident-response system in 2004 under the supervision of Timothy B. McDonald, Chief Safety and Risk Officer for Health

Affairs. The Center apportioned significant funding for patient safety and risk management efforts and began a complete restructuring of the incident-reporting and response process.[14] The resulting program implemented system-wide policies and procedures to effectively respond and handle incidents within the organization. The UIMCC defines the term *patient safety incident* as "an event or circumstance which could have resulted, or did result, in unnecessary harm to a patient"[14] By 2006, this program had been developed to incorporate processes by which the Center could practice full disclosure of unreasonable care that causes patient harm. The UIMCC's reasoning for the creation of this program was an inherent ethical obligation to fully disclose medical information to patients and facilitate prevention of future error in the healthcare setting.

Guiding Principles

The UIMCC adopted guiding principles very similar to those followed by the University of Michigan Health System and other institutions with full-disclosure programs. The guidelines are as follows:

1. We will seek to provide effective and honest communication to patients and families following patient safety incidents involving patient harm.

2. We will apologize and provide rapid compensation when inappropriate or unreasonable medical care causes patient harm and defend vigorously care that we believe was appropriate.

3. We will seek to learn from our mistakes.[14]

The UIMCC additionally transitioned to a "just culture" to offer provider protection for patient safety incidents that occur as a result of system failures. This safeguard was incorporated in anticipation of physicians' fear of participation and exposure to liability. To ensure that reckless behavior was appropriately addressed, however, UIMCC adopted two guiding principles for the professional-responsibility aspect:

1. Reckless behavior will be subject to corrective action.

2. We will provide support services for providers involved in patient safety incidents.[15]

Description of Program Elements

The UIMCC prides itself on its efforts to develop a comprehensive program that incorporates both full disclosure and a detailed process for responding to reported incidents. The UIMCC's approach includes seven pillars or layers of disclosure. In practice, these seven facets facilitate identifying medical errors in the early stages, recognizing necessary system changes to ensure patient safety, investigation of (and appropriate responses to) specific patient safety incidents, and maintaining open lines of communication with all parties involved.

Reporting
The first pillar of disclosure is reporting patient safety incidents. Ideally, reporting should occur immediately after the event is discovered or suspected. A risk manager is available at all times to respond to a report made by anyone at the facility, including patients and their families. Reporting may be done by telephone, letter, or online, and may be made anonymously.[15] The UIMCC recognizes that the success of a risk management and full-disclosure program is conditional upon prompt and regular reporting. The facility provides positive reinforcement for people who comply, and it penalizes those departments that fail to report patient safety incidents.

Preliminary Review and Investigation
The second pillar is a complete investigation of reported incidents conducted by the safety and risk management department. The initial review is referred to as a "rapid investigation,"

during which the responding risk manager determines the severity of harm to the patient and whether the incident should be categorized as either a sentinel event according to The Joint Commission, or a "never event" under the National Quality Forum guidelines. To promote uniform definition and reporting of these errors, the National Quality Forum has published 28 serious reportable adverse events with specific explanations included.[16] If no harm was caused to the patient, the incident information is recorded in the reporting database and will be further analyzed if determined a "near miss." If harm did occur, the Medical Staff Review Board of UIMCC is charged with overseeing the response process and protecting the information and results from discovery under the Illinois Medical Studies Act. The Act provides that all information and statements collected about a health professional's competence in the course of internal quality control, for the purpose of improving patient care, is privileged and confidential, and thus, not discoverable.[17] After an incident is determined to have caused harm, the chairperson of this committee is responsible for organizing a team to conduct a rapid investigation and root-cause analysis of an incident. These elements must be conducted within 72 hours of the initial reporting.

The UIMCC utilizes James Reason's algorithm of unsafe acts to initially determine whether the incident occurred because of failures in the system or as a result of an individual's negligent acts.[18] The algorithm includes five possible questions to consider. The first question asks whether the individual's actions were intended. If the answer is yes, then legal action is appropriate and the analysis is concluded. If the answer is no, the next question should ask whether there is evidence of substance abuse or illness. If neither situation is present, the third question is: Did the individual knowingly violate the policies and procedures of the institution? If the conduct is found to be a routine action, then the patient safety incident is attributable to the system rather than the individual. If the compliance analysis is inconclusive, the eval-

uator should ask whether similar errors have been made by like professionals at the facility. If the answer is affirmative, the incident was system-induced. In these cases, the final question to be asked is: Does the individual in question exhibit a pattern of unsafe behavior? At this point in the analysis, it is clear that the incident occurred as a result of failures in the system. The follow-up questions are intended to identify those professionals who need additional training in risk management and safety practices.[19]

The UIMCC offers provider counseling services during the entire process. The Center identifies health professionals as potential "second victims" who will additionally benefit from full disclosure of the facts and a safe environment. The Care for the Care Provider program has counselors available at all times to provide supportive care and conduct evaluations of future impact on health professionals. This program will likely be expanded to ensure the emotional and mental stability of the UIMCC faculty and staff.[20]

Communication and Full Disclosure

The third pillar of the UIMCC program is communication and disclosure with the patient. The facts of the incident revealed through the investigation process lay the foundation for future communication with the patient and the patient's family. To facilitate discussions, UIMCC created the Patient Communication Consult Service, a group of volunteer healthcare providers and administrators trained in disclosure. The Service additionally provides just-in-time coaching for professionals, if required.

Full-disclosure conversations involve sensitive information. The disclosure approach is based on the harm the patient suffered and whether the care was reasonable or unreasonable. If the care is assessed as reasonable, the team will provide full disclosure of the facts. Disclosure occurs through a series of meetings. Usually, the primary care provider is the main communicator with the patient and family. If appropriate, the provider will deliver an apology. The UIMCC employs Hickson and Pichert's "balance-beam approach" to communicating with the patient. This requires that a benefit-and-risk analysis be conducted considering alternative strategies before an approach is selected.* This method is used to prevent premature disclosures that may not be beneficial or accurate.

For all patient safety incidents at UIMCC, the rapid investigation team must determine that unreasonable care was provided before full disclosure to the patient will be accompanied by an apology and accountability. As guidance for effective disclosure, the UIMCC staff considers Stephanie P. Fein and her colleagues' findings regarding the six disclosure elements most desired by patients. These elements are an admission, a discussion of the event, a defined connection between the error and proximate effect, identification of the proximate effect, a link between the error and the harm suffered, and communication regarding any harm to the patient.[21]

Apology and Remediation

The fourth pillar is apology and remediation. The UIMCC considers this element to be essential in maintaining the trust of the patient and providing an adequate out-of-court remedy. The apology offers the patient and family regret for the harm caused and allows the health professional an opportunity to express remorse and apologize. If appropriate, the legal department will present an early offer of compensation. Additionally, the risk management team is authorized to provide remediation in the form of a waiver or hold on medical bills incurred while at the facility. This layer of the program is intended to introduce a remedial measure that provides an apology and financial relief in an effort to promptly address the concerns and needs of the patients and their families.

System Improvement

System improvement geared toward prevention of future errors is the fifth pillar of the UIMCC program. This layer serves as a proactive method for learning from past incidents and improving patient safety and risk management. The Medical Staff Review Board evaluates changes made to the system to ensure effectiveness. The risk managers at UIMCC are responsible for providing data that can be used to evaluate appropriate improvements. The UIMCC encourages patients and families involved in the process to contribute their recommendations as well.

Data Tracking and Performance Evaluation

The sixth pillar is the collection and analysis of performance data. The data recorded include the type of patient safety incident that occurred, the subsequent investigation, the disclosures made, implications for the medical center, system improvements, and communications with the patient. The Safety and Risk Management Department provides quarterly summaries to the UIMCC administration.

Education and Training

The seventh and final pillar of the UIMCC program is continuous education and training of health professionals to encourage compliance and transparency. This training involves communication coaching and evaluations. The UIMCC, as a teaching hospital, believes that it is important to introduce this education and training in the first years of medical school so that the students can become familiar and comfortable with full-disclosure methods and the UIMCC philosophy.[14] Clinicians are trained in reporting guidelines, full disclosure, patient safety, and identifying when a provider may benefit from the "second patient" program. Participation in counseling is encouraged following involvement in a patient safety incident.

Figure 18–2, a depiction of the seven pillars on which the program is based, details the process by which UIMCC responds when an unexpected adverse event is reported.

---

*Interview with Nikki Centomani, Director of Risk Management, University of Illinois Medical Center at Chicago, January 21, 2009.

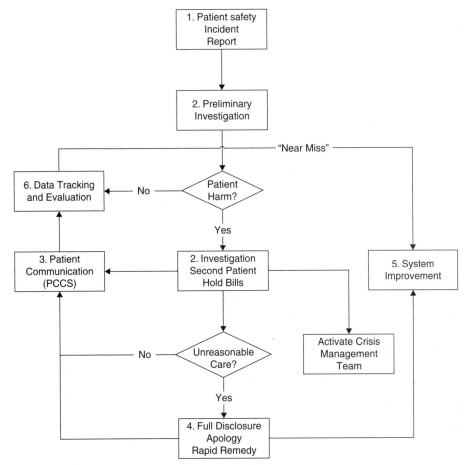

Figure 18–2 Comprehensive Process for Responding to Unexpected Adverse Events
These diagrams were created by the University of Illinois at Chicago and are used with their permission.

Programs at Other Facilities

Hospitals and health centers across the United States are implementing risk management and patient safety programs, and are now practicing full disclosure. The Johns Hopkins Hospital, one of the leading medical centers in the country and a prominent research facility, has been practicing full disclosure for decades. The Johns Hopkins Hospital and Johns Hopkins Health System staff are trained in responding to adverse events and supporting a culture of transparency at the hospital. The focus on patient safety was heightened after system failures resulted in the death of a young research participant in 2001.* Ellen Roche was involved in an asthma study focused on airway hyperresponsiveness. She received the drug hexamethonium to block neurotransmission by non-adrenergic, non-cholinergic nerves.[22] This drug was non-FDA approved and no

*Telephone interview with Margaret R. Garrett, Senior Counsel, Johns Hopkins Health System Legal Department, March 31, 2009

longer used in the clinical setting. The physician who conducted the study failed to fully disclose the potential health risks to the participants and failed to report Roche's symptoms of pulmonary toxicity. After her death, the federal Office for Human Research Protections conducted a review of the clinical research program and found significant deficiencies in the review of research protocols.

Johns Hopkins has subsequently developed an infrastructure dedicated to patient safety and quality improvements. The hospital follows new and innovative methods to avoid preventable medical errors. Critical care specialist Peter Pronovost has been at the forefront of the Johns Hopkins mission to improve patient safety. Recent winner of the MacArthur Fellowship (commonly known as the "genius grant"), Pronovost continues to develop creative procedures for decreasing mistakes in the healthcare setting. Pronovost's checklists of basic steps have been implemented in operating rooms and health centers across the United States and have significantly lowered infection rates.[23]

After reviewing the pioneering programs, Stanford University Medical Center (SUMC) launched a formal full-disclosure program in 2007. Jeffrey Driver, Chief Risk Officer at SUMC, describes the Stanford approach as optimistic and cautious.[24] Stanford's acronym for the program is PEARL, which stands for the process for early assessment and resolution of loss. PEARL encourages "transparency, integrity, fairness, and healing."[25] The program provides for an initial assessment to determine if the event was a preventable unanticipated outcome (PUO), telephone consultations for "concerning outcomes," just-in-time training for health professionals, and leadership in efforts to implement system improvements. In the case of a PUO, Stanford instructs its physicians and staff to stabilize the patient, ensure patient safety, promptly contact the PEARL risk and claims advisor, continue documentation, and record the advisor as the exclusive contact person regarding the event.[26] Coaching for a PUO will include

methods for practicing full disclosure and communicating with the patient and family. These discussions may be coupled with an early offer of compensation.[27] Stanford cautions health professionals and risk management officials against making assumptions, placing blame, and offering financial relief that has not been formally approved. (Chapter 19 provides a more in-depth discussion written by risk management staff at Stanford that describes their program and the need to move beyond the process of disclosure to early-offer remediation.)

Implementation of Your Program

A successful risk management and full-disclosure program requires well-defined policies and procedures for responding to preventable adverse events, coupled with a dedication to transparency. The process should be focused on fact finding and effectively and empathetically communicating known facts to the patient and family. There are two major components to these programs, which should be addressed separately. The first component is assigning staff responsibilities and creating checks to ensure that adverse-event response standards are met within the system. The second aspect is promoting transparency and enabling disclosure based on the patient's needs and preferences.

Staff Responsibilities and Adverse-Event Response

The first challenge is developing and distributing definitions of the program terminology and levels of event severity. The hospital or health system should distinguish between an adverse event and a medical error if pertinent to the type of response, as well as detail the added considerations when an event qualifies as a serious error or sentinel event. These definitions, along with the overarching principles for the program, should be included in physician and staff training. The general guidelines should address the components to the program and promote a just culture based on the health professionals' ethical responsibility to the patients. These programs are intended to preserve the sanctity of the relationship between patient and provider.

The American Society of Healthcare Risk Management recommends the following definitions:

> *Adverse Event:* An injury that was caused by medical management rather than the patient's underlying disease; also sometimes called "harm," "injury," or complication.
>
> *Medical Error:* The failure of a planned action to be completed as intended or the use of a wrong plan to achieve an aim. Medical errors include serious errors, minor errors, and near misses.
>
> *Serious Error:* An error that has the potential to cause permanent injury or transient but potentially life threatening harm.
>
> *Minor Error:* An error that does not cause harm or have the potential to do so.
>
> *Near Miss:* An error that could have caused harm but did not reach the patient because it was intercepted.
>
> *Preventable Adverse Event:* An injury (or complication) that results from an error or systems failure. Three recognized categories include: error by the attending physician, error by anyone else in the healthcare team, or systems failure with no individual error.[28]

Training is at the core of creating a culture that supports and complies with the program. In a study that surveyed physicians at three medical centers, only 62.3% of faculty and 49.5% of resident participants knew how errors were reported at their institution. Even fewer participants in these categories were aware of what kinds of errors should be reported. Of the respondents surveyed, 16.9% acknowledged a failure to report a previous minor error, and 3.8% admitted to not reporting a major medical error.[29] Ineffective or inadequate training can significantly damage the effectiveness of a risk management or full-disclosure program and prevent learning from near misses that may not otherwise be identified.

Once the principles and terms of the program are defined, the initial response process should be determined. Prompt reporting of *possible* events is the trigger for the response. Reporting methods should be convenient and accessible for patients and staff. Following a report, institutions should require actions to stabilize the situation to prevent additional harm, secure drugs, equipment, or records, and conduct a quick but comprehensive investigation. A risk management team or select group of individuals should perform the initial review. This team is often charged with determining the most appropriate communicator for discussions with the family. Once an initial chronology and set of facts are collected, a meeting with the patient should be scheduled. An exchange of communication early in the response process includes the patient and patient's family in the investigation and allows the patient to guide the process according to his or her needs. The proper method of communication must be case specific, but disclosure guidelines should be available.

The analysis phase begins with a determination of whether the event qualifies as a sentinel event. The Joint Commission allows each organization to define a sentinel event for its own purposes. This definition must be consistent with the general definition. If the incident qualifies, the institution is encouraged, but not required, to report the event to The Joint Commission and follow the mandated root-cause analysis and response process. A senior staff member should be appointed to oversee this analysis and ensure compliance.[30] Internal processes should be

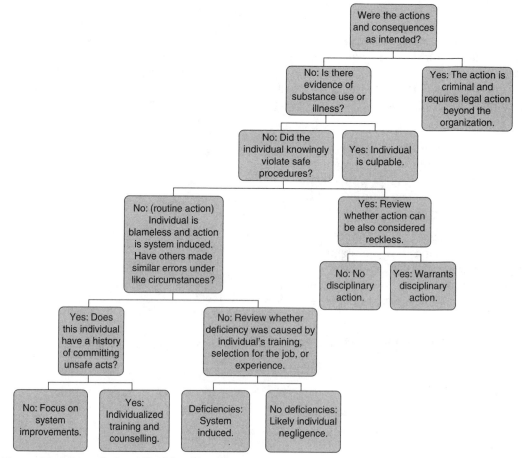

Figure 18–3 Unsafe Acts: Decision Tree Chart
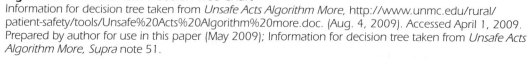
Information for decision tree taken from *Unsafe Acts Algorithm More*, http://www.unmc.edu/rural/
patient-safety/tools/Unsafe%20Acts%20Algorithm%20more.doc. (Aug. 4, 2009). Accessed April 1, 2009.
Prepared by author for use in this paper (May 2009); Information for decision tree taken from *Unsafe Acts
Algorithm More, Supra* note 51.

implemented to address less-severe events. The procedure should be tailored to the specific needs of the system and the types of patients seen. The analysis should allow for a thorough investigation of the event, evaluation of whether system failures or individual negligence caused the error, and continuous disclosure of confirmed facts.

The James Reason formula used in the University of Illinois Medical Center's analysis is an effective tool for distinguishing between individual and system failures. A decision tree that depicts this algorithm is given in Figure 18–3.

Documentation and data collection are essential for future institutional considerations. Proper documentation creates a clean record of actions taken by the hospital for use in potential litigation or review of how the case was handled. This information may also be important in the future treatment of the patient. The American Society for Healthcare Risk Management recommends that documentation include the objective details of the event, any subsequent conversations with the patient, the patient's condition and reaction, and questions posed by the patient or patient's family. The notating health professional should avoid including negative commentary on the treatment received or conduct of other providers.[31] Data collection can prove useful in the evaluation of potential system improvements and changes to response procedures. This information is also helpful in reviewing the overall effectiveness of these programs.

Throughout the response process, counseling services should be made available for all parties. Full disclosure and apology can prove therapeutic for the patient and provider, but the information discussed in these emotionally charged situations can be difficult to process. Although continuous training should be conducted, just-in-time coaching for health professionals should be available for a review of concepts or additional guidance.

Supporting Caregivers After an Adverse Event

The Brigham and Women's Hospital in Boston, Massachusetts, expanded its full-disclosure program to include supportive services for providers following an adverse event. The recently developed Office of Professionalism and Peer Support is composed of four components: peer support, professionalism training, disclosure and apology coaching, and a physician-defendant support group. The peer support section of the office, along with the Employee Assistance Program, oversees an ongoing pilot program in the operating room and other hospital departments. Previously trained staff members work closely with the Employee Assistance Program to identify affected staff members promptly after an adverse event occurs and convene a debriefing session. The risk management department will not only investigate the facts of the incident, but also the effect on the provider. The hospital takes a proactive approach to ensuring that the "second victim," the provider, has someone available for support. The goal is to arrange a conversation with a peer of the healthcare provider, rather than a mental health professional.* This is designed to assist the provider with his or her

emotional stability after an event. The intention is to provide an open forum for concerns and determine whether the provider needs time off of work or a change in assignment. The risk management department has continued to receive positive reactions from the physicians and staff regarding the program and the support available through the system.

Specific attention should also be given to patients' financial considerations. The risk management team or designee at the hospital may be authorized to suspend bills during the investigation process and reduce costs when appropriate. Financial issues are also present in funding for risk management programs. Both UMHS and UIMCC are privately insured institutions, with the ability to appropriate funding for development and implementation. Institutions with outside malpractice liability insurance or limited budgets should create a detailed financial plan to accompany the program proposal.

Full Disclosure

Currently, there is not a national consensus on how to effectively communicate with a harmed patient. This is partially a result of the case-by-case analysis required for each event. The method should always be tailored to the individual needs of the patient and the degree of harm. Studies have shown, however, that clinicians' varying interpretations of the term "full disclosure" may lead to partial transparency and the appearance of dishonesty.[32] Standards for disclosure, such as those issued by The Joint Commission, are simplistic and void of detailed guidance. The Joint Commission requires that: "Patients and, when appropriate, their families are informed about the outcomes of care, including unanticipated outcomes." The Joint Commission explains this standard as requiring that: "The responsible licensed independent practitioner or his or

---

*Interview with Janet N. Barnes, Executive Director, Clinical Compliance and Risk Management, Brigham and Women's Hospital, Boston, Massachusetts, April 30, 2009.

her designee clearly explains the outcome of any treatment or procedures to the patient and, when appropriate, the family, whenever those outcomes differ significantly from the anticipated outcomes."[33] Although this explanation served as a modest effort toward defining appropriate disclosure methods, the health professional is left with a vague understanding of how to "clearly explain" and what content is necessary. Health professionals are told that it is their ethical obligation to fully disclose, but they are offered minimal guidance on how to communicate empathy and sorrow to the patient while maintaining their composure as a medical professional.

In a study conducted by the University of Massachusetts and Fallon Foundation, five key elements of disclosure were identified. Researchers found that patients preferred disclosure containing (1) a definite statement that a mistake occurred, (2) a full description of the mistake and related health concerns, (3) how the mistake happened, (4) how the provider will prevent the mistake in the future, and (5) a meaningful and sincere apology.[34] The open communication between patient and provider begins in the informed-consent stage. In this early phase, the provider begins to learn the specific needs of the patient and the preferred disclosure strategies.

Health professionals are trained to continue an open dialogue throughout the care and treatment of the patient to maintain a trusting relationship and address any questions or concerns. Until recently, physicians were not offered training in disclosing unanticipated outcomes to patients or their families. The "deny-and-defend" culture, which in some contexts is so prevalent, focuses on preventing liability and deferring to counsel. Open-disclosure systems remove the health professionals from the safety of this protection. Promoters of full-disclosure programs ask for faith in the process while providing no assurances that the patient will not sue.

Full disclosure has been shown to elicit positive reactions from patients and decrease the likelihood that the patient will change physicians. The results of these programs have also shown a dramatic decrease in malpractice litigation.[34] Full-disclosure conversations, however, can be quite daunting for medical professionals, especially in states where the apology laws offer limited protections. In a study that surveyed pediatricians, researchers found marked variation in the physicians' intentions to disclose a potential medical error and the content of the discussions. The disclosure provided was often partial, defeating the intention of addressing all of the patient's needs following a traumatic event. Certain disclosure strategies can help the health professional become comfortable with disclosure while most effectively addressing the patient's needs and preventing litigation.

Full-disclosure programs introduce new and unfamiliar considerations. Health systems and hospitals should establish full-disclosure principles that guide physicians through the process while still allowing for a case-by-case approach. Programs should encourage the development of communication skills that convey empathy while calmly and comprehensively answering patient questions. Word selection can be extremely important for both the comfort level of the provider and the patient's interpretation of the event.

The health professionals and risk management team should be cognizant of the risks and benefits of these programs. This includes the effect that premature disclosure may have on the process. Although information and explanations should be promptly made available to the patient after an event occurs, the communicator should avoid stating assumptions or disclosing unconfirmed facts. The patient should be consistently reassured that all facts learned in the future will be disclosed and open lines of communication will be maintained. This is a balance-beam approach to disclosure that has been utilized by many of the nationally recognized programs. This method is recommended by Gerald B. Hickson and is taught at his primary institution, Vanderbilt University School of Medicine (Nashville, Tennessee). In simplest terms, the balance-beam approach holds that every strategy should be evaluated for its strengths and weaknesses before implementation. This concept ensures that every action is supported by an analysis and is a planned motion toward the intended result. Consideration should be given to how other health professionals in the field would respond to the proposed method and alternatives.[35]

Empathy

Conveying empathy is one of the greatest hurdles for health professionals in emotional disclosure discussions and is fundamental to the full-disclosure approach. The crucial element to expressing empathy is understanding the potential effect on the listener and framing the discussion to his or her needs. The challenge for health professionals is processing that patient's words and responding accordingly, rather than following a predetermined agenda. John Banja, a leading author in the field of disclosure, recommends that health professionals reflect on how they would respond if presented with a similar situation as a patient or family member.[36] Physicians should practice remaining attentive, silent if necessary, and aware of the other party's feelings.

To express empathy physically, the communicator should select a comfortable, relaxed environment for the meeting and avoid displays of superiority, such as standing or wearing a lab coat. The medical professional should prepare for the questions that may arise. The clinician must also be aware of his or her personal sensitivities and comfort level with admitting mistakes and accusations of care that is below the standard. Discussing future improvements is effective in addressing concerns that this mistake will reoccur and conveying the seriousness with which the system handles medical errors.

A common concern is that the patient or family will respond with anger. To anticipate this possibility, health professionals can set a reasonably limited period of time for each meeting, show feelings of empathy for the event, have someone trained in counseling patients present, detail the lessons learned from the mistake, and admit accountability for the error that occurred.[37] The clinician should try to diffuse the situation by using phrases such as "This must be (awful, dreadful, difficult) for you to hear"; or ask questions such as "How would you like me to proceed?" or "What would you like to have happen?"[38] Statements that allow the physician's emotions to interfere with those of the patient should be avoided. In addition, the patient's feelings should not be minimized to diminish the seriousness of the event.

Apology

An apology can be an essential element once an event is ruled a preventable medical error. An apology creates a connection between people allowing the parties to search for understanding, forgiveness, and redemption.[39] Health professionals generally avoid offering an explicit apology fearing that it will be used against them in subsequent litigation. In a study published by the American Medical Association, researchers found that physicians were almost twice as likely to express regret rather than clearly apologize.[40] If it is warranted, the forum should welcome a sincere apology regardless of what legal action the patient will take in the future. As Richard Boothman at the University of Michigan Health System stated, the patient and provider's interests at this juncture are the same: both face the prospect of litigation and want to avoid mistakes in the process.[41] If the health system is responsible for the medical error, the goal should be to resolve the claim with adequate compensation for the patient.

Apologizing in these situations allows the physician to therapeutically offer remorse while seeking forgiveness from the patient and family. Forgiveness on the part of the patient and family will ideally lessen their desire to seek justice and punishment for wrongdoing. As John Banja stated, "If justice is the sociocultural attempt to correct the imperfect revenge behavior, forgiveness provides complementary assistance in restoring psychosocial equilibrium so that a wrongful injury is absorbed into an individual's or society's memory in a way that no longer precipitates disturbance or disruption."[42] The individual who is usually most soothed by the apology is the forgiver. The health professional is asking the patient to reevaluate the adverse event and change his or her perspective of the physician. This encourages the patient to understand that the physician did not intend to commit the error and realize that the professional is forever changed by its occurrence.

Theorists have explained that a sincere and effective apology must include an identification of the error, an expression of remorse from the wrongdoer, a promise to prevent the error in the future, and an offer of reasonable compensation, if appropriate.[43] The first part of the apology signifies an acknowledgement and acceptance of the error. The second part should offer an explanation of the event and expression of regret. This portion includes the formal apology, which should be clearly articulated.

The third aspect is ensuring that this error will be prevented in future treatment of patients. The health professional should be encouraged to express remorse, shame, forbearance, and humility throughout the second and third stages.[44] The fourth element is an offer of compensation or financial relief. Although this aspect is not always necessary, many patients will require that a monetary response accompany the full-disclosure-and-apology process.

Table 18–1 is a chart that Gerald B. Hickson and James W. Pichert prepared that conveys the recommended elements of the disclosure-and-apology process and suggested communications with the patient. The discussion should flow based on the patient's individual needs, but this chart can be used as a general outline to ensure that the recommended elements are included.

Table 18–1 Suggested Communications Related to Disclosure and Apology

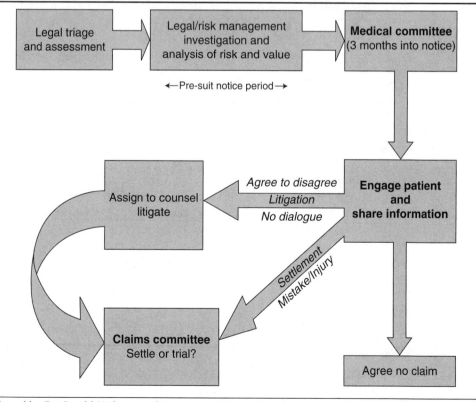

Developed by Dr. Gerald Hickson and James W. Pichert, PhD, for the National Patient Safety Foundation as published in *Disclosure and Apology* © 2007, and used with the permission of all parties.

Although more than half of the states have enacted apology laws, the protections vary. Health systems should review the laws in their respective states to ensure that the greatest protections are offered to those health professionals who apologize for errors. Identifying and explaining the pertinent protections before the apology allows the physician to fully disclose his or her remorse without a pressing fear of the outcome. Training should also explain the possibility that the patient or family will reject an apology and offer no forgiveness. There is no assurance that the full-disclosure-and-apology process will be successful and address all of the patient's needs. The patient's acceptance of remorse for the error is not the motivation for conducting such a program. The rationale is simply that the patient has a right to know and the health system has a responsibility to communicate.

RESULTS

The implementation of risk management and full-disclosure programs has resulted in a dramatic decrease in claims and litigation across the board. The data disprove the argument that full-disclosure methods expose health professionals to greater liability and encourage subsequent litigation; instead, these programs result in an overall decrease in medical errors, increase in patient satisfaction, improved quality of care, and a reduction in malpractice claims and suits brought against medical centers.

The result at University of Michigan Health System is dramatic. In 2001, when the transition to full disclosure began, UMHS had 262 open claims against the system and reserves valued at more than $70 million. Since 2001, the number of open claims has steadily decreased to 83 in 2007. The processing time for handling complaints has dropped from an average of 20.3 to 9.5 months. In addition, the total reserves for the system have been lowered by two thirds and the average litigation costs have been cut in half.[6] These changes have saved the system over $2 million dollars.[45] Additionally, the online reporting database has

allowed UMHS to capture and address three times as many potential claims. In a survey conducted at UMHS, 98% of the system physicians recognized a difference in the claims process since 2001. Over half of the participants felt that these changes contributed to their decision to remain at UMHS.[6]

The UMHS also surveyed the southeastern Michigan plaintiff's bar to evaluate attorney satisfaction. Of the attorneys surveyed, 100% rated UMHS as one of the best health systems for full disclosure and transparency. In addition, 81% of the attorneys stated that this change in approach had lowered their administrative costs, and 86% agreed that transparency encouraged better selection of malpractice suits to pursue.[6]

Similarly, of the 40 medical errors UIMCC identified in the first year of full disclosure, only one resulted in a lawsuit.[46] The UIMCC also reports a significant reduction in administrative and settlement costs as a result and continues to see a dramatic difference in the number of lawsuits and claims brought against the medical center. The full-disclosure method has not resulted in any increase in payment amounts.[7]

The Children's Hospital and Clinic of Minnesota, 28 hospitals in the Kaiser Permanente network, 16 Harvard-affiliated teaching hospitals, and many others have developed full-disclosure programs and have experienced similar results.[47] Insurance companies are beginning to notice the results and become involved. Catholic Healthcare West, a system comprised of 41 hospitals and medical centers, began a program in 1999. This system convinced its physicians' malpractice insurer, Physicians Reimbursement Fund, Incorporated, to implement a full-disclosure approach in 2002. By 2005, the group reported a 40% decrease in overall claims and payments distributed.[7]

One of the most notable private-sector examples is the COPIC Insurance Company's "3Rs" program. COPIC is a physician-directed liability insurer in Colorado. This company insures approximately 6000 physicians.[48] In 2000, COPIC created a program based on the "3R" principles: recognize, respond, and resolve. This concept was developed to identify harm through early event reporting, prompt response, and resolution of disclosure and compensation issues with the patient. COPIC's philosophy is to compensate for injury resulting from negligence, minimize the waste of resources in the tort system, and defend medicine that meets the standard of care. The program was developed in response to the overall ineffectiveness and inefficiency of the claims process.[49]

The 3R's program is designed as a non-fault system that prevents malpractice claims from entering the broken legal system. The response process is triggered when a physician in the program reports an event. The software flags the participant and trained administrators begin an investigation. If intervention is appropriate, the physician calls the patient to explain the situation and offers the 3R model of benefits to them. Through this program, the physician is able to explain the injury, express empathy, apologize, and answer the patient's questions in a no-fault context. Certain cases are not eligible for the 3R response; these include cases in which death occurs, attorneys have already been involved, a formal written demand for payment has been submitted, or an official legal document has been filed. The physician may also refuse participation.[50]

The COPIC program offers patients access to up to $30,000 in compensation for their healthcare expenses: $25,000 for out-of-pocket expenses and $5,000 for lost time. By 2005, the number of COPIC malpractice claims had decreased by 50% and settlement costs were lowered by 23%. In 2007, COPIC paid an average of $5,293 per verified claim. Since the program was implemented, no claims have proceeded to a jury trial.[48] Additionally, patient questionnaires after an event is resolved show positive perceptions of the process and preservation of the patient–provider relationship. The COPIC and Physician Reimbursement Fund programs signal a movement within the insurance industry to adopt full-disclosure policies. Without this transition, healthcare systems that are not self-insured will face barriers in having these alternative methods approved.

THE DISCLOSURE MOVEMENT

Apology Laws

One of the main concerns with full disclosure and apology is the discoverability of this information. To provide protections, many states have enacted laws that prohibit the use of a physician's apology in court. Pennsylvania was the first state to enact a so-called apology law. Unfortunately, not all of these state laws extend protection to information that accompanies an apology. Colorado's apology law, for example, prevents the discovery of all statements, gestures, and conduct that express some form of apology or fault. The law in Texas, however, only protects statements. Some states even limit the protection to oral expressions of regret.[6]

Various healthcare systems have chosen to ignore the discovery issues and trust that these disclosure programs will continue to prevent lawsuits from coming to fruition. The protections in Illinois are limited to expressions of grief, apology, or explanations made within 72 hours of when the provider knew, or should have known, of the cause of the unanticipated outcome.[51] Disclosure discussions at UIMCC realistically continue after this 72-hour period and discoverable apologies are given. The system's reasoning in those events where an apology is provided is that the hospital has recognized that the care was unreasonable and has already accepted liability; therefore, compensation is the only remaining issue, and an apology is not considered damaging. Seven of these states have intervened further and mandated disclosure to patients of severe unanticipated outcomes. These states include Nevada, Florida, New Jersey, Pennsylvania, Oregon, Vermont, and California.[50]

Nationwide Action

As mentioned in Chapter 17, The Joint Commission issued nationwide disclosure standards in 2001. These mandates require healthcare organizations to disclose all aspects of care, including unanticipated outcomes.[50] Although the standards failed to specify the method and content of disclosure, The Joint Commission's effort introduced national requirements for accredited hospitals.

In 2006, the Full Disclosure Working Group of the Harvard Hospitals published a consensus statement that describes the benefits and risks of open disclosure. The guiding principles for the paper were "medical care must be safe" and "medical care must be patient-centered."[28] The Group categorized full disclosure as an ethical responsibility engrained in the practice of medicine. The authors offered detailed explanations of effective responses to adverse events and recommendations on how disclosure communication should be conducted. This paper serves as a comprehensive manual on developing and implementing disclosure programs.

The Sorry Works! Coalition, launched in 2005, is an organization dedicated to promoting the use of full-disclosure-and-apology programs to battle the medical malpractice crisis.[52] Sorry Works! has become the leading advocacy group in the field. The organization's goals are to educate stakeholders, act as a leader and organizer in the movement toward full disclosure, and advocate for legislative assistance.[52] The recommended disclosure protocol is based on the Lexington Veteran Affairs Medical Center model. The organization's stance is that full disclosure is common sense and effectively addresses the deficiencies of the tort system. Sorry Works! recognizes the challenges of changing the culture of medicine, but they insist that it is a necessity.

Physician Response

The greatest hurdle may be receiving the support of medical professionals. Full disclosure may be interpreted as exposing the physician to liability and creating a record of admitted negligence. The success of these programs suggests that the probability of a lawsuit arising is dramatically decreased through the use of full disclosure; however, the potential still exists. To the skeptic, a "deny-and-defend" approach would offer greater protection. As studies have shown,

patients and families are more likely to seek legal counsel if the provider does not provide a sincere explanation for the outcome.

A study published by the American Medical Association researched what medical errors physicians would disclose to patients and what information they would provide.[53] The surveyed physicians and trainees practiced pediatric medicine. Participants were provided with one of two scenarios and were asked about the severity of the error, how responsible the physician was for the mistake, and whether the family should be notified. The first scenario involved an insulin overdose, which was presented as an apparent medical error. The second scenario was a failure to follow up on a laboratory test. Both hypothetical errors resulted in the hospitalization of the child.[53]

The results of the study showed that overall, 53% of participants would disclose the medical error and 58% would fully disclose the event details. Only 26% of respondents would provide an explicit apology. Half of the participants reported that they would discuss preventative measures for future patient care.[53] The most notable statistic is that twice as many physicians who received the scenario involving an apparent mistake would disclose the error to the patient's family. In addition, significantly more physicians in the apparent group would offer an apology. These findings suggest that the physicians surveyed did not view full disclosure as an ethical responsibility that applies to all errors that occur, but rather as being imperative only if the mistake is apparent to the patient or family.

This physician perspective was suggested in another study conducted in 2008. Researchers surveyed faculty and resident physicians regarding the likelihood of reporting errors and attitudes toward full disclosure. The results showed that although 84.3% of respondents agreed that reporting medical errors improves patient safety and the quality of care, 16.9% admitted that they had failed to report a minor error in the past, and 3.8% admitted a failure to report a major error.[29] When questioned about hypothetical disclosures, however, 73% of participants responded that they would likely report a minor error and 93% would report a major error. These findings show a philosophical inclination to disclose medical errors but a failure to consistently report when presented with an actual event. This discrepancy potentially exists because of a lack of training on how to report errors in the participants' respective institutions, and what events should be reported. When surveyed, only 62.3% of faculty and 49.5% of residents knew the process for reporting errors. In addition, only 53.6% of faculty and 30% of residents believed that they knew which errors should be reported. These responses highlight the importance of establishing and circulating reporting guidelines and providing clear definitions and expectations in the training of physicians. Hospitals and health systems should strive to inform health professionals of all aspects of a program and the benefits of compliance. The focus of disclosure coaching should be based on allowing the physician to feel comfortable in the communication and confident in the system's processes and outcomes.

CONCLUSION

The deficiencies in the United States healthcare and tort system have created a litigious medical-malpractice environment that is focused on monetary compensation rather than healing and improvement. As the Institute of Medicine report, "To Err Is Human: Building a Safer Health System," revealed, there are an alarming number of medical errors that cause injury each year in the healthcare setting. Patient safety practices and risk management techniques are intended to address these issues and prevent mistakes before they occur. As the pioneers of medicine first articulated, a physician's duty is to first "do no harm." In a high-risk setting, however, mistakes do occur. Remedial measures should rectify the situation by fulfilling the needs of the patient and the provider. The process

should appeal to the human element and offer emotional, intellectual, and psychological responses in addition to financial relief or compensation. This can be accomplished through the use of humanistic approaches, such as full disclosure, apology, and expressions of empathy or remorse.

Risk management and full-disclosure programs are being developed nationwide. The healthcare industry is starting to embrace a culture of patient safety and transparency in response to the reality of medical error. Disclosure policies and procedures in response to adverse events are the first step toward identification and prevention of system failures. National organizations and legislators are recognizing this transition and are striving to accomplish widespread change in the healthcare delivery system.

Risk management and full-disclosure programs are a moderating solution to the tort system that address the concerns associated with the present medical-malpractice crisis. An effective malpractice claims system must accomplish four goals: minimize the number of preventable medical errors, foster open and honest communication between patients and providers, provide patient access to reasonable compensation for injuries caused by malpractice, and reduce insurance premiums.[54] Caps on non-economic damages only target one element and have no impact on future prevention. Similarly, the traditional "deny-and-defend" culture hinders the potential for system improvement, forces the patient to handle malpractice claims outside of the institution, and disrupts the communication and relationship between patient and provider. As Richard Boothman at the University of Michigan Health System simply stated: "Improving patient safety and patient communication is more likely to cure the malpractice crisis than defensiveness and denial."[55]

Working together, healthcare providers and the patients they serve can take this problem to the solution stage.

APPENDIX 18–A: THE UNIVERSITY OF MICHIGAN HOSPITALS AND HEALTH CENTER FLOWCHART FOR REVIEW AND ANALYSIS OF PATIENT SAFETY REPORTS

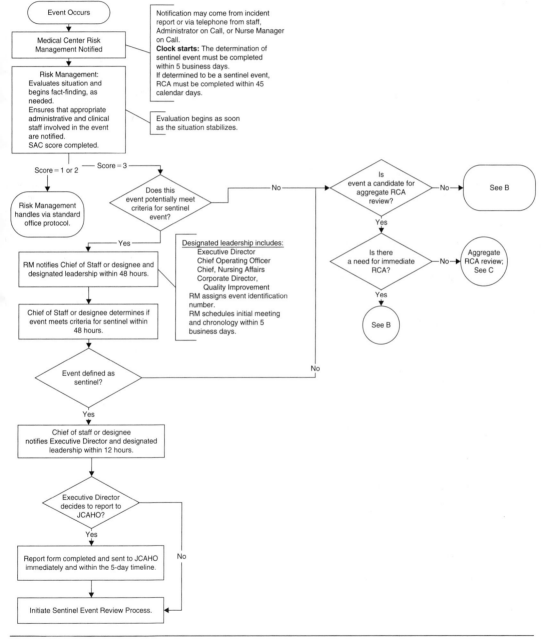

These diagrams were created by the University of Michigan Health System and are used with their permission.

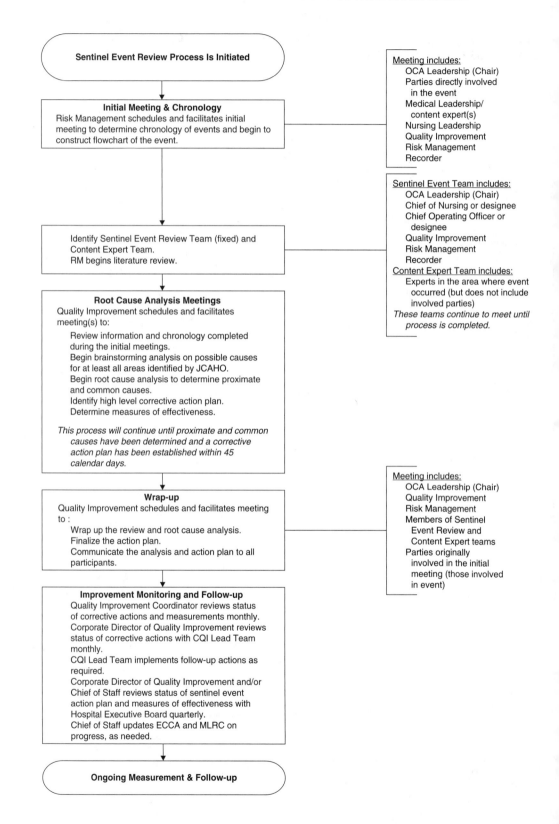

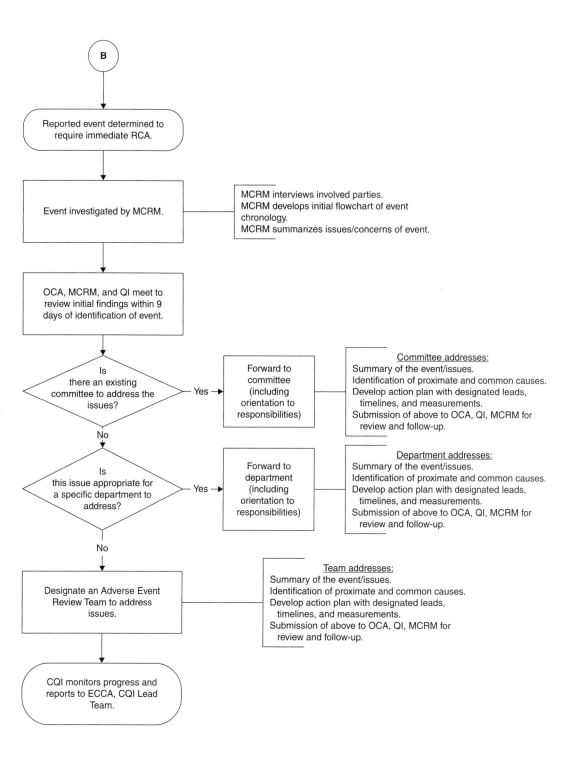

B

Reported event determined to require immediate RCA.

Event investigated by MCRM.

MCRM interviews involved parties.
MCRM develops initial flowchart of event chronology.
MCRM summarizes issues/concerns of event.

OCA, MCRM, and QI meet to review initial findings within 9 days of identification of event.

Is there an existing committee to address the issues?

Yes →

Forward to committee (including orientation to responsibilities)

Committee addresses:
Summary of the event/issues.
Identification of proximate and common causes.
Develop action plan with designated leads, timelines, and measurements.
Submission of above to OCA, QI, MCRM for review and follow-up.

No

Is this issue appropriate for a specific department to address?

Yes →

Forward to department (including orientation to responsibilities)

Department addresses:
Summary of the event/issues.
Identification of proximate and common causes.
Develop action plan with designated leads, timelines, and measurements.
Submission of above to OCA, QI, MCRM for review and follow-up.

No

Designate an Adverse Event Review Team to address issues.

Team addresses:
Summary of the event/issues.
Identification of proximate and common causes.
Develop action plan with designated leads, timelines, and measurements.
Submission of above to OCA, QI, MCRM for review and follow-up.

CQI monitors progress and reports to ECCA, CQI Lead Team.

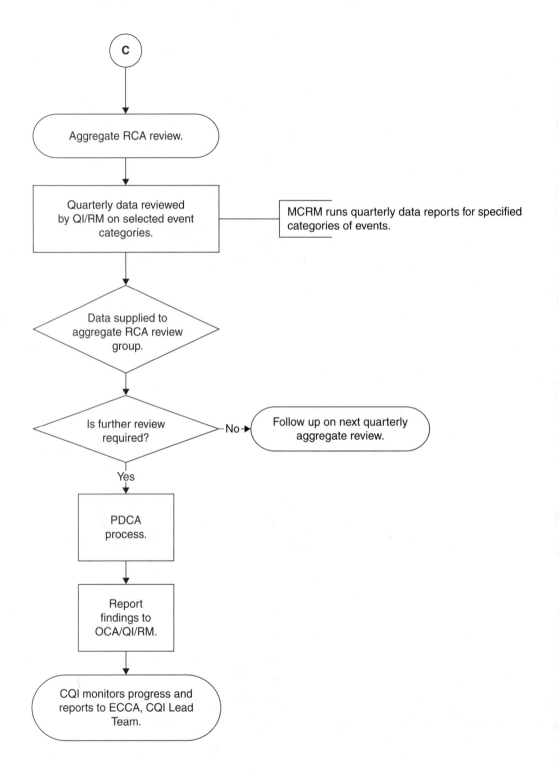

Disclosure Element	Suggested Communications
1. Offer apology (be *precise*), and explain nature of error, and harm.	Mr./Ms.____, I'm sorry to report that [nature of error and specific outcome]. On behalf of us all, I apologize for the [error and outcome].
2. Explain when and where error occurred.	Here's what happened . . . [explanation appropriate for patient/family understanding of medical facts]
3. Explain causes and results of harm, actions taken to reduce gravity of harm, and actions to reduce or prevent reoccurrence.	The error occurred because [explain briefly in non-technical language]. As a result, what happened to you is [again, explain briefly]. Once we realized the error, we [explain actions taken to address that patient's needs, if applicable]. We have a team that reviews error and recommends how to prevent recurrences.
4. Explain who will manage ongoing care.	If you allow me to continue, I will work [together with other team members and administrators] on your care.
5. Describe error review process and reports to regulatory agencies, and how systems issues are identified.	We take mistakes very seriously. Everything will be reviewed by experts. The results will be reported to me [and, if applicable, to the ____Agency]. If the review reveals ways we can better care for our patients, we will work to make those changes.
6. Provide contact info for ongoing communications.	I [or Dr.____] will communicate about your continuing care. When questions arise, please have me paged. Or call my assistant, [name] who can help or find me.
7. Offer counseling and support if needed.	People in the ____office can talk with you and connect you with support services. Here's their card. May I call them or anyone else for you?
8. Address bills for additional care.	The review I requested will fairly address the charges resulting from the error. The focus now is [returning you to health, restoring function, assist with grieving process. . . .]

References

1. Kraman, S.S. & Hamm, G. (December 12, 1999). "Risk Management: Extreme Honesty May Be the Best Policy." *Ann Intern Med 131*(12), 963–967.

2. Kauman, Doug. (April 30, 2004). *Apologizing and offering fair compensation can circumvent malpractice suits*, http://sorryworks.net/media4.phtml/. Accessed April 15, 2010.

3. Kauman, *supra* note 19.

4. University of Michigan Health System. (2008). *Facts and figures, FY2008.* http://www.med.umich.edu/1busi/facts.html/. Accessed April 2, 2009.

5. University of Michigan Health System. (2009), *Medical malpractice and patient safety at UMHS.* UMHS Newsroom. http://www.med.umich.edu/news/newsroom/mm.htm/ Accessed February 12, 2009.

6. Boothman, R.C. (2006). *Medical justice: Making the system work better for patients and doctors*, testimony of Richard C. Boothman, Chief Risk Office, University of Michigan Health System before the United States Senate Committee on Health, Education, Labor, and Pensions (June 22, 2006).

7. Boothman, R.C., Blackwell, A.C., Campbell, D.A., Jr., et al. (2009). A Better Approach to Medical Malpractice Claims? The University of Michigan Experience. *J Health and Life Sci Law, 2*(2): 137.

8. The University of Michigan Health System. (2009). *Approach to malpractice claims.* UMHS Newsroom. http://www.med.umich.edu/news/newsroom/mm.htm#summary/. Accessed February 12, 2009.

9. University of Michigan Hospitals and Health Centers. (2001). *Policy 03-07-011. Disclosure of*

unanticipated patient outcomes. http://www.med
.umich.edu/patientsafetytoolkit/disclosure/
disclosure.pdf/. Accessed April 1, 2009.

10. University of Michigan Hospitals and Health
Centers. (n.d.). *Flowchart for review and analysis of patient safety reports.* http://www.med
.umich.edu/patientsafetytoolkit/events/review
_analysis.pdf/. Accessed April 1, 2009.

11. The Joint Commission. (2007). *Sentinel events
policy and procedures.* http://jointcommission
.org/SentinelEvents/PolicyandProcedures/.
Accessed April 1, 2009.

12. University of Michigan Hospitals and Health
Centers. (2009). *Adverse event—initial meeting: Agenda.* http://www.med.umich.edu/
patientsafetytoolkit/events/initial_mtg_agenda.
pdf/; UMHHC. *Policy 03-07-004. Sentinel and
serious adverse event reviews.* http://www
.med.umich.edu/patientsafetytoolkit/events/
se_review.doc/. Accessed April 1, 2009.

13. Boothman, R.C., Blackwell, A.C., Campbell,
D.A., Jr. et al. (2009). A Better Approach to
Medical Malpractice Claims? The University of
Michigan Experience. *J Health and Life Sci
Law, 2*(2): 140.

14. McDonald, T., Helmchen, L.A., Smith, K.M.,
Centomani, N., Gunderson, A., Mayer, D., &
Chamberlin, W.H. (2009). Responding to
patient safety incidents: The seven pillars.
Qual Saf Health Care 0: qshc.2008.031633v1-
qshc.2008.031633.

15. McDonald et al., *supra* note 42.

16. National Quality Forum. (2006). *Serious
reportable events in healthcare, 2002. Consensus
report.* http://www.premierinc.com/all/safety/
topics/guidelines/downloads/nqf-serious-
reportable-events-10-15-06.pdf. Accessed
April 5, 2009.

17. The Illinois Medical Studies Act, 735 ILCS 5/8-
2101 (Westlaw 2008).

18. Reason, J. (1997). *Managing the risks of organizational accidents.* Surrey, UK: Ashgate Publishing.

19. Index of Rural Patient-Saftey Tools. (August 4,
2009). *Unsafe acts algorithm more.* http://www
.unmc.edu/rural/patient-safety/tools/
Unsafe%20Acts%20Algorithm%20more.doc.
Accessed April 1, 2009.

20. Hickson, G.B., Pichert, J.W., Webb, L.E., &
Gabbe, S.G. (2007). *A complementary approach
to promoting professionalism: Identifying, measuring, and addressing unprofessional behaviors, Acad Med 82*(11): 1040–1048, 1047.

21. Fein, S.P., Hilborne, L.H., Spiritus, E.M., Sey-
mann, G.B., Keenan, C.R., Shojania, K.G., et
al. (2007). The many faces of error disclosure:
A common set of elements and a definition.
Journal of General Internal Medicine, 22(6),
755.

22. Steinbrook, R. (2002). Protecting research
subjects: The crisis at Johns Hopkins. *New
England Journal of Medicine, 346*(9), 716.

23. Johns Hopkins Medicine. (n.d.). Peter
Pronovost's seemingly simple ideas are changing the face of patient care. http://www
.hopkinsmedicine.org/quality/safety/pronovost
/index.html/. Accessed April 1, 2009.

24. Driver, J., & Johnson, S. (2008). *Disclosure and
risk management in HSCT.* http://bmt.stanford
.edu/documents/symposium2008/driver
.pdf, PowerPoint presentation, Stanford University, Palo Alto, Calif.

25. Ibid, p. 7.

26. Ibid, p. 12.

27. Ibid, p. 11.

28. ASHRM. (2006). *When things go wrong:
Responding to adverse events.* A consensus
statement of the Harvard Hospitals. ASHRM
survey definitions (Vol. 2004). http://www
.premierinc.com/quality-safety/tools services/
safety/safety-share/tool-list-by-category.xls.
Accessed April 1, 2009.

29. Kaldjian, L.C., Jones, E.W., Wu, B.J., Forman-
Hoffman, V.L., Levi, B.H., & Rosenthal, G.E.
(2008). Reporting medical errors to improve
patient safety: A survey of physicians in
teaching hospitals. *Archives of Internal Medicine, 168*(1), 40.

30. Kaldjian et al., *supra* note 66.

31. ECRI Institute. (n.d.). *Healthcare risk control:
Executive summary.* https://www.ecri.org/
Documents/Patient_Safety_Center/HRC
_Disclosure_Unanticipated_Events_0108.pdf/.
Accessed April 1, 2009.

32. Fein, S.P., Hilborne, L.H., Spiritus, E.M., Sey-
mann, G.B., Keenan, C.R., Shojania, K.G.,
Kagawa-Singer, M., & Wenger, N.S. (June 2007).
The many faces of error disclosure: A common
set of elements and a definition. *J Gen Intern
Med 22,* (6): 755–761.

33. Banja, J. (2005). *Medical errors and medical
narcissism.* Sudbury, MA: Jones and Bartlett
Publishers.

34. Mazor, K.M., Reed, G.W., Yood, R.A., Fischer,
M.A., Baril, J., & Gurwitz, J.H. (2006). Disclo-

sure of medical errors: What factors influence how patients respond. *Journal of General Internal Medicine, 21,* 704.

35. Hickson, G.B., & Pickert, J.W. (2007). *Disclosure and apology.* Boston: National Patient Safety Foundation.

36. Banja, J. (n.d.). *Discussing unanticipated outcomes and disclosing medical errors.* Georgia Hospital Association. http://www.gha.org/phaold/video/medical.mpg/. Accessed April 13, 2009.

37. Woods, J.R., & Rozovsky, F.A. (2003). *What do I say? Communicating intended or unanticipated outcomes in obstetrics.* San Francisco: Jossey-Bass.

38. Banja, J. *Discussing unanticipated outcomes. supra* note 76.

39. Hilfiker, D. (January 12, 1984). Facing our Mistakes. *N Engl J Med, 310*(2):118–122.

40. Gallagher, T.H., Garbutt, J.M., Waterman, A.D., Flum, D.R., Larson, E.B., Waterman, B.M., et al. (2006). Choosing your words carefully: How physicians would disclose harmful medical errors to patients. *Archives of Internal Medicine, 166*(15), 1585.

41. Richard C. Boothman, *Medical Justice, supra* note 26.

42. Banja, J. (2005). *Medical Errors, supra* note 72, at 111.

43. Hoffman, L. (2008). *An apology is a powerful statement.* University of Michigan Health Law Section. Winner of 2008 writing competition.

44. Lazare, A. (2006). Apology in medical practice: An emerging clinical skill. *Journal of the American Medical Association, 296,* 1401.

45. Sixwise.com. (n.d.). *The full disclosure/early offer movement: What it could mean for you if you ever suffer a medical mistake.* http://www.sixwise.com/newsletters/07/09/12/the-full-disclosure-early-offer-movement-what-it-could-mean-for-you-if-you-ever-suffer-a-medical.html/. Accessed April 1, 2009.

46. Graham, J. (2007, August 19). Admitting mistakes not just right thing to do, medical community finds it may prevent malpractice suits. *Chicago Tribune.* http://www.sorryworks.net/tribune.phtml/. Accessed April 1, 2009.

47. Harvard Public Health Review. (2007). *We're sorry.* http://www.rmf.harvard.edu/files/documents/reviewfall07/APOLOGY.pdf/. Accessed March 30, 2009.

48. Gallagher, T.H., & Quinn, R. (2006). *What to do with the unanticipated outcome: Does apologizing make a difference? How does early resolution impact settlement outcome?* Medical liability and health care law seminar. Phoenix: Defense Research Institute.

49. Quinn, R. (n.d.). *COPIC's 3Rs program: Recognize, respond to and resolve patient injury.* PowerPoint presentation. http://www.sorryworks.net/copic.phtml/. Accessed April 13, 2009.

50. Gallagher, T.H., Studdert, D., & Levinson, W. (2007). Disclosing harmful medical errors to patients. *New England Journal of Medicine, 356*(26), 2713.

51. American Medical Association. (2007). *I'm sorry laws: Summary of state laws.* http://www.physicianspractice.com/images/publication/charts/11_2007_TheLaw_Chart1.pdf/. Accessed April 14, 2009.

52. Qojcieszak, D., Banja, J., & Houk, C. (2006). The Sorry Works! Coalition: Making the case for full disclosure. *Journal on Quality and Patient Safety, 32*(6), 344.

53. Loren, D.J., Klein, E.J., Garbutt, J., Krauss, M.J., Fraser, V., Claiborne Dunagan, W., et al. (2008). Medical error disclosure among pediatricians: Choosing carefully what we might say to patients. *Archives of Pediatrics & Adolescent Medicine, 162*(10), 922.

54. Clinton, H.R., & Obama, B. (2006). Making patient safety the centerpiece of medical liability reform. *The New England Journal of Medicine, 354*(21): 2205–2208.

55. Sack, K. (2008, May 18). Doctors to say 'I'm sorry' long before 'See you in court.' *New York Times.* http://www.nytimes.com/2008/05/18/us/18apology.html/. Accessed February 22, 2009.

19

DEVELOPING EARLY-OFFER PROGRAMS FOLLOWING DISCLOSURE

Renée Bernard, JD
Jeffrey F. Driver, JD, MBA

INTRODUCTION

The staggering number of injuries and deaths caused by medical error, reported by the Institute of Medicine (IOM), far surpassed the most commonly discussed causes of death and injury, such as motor vehicle accidents, breast cancer, and AIDS. As of 1999, between 44,000 and 98,000 deaths, and more than 900,000 injuries, were occurring annually in American hospitals.[1] The IOM released a follow-up report in 2006 stating that approximately 400,000 patients per year are injured or killed by medication errors in American hospitals.[2] It also estimated that $1–$3 million in excess costs in average-size hospitals can be attributed to complications from medical errors.[3]

Sweeping changes have taken place in the healthcare industry to begin rectifying these tragic statistics. One important change is that healthcare institutions have now distinguished unanticipated outcomes that are not preventable (complications) from those that are preventable (medical error) and have adopted full and transparent disclosure policies following unanticipated outcomes. In the case of a preventable unanticipated outcome or medical error, a full, transparent disclosure will include (1) explaining what error has caused the outcome, (2) apologizing for the error, (3) telling the patient exactly what changes will or have been made to assure that the error does not happen again to another patient in a similar situation, and (4) in some institutions, such as Stanford University Medical Center through its formal PEARL program, the offer of reasonable and early compensation outside of a legal proceeding.* The principle at work in full and

---

*Stanford's PEARL program was adopted in 2007 by its wholly owned captive insurance company, the Stanford University Medical Indemnity and Trust Insurance Company. PEARL stands for the Process for the Early Assessment and Resolution of Loss and is known nationally as a "disclosure and offer" program.

transparent disclosure policies is that only by exposing medical errors can a medical system learn from them and take steps to assure that they be prevented in the future.

This chapter moves beyond the concept of disclosure as described in Chapters 17 and 18 to acknowledge the fact that once errors are disclosed, patients may seek, and indeed are entitled to, some form of remediation. The chapter describes the work being done at Stanford University Medical Center to go further than disclosure by addressing the subsequent needs of the patient in an attempt to make the patient whole again.

THE POWER OF DISCLOSURE AND OFFER PROGRAMS

Recommendations from professional organizations and regulatory mandates support disclosure and transparency as a matter of healthcare policy by addressing the occurrence of medical error with the patient and/or family directly. The American Medical Association, American College of Physicians, and the American Nursing Association urge disclosure and transparency as an ethical obligation of the care provider.[4] Disclosure and transparency is now listed as a safe practice as well: In 2007, the National Quality Forum, which develops consensus standards for healthcare delivery, added disclosure to its list of safe practices.[5] The Joint Commission, which sets standards and accreditation for healthcare organizations, issued a standard in July 2001 that requires transparent disclosure of unanticipated outcomes.[6]

The next generation of transparent disclosure policies and programs includes an early offer of compensation when a patient is harmed by a preventable unanticipated event or medical error. These formal programs and policies are now becoming known as "full-disclosure" or "disclosure-and-offer" programs. For the purposes of this chapter, we blend these terms and call the programs

"full-disclosure-and-offer" programs. (More traditional disclosure programs that do not include a formal mechanism for early compensation are often called "partial-disclosure programs.")

An early offer of compensation is just the final step in the otherwise transparent disclosure process that a patient deserves after experiencing a preventable adverse outcome in the course of care. Less than a dozen private and governmental institutions, including hospitals and insurance companies, are on the forefront of next-generation formal full-disclosure-and-offer policies and programs, but there are early reports from these programs that the impact includes reduced claim costs, increased patient and family satisfaction, as well as hospital and medical-staff satisfaction with the process.

Industry standards for resolving a claim for compensation average 5 years.[7] This time frame is due to extensive and time-consuming litigation. In reality, very often these matters can be resolved without need for litigation by using an early-offer compensation process. Managed correctly, the early offer of compensation for a patient's injury or death due to medical error affords the healthcare organization and patient the opportunity for a timely, empathetic, and reasonable resolution

There is also evidence of direct financial savings when an adverse event is addressed with an early assessment and resolution process. The costs to an organization of defending a typical medical-malpractice lawsuit can run into tens of thousands of dollars due to administrative costs and, in some cases, can include the additional cost of a compensation award to the patient and/or family. (The greatest financial cost to the plaintiff is the attorney-contingency fee.) These costs may be justified when the facts reveal that the care rendered to the patient was appropriate; however, there is little or no justification for promoting this course of resolution where the care was questionable or clearly below standards.

Quality of Disclosure Matters

An empirical examination of the effect of apology in the course of disclosure found that quality of the disclosure affects the ability of an organization to resolve patient claims for compensation related to medical error. The study, reported by Jennifer K. Robbenolt in 2003, concluded that the nature of apology, whether full or partial, influences the patient's willingness to accept an offer of compensation as resolution.[8] A poorly executed disclosure will impact an early-offer process negatively but does not mean that the door closes on the ability to settle out of court.

While this chapter does not address the types of apologies and apology laws, it should be noted that the content of a disclosure paves the path toward resolution and actions can be taken to ensure that the path is more smooth than rocky. The study found that the more full and transparent the disclosure and apology, the more likely a patient and/or family will be inclined to accept an offer of compensation and settle the matter with the organization without litigation: 73% of the study participants stated that they would be inclined to settle the event with the organization directly; less than 15% were either inclined to reject the offer or remained unsure as to what they would do.[8] Interestingly, the amount of the settlement that a recipient is likely to accept does not appear to be affected by the quality of disclosure and apology; yet, the studies associated with these findings merely assessed the participant's propensities to accept or reject a specific settlement offer.

The transparency and accuracy that quality disclosures provide may directly affect the ability of the risk manager or organization's claims representative to foster and continue ongoing settlement discussions. It is human nature to attempt to arrive at a speedy conclusion and communicate that an outcome was due to medical error, and how it

---

VIGNETTE

A terminally ill patient dies from complications related to underlying pathology. If the patient had been treated sooner, arguably the patient might have survived longer. The complication had been, in fact, recorded in routine lab test results but not acknowledged by the receiving practitioner. The hospital takes proactive steps to make timely disclosures, waive bills for hospitalization related to the complication, and offers assistance to the family while the investigation is ongoing. The family contacts the primary physician, and in the course of their discussion, the family asks what the "mistake" is worth in the physician's opinion. The physician, angry at the nurse practitioner, states to the family, without consulting with risk management, that the physician would ask for a sum in the millions. The physician expresses disbelief that another practitioner did not check the lab results and is angry because this outcome has never happened to the physician.

The physician likely felt better; however, the settlement discussion—formerly at an appropriate amount consistent with state tort caps—must now be carefully explained back down from millions. The entire early-offer process was disrupted to the benefit of no one involved.

Robbenolt believed that further empirical study was necessary to explore the extent to which potential litigants' monetary expectations of settlement are affected by apology—in other words, in sincere and transparent communication. However, risk managers can reasonably infer that a sincere and quality disclosure process without blame and defensiveness will reduce the likelihood of higher financial expectation on the part of a potential litigant who is harboring anger and disappointment at the organization and care providers. Additionally, considering the direct (personnel, internal legal counsel, etc.) and indirect (loss of goodwill, public-relations hit, etc.) costs associated with the time it takes to address anger in a potential litigant who feels stonewalled or treated insincerely, one can also infer that transparency is smart business practice in the long run.

occurred, in a single disclosure conversation with a patient. However, more often than not, adverse events do not lend themselves to quick understanding and require a thoughtful and methodical investigation to gain a complete understanding; thus, sequential discussions with a patient allow more accurate information to be provided by the organization for consideration by the patient and/or family. In an effort to promote a smooth early-offer process, it is recommended that disclosure discussions follow the maxim, "Better late than early," because sometimes what appears at first to be a medical error may in fact be an unanticipated outcome that could have occurred under the best of care. An erroneous disclosure conversation later retracted by a healthcare provider or institutional representative will more often than not be greeted with mistrust leading to a breakdown of, or complete disruption of, the disclosure process.

A poorly executed disclosure can occur for many reasons. For example, one physician blaming another physician results in "jousting" between the physicians and appears unprofessional when witnessed by the patient and/or family. This scenario reinforces the common complaint of "one hand did not know what the other was doing," and can increase the financial expectation of the patient and/or family toward the organization. A helpful adage to impart to physicians is that while standing in the same boat (the organization), one physician should never point the finger at another and state "you sank the lifeboat," because in this kind of situation everyone is going to drown.

Are Early-Offer Processes Financially Feasible?

Studies such as Robbenolt's study, as well as experts in the field, support the findings that patients who experience medical error:

1. Sue if they are not given sufficient information about the event

2. Desire communication that the organization is taking responsibility for what has occurred
3. Tend not to sue when their expectations are met

The Harvard Study was conducted to test the theory that disclosure programs can reduce litigation costs to practicing organizations.[9] The study hypothesized that the quantity and cost of prompted claims revealed by rigorous disclosure programs would "trounce" any deterrent effects that healthcare organizations could expect from proactive disclosure programs.[10] It predicted that the forecasts of reduced litigation costs would not be realized and the costs would likely increase.[11]

The study concluded that healthcare institutions practicing rigorous disclosure practices can expect an increase in litigation volume and costs, because rigorous disclosure of unexpected medical injury will reveal a pool of patients who would not consider bringing suit based on their care outcome if not for the disclosure. This situation is referred to as "the great unlitigated reservoir."[12] The researchers found that approximately 8 of 10 serious injuries are in fact due to negligence, and more than 9 of 10 serious injuries never trigger litigation.[12] Because the number of unlitigated injuries vastly outnumber litigated ones, disclosure of injuries that would have otherwise remained undiscovered by the patient will likely lead to an increase in claims and litigation costs.[12]

The Harvard researchers stated that the problem with the risk management hypothesis that disclosure is smart business practice is that it "misreads and overreaches the available evidence."[12] The current evidence related to disclosure consists of studies done with data gathered retrospectively from a combination of sources such as surveys submitted to plaintiffs at the end of the process, closed claims files, and analysis of characteristics of physicians who were sued or escaped litigation, as well as analysis of breakdowns in communication that occurred between the patient and physician.[13] They suggested that more reliable data would come from a study of decision making immediately after the injury, specifically accounting for the possibility that without a disclosure the patient may not have discovered the injury or its cause.[13] As the study points out, to date, evidence of this research has not been reported.[14]

The Harvard Study posited that the movement toward transparency about medical injuries will expose tension between doing the right thing—disclosing medical error—and managing the cost of such a disclosure. That being the case, risk managers have been encouraged to engage in prudent financial planning as they engage in transparent disclosure practices.

After a searing response from experts in the field from the United States to Australia regarding the methodology used to come to their conclusion, the Harvard researchers stated that "responsible health care institutions will not use our study findings as a reason to violate regulatory and professional ethical mandates to disclose injuries."[14,15]

Response to Harvard Study: Risk Managers Should Not Be Deterred

> Rely upon your own judgment as there will be those who tell you that you are foolish; that your judgment is faulty, but heed them not. If what they say is true, the sooner you, as a searcher of wisdom, find it out the better, and you can only make that discovery by bringing your powers to the test. Therefore, pursue your course bravely.
>
> —James Allen

Experts in the field of healthcare risk management have considered the prediction of increased litigation costs reported in the Harvard Study, and they still do not agree.

Early field reports of disclosure-and-offer-program outcomes, at least thus far, indicate reduced litigation costs and liability-insurance-premium relief. Only time and further study of pioneering disclosure-and-offer-program outcomes will reveal the truth about the financial viability of disclosure-and-offer programs.

The methodology used by the Harvard researchers relied on the use of legal, medical, and insurance professionals who cannot simulate the emotional response brought about by transparent communication with an injured patient and/or their family. The responses captured by the experts used were possibly based on the old school of thought that malpractice resolution is all about money. In fact, disclosure engages the human aspects of medical error, such as trust, compassion, understanding, forgiveness, and mitigation of anger. Patients and families are often first interested in ensuring that the medical error does not happen to another patient; thus, disclosure of steps taken to improve patient safety, which include the family's input and ability to tell their story, often allows the parties involved to gain significant ground toward resolution. The assumption that money is the key factor in disclosure exhibits a lack of understanding of what patients and families desire in the wake of an adverse medical event.

On the other hand, the "unlitigated reservoir" is no more frightening than the dark "deny-and-defend" regime from which risk management is emerging. Transparency brings new and unexpected aspects of patient care and risk management to light, and risk managers must rise to the occasion and navigate the labyrinth of actions and reactions. As often is the case in risk management, the lessons will be learned on a case-by-case basis.

Institutions with transparent disclosure practices continue to report success in resolving adverse medical outcomes. The success is seen in the decreased amount of time that such events are resolved, the ability to work with the patient or family directly, and—due to both of these aspects—an overall decrease in litigation costs.

PEARL: PROCESS FOR EARLY ASSESSMENT AND RESOLUTION OF LOSS

Stanford University Medical Center's captive lies at the heart of its risk management strategy. The captive, Stanford University Medical Indemnity and Trust (SUMIT), was established in the early 1980s to cover medical-malpractice claims.[16] SUMIT established the Process for the Early Assessment and Resolution of Loss (PEARL) in 2007 to implement an institution-wide system of early assessment of "concerning outcomes," open disclosure of preventable unanticipated outcomes, compensation when warranted, and turning the learning lessons of these concerning outcomes into performance-improvement opportunities.[17] The process fosters not only early analysis of unforeseen medical events but also helps create a team atmosphere with the patient or family through consistent and open communication intended to provide desired and needed information after such an event.

Documented Success of PEARL

A PEARL case is ideally reported after a concerning outcome is reported to the risk management office. The average time for a claim to come to the attention of SUMIT Risk Management in non-Pearl cases is 11 months, and these typically take the form of a written claim or lawsuit.[17] In PEARL matters, however, SUMIT Risk Management often can be involved only hours, or a few days, after the event, which allows for more in-depth review and assistance to the patient and medical staff at the critical time of care.[17]

Additionally, industry standards for resolving a claim file from date of opening the file to closing the file average 5 years.[17] Extensive and time-consuming litigation is often the cause of this lengthy period, which also adds to the emotional and financial cost to all involved. Of a number of PEARL files recently analyzed, the average time frame for resolution and closing the file was 6 months.[17] Very often these matters can be resolved without need for litigation, which results in a tremendous savings in the emotional and time costs to all involved.

There is evidence of direct financial savings when a concerning outcome is addressed within an early-offer-and-disclosure process. By directly engaging the patient and/or family in the process of understanding what has occurred, how the matter can be resolved for the patient and, if applicable, avoided for other patients, the need for retained legal representation for both parties is significantly reduced. Not only have PEARL outcomes shown a marked decrease in the overall claim costs when compared with litigated cases, but the expenses involved in a PEARL review can be as low as 5% of the average cost of a litigated case.[17] PEARL is a successful process for both the clinician and the patient. Its benefits have been demonstrated, from defending staff aggressively based upon early findings of no negligence, to open and honest evaluation and disclosure of human error, to lessening the emotional toil and time consumption related to adversarial litigation.

CARE COSTS THAT FLOW FROM MEDICAL ERROR ARE THE INSTITUTIONS' RESPONSIBILITY

As the largest insurer in the United States, The Centers for Medicaid and Medicare Services (CMS) decision not to pay for medical error will influence how public and private institutions manage costs associated with inappropriate care. In October 2008, CMS formally announced that it will no longer pay for specified, reasonably preventable hospital-acquired conditions (HAC) that occur to a Medicare beneficiary as an inpatient.[17] The CMS policy is based on providing incentive for institutions to improve patient safety systems and to place appropriate institutional accountability for the costs that stem from unanticipated, reasonably preventable medical outcomes.[18] See Chapter 7 for a detailed discussion of these programs.

Specifically, the final acute-care inpatient prospective payment system (IPPS) rule published by CMS includes nine potential categories of conditions for 2008: six are finalized, and three are being considered for finalization.[18] Hospitals that treat Medicare beneficiaries as inpatients can expect not to receive payment for the following HACs:[18]

- Foreign object retained after surgery
- Air embolism
- Blood incompatibility
- Stage-III and stage-IV pressure ulcers
- Fall or trauma resulting in serious injury
- Catheter-associated vascular injury
- Urinary tract infections

Additionally, the following HACs are under consideration for non-payment:[18]

- Surgical-site infections following certain elective procedures, including certain orthopedic surgeries and bariatric surgery for obesity
- Certain manifestations of poor control of blood-sugar levels
- Deep-vein thrombosis or pulmonary embolism following total-knee replacement and hip-replacement procedures

Additionally, Medicaid programs and some of the country's largest insurers have announced that they will not pay for at least 28 "never events" in several states.[18] For example, in April 2008, Maine became the first state to ban the practice of billing for medical errors.[18]

Where responsibility for an adverse care outcome is the result of medical error, the full responsibility for the costs associated with the care should rest with the organization. Risk managers should engage their process for capturing or holding costs associated with suspected medical error while the course of care is investigated. Once it is determined that the costs, in fact, flow from the medical error, then risk management should ensure that such costs be absorbed by the organization as opposed to being submitted to insurance. In situations that do not involve "never events" or do not appear to have been caused by medical error, risk managers should look to the practice of their organization to determine if there are bills that should be waived solely as a matter of customer service.

CASE-STUDY ILLUSTRATION OF THE EARLY-OFFER PROCESS

As seen in the examples of early-offer programs discussed previously, the nuts and bolts of creating and managing an early-offer process may vary according to institutions and their respective legal jurisdictions. The vignette presented on the following page is a fictitious case-study illustration of how an early-offer process works to reveal facts, shape disclosures, and resolve care matters in a timely manner to the benefit of both the patient and the organization.

ACTIONS THAT SHOULD FOLLOW AN UNANTICIPATED MEDICAL EVENT

Immediate Counsel After an Event

Care providers should be encouraged to contact risk management no more than 4 hours after an unanticipated medical event. Involving risk management as early as possible creates a collaborative effort toward understanding the cause of the event. Risk management's role is to review the event facts to confirm severity and causation in collaboration with quality, internal or external experts, and legal counsel. The risk manager should engage legal counsel to provide attorney–client protections to the investigation and management of the matter. Further confidentiality may be provided by engaging the peer-review process depending on the laws of peer review in the jurisdiction.

VIGNETTE

A 42-year-old insurance executive and weekend athlete presented to the emergency department via ambulance following multi-trauma during the bicycling portion of a triathlon race. The primary injury appeared to be to the left shoulder, and radiographs confirmed non-displaced fractures of the scapula and comminuted fracture of the humerus. The emergency department attending physician also ordered chest and spine films, which were negative for fractures or other significant findings. The patient also had abrasions of both lower legs and complained of left-calf pain, but lower-extremity X-rays were negative for injury as well. Following an orthopedic surgery consult, the patient was taken to the operating room for open reduction–internal fixation of the humerus fracture. On postoperative day one, the patient complained of chest pain radiating to the left (post-surgical) shoulder and arm. Blood was drawn to check for cardiac enzymes and results showed an elevated enzyme level consistent with the leg-muscle injury from the bike accident. The patient's postoperative pain medication was increased. On night nursing rounds, the patient was found in his bed without respiration or pulse. Resuscitative efforts were unsuccessful. The case was referred to the county medical examiner. The care team consulted risk management.

Risk management recommended that the physician meet with the patient's wife as soon as possible, and after empathizing with, and listening to, the wife, disclose known facts, explain that the actual cause of the patient's death was currently being investigated because it was not clear, and provide contact information of the individual so that the wife could follow up should she have more questions prior to the next meeting.

A root cause analysis (RCA) was held the morning following the patient's death. The RCA revealed that an electrocardiogram performed after the onset of left chest pain was normal except for tachycardia to a rate of 120. Blood was drawn to check for cardiac enzymes, and results showed elevated enzyme levels consistent with the muscle injury from the bike accident. The patient's oxygen level was low and his respiratory rate was high, but the symptoms were attributed to pain. A pulmonary ventilation/perfusion scan to rule out pulmonary embolism was ordered for the following morning. An emergency room physician stated that he did not appreciate hearing that a surgical staff member told the wife that her husband's calf pain should have been evaluated further in the emergency department because clearly the embolism had occurred on the surgical team's watch.

One month after the event, the wife agreed to meet to discuss the findings of the investigation. She expressed anger and sadness as well as a desire to understand how this could have happened, because one of the physicians stated that it was an obvious mistake. She wanted to know what was being done to prevent this in the future. She asked what the hospital would do to make amends. Risk management explained how the care decisions were made and why a pulmonary embolism could have been, but was not, considered. Risk management carefully explained the tort-reform cap on damages and made a fair and reasonable offer of compensation. The wife was offended, stating that she and her two children relied on her husband for their income. Risk management recommended that in the event that a financial agreement could not be reached between them, the organization would pay to have the matter mediated by an unaffiliated, third-party mediator. The wife asked if she could involve an attorney.

Internal peer review of the matter revealed that the patient's death was likely preventable. A letter was sent by risk management communicating sympathy, assurance that the organization was actively responding to this incident, and a desire to meet with the patient's wife when she felt she was ready. In the weeks prior to the wife's response, the medical examiner's report confirmed that the cause of death was pulmonary embolism.

The wife took more time to think about the offer and discussed the matter with the rest of her family. She decided that her husband would have wanted her to ensure that the organization could change its practice to protect other patients. Within 3 months, she communicated that she wanted the proposed offer and an opportunity to tell her husband's story. Risk management offered to collaborate with her to create education on the topic in her husband's name.

Disclosure Consultation

Risk managers are an important consultative resource for care providers who treat a patient who has experienced a medical event. Disclosure conversations can be awkward and difficult, and therefore it is imperative that care providers receive consultation in preparing for, and conducting, the disclosure to the patient, and if appropriate, the patient's family.

Just-in-Time Coaching Prior to Disclosure

In addition to investigation of serious medical events, the Anesthesia Patient Safety Foundation (APSF) and The Joint Commission require that institutions disclose an unexpected outcome to the patient with the help of a risk manager. Risk management's role is to shape the disclosure conversation into one that is forthright and reassuring, but which does not exacerbate the situation. One of several disclosure methods is called the just-in-time model. The just-in-time model approaches disclosure of an unexpected outcome through the individual practitioner, who discloses to the patient facts as they are known, at the site of the event. The discloser is any physician or care provider who has the strongest relationship with the patient or family, depending on the significance of the event and seriousness of the outcome. The American Society of Healthcare Risk Management suggests that this approach is the "ultimate in mature patient/family partnering." The approach focuses on the importance of maintaining patient trust in the individuals who have been most responsible for care.

Early-Assessment Period

The early-assessment period of an early-offer process is key to a timely determination of the facts of the event, understanding severity, and planning of the next steps. Early assessment begins at the point of notification of an event to risk management. Ideally, the early-assessment period spans no more than 5–10 days. To maintain this time frame, a 7-day multi-level assessment that involves quality review in the form of a root-cause analysis, review by internal and external experts, and legal analysis of the potential for a medical-malpractice claim as a result of the event is recommended.

Internal and External Expert Review

In matters that involve complex medical complications, immediate expert review is recommended. Risk management may engage physicians who serve on the facility's internal peer-review committees for review of the medical-care decisions tied to the event. Such engagement allows expert review of the care provided while adding the legal protection afforded to the peer-review process by the jurisdiction within which the event took place.

It is also recommended, where feasible, that an external-expert review of the matter be obtained in cases that involve complex medical issues. Maintaining legal protection of the external review is achieved by having legal counsel manage the hiring and communications between the organization and the medical expert.

Factual Assessment of the Event

Within 1 week, using an early-assessment process, a clear picture of what actually gave rise to the event will emerge. Using this information, legal counsel in collaboration with risk management will determine whether the standard of care was met and the event was unpreventable. If the standard of care was not met, the next determination is whether the breach in standard of care actually caused the injury experienced by the patient; if it did, then legal counsel will need to determine both the general and special damages that flow from the injury.

Setting Claim Reserves

Upon notice of a potentially compensable event, the claims representative will set reserves. The reserves will be based initially on general damages. In cases involving the death of a patient, the reserve should reflect any tort-reform limits set by state law as the ceiling on reserves for general damages. Special damages tend to be subjective and include consideration of absolute liability, egregiousness of the facts, any past-experience valuation of the same type of injury, provable lost income, and leaving room for unknown factors that may be discovered later.

Advising Patients or Their Families to Seek Legal Counsel

Understanding that patients and their families may lose trust in the organization in the course of a medical error, they will often ask if they can or should seek legal counsel. It is recommended that the risk manager empathize but also state that the risk manager cannot provide such legal advice and will abide by whatever the patient or family decides to do; however, it should be made clear that once the patient is represented, the risk manager can no longer communicate on the matter directly with the patient. Additionally, the risk manager should assure the patient that in any case, the intent of risk management is to resolve the matter in a fair manner.

Sponsored Mediation

When discussions with the family are not fruitful, it is recommended that the risk manager offer sponsored mediation. Sponsored mediation offers another opportunity to convey a good-faith effort to resolve the matter out of court. The patient or family can be offered a choice of several mediators in the area from which to choose after doing research, if desired. The mediators should be well versed in the law of the state and have a good reputation in the industry. The costs of mediation are covered by the organization.

Settlement Agreements

Legal counsel should be engaged in drafting a settlement agreement that is designed to prevent the ability to further litigate the matter and to create a confidentiality contract between parties. The patient or family must be provided the document with time to review and evaluate it prior to signing. In some cases the confidentiality agreement will not be straightforward and will need to be crafted to fit the agreement reached by the parties.

Managing Media Involvement

The organization should have a policy regarding who will respond to media matters. This individual or department will require a clear understanding of the facts of the matter and the goal of communications on the matter from the organization.

References

1. Kohn, L., Corrigan, J., & Donaldson, M. (Eds.). (2000). *To err is human: Building a safer health care system.* Committee on Quality of Health Care in America, Institute of Medicine. Washington, DC: National Academy Press.
2. The Stanford University Medical Indemnity and Trust Insurance Company. (2008). Process for the Early Assessment and Resolution of Loss, PEARL. Board of Trustees of the Leland Stanford Jr. University, p. 3.
3. Stanford University Medical Center. (2007). *Risk Management Advisory, 3*(2).
4. American Medical Association of Medical Ethics. (2004). *Code of medical ethics. Opinion 8.12—patient information.* http://www.ama-assn.org/ama/pub/physician-resources/medical-ethics/code-medical-ethics/opinion812.shtml/. Accessed July 15, 2009.

5. National Quality Forum. (2007). Safe practices for better health care: 2006 update. A consensus report, p. 77.

6. The Joint Commission. (2007). Hospital accreditation standards, 147. Standard RI 2.90.

7. Studdert, D.M. (2009). *Malpractice Insurers Medical Error Surveillance and Prevention Study.* http://www.rmf.harvard.edu/research -resources/research-studies/MIMESPS -study.aspx/. Accessed July 15, 2009.

8. Robbenolt, J.K. (2003). Apologies and legal settlement: An empirical examination. *Michigan Law Review, 102,* 460.

9. Ibid, p. 487.

10. Studdert, D., Mello, M.M., Gawande, A.A., Brennan, T.A., & Wang, Y.C. (2007). Disclosure of medical injury to patients: An improbable risk management strategy. *Health Affairs, 26*(1),215–226. http://content.healthaffairs.org/ index.dtl/. Accessed July 15, 2009.

11. Ibid, p. 216.

12. Ibid. p. 222.

13. Ibid, p. 223.

14. Ibid, p. 224.

15. Kraman, S.S., & Hamm, G. (2007). Bad modeling? *Health Affairs, 26*(3), 898–905. http://content.healthaffairs.org/index.dtl/. Accessed July 15, 2009.

16. Boothman, R.C. (2006). *Medical justice: Making the system work better for patients and doctors.* Testimony of Richard C. Boothman, Chief Risk Officer, University of Michigan Health System, before the Senate Committee on Health, Education, Labor and Pensions, June 22, 2006. http://www.yellowdocuments .com/10146167-testimony-of-richard-c- boothman. Accessed April 20, 2010.

17. Stanford University Medical Indemnity & Trust Insurance Company, et al. (2007). Process for Early Assessment and Resolution of Loss (PEARL).

18. Centers for Medicare and Medicaid Services. (2009, April 18). *Medicare and Medicaid move aggressively to encourage greater patient safety in hospitals and reduce never events.* Press release. http://www.cms.hhs.gov/. Accessed July 15, 2009.

20

CRIMINALIZATION OF HEALTHCARE NEGLIGENCE

Deb Ankowicz, BSN, RN, CPHQ, CPHRM

INTRODUCTION

The Patient Safety movement in the United States has been driven by accreditation organizations and the public's expectations that healthcare providers should always deliver perfect patient care or zero defects (to borrow a term from the manufacturing industry). Is such a thing humanly possible? Humans currently delivering health care increasingly must interact with technology to deliver, monitor, and record interventions taken and care delivered. Moreover, while the technological trend is seen as a positive means to reduce human error, as evidenced by the use of bar-code scanning of medications at the bedside, robots to perform surgery in the operating room, the implementation of "smart pumps" to deliver intravenous (IV) medications, and the nationwide push toward the adoption of the electronic medical record, the interface between man and machine introduces new and often unanticipated risks.

The field of Human Factors Engineering is making great strides to identify and mitigate the risks that these human–equipment interface errors introduce by studying healthcare work flows and how humans interact with technology. Only by understanding human behavior and current models for healthcare delivery are we able to begin to anticipate and understand the creative work-arounds that providers discover to get the job done when technology poses perceived barriers. When medical-equipment engineers understand the nature of interface errors, they are able to design technology to reduce the errors to make healthcare delivery safer; however, we have a long way to go before we can ensure that health care will be 100% error free. Indeed, as long as humans are involved, zero defects may be only a dream.

Are we expecting the impossible from our healthcare system and our healthcare providers? Who will want to enter the inherently high-risk healthcare professions in the future if this small but growing trend toward criminal prosecution of those whose intention it is to heal rather than harm continues? What has happened to the concept of criminal intent? To achieve the goal of transparency and a culture that fosters open reporting of unintended outcomes, we must strike a balance that allows providers to feel safe reporting errors and free from the fear of frivolous civil litigation and criminal prosecution in the absence of premeditation or willful, reckless endangerment. Only by achieving this balance will we be able to aggregate and analyze these data to better understand the complex nature of healthcare delivery and make the systems safer for both the patients and providers.

Additionally, manufacturers and equipment suppliers must assist in this effort and standardize equipment and products so that human error can be minimized. Until the equipment with which physicians, nurses, and other healthcare workers interact to deliver care are standardized, variations in product design will continue to allow even the most diligent practitioner to make an unintended error if certain conditions are present. The recent rise in the number of safety alerts and device-recall notices being distributed by medical-device manufacturers to healthcare facilities and providers shows a growing recognition of liability issues surrounding the use of medical devices and the attempt to shift the liability from the manufacturer to the facility or provider using the device. The next step is for the manufacturing industry to partner with the healthcare industry by employing the science of human-factors engineering principles in the research, development, and design phases of medical-device production to prevent human errors from being able to occur (e.g., tubing misconnections) with device use.

Finally, circumstances such as an inadequate number of staff or inadequately trained staff in facilities that provide around-the-clock care (e.g., hospitals and nursing homes) are common in our facilities today and may get worse as the nursing work force

ages. Working too many hours in a row, working too many hours in a pay period, or doubling back from nights to days may lead to sleep deprivation. Sleep deprivation is known to be dangerous and has led to work rules that limit the hours that can be worked in other industries, such as the airline and over-the-road trucking industries. Residents-in-training now have similar limitations in the number of hours that they are allowed to work, and some states have followed suit by passing legislation to limit nursing hours to help prevent fatigue-related errors from occurring. These limitations address the fatigue issue, but the resulting increase in the number of hand-offs presents new communication challenges and new opportunities for errors to occur.

INCIDENT REPORTING, LEGAL PROTECTIONS, AND EFFECTS ON CULTURE OF SAFETY

To gain a better understanding of what type of errors occur in health care, it is necessary to collect data. Incident reporting was one of the first risk management tools developed by the insurance industry for insureds to report a claim. In the beginning, reports were simple narrative accounts of the facts of the incident. Only when reporting formats became more standardized, collecting information by incident type as well as contributing factors with information recorded in databases, were trends and opportunities to prevent similar occurrences from happening in the future identified. Incident reporting became more than just a method to report a claim; it also became a useful tool to be used by the quality assurance/improvement department to look at system-improvement opportunities. Risk and quality have been sharing this factual data-collection tool since then. A trend toward on-line reporting in recent years has allowed for more information to be gathered on actual and near-miss events with greater opportunity for timely analysis of the information to examine potential system failures and the ability to take quicker action to remedy or mitigate a situation that has been reported.

Protecting the information contained in incident reports from discovery in civil litigation has been very important toward encouraging the reporting of errors. Only when providers feel safe completing an occurrence report have we seen reporting rates of actual events, near misses, and unsafe conditions improve. Overall organizational reporting rates generally correlate with how safe providers feel, and self-reporting of healthcare errors absolutely requires a mature culture of safety. It has been repeatedly demonstrated that when providers fear litigation, reporting rates decline.

The Agency for Healthcare Research and Quality (AHRQ), Press Ganey Associates, and other patient safety organizations encourage conducting a periodic culture-of-safety survey and have developed standardized tools for use to better understand the reporting culture of an organization over time as well as compared with other similar organizations. Recent reports from these safety-culture surveys consistently demonstrate that fear of information being used in a punitive manner drives down reporting.[1] Our goal, therefore, must be to continue to do everything we can to foster a culture of open and honest reporting as well as trust in leadership.

Figure 20–1 illustrates typical responses from healthcare providers that explain their reluctance in reporting medical errors.

Early in the patient safety movement, a "no-blame" culture was encouraged and there was a focus on system errors instead of a focus on the traditional model of identifying the "bad-apple" provider. Over time, this systems-thinking approach was balanced with individual accountability. Now we strive for a "just" culture, one where individuals are held accountable for knowing and following organizational policies and procedures, and yet, if while doing so they commit an unintended error, they can feel safe reporting the error, knowing that systems will be examined to help minimize the chance that others will make the same mistake. They do not fear termination or retaliation for reporting the event, because they know that they will be treated fairly by the employer. A "just" culture provides a balance that allows for personal accountability for an individual's actions while learning from a non-punitive examination of the systems that allowed the error to occur in the first place.[2] There are essentially three types of behaviors that are considered in applying the principles of a just culture: human error, at-risk behavior, and reckless behavior (Figure 20–2). This "Guide to Just Decisions about Behavior," developed by the Missouri Baptist Medical Center, provides a

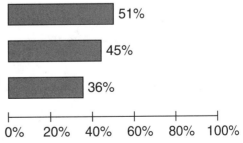

1. Staff feel like their mistakes are held against them. 51%
2. When an event is reported, it feels like the person is being written up, not the problem. 45%
3. Staff worry that mistakes they make are kept in their personnel file. 36%

0%   20%   40%   60%   80%   100%

Figure 20–1 Nonpunitive Response to Error
Source: AHRQ Hospital survey on patient safety culture: 2008 comparative database report (online). http://www.ahrq.gov/qual/hospsurvey08.

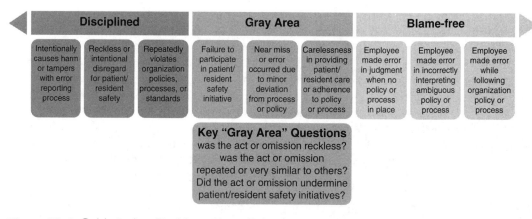

Figure 20–2 Guide to Just Decisions About Behavior

roadmap for employers and employees alike to make informed decisions in a "just" and fair culture of accountability and safety.[3]

The Joint Commission (TJC) requires accredited organizations to analyze significant errors, to identify and understand the "root cause" of an incident, and to put into place measures that address the root cause, in order to prevent repeat occurrences. The voluntary reporting of root-cause-analysis (RCA) findings to TJC has resulted in the release of numerous TJC sentinel-event alerts that help the industry proactively learn from system failures identified by others. We know that the ability to analyze and understand the causes of error is helpful, but the voluntary system that TJC has in place is only a beginning. The Joint Commission has recognized the limitations of a voluntary reporting system, as evidenced by the relatively low numbers of sentinel events reported annually; however, aggregate data collected over the years have proved invaluable toward understanding specific types of healthcare errors. Many states are following suit, now requiring mandatory reporting of specific event types to further foster the sharing of lessons learned. Despite this shared learning, we still have medical errors occurring in our hospi-

tals and clinics every day. Why the low number of voluntary reports, and why do we keep making the same or similar types of errors?

Many organizations do not voluntarily report to TJC due to the patchwork of legal protections provided by individual state laws. Some states have mandatory reporting of errors along with essential legal protections for providers to prevent information from being used against them in civil litigation. Other states with mandatory reporting of errors, but not the same legal protections, experience higher malpractice claim rates. Provider shortages also seem to be endemic in these states, as the cost and fear of litigation drive providers to seek employment in less litigious environments. This paradox unfairly punishes while driving reporting of occurrences down. Until we reform our malpractice system nationally, we will continue to see variances in reporting and barriers to learning from the medical errors of others.

Passage of the Patient Safety and Quality Improvement Act of 2005 (Patient Safety Act) and issuance of the final rule for Patient Safety Organizations on January 19, 2009, governing the development of Patient Safety Organizations (PSOs), affords additional protection for some incidents reported through

PSOs (see Chapter 8). Over time, the hope is that by organizational reporting of event data and event analysis collected through PSOs in a uniform format, lessons learned will be able to be shared with the entire healthcare industry to help others avoid the same or similar errors. Time will tell how much additional protection from civil litigation, and perhaps criminal prosecution, organizations that report to PSOs will experience.

THE HUMAN FACTOR IMPACT ON HEALTHCARE DELIVERY

It is helpful to analyze the potential risks of a new technology before it is introduced by conducting a proactive risk assessment using a tool such as a Failure Modes Effects Analysis (FMEA) or other similar tool. By identifying the potential failure points of a system prior to an actual event occurring, mitigation strategies may be deployed in anticipation of incidents to prevent them from happening; however, no matter how robust and how thoroughly conducted an FMEA may be, humans are not predictable, and creative solutions to performing the job duty may introduce unintended errors based on unanticipated work flows. Technology may be helpful, but it also may be cumbersome and time-consuming, causing the provider to develop creative work-arounds that may also produce unintended consequences.

Understanding why humans make errors is a fascinating and evolving area of behavioral science. In the book, *Why We Make Mistakes,* Pulitzer Prize-winning journalist and former Nieman Fellow at Harvard University, Joseph T. Hallinan, examines the factors that contribute to human errors.[4] Many of the factors that he has identified help to explain why errors may continue to occur in the delivery of health care. For example, the more familiar we are with a process, the more shortcuts we take. We look, but we do not necessarily see what we need to see to prevent an unintended outcome because we perceive what we *expect* to see, which may explain why

patient-identification errors continue to occur. We recall events in a more favorable light when asked to reconstruct them, which may explain why events continue to occur even after conducting an RCA and system changes have been made to reduce the likelihood of a repeat occurrence. When we multitask, our brains slow down, but still we expect our healthcare providers to deliver complex treatments and perform technically complicated interventions while enduring multiple interruptions and distractions. When we are fatigued, we also do not respond as quickly or think as clearly as when we are well rested, yet staffing shortages encourage overtime use, which may result in a fatigued healthcare work force. Unfortunately, we expect our healthcare colleagues to always identify potentially harmful occurrences before causing patient harm, when perhaps the best we can hope for is that the most important errors will be identified. Understanding and accepting our humanness and how it affects our work environment is an important step in understanding our ability to apply solutions to prevent unintentional patient harm.

The Joint Commission also has accreditation standards for hospitals that require disclosure of unanticipated outcomes to patients. Other organizations, such as the Leapfrog Group for Patient Safety and the Institute for Healthcare Improvement (IHI), have similar recommendations. Moreover, while most providers will agree that disclosure is the right thing to do, their professional-liability insurance carriers may not necessarily share the same view; thus, providers involved in an unanticipated patient outcome must carefully choose their words when disclosing the facts of an event so as not to admit liability, which in turn could potentially void any coverage in the event of civil litigation. If there is a death involved or substantial permanent patient harm and the potential for criminal prosecution, the risk of negative consequences for the provider may increase when events are reported and disclosed if not done thoughtfully and carefully. Criminal-liability defense may be covered by a professional-liability policy, but many policies do not include such coverage. Directors and Officer (D&O) policies also may afford criminal defense coverage, but again, coverage will most certainly end if there is a finding of criminal action, with some policies requiring a funds "pay back" if that is indeed the case. Most liability policies, however, have no provision for defense costs, and personal assets may be at risk in such instances, leaving providers worried about the cost for the defense of a criminal case and its impact on their family's financial security even if they are found to be innocent of the charges. If the provider is found guilty of criminal charges, he or she could be facing jail time instead of just a monetary penalty, as in a civil case, and in addition, the criminal-defense costs.

DIFFERENCES BETWEEN CIVIL AND CRIMINAL LITIGATION

Legally, the term "civil" refers to private rights and remedies that are sought by action or suit.[5] Malpractice litigation is a civil matter and the action or suit is brought by an individual against a provider or organization that seeks to resolve a legal dispute. If the provider or organization is found to have behaved in a negligent manner in judgment or performance of a procedure, the provider and/or the organization would be subject to civil money penalties. The standard for medical malpractice is that the plaintiff must prove by a preponderance of evidence that the defendant had a duty to the plaintiff, was responsible for the plaintiff's alleged injury by performance of an act or by an omission that fell below the standard of care (as proved by expert testimony), and that the injury caused damages. Evidence is controlled by the parties involved and is obtained through the discovery process in preparation for trial. The case is heard by a jury at a trial, a verdict is reached, and com-

pensation for damages is awarded. In some states, punitive damages are allowed, whereas in others they are not. In some states there are caps on non-economic damages. Professional-liability policies cover damages within the policy limits and often attorney fees as well, depending on the policy terms. Excess coverage or umbrella policies are often purchased to cover the "big-dollar" cases, and personal assets are only at risk in certain circumstances where the award exceeds limits or in states that allow providers to "go bare," or in other words, to not purchase professional-liability insurance. The majority of states now require the provider be covered by professional-liability insurance to protect the rights of injured patients. Either the defendant or the plaintiff may appeal the verdict in a civil case.

Criminal litigation applies different legal standards. Charges are brought by a state prosecutor against the defendant and evidence is controlled by the prosecutor's office. There is a higher burden of proof than in a civil case, and findings must be beyond a reasonable doubt before the defendant is found guilty of the charges. If the defendant is found to be guilty, he or she faces monetary fines, prison time, and often probation. Only the defendant has a right to appeal the verdict in a criminal case. No insurance policy covers these types of monetary fines and criminal-defense fees are usually excluded from professional-liability policies.[6]

A key difference between civil litigation and criminal prosecution is to whom the defendant must pay: the injured victim or society. In a civil healthcare negligence case, the defendant is required to pay the plaintiff for negligent performance of a medical act or omission, whereas in a criminal case the defendant owes a debt to society at large. Another key difference is that in a criminal case, prosecution is intended to deter performance of the criminal act with retribution through punishment, whereas in a civil case the defendant is ordered to pay a monetary penalty to make the plaintiff whole.

In the case of healthcare negligence due to complex and confounding human factors, such as fatigue or system failures (e.g., different types of medical tubing that can easily be misconnected), the question becomes, "Would criminal prosecution achieve the desired effect of deterrence?" Perhaps, by asking this question as each case presents, a reasonable standard of when to pursue civil litigation versus criminal prosecution can be established, particularly when the case is in the "gray zone" between clear-cut medical error and cases with willful criminal intent. Additionally, at the heart of civil malpractice litigation are the objectives to reimburse the injured patient and to monitor the quality of health care provided. When these objectives are not met by malpractice litigation, the public questions the effectiveness of civil litigation and may demand punishment, a remedy that may only be available through criminal prosecution.[7]

THE BEGINNING OF THE TREND: CRIMINAL NEGLIGENCE IN MOTOR VEHICLE CASES

Auto accidents with fatalities began to be prosecuted as vehicular homicide when individuals knowingly took an unacceptable risk, showing a blatant disregard for human life, such as driving drunk. Society demanded that these individuals be punished for their acts, even though there was not intent to harm, because the act of drinking and driving was seen as a blatant disregard for life. In *State v. Barman* (183 Wis.2d 180 [1994] 515 N.W.2d 493), the defendant was convicted of homicide by negligent operation of a motor vehicle because he had failed to observe a stop sign, entered an intersection without stopping, and collided with another vehicle, killing three of its passengers. It was later determined that he had likely fallen asleep at the wheel. He lost on appeal and the standard for criminal negligence in Wisconsin was determined to be an objective one: a defendant's conduct is judged from the perspective of a reasonably prudent person. The objective standard has been applied to numerous cases since that time, meaning that the state does not need to prove why a defendant crossed the centerline of a highway, which is a subjective determination, but rather, a reasonably prudent person knows that crossing the centerline of a highway at high speed creates a situation of unreasonable risk and high probability of death, great bodily harm, or bodily harm to others. The trend toward criminal prosecution of negligent behavior in auto-accident cases, even without clear-cut evidence of reckless disregard, has continued because the public outcry in vehicular homicide cases has continued. For example, a case where a truck driver reached down to pick up a pack of cigarettes that he had dropped, causing him to accidentally rear-end a stopped vehicle, killing a mother and her children, resulted in criminal charges. This unintentional act resulted in deaths, but the driver of this vehicle never intended any harm. (Interestingly, accident reports are not allowed to be used in court against the defendant in vehicular homicide cases, whereas the same is not true in criminal prosecution of healthcare negligence.)

One of the greatest impediments to preventing errors is that errors frequently are not reported due to fear of punishment. Lucian Leape, adjunct professor of health policy, Harvard School of Public Health, Harvard University, Boston, has stated that the single greatest impediment to error prevention is that "we punish people for making mistakes."[8] Treating unintentional mistakes non-punitively has enabled industries as diverse as aviation and anesthesiology to make great strides in safety improvements. If the airline industry had similarly prosecuted pilots who committed unintentional negligent errors that resulted in passenger deaths, would we have made as much progress as we have in making airline travel safer? If we had criminally prosecuted anesthesiologists for hooking up the wrong gases during surgery, rather than letting civil malpractice claims be filed, allowing later analysis of closed claims to determine the root causes of these events, it is unlikely that the manufacturers of anesthesia equipment would have been forced to standardize the hookups to prevent this type of error from occurring. This difference has made the practice of anesthesiology much safer, as evidenced by the drop in malpractice-insurance premiums that has resulted from the drop in anesthesia-related claims throughout the United States.

Criminal law overall is premised upon the fact that guilt is individual, and that an individual is entitled to advanced notice that one's actions could be criminal. The law must give a person of ordinary intelligence a reasonable opportunity to know what is prohibited, so that he or she may act accordingly. Strict liability means that no intent is required, such as operating while intoxicated, parking citations, speeding citations, and statutory rape. Criminal negligence is defined as ordinary negligence to a high degree, consisting of conduct that the actor should realize creates a substantial and unreasonable risk of death or great bodily harm to another person. To prove criminal negligence, the state must satisfy jurors beyond a reasonable doubt that the defendant engaged in harmful conduct, which, under all of the circumstances present, the defendant should have realized would create a substantial and unreasonable risk of death or great bodily harm to another person.[9]

CRIMINAL PROSECUTION OF HEALTHCARE NEGLIGENCE

Criminal prosecution of healthcare negligence was historically reserved for intentionally ending a person's life through euthanasia, or in "angel-of-death" cases, where a provider decided to play God, or in cases where the provider would benefit from the death through personal gain (doctor killing his wife for the life-insurance money). A surgeon who operates on an individual while intoxicated similarly results in criminal

charges, as this act demonstrates intentional disregard for human life.

It is one thing to get sued for malpractice and quite another to go to jail for doing your job and becoming a victim ("second victim") of a healthcare delivery system that allowed you, the healthcare provider, to make an unintended mistake. To what can we attribute this shift toward criminal prosecution of unintentional healthcare negligence? Since the 1990s, there has been an increased public awareness of healthcare errors. While quality-improvement efforts have shifted away from the search for the "bad-apple" approach of early quality-assurance programs toward efforts to improve the healthcare delivery systems that allow errors to occur, it is clear that the legal system has not yet recognized a systems approach to dealing with healthcare error. Criminal prosecution conflicts with a system-based approach to discourage error reporting.

During the hurricane Katrina disaster, a physician and two nurses were arrested in New Orleans and were criminally prosecuted for the deaths of stranded critically ill hospitalized patients. Charges against them were subsequently dropped after a grand jury in New Orleans declined to indict them for alleged mercy killings, but the chilling effect of the year-long prosecution remains in the minds of providers.[10] If that doctor and those nurses had been found guilty, the ramifications could have been far-reaching, and may still have an unanticipated negative impact on response planning for future disasters where we will need to elicit the assistance of medical professionals in these efforts (see Chapter 21).

Our overburdened emergency-care system is continually placing increasing demands for healthcare providers to do more with fewer resources. In 2007, in Waukegan, Illinois, a triage nurse was criminally charged with homicide in the death of a woman who died in the emergency department (ED) waiting room. She had been triaged inappropriately in the ED during a particularly busy shift and suffered a heart attack while waiting her turn for treatment. While prosecutors ultimately decided not to bring charges, a coroner's inquest ruled the death a homicide.[11] Was this criminal neglect or negligent triage resulting in a delay in hospital treatment due to an overburdened environment?

An Ohio pharmacist was found guilty of involuntary manslaughter in May 2009 for a medication error that subsequently led to the death of a 2-year-old girl who received a lethal dose of saline solution with her chemotherapy agent. The bag of chemo was to be mixed in a 1% saline solution when in fact it contained 23%—an error made by a pharmacy technician, not caught by the pharmacist who was ultimately responsible, when checking the chemo agent prior to administration to the child. The pharmacist lost his license in 2007 as a result of the prosecution, eventually pleaded no contest to the charge, and is awaiting sentencing. The maximum sentence is 5 years in prison and a $10,000 fine. In addition, Ohio passed Emily's Law, a set of guidelines and educational and testing requirements that govern pharmacy technicians, and there is also a movement to require national regulations for pharmacy technicians.[12]

In a 2006 Wisconsin case, a nurse was charged with criminal neglect of a patient by causing great bodily harm in the medication-error-related death of a young woman during child birth. The criminal complaint alleged that the nurse failed to follow the "five rights" of medication administration (right drug, right patient, right route, right time, and right dosage), and that she did not use an available bedside bar-coding system. Instead of the case going forward as a civil suit and allowing the Department of Regulation and Licensure (DRL) to attend to the matter as a usual course of business, the nurse was charged with a felony for an unintended healthcare error by an overzealous and creative junior prosecutor. For whatever reason, be it fear of the loss of federal funding or a lack of a proactive, supportive patient safety culture, the nurse involved did not feel supported by the organization that employed her during this difficult ordeal; instead, she was fired for not following hospital policy for properly dispensing medications. Fatigue and a number of other contributing factors played a significant role in this unfortunate event. Because the nurse was accused of a criminal act and was no longer employed by the facility, the hospital's malpractice coverage afforded the nurse no defense assistance and she had to hire a criminal-defense attorney at her own expense. The case involved the death of a young patient, and the experienced nurse was understandably distraught. She participated fully with the investigation of the facts of the event, and unfortunately, her statements and the hospital's internal incident report were subsequently used against her in the criminal case.

In this case, the Wisconsin Board of Nursing was doing its job parallel to the ongoing criminal proceedings. A day before her court appearance, the Wisconsin DRL suspended the nurse's license. The case went the criminal route, and only when the criminal charges were reduced from a felony to a misdemeanor plea to two counts of illegally administering prescription medications was the licensing board able to proceed with disciplinary actions.

In this case, the Wisconsin Board of Nursing's Order in the Disciplinary Proceedings (December 14, 2006) against the nurse found that her conduct violated the minimum standards of the nursing profession necessary for the protection of the health, safety, and welfare of a patient or the public, which indicated unprofessional conduct, and her license was suspended for 9 months. She was also required to complete an educational program, which addressed the roles of individuals and systems in preventing medication errors and healthcare errors. Within 90 days of completing the educational programs, she was required to make presentations to groups of nurses or nursing students on the topic of the roles of individuals and systems in preventing medication errors and healthcare errors. She was also required to pay the department's costs of the proceedings.[13]

THE ROLE OF LICENSING AND MEDICAL EXAMINING BOARDS

The trend toward criminal prosecution of healthcare negligence may be due, in part, to the fact that licensing boards and medical examining boards historically have not protected the public from bad providers as well as they might have. The licensing authorities have different legal objectives than those of criminal courts. Licensing boards' primary purpose is to discipline a provider to protect the public, to rehabilitate the licensee, to deter the licensee from engaging in similar conduct in the future, and to deter other licensees from engaging in similar conduct. Disciplines that may be imposed by the licensing authority include revocation, suspension, limitation, reprimand, and forfeiture.[14] In recent years, state medical examining boards and licensing boards for nursing and other professions have become more visible in their enforcement efforts to change the public perception of leniency. State governmental budgetary cuts, staffing shortages, and case backlogs continue to be problematic in some states, however, which may be contributing to the trend toward criminal prosecution of negligence.

FEDERAL RAMIFICATIONS AND OTHER CONSEQUENCES

The ramifications of criminal prosecution for healthcare negligence are far greater than jail time and monetary penalties. In the case of the Wisconsin nurse discussed previously, the federal government later imposed sanctions that prevented the nurse from working for any federally funded healthcare organization for 5 years.[15] This essentially meant that she was unable to work as a nurse in any hospital or clinic that received Medicare or Medicaid, thus ending a life-long nursing career, which was her livelihood.

The nurse went to work with Dr. Charles Denham, founder and director of the Texas Medical Institute of Technology, joining his team to work with patient safety leaders in the United States to help further the adoption of patient safety best practices. Now a certified patient safety officer, Julie Thao gives talks around the country on patient safety and her experience as a second victim, helping caregivers to avoid medication errors and educating hospital leadership teams on how important it is to support the practitioner when such unintended errors occur. She explains that the emotional impact on her life was devastating and far greater than the financial ramifications. Although she was prosecuted for not following the Five Rights of Medication Administration, she now lectures on this emotional impact and on TRUST: the Five Rights of the Second Victim. These Five Rights are:

1. Treatment that is just (fair)
2. Respect
3. Understanding and compassion ("The instant preventable and unintentional harm occurs to a patient, their caregivers become patients." —J. Thao)
4. Supportive care
5. Transparency and opportunity to contribute

Without stronger protections for our healthcare providers, this need to contribute toward understanding why an event occurred is stifled because peer-review laws are variable from state to state. Tort reform and legislative efforts to strengthen legal protections are often initiated in states following criminal prosecution of healthcare negligence.

The American Medical Association (AMA) has developed position statements against the criminalization of medical judgment and the criminalization of healthcare decision making in response to the current trend toward criminalization of malpractice. The Association of periOperative Registered Nurses (AORN) also published a position statement in April 2008 on the criminalization of human errors in the periOperative setting, strongly opposing attempts to criminalize unintended errors.[16] With national healthcare reform looming before us, the AMA and other groups that represent healthcare providers nationwide are hoping to educate opinion leaders, elected officials, and the media regarding the detrimental effects on health care that results from the criminalization of healthcare decision making.

LEGISLATIVE EFFORTS (WISCONSIN LEGISLATION, PSO PARTICIPATION, ROLE OF INTENT)

Legislative strategies have emerged to address criminalization of unintended healthcare errors and the need to restore trust in order to maintain an effective culture of patient safety, which includes an effort to redefine and clarify non-criminal and criminal conduct. The criminal prosecution of the Wisconsin nurse rocked the Wisconsin healthcare community, and on December 20, 2006, a coalition of interested healthcare providers and payers, employers, patient safety organizations, attorneys, risk managers, and others met to define and consider the issues presented by the Wisconsin Department of Justice's decision to criminally charge a Wisconsin nurse for negligent administration of medication that caused a patient's death. A smaller group of individuals were charged with further consideration of the issues and to prepare options and recommendations for the coalition to consider. AB 863 was introduced relating to confidentiality of healthcare services reviews; use as evidence of information regarding healthcare providers; homicide or injury by negligent handling of a dangerous weapon, explosives, or fire; criminal abuse of individuals at risk; and criminal abuse and neglect of patients and residents. The Wisconsin Nurses Association supported this legislation because it addressed decriminalization for unintentional medical errors caused by nurses and other healthcare professionals. It was

approved by the Assembly but stalled in the Senate. Efforts to enact protective legislation in Wisconsin continue, and 2009–2010 efforts have focused on amending criminal-conduct statutes (if the act was not intentional, then no criminal charge can be brought) and replicating motor vehicle statutes that prohibit accident reports from being used in court against the accused. Other states may have similar legislative efforts in motion.

FEDERAL PROSECUTION OF MEDICAL NEGLIGENCE

Another recent approach to treating medical negligence as a crime is federal prosecution when a bill is sent to Medicare or to Medicaid for a procedure in which negligence occurred, alleging that fraud has been committed because the government paid for a service that was not received as promised. This trend has recently emerged in the nursing-home industry, and in at least one case in Michigan, it was used against a physician and the hospital in which he practiced. In these cases, the Department of Health and Human Services has been forwarding instances of negligence to the Attorney General's Office for investigation and prosecution. Because fraud is much easier to prove than a criminal-negligence case, the trend likely may continue. Time will tell what this may mean for hospitals and providers. Are we next going to see criminal prosecution for fraud in cases where a hospital or physician bills for a condition on the list of hospital-acquired conditions? Time will tell.

RISK MANAGEMENT STRATEGIES

Risk managers may find themselves in a difficult position when a medical-negligence case is criminally prosecuted. If the risk manager is working for a hospital or a healthcare system governed by accrediting-body standards, she or he knows that disclosure and event analysis are mandated to occur. The balancing act of doing the investigation and event analysis while protecting the organization and the healthcare provider involved in the incident from having statements and facts used against them in the criminal matter can be challenging. So what advice does one offer to a doctor, nurse, pharmacist, or other healthcare provider involved in a devastating event, particularly when a death occurs? Until stronger, uniform protections are in place to allow providers to freely report errors and participate in the root-cause investigation without fear, each case must be individually evaluated to determine the best advice for the risk manager to give to those involved; however, the basic advice is the same for all:

1. In cases where the patient dies or suffers great bodily injury, notify your risk manager or legal counsel immediately. They will assess the situation and advise you to seek the advice of a criminal-defense attorney immediately if the case is potentially a criminal matter.

2. Be objective and factual when completing an incident report of an event, avoiding self-incriminating statements.

3. Be cooperative, but only talk to anyone about the facts of the matter with your criminal-defense lawyer present if there is potential for criminal prosecution.

4. Do not participate as a member on the RCA team. The facts of the event, gathered during the investigation conducted with your defense attorney present, will be protected from discovery if a criminal case ensues but will still be able to be used to complete the event RCA.

What can risk managers do to protect their organizations in instances where criminal prosecution of a negligent event is going to occur? Proactive strategies include the following:

1. Explore adding a Criminal Defense Extension Endorsement to your entity's professional-liability policy to include defense costs incurred in defending any

criminal proceeding brought by a federal, state, or local government, or governmental agency, against an insured officer, director, manager, administrator, medical director, department head, or supervisor of an insured entity acting in his or her capacity as such and alleging violation of any federal, state, or local law, ordinance, rule, or regulation that pertains to the operation of an insured facility and arises out of a medical incident during the coverage period of the policy. The endorsement would need approval from the state's insurance commissioner and could not erode the underlying limits. Defense would be provided only until there was adjudication, plea, or another finding that the criminal conduct had in fact occurred.

2. Develop a second-victim support program so that when healthcare providers are involved in a tragic error they are treated with respect, compassion, and understanding.

3. Limit organizational use of overtime to ensure patient and provider safety, and educate all employees and physicians that they are responsible for knowing when fatigue could impact personal performance.[17]

4. If a significant event occurs that could appear in the media, notify your public affairs department and the governing board.

5. Prepare the organization for a regulatory visit, which could likely follow a significant event.

6. Develop safe healthcare delivery systems. Analyze significant near-miss events (as time allows) to continually strive to improve systems.

7. Set clear expectations for staff performance and emphasize the need to understand why, not just what, to encourage the development of critical-thinking skills.

8. Perform FMEAs prior to introducing new programs, procedures, or technology.

9. Error-reduction toolboxes and other strategies should be utilized whenever possible to reduce the likelihood of human-error occurrence, such as the following:
   a. Encourage the use of situation, background, assessment, recommendations (SBAR), and hand-off forms to standardize communications.
   b. Use checklists, such as the Surgical Safety Checklist, which outlines essential standards of surgical care and is designed to be simple, widely applicable and capable of addressing common and potentially disastrous lapses.
   c. Develop line-reconciliation and tube-reconciliation policies.
   d. Implement bar-code scanning of medications.
   e. Conduct downtime procedure drills to ensure that when technology fails, your staff is able to deliver effective care (e.g., dispensing medications, hanging IVs), without the availability of pumps and scanners. How will staff document patient care during extended electronic-medical-record downtime?
10. Utilize the Just-Culture Checklist—tips to assist your organization in becoming a fair, accusation-free environment:
   a. Avoid blame.
   b. Work on fixing the system, not the person.
   c. Steer clear of complexity in process design.
   d. Include redundancy, especially in high-risk procedures (checks and rechecks).
   e. Make expectations clear.
   f. Work to mitigate risk, such as fatigue, distractions, overload, and complexity.
   g. Always involve staff before making changes.
   h. Focus on process and behaviors, not on the outcome.
   i. Use coaching to correct knowledge deficit and risky behaviors.
   j. Use discipline for reckless behavior that puts patients at risk.
   k. Address skill issues; competency is not optional.
   l. Use errors as a learning experience.
   m. Ensure solid orientation for new staff.
   n. Make sure that all staff members are up to date on practice issues and improvements.
   o. Be vigilant for system weaknesses.
   p. Proactively address system short- and long-term solutions.
   q. Remember that neither people nor systems are perfect.
   r. Talk about patient safety at every staff meeting.
   s. Staff "right" and provide contingency safety help if staffing is not optimal.
   t. Consider why rules may be broken; maybe they are bad rules or there is pressure to work around the rule.
   u. Measure it.
   v. Emphasize that safety is everyone's job.
   w. Instead of demanding perfection, we must continue to design safe systems for healthcare delivery and recognize that all systems, like all humans, are not perfect.[18]

We can perform proactive risk assessments or FMEAs to try to identify the potential sources of problems, and by analyzing actual events to determine the root causes and improving the delivery systems, we can reduce errors; however, health care, by its very nature, is a high-risk field, and providers put themselves at risk when choosing a healthcare profession. We must continue to involve patients in patient safety activities and educate patients to be partners in their care. Until legislation and laws are enacted to better balance the risk to those who pledge to heal rather than harm are in place, we must continue to strive for a more robust culture of safety so that we can learn from events reported and continue to improve our healthcare delivery systems, making the system safer for providers and patients alike.

References

1. Press Ganey. (2009). Pulse report 2009. Safety culture, staff perspectives on American health care. Agency for Healthcare Research and Quality (AHRQ). Hospital survey on patient safety culture: 2009. Comparative database report.
2. Marx, D. (2007). *Patient safety and the "just culture."* http://www.health.state.ny.us/professionals/patients/patient_safety/conference/2007/docs/patient_safety_and_the_just_culture.pdf. Accessed April 20, 2010.
3. Fitzpatrick, D. (2009). Strategies for implementing a just culture. *WiscRisk, 11*(1).
4. Hallinan, J.T. (2009). *Why we make mistakes.* Portland, OR: Broadway Books.
5. Garner, B.A. (1999). *Blacks law dictionary* (7th ed.). St. Paul, Minnesota: West, 238(s).
6. Youngberg, B. (2004). *The Patient Safety Handbook.* Sudbury, MA: Jones and Bartlett Publishers, 734.
7. Monico, E., Kulkarni, R., Calise, A., & Calabro J. (2007). The criminal prosecution of medical negligence. *The Internet Journal of Law, Healthcare, and Ethics.* http://www.ispub.com/journal/the_internet_journal_of_law_healthcare_and_ethics/volume_5_number_1_45/article_printable/the_criminal_prosecution_of_medical_negligence.html. Accessed April 20, 2010.
8. Leape, L. (2001). Testimony before Congress on health care quality improvement. http://md-jd.info/leap2001.html. Accessed April 29, 2010.
9. Hurley, S.P., & Berghahn, M. (April 2010). Medication Errors and Criminal Negligence: Lessons from two Cases. *Journal of Nursing Regulation 1*(1), National Council of States Boards of Nursing, Chicago, 29.
10. Blesch, G. (2007). *Charges of a different kind.* http://www.ModernHealthcare.com/. Accessed May 22, 2010.
11. Sorrel, A.L. (2006). Woman's death in hospital emergency department ruled a homicide. *American Medical News.*
12. Mentrek, M. (2009). Ex-pharmacist Eric Cropp found guilty in medication death of Emily Jerry, 2. http://blog.cleveland.com/metro/2009/05/expharmacist_eric_cropp_found.html. Accessed May 22, 2010.
13. Wisconsin Board of Nursing. (2006). WI Board of Nursing's order in the disciplinary proceedings.
14. Zwieg, J.R. (2007). The role of the Department of Regulation and Licensing in addressing medical errors. Spring Conference Speaker at meeting sponsored by the Wisconsin Society of Healthcare Risk Management, April 27, 2007
15. Lillesand, K. (November 2007). Julie Thao Update, It is not over. *Nursing Matters.* http://www.nursingmattersonline.com/nursingmattersonline/newsdetail.asp?newsid=1722. Accessed April 21, 2010.
16. Association of periOperative Registered Nurses (AORN). (2008). Position statement on criminalization of human errors in the perioperative setting. Denver, CO: AORN.
17. Denham, C.R. (2007). TRUST: The 5 rights of the second victim. *The Journal of Patient Safety, 3*(2): 107.
18. Pastorius, D. (October 2007). *Nursing Management, 38*(10), 18–27.

21

Preparing for and Limiting Potential Liability for Medical Care Provided During Disaster Events

Margaret L. Begalle, JD

INTRODUCTION

In the wake of September 11, hurricane Katrina, and more recently, the outbreak of the H1N1 virus, there is a strong interest in the role of medical professionals during disasters and epidemics. More specifically, the interest lies in the liability that healthcare professionals may face resulting from the care they provide during disasters and emergencies. While the standard of care expected from physicians and other medical professionals should be considered based on the specific circumstances, it is not always clear what standard is expected and the possible consequences for failing to meet that standard.

This chapter discusses the events that occurred at Memorial Medical Center ("Memorial") after hurricane Katrina struck New Orleans in late August 2005. In the days that followed hurricane Katrina, Memorial experienced a loss of resources, deteriorating conditions, and sporadic help from outside the hospital walls. All of these factors com-bined contributed to a high number of patient deaths, followed by the arrests a year later of a prominent Memorial physician and two nurses on charges of second-degree murder. This chapter then considers the existing federal and state statutory framework aimed at protecting healthcare professionals from liability resulting from the care they provide during disaster and emergency situations. While some federal and state laws provide liability protections for healthcare professionals who respond to disaster events, the current framework is fragmented and varies in terms of when, and to what extent, the protections apply. The concern in not having uniform liability standards is that healthcare professionals may not be willing to provide care in disaster situations for fear of liability; thus, it is desirable to develop uniform liability standards for healthcare professionals who respond to disaster situations.

In addition to consistent liability standards, many medical professionals are lobbying for altered standards of care during disaster events. The development of altered standards of care requires cooperation from all levels of government. Furthermore, any altered standards should be consistent, fair and equitable, and grounded on solid legal and ethical principles. Although altered standards of care are worthy of discussion, most state and local governments have yet to develop and implement such standards.

The need to educate and train healthcare professionals in responding to disaster events is evident. Proactive planning and implementation of comprehensive risk management and patient safety policies and procedures for disaster events will provide healthcare professionals with the skills they need for treating patients under such circumstances and may help to head off liability concerns.

THE EVENTS AT MEMORIAL MEDICAL CENTER FOLLOWING HURRICANE KATRINA

In the early hours of Monday, August 29, 2005, hurricane Katrina struck New Orleans with a fury. By all accounts, the storm reduced the city to what looked like a war zone. At the time, more than 2,000 people were taking shelter from the storm at Memorial, including more than 200 patients and 600 healthcare professionals and staff.[1] Around five o'clock that morning, city power to Memorial was exhausted and the auxiliary generators kicked in, which allowed for the operation of emergency lighting, critical equipment, and a handful of outlets on each floor. At the same time, Memorial lost the use of its air conditioning system.[1] The events at Memorial during and after hurricane Katrina illustrate the complications and potential liabilities that can arise when physicians and other healthcare professionals provide care during disasters.

Although the hurricane caused some damage to the hospital and surrounding areas, as we now know, the breach of the levies caused much more damage to New Orleans than the storm itself. On Tuesday, August 30, after the floodwaters from the storm initially receded at Memorial, the breach of the levies soon caused the streets surrounding Memorial to flood. The rising waters caused Memorial's staff to become concerned about the power supply to the hospital.

While Memorial had drafted an emergency plan, the plan failed to address how to deal with a complete loss of power or how to evacuate in the midst of rising floodwaters.[1] Memorial's staff began to discuss how to evacuate the hospital and decided that babies in the neonatal intensive care unit, pregnant mothers, and critically ill patients in the intensive care unit would be evacuated first due to the risks posed to those particular patients from the extreme heat in the hospital.[1]

In addition to the Memorial patients, the seventh floor of the facility housed LifeCare Hospitals ("LifeCare"), a healthcare company that treated critically ill patients in need of intensive around-the-clock care.[1] LifeCare had its own credentialed physicians, administrators, nurses, pharmacists, supplies, and even its own "incident commander."[1] More than 50 LifeCare patients were being treated on the seventh floor of Memorial. Most of LifeCare's patients were bedbound and many required ventilators.[2] LifeCare's incident commander requested that the LifeCare patients be included in any evacuation plans. According to LifeCare's incident commander, however, such a request apparently required approval from Memorial's corporate owner.[1]

On Tuesday afternoon, Coast Guard helicopters arrived to begin the evacuation of Memorial.[1] The helicopters used a helipad on the top of a parking garage next to Memorial. Evacuation required Memorial staff to guide patients down a stairwell and through hallways to the only working elevator, and subsequently pass the patients through a 3 × 3-foot hole in the wall that accessed the parking garage. From there, Memorial staff transported patients by truck to the roof of the parking garage where two flights of stairs led to the helipad.[1] As it became dark, the evacuations ceased for the day, leaving approximately 130 patients still stranded at Memorial, not to mention the hundreds of people who had taken shelter there after the storm. All 52 of the LifeCare patients remained on the seventh floor of the hospital.[1]

The rising waters eventually disabled Memorial's backup generators in the early hours of Wednesday, August 31. The total power outage occurred approximately 48 hours after hurricane Katrina initially hit New Orleans.[1] The power failure left Memorial staff "to care for critically ill patients in a dark building with no electric power, no fresh water, a flooded first floor, a nonfunctional sanitation system, and an interior temperature above 100°F."[2] Ventilators stopped and Memorial staff, including Memorial cancer surgeon Dr. Anna Pou, began manually helping the LifeCare patients who could not breathe on their own. The Coast Guard was able to evacuate a handful of critical patients, but three patients who relied on ventilators died that morning.[2]

With more than 100 patients still at Memorial, and the Coast Guard too busy with evacuations in other parts of the city, the staff decided to place patients in one of three groups to aid the evacuation efforts. Dr. Pou agreed to help assign the patients to groups. Group-1 patients consisted of those who could sit up or walk on their own and were otherwise in fairly good health; they were to be evacuated on rescue boats that had started to arrive at the hospital.[2] Group-2 patients were those who needed more assistance during the evacuation, and the staff determined it was necessary to evacuate group-2 patients by helicopter.[2] Finally, group-3 patients, the most critical patients left at Memorial, including the LifeCare patients, would be evacuated last.[2] Group-3 patients were those with the least chance of survival. Thus, with little guidance, Memorial's medical staff created a makeshift triage system. It is important to note that the physi-

cians and staff had never received training for the circumstances they faced in the days following hurricane Katrina.

The evacuations picked up again on Thursday, September 1, approximately 72 hours after hurricane Katrina rolled through New Orleans; however, by that time some physicians and other hospital staff, who had been working at Memorial since Monday, knew it would be difficult, if not impossible, to evacuate all of the remaining patients, including the LifeCare patients, many of whom were in critical condition.[2] Resources were clearly limited, physicians and staff were exhausted, and the conditions, which had been constantly deteriorating for 4 days, were horrendous. In addition, communications with the outside world and even within the walls of Memorial had broken down. Many of the decisions made with respect to triage and evacuation were made without consulting the LifeCare administrators and staff.

Although reports vary, at some point during the afternoon of September 1, Memorial apparently received word that no more evacuations would be performed that day. At that time, Memorial's medical staff made the decision to give certain patients, including a number of LifeCare patients, a combination of morphine and midazolam, a sedative.[2] Dr. Pou was put in charge of administering the drugs. According to Dr. Pou the intention was only to "help the patients that were having pain and sedate the patients who were anxious because we knew they were going to be there another day, that they would go through at least another day of hell."[2] Evacuations resumed, however, and by early Thursday evening, all remaining patients were evacuated.[2] The patients who received the morphine and midazolam combination died at Memorial.[2]

At least 34 patients died at Memorial in the wake of hurricane Katrina; more than any other comparable hospital in New Orleans.[2] Stories began to emerge that Dr. Pou and others euthanized some of the patients at Memorial.[2] These rumors eventually led to an investigation by Louisiana's attorney general and the subsequent July 2006 arrest of Dr. Pou and two nurses from Memorial on charges of second-degree murder.[3] The State of Louisiana eventually dropped the charges against the two nurses in return for their testimony to the grand jury.[3] In July 2007, a grand jury refused to indict Dr. Pou on nine murder counts stemming from the events that occurred at Memorial following hurricane Katrina.[3] Dr. Pou still faces civil liability.

LIABILITY AND STANDARD-OF-CARE ISSUES ARISING FROM DISASTER EVENTS

Although the district attorney believed that the actions of Dr. Pou warranted her arrest for second-degree murder, many in the medical profession disagree. The medical community sympathizes with Dr. Pou and believes that it was more likely that, when faced with the decision of abandoning patients who could not be evacuated,* she chose the only available option—to offer palliative care for her patients.[4] Healthcare professionals believe that the threat of criminal prosecution for providing medical care in times of extreme disaster will have a "chilling effect on the willingness of medical professionals to volunteer during disasters."[4]

The events that unfolded at Memorial in the wake of hurricane Katrina demonstrate the extremely difficult decisions physicians must make during disaster events, and the potential liability stemming from those decisions. In disaster situations, specific hospital policies and protocols are often lacking, and physicians and other medical staff are often faced with circumstances beyond any training or education they may have received and with-

out many of the resources that they use in their everyday practice; yet, they are expected to maintain a certain level of care for their patients. As James G. Hodge, Jr., states:

> Hospitals [and healthcare professionals] owe duties of care to their patients that stem from the relationship that is formed when the patients present for care. Patients arrive at a hospital with reasonable expectations that the hospital and its staff will provide adequate, competent, and quality care. During an emergency, a patient's expectations may change as standards of care may be altered, but the duty to provide some level of care remains.[5]

When physicians fall below the expected level of care, they may find themselves facing civil lawsuits or even criminal prosecution.

Legal standards of care are actually flexible and are based on whether the practitioner acted as would a reasonable practitioner under similar circumstances; however, while "[f]lexibility of the legal standard of care may be beneficial in emergencies, [that same flexibility] does not always lend [itself] to predicable outcomes when legal disputes arise."[6] This uncertainty may cause healthcare professionals to shy away from providing care in disaster situations for fear of liability; thus, it is important to have legal protections available for healthcare professionals responding to disaster events. But what standard of care should the public expect from medical professionals in disaster situations and what liability should those professionals face if they fail to meet the expected standard of care?

THE LEGAL LANDSCAPE OF LIABILITY IN DISASTER EVENTS

The destruction caused by hurricane Katrina, and the flooding that followed, has drawn comparisons to a military war zone. It is interesting to note that in military situations, the standard of care is much lower than that

---

*Many of the patients who received the morphine and midazolam drug combination were already extremely ill, and in a number of cases, patients could not be easily transported and maneuvered through the hospital for evacuation due to their medical condition, body weight, or both.

which is expected from civilian physicians and medical staff. In addition, military physicians have broad-based immunity from liability. Under the Federal Tort Claims Act (FTCA) and the Gonzalez Act, military physicians are protected from personal liability for any injury that results from the care they provide. Under the Gonzalez Act, the FTCA provides the only means of recovery for an individual injured by a military physician.[7] An injured party's only recourse is to seek recovery from the United States government. "[H]ealthcare providers are immune from liability for care given while acting within the scope of their duties or employment."[7] The Supreme Court has confirmed that military physicians enjoy absolute immunity from claims arising from the care they provide during the scope of their employment.[8]

Civilian healthcare professionals often do not receive the same liability protections even when the circumstances resemble military-like conditions; thus, the fear of liability is a major concern among healthcare providers.[9] "Potential liability claims against [healthcare] practitioners and entities can result from alleged civil, criminal, and Constitutional violations" and "may arise from claims of medical malpractice, discrimination, invasions of privacy, or violations of other state and federal statutes."[10]

The concern about liability is likely to deter physicians and other healthcare professionals from providing care in disaster situations. Understandably, without some sort of guaranteed protection from civil liability and criminal prosecution, healthcare providers may simply choose not to provide care during disaster events. A 2006 survey by the American Public Health Association reported that "[a]lmost seventy percent of [clinicians] answered that immunity from civil lawsuits would be an important (35.6%) or essential (33.8%) factor when considering whether to volunteer in an emergency."[11]

While various state and federal statutes exist for limiting the liability for healthcare professionals in disaster situations, commen-

tators frequently describe the liability protections as "patchwork" in terms of when they apply and whom they protect.[12] In response to a declared emergency, "an array of state and federal liability protections exist for providers—particularly volunteers and government entities and officials acting in their official duties—who act in good faith and without willful misconduct, gross negligence, or recklessness."[13] However, paid healthcare providers (non-volunteer and nongovernmental workers), are largely unprotected from liability under state and federal statutes;[14] yet, paid healthcare professionals are the most vulnerable to liability in disaster situations, because they are likely to be some of the first responders. Thus, the "existing patchwork of liability protections can complicate planning and response efforts and deter emergency-response participation."[15]

The so-called patchwork of liability protections includes Good Samaritan laws and the Volunteer Protection Act of 1997 (VPA). Various Good Samaritan laws and the VPA typically protect volunteers who respond to a disaster or emergency from liability for injuries that may result from the care they provide.[16] Many states have enacted Good Samaritan laws, which shield healthcare professionals from liability for negligently causing injury while providing care in response to emergencies. Such statutes, however, are generally limited to volunteers; thus, under most Good Samaritan laws, paid healthcare professionals do not enjoy the same protections as volunteers when responding to a disaster or emergency. Additionally, most Good Samaritan laws do not shield from liability any injury caused by willful or wanton conduct, or gross negligence.[17] For example, section 25 of the Illinois Good Samaritan Act provides an exemption from civil liability for physicians who provide care without compensation, and in good faith:

> Any person licensed under the Medical Practice Act of 1987 or any person licensed to practice the

treatment of human ailments in any other state or territory of the United States who, in good faith, provides emergency care without fee to a person, shall not, as a result of his or her acts or omissions, except willful or wanton misconduct on the part of the person, in providing the care, be liable for civil damages.[18]

Similarly, the Volunteer Protection Act is a federal statute that also protects volunteers from liability arising out of medical care provided in response to an emergency. Again, the VPA is limited to volunteers, meaning that individuals who receive compensation for providing medical care during an emergency or disaster do not receive the same protection from liability.[19]

Several states have also enacted emergency response statutes that provide different protection for emergency responders. Some state statutes provide immunity to healthcare professionals if they are acting under the command of the government in the event of a public health emergency. For example, in Wyoming, healthcare professionals who follow the instructions of a state health officer during a public health emergency are not liable for any injury caused while acting in compliance with those instructions.[20] Other state statutes are broad in their liability protections for healthcare professionals. In California, all healthcare professionals who render services during a state of emergency receive liability protection, unless their acts are willful.[21]

After Dr. Pou's arrest on charges of second-degree murder, Louisiana worked to enact a number of statutes aimed at protecting healthcare professionals from liability arising from the care they provide during disasters such as hurricane Katrina.[22] One such statute provides immunity for healthcare professionals who perform evacuations or medical treatment during a declared state of emergency. Under this statute, healthcare profes-

sionals cannot be held "liable for any civil damages to a person as a result of an evacuation or treatment or failed evacuation or treatment conducted in accordance with disaster medicine protocol and at the direction of military or government authorities, unless the damage or injury is cause by willful and wanton misconduct."[23]

A second Louisiana statute limits the liability of healthcare professionals who, in good faith, provide healthcare services during a declared state of emergency, regardless of whether or not the healthcare professional receives compensation for such treatment.[24] The limitation of this statute is that healthcare professionals are not protected from liability if their care, or failure to provide care, is "caused by gross negligence or willful and wanton misconduct."[25]

A third Louisiana statute addresses potential criminal prosecution arising from medical care provided during a state of disaster or emergency. The bill requires the assembly of a medical review panel prior to any criminal prosecution of a healthcare professional "for acts arising out of the rendering of, or failing to render, medical services during a state of disaster or medical emergency."[25] The panel reviews the healthcare professional's clinical judgment regarding the services rendered and determines whether such judgment meets the appropriate standards under the specific circumstances.

The statute actually prohibits the prosecuting authority from arresting a healthcare professional on criminal charges until the panel's investigation is complete. The panel is to submit a written report to the prosecuting authority with its conclusions as to whether or not the healthcare professional in question exercised good-faith clinical judgment under the circumstances; however, the panel's opinion is advisory only, and the statute does not require the prosecuting authority to follow the advice of the panel. "Upon receipt of the advisory opinion from the panel, the prosecuting authority, after giving due consideration to the panel opinion, may proceed in accordance with the United States constitution and laws of this state to prosecute conduct which, in the prosecuting authority's sole discretion, is deemed actionable."[26] One important note is that the bill protects both paid healthcare workers and volunteers.

Given the patchwork landscape of federal and state laws that exist in disaster situations, it is easy to understand the reluctance of healthcare professionals in responding to disaster events. Many of these laws only take effect after an official state of disaster or emergency is declared. Some states protect volunteers only, while others also protect paid healthcare professionals. Some states provide protection against both criminal prosecution and civil liability, while other states limit liability only for civil actions; thus, healthcare professionals may not always be clear on when, where, and how such laws apply. With such a patchwork of laws, the government is leaving it up to healthcare professionals to know which laws apply, when they apply, and to what extent they apply under any given circumstances. In disaster situations, however, it seems more prudent for healthcare professionals to focus on the best care they can give to their patients, and not on the fear of what might happen if they are unable to meet the normal standard of care under the circumstances.

THE DEVELOPMENT OF ALTERED STANDARDS OF CARE

Because of the patchwork system of liability statutes, many healthcare professionals are lobbying for altered standards of care in disaster situations. This concept relates to liability because the issue becomes one of not only a modified standard of medical care, but also standards of care in the legal sense that support the modified medical standards. Modification of the medical standards alone will do nothing to alleviate the risk of civil liability or possible criminal prosecution if the legal system fails to recognize the need for modified medical standards.

In a disaster event, healthcare resources will reach their capacity and eventually become strained and, in some instances, unavailable. This strain will almost certainly decrease the ability of healthcare professionals to provide the type and quality of care they provide under normal circumstances. Recognizing the need to prepare in advance for disaster situations, the Institute of Medicine (IOM) recently convened a "committee to develop guidance that state and local public health officials and health-sector agencies and institutions can use to establish and implement standards of care that should apply in disaster situations—both naturally occurring and manmade—under scarce resource conditions."[26]

The IOM focused on establishing a framework for developing and implementing what they call "crisis standards of care," but they did not go so far as to establish or define what exactly the crisis standards of care should be.[27] In other words, the committee set forth the key factors for governments and healthcare providers to consider when developing crisis standards of care, but they did not set forth the actual standards. The IOM defines crisis standards of care as:

> [a] substantial change in usual healthcare operations and the level of care it is possible to deliver, which is made necessary by a pervasive (e.g., pandemic influenza) or catastrophic (e.g., earthquake, hurricane) disaster. This change in the level of care delivered is justified by specific circumstances and is formally declared by a state government, in recognition that crisis operations will be in effect for a sustained period. The formal declaration that crisis standards of care are in operation enables specific legal/regulatory powers and protections for healthcare providers in the necessary tasks of allocating and using scarce medical resources and implementing alternate care facility operations.[28]

The goal of the IOM's report is to help federal policymakers as well as state and local governments develop consistent crisis standards-of-care policies and protocols that apply to every disaster situation, whether manmade or natural. The IOM's "vision" for crisis standards of care requires: (1) standards that are fair to all those affected by them; (2) equitable implementation of the standards; (3) involvement of the community in developing the standards; and (4) a legal framework that allows for an appropriate response in disaster events and supports the crisis standards of care.

To accomplish this vision, the IOM report discusses a broad process to use as a starting point for developing crisis standards of care. Specifically, the IOM report sets forth six recommendations to follow in developing crisis standards-of-care protocols. Firstly, the IOM recommends developing consistent state crisis standards of care protocols that include the following key elements: (1) a strong ethical grounding; (2) community and provider engagement and communication; (3) assurances regarding the legal environment and framework; (4) clear indicators and triggers; and (5) evidence-based clinical operations.[29] The IOM believes that incorporating these elements into the development of crisis standards of care ensures a response in disaster events "that is ethical, legal, and consistent within and across state borders."[30] These five key elements form the basis for the IOM's remaining recommendations, which include adhering to ethical norms, seeking community and provider engagement, providing necessary legal protections for healthcare practitioners and institutions implementing crisis standards of care, ensuring intrastate and interstate consistency between neighboring jurisdictions, and ensuring consistency in crisis standards of care implementation.

The IOM places a significant amount of emphasis on ethical considerations in developing crisis standards of care. The IOM stresses that practitioners, even during disaster situations when resources are scarce, must adhere to ethical norms; it is the situation that changes during a disaster, not the ethical standards.[31] Crisis standards of care protocol should consider the fairness of the standards, the duty to provide care, the duty to allocate and conserve resources, transparency as to how the standards will apply, consistency in application of the standards, standards that are proportional to the situation, and appropriate levels of accountability before, during, and after the disaster.[32]

Next, the IOM believes that community involvement is critical in developing crisis standards of care. Such involvement allows the community to understand "why such standards are necessary and how these standards will apply in response to a disaster."[33] Community involvement and education allow everyone "to be on the same page," and the community will gain a level of trust that the standards are fair and equitable.

The legal framework must support the use of crisis (or altered) standards of care during disaster events. The IOM report encourages federal, state, and local governments to "[r]eview existing legal authority for the implementation of crisis standards of care and address legal issues related to the successful implementation of these standards, such as liability protections . . . [and] [r]evise and reform laws (statutory, regulatory) or policies as necessary."[34] The IOM hopes to influence lawmakers to prepare for disaster events not only by addressing the need to develop fair and equitable standards of care in disaster situations, but also by developing a consistent legal framework in which healthcare professionals can use crisis standards of care without the fear of civil liability or criminal prosecution.[35] The IOM specifically recommends that in disaster situations, state and local governments "provide necessary legal protection for healthcare practitioners and institutions implementing crisis standards of care."[36]

The IOM also recommends knowing what indicators and triggers may signify the need to switch to crisis standards of care. Indicators are measurements that are "used to recognize capacity and capability problems within the healthcare system, suggesting that crisis standards of care may become necessary and requiring further analysis or system actions to prevent overload."[37] Indicators may include monitoring bed availability and availability of critical equipment and medication. When such resources become scarce, it may be necessary to implement crisis standards of care protocols. "Trigger events revolve around changes to staff, space, and supplies that constitute a change in standard practices such that morbidity and mortality risks to the patient increase (i.e., to the crisis standards of care)."[38] According to the IOM, a facility reaches its trigger point when it no longer has the ability to accommodate demand; thus, crisis standards-of-care protocols are triggered when staff, space, and supplies are unable to accommodate the demand such that patient morbidity and mortality risks increase.

The IOM's discussion of clinical process and operations has many elements, and includes interstate and intrastate development and communication of crisis standards of care, the development of strategies to deal with resource shortages and coordination of such resources, and the development of triage standards. The IOM recognizes the importance of interstate and intrastate development and communication of crisis standards of care. The IOM recommends that the development of crisis standards include various levels of authority to ensure consistency in implementation. On an interstate level, "[s]pecific efforts are needed to ensure that Department of Defense, Veterans Health Administration, and Indian Health Services medical facilities are integrated into planning and response efforts."[39] On an intrastate level, state departments of health should work with other state and local agencies to develop and implement crisis standards of care. Among other things, the IOM suggests "using 'clinical care committees,' 'triage

teams,' and state-level 'disaster medical advisory committee(s)' that will evaluate evidence-based, peer-reviewed critical care and other decision tools and recommend and implement decision-making algorithms when specific life-sustaining resources become scarce."[40] Such algorithms will provide guidance with respect to resource allocation and triage decisions.

While the IOM's guidance on planning and development of crisis standards of care is helpful, such standards and the corresponding legal protections are still in development in most states. The process of developing and implementing crisis standards of care for disaster events will not happen overnight. Much planning and coordination must take place before such standards become commonplace and consistent from state to state. Thus, while consistent standards of care and liability protections may aid healthcare professionals once such standards and protections are in place, until then it is possible that other healthcare professionals will find themselves in the same position as Dr. Pou if faced with a disaster situation.

In the meantime, it may be up to individual healthcare facilities and professionals to acquire training and education on how to respond and provide medical care in disaster situations. Training and education is no guarantee that healthcare professionals will avoid liability stemming from the care they provide in response to a disaster; however, healthcare professionals will be better prepared to respond, and that preparation may help limit any potential liability issues and concerns.

PROACTIVE PREPARATION FOR DISASTER EVENTS

Although it is important to develop more uniform liability standards for healthcare providers during disaster and emergency situations that will ensure their participation under such circumstances, it is equally, if not more, important to consider how to proactively minimize the risk of any potential liability, irrespective of state and federal statutes limiting liability. Any appropriate training and education prior to a disaster event will allow healthcare professionals to focus on the task at hand, i.e., effectively caring for patients, rather than worrying about potential liability issues that may plague them when normalcy resumes. "In emergencies . . . , one of the most effective strategies to limit liability in hospital settings is to prevent the conditions under which [liability] may arise. Effective planning can be a preventative remedy for the ills of liability."[41]

LACK OF EDUCATION AND TRAINING FOR DISASTER EVENTS

Dr. Pou herself has stated that more focus needs to be placed on the issues that were brought to light during hurricane Katrina, including "inadequate preparation and a systems failure at every level":[42]

> Issues that need to be addressed include the training of civilian physicians and others in disaster or battlefield triage; education of the public and medical personnel regarding military evacuation protocols; the need for hospital owners (corporations) and administrators to have a feasible and tested plan that is actually followed at the time of crisis, including the possibility of total hospital evacuation; the need for federal, state, and local governments to plan, test, and coordinate their response efforts; . . . and finally, the need for medical and ethical guidelines for disaster care.[42]

A recent report by the Council on Medical Education researched current medical school curricula related to disaster medicine and public-health preparedness and found training in these areas to be insufficient.[43] The IOM has also recognized the need to include disaster preparedness and emergency-care

competencies as part of the curricula for all levels of healthcare professionals.[44]

Many entities, including the American Medical Association (AMA) and the federal government, have attempted over the years to encourage, and in some cases even fund, disaster medicine and public-health-preparedness education and training. For example, in 2003 the AMA began working on a "training initiative called the National Disaster Life Support Program™ (NDLS™) to provide physicians, medical students, other health professionals, and other emergency responders with a fundamental understanding and working knowledge of their integrated roles and responsibilities in disaster management and response efforts."[45]

The disaster-preparedness curriculum in medical schools and other healthcare programs is spotty at best, and most recent medical school graduates are wholly unprepared to deal with disaster situations on the scale of the September 11 terrorist attacks or hurricane Katrina. In a recent survey, almost half of the medical school students surveyed stated that they are inadequately prepared during medical school to respond to disaster events.[46] In another survey, 96% of medical students stated that they are willing to provide care during a disaster event, yet only 17% of those students actually believed that they had received the appropriate training and education to do so.[47]

PLANNING AND IMPLEMENTING A DISASTER-RESPONSE PLAN

As part of a comprehensive risk management and patient safety plan, hospitals and other healthcare facilities should develop and implement plans and strategies for providing care in extreme disaster events. The plan should address issues of internal and external communications as well as chain of command and triage, and it should acknowledge both the vulnerabilities of patients and staff during times of crisis. Although Memorial had an emergency plan in place, that plan clearly fell short of educating and training its physicians and staff on how to respond during a disaster of the magnitude of hurricane Katrina.

The facility must clearly communicate the disaster plan to all physicians and staff. All physicians and staff should know that the plan exists, be required to review the plan, and be familiar with the policies and procedures of the plan. They must have a clear picture of when and under what circumstances the policies and procedures apply. For example, the plan should include specific triggers and indicators, such as capacity and capability limitations.

Planning and communication, however, are not enough. It is necessary for physicians and staff to receive appropriate training to be able to perform their duties according to the disaster plan's policies and procedures. At a minimum, training should include procedures for the coordination of staff, resources and supplies, patient triage, palliative care, and evacuation procedures. Proper coordination and training of staff will allow everyone to know the role that they will play during a disaster event and limit the amount of chaos that is likely to be present during such an event. Coordination of resources and supplies will also help physicians and staff to work more effectively and efficiently to allocate limited resources to those patients who need them most. Training can occur through continuing education-type seminars. In addition, simulated exercises of disaster events may add immense value and knowledge to the disaster preparedness of healthcare professionals.

Management should make sure to update the plan as necessary and communicate any updates to all healthcare professionals in the facility. To the extent possible, the facility should work with state and local agencies in developing a disaster-response plan. Physicians and staff should be made aware of any state and local initiatives and how those initiatives relate to the disaster management and patient safety plan of the facility, including any liability protections offered by the state.

CONCLUSION

Hurricane Katrina and the events that followed at Memorial Medical Center, including the arrest of a prominent doctor on charges of second-degree murder, highlight the problems that physicians and other healthcare professionals may encounter when providing medical care in disaster situations. To ensure that healthcare professionals continue to provide necessary medical care in response to disasters, federal, state, and local governments should consider developing consistent crisis standards of care and a corresponding legal framework that supports such standards. Until consistent standards are developed, however, individual facilities must take the initiative to develop and implement policies and procedures, and train and educate physicians and staff on how to respond to disaster events. A comprehensive and well-conceived risk management and patient safety plan will help limit potential liability issues and allow physicians and staff to focus on providing patient care.

References

1. Fink, S. (2009, August 30). Strained by Katrina, a hospital faced deadly choices. *New York Times.* http://www.nytimes.com/2009/08/30/magazine/30doctors.html?pagewanted=print/.
2. Okie, S. (2008). Dr. Pou and the hurricane: Implications for patient care during disasters. *New England Journal of Medicine, 358*(1), 1.

3. O'Reilly, K.B. (2007, August 13). Grand jury clears Dr. Pou; medicine wants to protect future disaster responders. *American Medical News.* http://www.ama-assn.org/amednews/2007/08/13/prl20813.html/. Accessed April 18, 2010.
4. Supra note 2, p. 4.

5. Hodge, J.G. Jr., Calves, S.H., Gable, L., Meltzer, E., & Kraner, S. (2006). Risk management in the wake of hurricanes and other disasters: Hospital civil liability arising from the use of volunteer health professionals during emergencies. *Michigan State University Journal of Medicine & Law, 10,* 57, 69.

6. Institute of Medicine. (2009). *Guidance for establishing crisis standards of care for use in disaster situations: A letter report 45.* http://www.nap.edu/catalog/12749.html/. Accessed April 18, 2010.

7. Homeland Security Institute. (2004). Smallpox strikes Puerto Rico in bioterrorism exercise lessons learned from exercise blue advance. *Journal of Homeland Security.* http://www.homelandsecurity.org/journal/Default.aspx?oid=108&ocat=1/. April 18, 2010.

8. See U.S. v. Smith, 499 U.S. 160 (1991).

9. Supra note 6, p. 45.

10. Supra note 6, p. 48.

11. Hoffman, S. (2008). Responders' responsibility: Liability and immunity in public healthy emergencies. *Georgia Law Journal, 96,* 1913, 1925–1937.

12. Supra note 11, p. 1917.

13. Supra note 11, pp. 1950–1954; see also supra note 6, p. 49.

14. Supra note 6, p. 48.

15. Supra note 11, p. 1953.

16. Supra note 6, p. 49.

17. Supra note 11, pp. 1943–1945.

18. Ibid, p. 1943.

19. 745 ILCS 49, § 25 (1998).

20. 42 U.S.C. § 14505(6) (2000).

21. Wyoming Stat. Ann. § 35-4-114 (2007).

22. California Government Code § 8659 (2005).

23. Worth, T. (2008). Disaster legislation shields healthcare workers in Louisiana. *American Journal of Nursing, 108,* 20. http://www.nursingcenter.com/pdf.asp?AID=818847/.

24. R.S. 29, § 735.3 (La. 2008).

25. R.S. 37, § 1731.1 (La. 2008).

26. R.S. 29, § 735.4 (La. 2008).

27. Supra note 6, p. 1.

28. Ibid, p. 10.

29. Ibid, p. 18.

30. Ibid, p. 20.

31. Ibid, p. 20.

32. Supra note 6, pp. 5–6, 35.

33. Ibid, pp. 28–33.

34. Ibid, p. 37.

35. Ibid, p. 24.

36. Ibid, p. 49.

37. Supra note, pp. 7, 47.

38. Ibid, p. 61.

39. Ibid, p. 63.

40. Ibid, p. 75.

41. Ibid, p. 89.

42. Supra note 11, p. 82.

43. Pou, A.M. (2008). Hurricane Katrina and disaster preparedness. (Letter to the editor.) *New England Journal of Medicine, 358*(14), 1524.

44. American Medical Association Council on Medical Education. (2009). *Education in disaster medicine and public health preparedness during medical school and residency training.* http://www.ama-assn.org/ama1/pub/upload/mm/377/cme-report-15a-09.pdf/. Accessed April 18, 2010.

45. Ibid, p. 4.

46. Ibid, pp. 3–4.

47. Ibid, p. 6.

PROACTIVE LOSS CONTROL: APPLYING PRINCIPLES OF RISK MANAGEMENT AND PATIENT SAFETY TO CHANGE THE ENVIRONMENT

22

CREATING SYSTEMIC MINDFULNESS: ANTICIPATING, ASSESSING, AND REDUCING RISKS OF HEALTH CARE

Barbara J. Youngberg, JD, MSW, BSN, FASHRM

INTRODUCTION

In this chapter and the chapters that follow the reader will be exposed to a number of concepts that present a different approach for dealing with the common and root causes of error. It is this risk management function (which really is more akin to a tool kit of approaches) that has changed most dramatically following the release of the Institute of Medicine's (IOM) report and that often requires that risk managers obtain additional training and alter the manner in which they previously performed their work. Risk managers who have worked in the field for a number of years no doubt appreciate that the investigations following an event were often done in anticipation of having to defend a provider who, because of the event, became a defendant in a lawsuit. Typically, the risk manager looked at the specific actions of the individual and whether or not they fell below the standard of care. Further analysis as to how those events might have

occurred, and recognition that the root causes that contributed to one type of event might exist elsewhere and cause additional harm to other patients, was often not appreciated. In addition, because the focus of the investigation was often "in anticipation of litigation," what was learned was often buried in the legal file and never used to more fully understand the etiology of error, to drive educational efforts, or to create the case for much-needed change.

When risk management became more than merely a risk-financing and claims-management function, it was logical to start by developing proactive risk-avoidance plans by looking retrospectively at the areas where claims were either highest in frequency or were costing the organization or the insurance provider the greatest amount of money. It was not surprising that the areas of obstetrics and neonatology, anesthesia, and emergency medicine were those clinical areas where early risk-modification efforts occurred. In those areas, patients were often highly vulnerable to errors; providing care was complicated and often included the use of complex technology. The injuries suffered due to this complexity and the critical nature of the patients' condition were significant and often fatal. These early approaches focused not on the underlying factors that might have been present in all events (such as poor communication, inadequate transfer of care from one provider to another, or fatigue) but instead on the specific and unique factors associated with caring for specific patients presenting with specific clinical conditions. It was often the case that the investigation looked at the behavior of the caregiver involved in the error and perhaps the judgment that he or she evidenced, but it often failed to appreciate the systemic processes that set that individual up for that particular error at that particular time and place. Clearly, it is still important that risk management and patient safety experts recognize the unique risks and challenges that might be present in a specific environment, but if that is as deep as their investigation goes, they are likely to miss much-needed additional information.

Chapter 23 begins the process of proactive risk management by looking at the specific risks inherent in selected high-risk hospital departments. I am grateful to Alice E. Epstein and Gary H. Harding for allowing me to use their chapter, which first appeared in *Risk Management in Health Care Institutions: A Strategic Approach* (second edition). In my mind, this is where the process must begin.

WHAT WE CAN LEARN FROM OTHER INDUSTRIES

The IOM report and subsequent research into the science of safety has provided us with many examples, notably from non-healthcare organizations, as to how the risk management process should change given the nature of the work that we do and the relative lack of success that we have had in doing it. Clearly, the punitive culture of health care has ham-

pered our ability to learn, but our lack of systems thinking and organization commitment to a culture of safety has also limited our progress, in addition to thinking of health care as a totally unique function unable to learn from other equally hazardous industries and complex organizations, about the etiology of errors and possible strategies to prevent them. Furthermore, our progress has been limited in understanding—for example, the impact of fatigue on cognitive thinking, the impact of hierarchy on culture, and the value of well-defined processes and checklists to avert potential errors—because we are unable to acknowledge that what has been learned in fields such as aviation and nuclear power might actually provide great value for health care.

CREATING HIGH-RELIABILITY ORGANIZATIONS TO PROMOTE PATIENT SAFETY AND REDUCE HEALTHCARE RISK

Health care, especially the complex hospital care required to treat serious diseases, falls into the category of a "high-hazard industry."[1] These industries involve potent activities with the power to kill or maim. Our society depends on our technologically advanced system of health care but increasingly demands that the care be safe and effective as well. The focus on patient safety, which emerged following the IOM's pioneering work detailed in two broadly distributed reports on patient safety,[2,3] stresses the importance of developing a new infrastructure to support the activities that create understanding and foster improvement. One of the management theories that has been shown to yield positive results in other high-hazard industries is known as high-reliability organizational theory (HROT). Its characteristics are described in this chapter, and its particular relevance to risk management and patient safety are also discussed.

A high-reliability organization (HRO) is a highly complex high-hazard organization that is prone to unexpected error or injury; however, it continues to operate effectively and consistently despite a high potential for system failure and other catastrophic outcomes associated with error. In fact, HROs have evolved to become virtually 100% reliable and virtually error free. Errors are rare, and almost never fatal, to the continued functioning of the organization as a whole due to the implementation of sophisticated methods of predicting, recognizing, and responding to error, and solid leadership. Performance levels remain high despite this high potential for error. An HRO can operate without error for extended periods of time. Failure-free operation is the goal of every HRO when faced with the unexpected. Some examples of HROs are aircraft carriers, nuclear power plants, air-traffic control, and electric companies. Some studies have been done to evaluate the potential for schools as HROs. The medical setting is optimal for the implementation of an HRO structure, because a healthcare delivery system (such as a hospital) must maintain high levels of reliability and safety despite significant error potential, and because safety is the hallmark of every HRO's organizational culture.

The focus of this chapter is on the infrastructure or cultural changes that must occur in an organization, and indeed in the traditional risk management process, to not only reduce errors but to render high reliability and to enhance the overall culture of safety. More importantly, the cultural and foundational competencies established by these new processes are necessary to support and empower the individual stakeholders in the organization so that they remain committed to moving the risk management and patient safety agenda forward. All of the changes must be endorsed and supported by the leadership of the organization and may impact the process of risk management as it currently exists.

The HROT view is that proper organization of people, technology, and processes can handle complex and hazardous activities at acceptable levels of performance.[4] In high-reliability organizations, safety is the hallmark of organizational culture and professional behavior. Safety is spoken, always considered, and has at least as high a priority as all other aspects of operational decision making. All decisions and actions that impact clinical care rendered to patients include an analysis of the safety implications associated with that decision proactively and when systems fail retrospectively to assure that contributing, underlying system issues are corrected so that errors are not replicated and error-prone behaviors are eliminated. Team interaction is collegial rather than hierarchical, and each team member has an obligation to speak up if a question of safety arises.[5] In addition, all team members have an obligation to listen when another does identify an issue of concern, and to respond appropriately. Communication (including reporting of accidents and near misses) is highly valued and rewarded. It is understood that when team members fail to engage in respectful interactions, errors can occur.[5] Emergencies are rehearsed and the unexpected is practiced. Successful operations are viewed as potentially dangerous because success leads to system simplification and shortcuts.[6] Preparation, practice, and revaluation of team decision making and resulting consequences are a constant feature of day-to-day operations. In addition, the need for open and forthright discussion about errors, including having those discussions with patients or their families, is paramount.

It is hypothesized that increased patient safety would result if the principles of teamwork and high reliability could be more widely accepted and applied in all aspects of clinical care. It is recognized, however, that some of what is required will mandate that the organization and its risk manager think differently about the work that they do. This chapter describes the characteristics of high reliability and, for each one, the tension or the opportunity that the organization's risk manager might experience. The characteristics of HROs are complex, because they are both centralized and decentralized, hierarchical and collegial, rule bound and learning centered.[7]

The platform for patient safety and the rationality for promoting a culture of high reliability is predicated on multiple important competencies:

- The ability to reinforce the systems and structures to promote safety based on evidence drawn from the science of safety (in fields such as aviation, nuclear power, fire fighting, and manufacturing)
- The ability to create a culture that develops and supports those who provide care and services to allow for greater capacity for teamwork, risk awareness, risk mitigation, and resiliency
- The ability to focus and align resources to create and promote advancements in safety
- The commitment to assure that evidence-based, patient-centered, and system-centered work is done
- The promise to all concerned that honest, ethical dialogue with patients is necessary when breaches in safety occur

Building systems that reduce the probability of accident and harm requires recognition and understanding of four basic concepts, which are as follows:[8]

1. Health care is a complex system, and complex systems are inherently risk prone, particularly operating rooms, intensive care units, and emergency rooms, where teamwork is essential and crises are common.
2. People, no matter how competent and vigilant, are fallible because they are human and therefore physically and psychologically limited in memory capacity and the ability to deal with simultaneous multiple cognitive demands. Fatigue caused by long and stressful work hours further exacerbates these problems.
3. People create safety by defending against risk and intercepting error before it reaches the patient. They are also perpetrators of risk due to their being human, and are therefore subject to stressors such as fear, fatigue, and social factors that impair cognitive and motor function.
4. Safety is a system and can pose threats of failure from inadequate or clumsy equipment, fatigue-inducing schedules, flawed or incomplete procedures, excessive incentives for production, and risk-prone professional and organizational cultures often associated with faulty communications.

Given the competencies articulated and the restraining paradigms delineated above, where and how do we begin to move our healthcare organizations forward in order to make them more highly reliable?

The culture of health care uses the framework and blueprint upon which all systems are built. It is thus a change in the culture that must occur if we are to succeed in making our organizations HROs. In order to achieve an HRO, it is important to understand the characteristics of high reliability and the risk manager's relationship and responsibility toward them. The key characteristics of high reliability are:[9]

- Trust and transparency
- Reporting
- Flexibility in hierarchy
- Organizations perceived to be just and accountable
- Engagement and dedication in terms of continuous learning

Trust and Transparency

The concepts of trust and transparency help to define the ethical framework of HROs. The patient-centered ethic underscores the provider's obligation to inform the patient of potential adverse outcomes as well as solicit and take seriously the patient's self-assessment regarding unacceptable risk.[10] These concepts also relate to the employees of the organization, who must believe that the organization values open and honest discussion and recognizes that it is the only mechanism for rooting out systemic problems.

Risk managers often struggle with the concepts of trust and transparency, particularly in light of today's highly litigious society and a tort system in need of reform. Although the standards of The Joint Commission require that organizations have a policy in place related to the disclosure of error, it remains unclear how many organizations actually do have these discussions with patients and what indeed is disclosed. For example, when a patient is given the wrong drug in error, is the disclosure that the patient "reacted poorly to the drug and we are investigating," or is it that "the nurse gave the patient a drug that was meant for another patient because the system of double-checking failed"? Also, when a patient does poorly in surgery because the surgeon failed to appreciate the extent of his vascular disease, are the facts as revealed through a true and accurate disclosure blamed for the outcome, or is the patient's own condition blamed? Often attempts are made to justify the lack of transparency regarding a person's right to privacy, or unjustifiable and often paternalistic concerns about the repercussions of open and honest dialogue and the patient's ability to handle the truth, particularly as it might relate to the fueling of litigation. What healthcare professionals often fail to realize is that an event that requires disclosure may indeed be one where compensation should be paid, and the more positive the conversation in terms of openness about the event, the more manageable the compensation is likely to be.

Transparency is discussed in greater detail in prior chapters because it relates to disclosure to patients, but in the HROT context, it also refers to openly discussing errors throughout the organization in an effort to facilitate learning.

Reporting

High-reliability cultures encourage and reward reporting. They recognize that valuable information can come from any source within the organization, and that each reporter has a perspective that is valuable and must be heard. Health care as a national system currently has a relatively weak, mostly local, system for investigating and reporting adverse events. The bulk of reporting is generally within the hospital-system-incident or event-reporting system, but only a handful of events are officially reported via the quality-management system.[9] Despite the call for mandatory reporting in the IOM report that began the national discussion on patient safety,[2] organizations remain reluctant to share their error data, unless such sharing is mandated by the state in which the hospital does business. Although organizations continue to review their data (in standard mortality and morbidity conferences, pharmacy and therapeutic committees, infection control committees, etc.), few have fully integrated and highly effective processes whereby risk management, quality management, and near-miss data are evaluated with the same rigor and with the hopes of identifying problematic, but correctable, trends. Also, many organizations have yet to grasp that the more reporting that occurs in the organization, the more likely that organization will understand the etiology of the problem and the best manner in which to resolve it.

Risk managers often thwart effective reporting systems. The tension between preserving historic practices (sequestering and protecting any and all incident reports and actual and potential lawsuit information) and promoting a sharing of information through other channels in their organization remains a significant problem. This reluctance to share information is heightened by the current dire malpractice crisis and the feeling that state tort systems are out of control. Risk managers, eager to be part of an HRO, need to think differently about their responsibilities to the organization and perhaps to its patients. At some point, one must ask if it is worth protecting information learned in the process of building a defense in one lawsuit, if additional patients are injured as a result of the same systemic and contributing factors, which fail to get shared because they are shrouded under the attorney–client privilege? Although many organizations continue to struggle with how to integrate quality improvement, risk management, and safety and near-miss data, certainly there are enormous benefits for doing just that. Recognizing that state peer review or medical-studies acts may allow broader protection may, in some states, provide a good place to begin.

Flexibility in Hierarchy

Most high-hazard industries are extremely centralized. The aircraft-carrier flight deck, nuclear power in the United States, and to a lesser extent, commercial aviation, are all examples of centralized operations where clear rules and procedures govern. In contrast to these industries, health care is extraordinarily decentralized. There are hundreds of thousands of doctors' offices (over 470,000 physicians are identified as involved in "office-based" patient care),[12] which are increasingly becoming the site for invasive procedures.[13] There are a number of hospitals, many of which are in the process either of merging with others or de-merging, when relationships once thought to be advantageous turn out to be unworkable. Although regulatory and accrediting agencies do play a role in standardizing operations, clinical care and clinical decision making remain highly decentralized.

Although usually risk managers can do little to influence physicians' clinical judgment and behaviors, they often are in a position to address the issue of the benefits of a highly centralized work environment for the rest of the care providers (nurses, pharmacists, lab technicians). Pushing for standardization of work processes and equipment, as well as for standardized protocols to govern specific types of patient-care encounters, can have a positive impact on creating greater reliability in the care provided. Furthermore, risk managers might see enormous benefit if they enhance their current processes of data collection. These enhancements would allow for the tracking of systemic and contributing factors associated with harm (such as human factors, environmental factors, and team factors) so that reviewers can focus their efforts on those factors that will yield the greatest benefit.

It is possible that the Patient Safety and Quality Improvement Act of 2005 and the subsequent Patient Safety Organizations legislation described in Chapter 8 will assist in moving this process along, but at this point it appears to be too early to tell.

Perceived to Be Just and Accountable

Much has been written about the non-punitive culture in other industries that is required to support the culture of safety. This non-punitive concept does not seek to turn a blind eye to holding individuals accountable for their professional actions but rather to understand that often—and most people would say too often—the environments in which we place professionals to work sets them up for failure. In an organization that sets out to be fair, one must always ask how it was that the error was allowed to happen? How could better systems, better structure, and better technology have assisted these individuals so that they could have done their job as intended? In addition, risk managers should become familiar with the concept of "just culture," which was developed by David Marx and his colleagues[14] and which helps to differentiate between how systems fail healthcare providers and how providers can make decisions that render them accountable for an untoward outcome. The work of Marx and colleagues clearly lays out the appropriate risk responses depending on whether the system was at fault or whether the person working in that system either consciously or unconsciously drifted into error-prone behaviors.

Engaged and Committed to Safety and Dedicated to Continuous Learning

High-reliability organizations always recognize that safety is fundamental to their operations and core to their business strategy and mission. The risk manager may play an important role in the organization to "hardwire" patient safety into the daily lifeblood and operations of the organization, but the business choices made by the senior leadership team will not only assure the success of patient safety but also allow staff to recognize its importance. Embracing and applying lessons learned from leaders in other industries, such as aviation, nuclear power, fire fighting, and manufacturing, can inform and accelerate action. There are known safety principles from industry to incorporate into daily work. Those principles include:[15]

- An employee-training process that trains staff in effective teamwork, decision making, risk awareness, and error management, as well as in the technical aspects of the job.
- Policies and procedures that simplify and standardize work processes and products, such as the use of a consistent monitoring system with consequences when employees knowingly drift away from adherence to these procedures.
- A commitment to designing self-correcting systems or redundant systems that make it difficult to do the wrong thing, such as verifying messages about who will take what action when, or using technical monitors to complement judgment.
- Systems and processes that reduce reliance on human memory through protocols, checklists, and automated systems, and that enhance communication among colleagues.

- Appropriately using automation to support and enhance manual processes that can reduce specific types of errors.
- A commitment to drive out fear of blame in error reporting and systems that facilitate the collection of data that can assist in learning about error and near-miss events or unsafe situations or circumstances. The risk should be in failing to report, not in the act of bringing bad news.
- Increased leadership awareness regarding unit-level concerns facilitated by leaders becoming more visible within the organization. This can be accomplished through regular "town hall" meetings, unit walk-arounds, or more flexible open-door policies.
- Reacting to what is learned and conveying to staff that they have been heard. When processes need correction, take action.
- Systems and processes that do not tolerate violation of standards or failure of staff to take available countermeasures against error (such as input from colleagues, use of checklist) and hold people accountable for their actions.

Flexibility in Work Structure

A flexible structure is needed to allow for rapid movement from bureaucratic tight coupling to a more malleable form as conditions warrant.[16] There are several essential and unique characteristics of any HRO. Firstly, HROs use a systems approach to error rather than an individual approach (called human error). This means that when an error occurs within an HRO, the entire organizational system is at fault and subject to review. Individual responsibility is not the focus, and blame shifting is therefore discouraged. This promotes progress within the organization. Decision making is accomplished using a flexible hierarchy model—that is, members of staff most qualified to make decisions can make them regardless of rank. This strays from the traditional method of decision making, which defers to a strict hierarchy and leaves decisions in the hands of upper management, who may have no concept of critical issues on the frontlines of the organization. An HRO setting employs an empowered and informed staff at all levels. Management is aware of the big picture but is not always needed for a final decision to be made. In addition to a flexible hierarchy, all HROs have standard operating procedures in place to deal with routine matters. These procedures are developed using formal logical decision analysis to identify processes and particular tasks involved in an error event. "Some things must be universal" to ensure success, increase safety, and reduce error.

Emphasis on Reliability Over Efficiency

High-reliability organizations promote reliability over efficiency. Because of this, HROs possess top-of-the-line equipment as well as sophisticated databases. Furthermore, there is a level of redundancy within every HRO. This means that material is repeatedly checked and errors are constantly discussed and corrected. Another method of promoting reliability is through extensive training and education, heavy recruitment, and regular staff evaluations. Each member in an HRO has knowledge of his or her individual role as it relates to the big picture, the team mission. Teamwork is essential to success. Effective modes of communication and interaction, due to monitoring practices between staff, facilitate team strength.

High-reliability organizations use an incentive system as a means of encouraging optimal safety-promoting behavior. Recognition in an HRO's newsletter or at an awards ceremony motivates positive change and maintains high morale within the organization. Punishment has the opposite effect and leads to a reduction in reliability, which in turn can compromise safety. Furthermore, rewarding performance demonstrates public commitment to the safety of, and loyalty toward, the organization.

Command and Control

Formal rules and procedures are necessary; these are not to be confused with creating bureaucratic complexity, but instead exist to ensure adherence to the standards and shared knowledge of best practice. This implies intelligent and thoughtful application of rules and procedures, not routinized compliance. The rules and procedures should foster knowledge-based decisions in which experts can determine when a variation or innovation is required due to a unique condition. This factor is expanded by Libuser and Roberts, who outline the following command-and-control elements:[17]

- Migrating decision making. The person with the most expertise makes the decision.
- Having redundancy. Backup systems are in place, whether they consist of people or technology support.
- Seeing the "big picture." Senior managers see the big picture and therefore do not micro-manage, but they attend to patterns and systems.
- Establishing formal rules and procedures. There is hierarchy with procedure and protocol based on evidence.
- Conducting ongoing training. Investment is made in the knowledge and skills of workers at the front line. This includes training in teamwork, such as crew-resource and management-team practices.

Finally, HROs have unique methods for identifying a risk and reacting effectively and rapidly to contain that risk. There exists a complex reporting system, a highly organized team structure, and effective error-recording methods using a non-punitive system. Feedback is given regularly, and corrective actions are taken and monitored to promote a continual learning environment with the goal of producing a completely error-free system.

The healthcare system stands to benefit from the systems approach to error reduction that is used by HROs. The usual approach to addressing errors within the healthcare field has been to stress individual responsibility and to center on improving an individual provider's performance. In the complex world of medicine, this approach is too simplistic and fails. It is essential to assess the origins of adverse events deeply rooted within the healthcare system in order to forge ahead with the patient safety movement. This has only recently begun to be addressed by medical journals and the like. By comparing other non-medical HROs' approaches to error theory and accident causation, a broader understanding of the context in which errors occur in healthcare delivery can be reached. For example, methods of critical-incident analysis used in the aviation field can also be used to assess incidents that involve medical accidents. Furthermore, causation in these highly complex systems is often multi-factorial, resulting from a chain of events and necessitating an overhaul in the system's training programs, equipment, and management. An analysis of contributory team factors to assess reliability is also essential, because one person cannot run an HRO. In order to create a safety culture within the realm of health care, there must exist a culture of reporting, flexibility, learning, and trust. High-reliability organizations' approach to safety culture allows them to reconfigure operations in the face of danger without compromising productivity and system continuity. The healthcare delivery system cannot afford such compromises. Evidence of poor design and poor maintenance must be addressed system-wide in order to ensure a virtually error-free climate. Near misses must no longer be considered successes within the healthcare field; instead, they should be viewed as potential failures requiring immediate analysis, much like what is done in air-traffic-control risk management or nuclear-power safety systems.

Viewing the healthcare system as an HRO is a step in the right direction when it comes to improving the quality of health care. No progress can be truly accomplished until all stakeholders become involved in this common goal of safety and begin to embrace the concept of high reliability.

Root-Cause Analysis: Learning Well from Mistakes

Along with fostering an environment of transparency and trust where apologies for medical errors can happen, an HRO takes advantage of its mistakes and medical errors by performing a meaningful root-cause analysis (RCA) and failure mode and effects analysis (FMEA). A root cause is the most basic causal factor or factors that, if corrected or removed, will prevent recurrence of a situation.[18] An RCA is a formal investigation of an adverse event, or a potentially adverse event, designed to address the event's root cause.[18] Root-cause analyses are not opportunities to place blame, but instead are programs that rely on rational decision-making processes to provide impartial, analytical tools for adverse-event analysis.[18] Moreover, RCA is a questioning process that provides a structured method to enable people to recognize and discuss the beliefs and practices in an organization. Root-cause analysis is a potentially effective tool because root causes reside in the values and beliefs of an organization. The fact that meaningful RCAs have the potential and purpose to affect an institution this significantly is the reason that RCAs should be a part of any high-reliability nursing home.

Root-cause analyses help foster the development of HROs because they require a culture of reliability and mindfulness in order to be effective. Also, RCAs are consistent with HROT because they force an institution to focus on potential adverse events, not just past injuries.[19] Root-cause analyses also promote high reliability because they help to foster communication across all levels of a healthcare institution, because RCAs have the potential to place members of management at a table with members of the healthcare team to discuss how the institution's culture may need to change.[19]

Principles of High Reliability Present in High-Performing Healthcare Organizations

In a quality and accountability study performed by the University Healthsystem Consortium (an alliance of 100 academic health centers throughout the United States), the attributes that existed in the top-performing organizations were identified and described.[20] Using the process developed by Jim Collins in his study of top-performing Fortune 500 companies,[21] a study team first performed an analysis of important metrics of performance that were identified as valuable among healthcare consumers and providers. Factors such as mortality rates, complications rates, adherence to patient safety practices and evidence-based practice, and equitable treatment for all patients were compiled in a composite scorecard, and organizations having the highest scores, average scores, and low scores were all visited. Through a rigorous process of data collection and analysis, coupled with comprehensive site visits of both top performers and those performing less well, the site-visit team recognized that many of the attributes found in top-performing healthcare organizations (but absent in healthcare organizations performing less well) were consistent with those identified in HROT. The following attributes were consistently present in the top-performing healthcare organizations:

- A shared sense of purpose where there was clarity regarding the mission and vision of the organization and where leaders worked collaboratively to advance quality and safety in patient care.
- A leadership style that was authentic and hands-on. Staff described how the actions of leaders were consistent with what they said and that leaders demonstrated their commitment to quality and safety in all of their actions and business decisions.
- The presence of an accountability system for quality, safety, and service that blended centralized and decentralized processes. Each of the top performers were highly transparent, data driven, and held staff to specific standards of performance.
- A clear focus on results, which provided clarity regarding expectations and encouraged transparency.
- A culture that was collaborative, respectful, and with limited hierarchy. This fostered open communication and team-work.

In the remaining sections of this book, specific strategies are presented to allow risk managers to view error through a safety-focused or HROT lens. Each chapter was selected because of research that points to the benefits that many healthcare organizations and providers have experienced by applying best practices to their work.

References

1. Gaba, D.M. (2000). Structural and organizational issues in patient safety: A comparison of health care to other high hazard industries. *California Management Review, 43*(1), 83–102.
2. Kohn, L., Corrigan, J., & Donaldson, M. (Eds.). (2000). *To err is human: Building a safer health care system.* Institute of Medicine, Committee on Quality of Health Care in America. Washington, DC: National Academy Press.
3. Institute of Medicine, Committee on Health Care Quality in America. (2001). Crossing the quality chasm: A new health care system for the 21st century. Washington, DC: National Academy Press.
4. Supra note 1, p. 86.
5. Knox, G.E., Kelley, M., Simpson, K.R., Carrier, L., & Berry, D. (1999). Downsizing, reengineering and patient safety: Numbers, newness and resultant risk. *Journal of Healthcare Risk Management, 19*(4), 18–25.

6. Roberts, K.H. (1990). Some characteristics of high reliability organizations. *Organization Science, 1*(2), 160–176.

7. Libuser, C.B., & Roberts, K. (1998). *Risk mitigation through organizational structure.* Presented at the Annual Meeting of the Academy of Management, August 1998, San Diego, California.

8. Helmreich, R., & Merritt, A. (1998). Culture at work in medicine and aviation: National organizational and professional influences. Aldershot, UK: Ashgate

9. Hatlie, M. (2000). *Patient safety collaborative lecture series.* Regional collaboratives. Voluntary Hospitals of America, Waltham, Massachusetts.

10. Youngberg, B.J., & Hatlie, M.J. (Eds.). (2004). *The patient safety handbook.* Sudbury, MA: Jones and Bartlett Publishers.

11. Cullen, D., Bates, D., Small, S., Cooper, J., Nemeskal, A., & Leape, L. (1995). The incident reporting system does not detect adverse drug events: A problem for quality improvement. *Joint Commission Journal for Quality Improvement, 21,* 541–548.

12. American Medical Association. (2000). *Nonfederal physicians in the United States and possessions by selected characteristics.* http://www.ama-assn.org/phys-data/physnow/nowgraf1.htm/.

13. Morell, R. (2000). OBA questions, problems just now being recognized, being defined. *Anesthesia Patient Safety Foundation Newsletter, 15,* 1–3.

14. Marx, D. Patient Safety and the Just Culture. http://www.health.state.ny.us/professionals/patients/patient_safety/conference/2007/docs/patient_safety_and_the_just_culture.pdf. Accessed April 20, 2010.

15. Nance, J.D. (May 1997). Managing human error in aviation. *Scientific American,* 62–67.

16. Roberts, K.H. (1990). Some characteristics of one type of high reliability organization. *Organizational Science, 1,* 160–176.

17. Libuser, C.B., & Roberts, K. (1998). Risk mitigation through organizational structure. Paper presented at the Annual Meetings of the Academy of Management, San Diego, CA, August 1998.

18. Dew, J.R. Using root causes analysis to make the patient care system safe. http://bama.ua.edu/ ~ st497. Accessed May 5, 2010.

19. Supra note 18, p. 1669.

20. Keroack, M.A., Youngberg, B.J., Cerese, J.L., Krsek, C., Prellwitz, L.W., & Trevelyan, E.W. (2007). *Academic Medicine, 82*(12), 1178–1186.

21. Collins, J. (2001). *Good to great: Why some companies make the leap and others don't.* New York: HarperCollins Publishers.

RISK MANAGEMENT IN SELECTED HIGH-RISK HOSPITAL DEPARTMENTS*

Alice L. Epstein, MHA, CPHRM, CPHQ, CPEA
Gary H. Harding, BS, BMET

INTRODUCTION

Each clinical-care area and medical specialty brings to patients the hope and promise of successful medical intervention, as well as the potential for poor outcomes and unexpected complications. There are management issues applicable to all clinical departments that are relevant to the delivery of safe and effective patient care. For example, medical-record documentation, competency of staff, and credentialing to perform the tasks necessary to care for the patient are important regardless of the department or medical specialty. Patient-monitoring capabilities and technical equipment must be in place and be effective so that staff is always aware of the physiological condition of the patient and is prepared to intercede if and when necessary.

Departments such as pharmacy, radiology, pathology, and laboratory typically do not have their own patients, but they interact with other specialty departments. In many cases, the challenge is even more difficult for the support departments, since requests for services are referred from outside the department. Accurate and timely communication among the departments and the referring physicians is essential. Without effective communications, laboratory tests may be ordered incorrectly, the wrong patient may be identified for a test, test results may be interpreted inappropriately, and needed intervention may be delayed.

Regardless of the clinical specialty, the risks and risk management interventions are often specific to the clinical specialty. Liabilities are inherent within select clinical specialties, particularly those that the medical literature and insurance data identify as posing heightened risk to patients, institutions,

*Originally appeared in Florence Kavaler and Allen D. Spiegel's *Risk Management in Health Care Institutions: A Strategic Approach, Second Edition.* Jones and Bartlett Publishers, Boston, 2003.

and professionals. It is important to note that a recent analysis of claims[1] indicates that new patterns of high risk are emerging. The nursing/patient care category (which includes medical, surgical, and intensive care) is now the leader for total dollar losses, outpacing perinatal, surgery, and emergency services. The analysis suggests that by improving just a few specific risk management practices, patient safety is improved and the cost of claims is lowered. The following selected high-risk departments within clinical care deserve special attention: emergency medicine, obstetrics and neonatology, and surgery and anesthesia.

EMERGENCY MEDICINE

Emergency departments care for more than 100 million patients annually and provide accurate and effective diagnoses in well over 99% of cases.[2] Emergency medicine has a unique set of inherent risks. Most patients who arrive at an emergency department are in a medical crisis; however, some patients who come to the emergency department are overreacting to a nonemergency situation and thus are not appropriately accessing the medical system—that is, through a primary-care provider. As a result, there are problems with the allocation of resources.

According to the American College of Emergency Physicians (ACEP), the most common allegations of malpractice involve the failure to diagnose the following:[3,4]

- Fractures
- Foreign bodies in wounds
- Myocardial infarctions
- Complications of lacerations, including tendons and nerves

The most costly malpractice allegations involve the following conditions:

- Myocardial infarctions
- Meningitis
- Fractures
- Ectopic pregnancies

STANDARDS AND GUIDELINES

Many professional medical organizations developed standards and guidelines regarding the safe and effective delivery of health care in the emergency setting. Such organizations include the American College of Emergency Physicians, American College of Osteopathic Emergency Physicians, Committee on Trauma of the American College of Surgeons, Emergency Nurses Association, Emergency Department Nurses Association, and the National Association of Emergency Medical Technicians.

According to the American Hospital Association, a true emergency is "any condition clinically determined to require immediate medical care."[5] Some courts have defined an emergency as existing when treatment is necessary to alleviate severe pain or to prevent further deterioration or aggravation of the patient's condition. Federal legislation defines an emergency condition as manifested by acute symptoms of sufficient severity that the absence of immediate medical attention could reasonably be expected to result in serious jeopardy to an individual's health, serious impairment to bodily functions, or serious dysfunction of any body organ or part.

All patients, regardless of economic issues, have a right to receive needed emergency care. In 1986, Congress passed the Consolidated Omnibus Reconciliation Act (COBRA), which contains a section titled the Emergency Medical Treatment and Active Labor Act (EMTALA). This legislation was designed, in part, to prevent patients from being transferred solely for economic reasons. COBRA provides that any hospital that receives Medicare funds and has an emergency department must provide appropriate medical screening to determine if a medical emergency exists or if the patient is in active labor.[5] If possible, the patient must then be examined and stabilized prior to transfer or discharge.

Whereas clinicians and risk managers tend to define emergencies as "life-threatening" situations, lawyers and courts may take a more liberal view. Merely the existence of an emergency department implies an implicit duty to treat any patient who arrives needing immediate attention. Courts have found that a patient–physician relationship commences as soon as the emergency department is offered as a source of treatment to the general public and the public it seeks to serve. An insurance study has demonstrated a 600% increase in the cost of an ER claim when risk management practices are not followed.[6]

PREHOSPITAL SERVICES

Time is of the essence in emergency situations. The more rapidly that medical intervention occurs after the medical condition is discovered, the more likely the results will be positive. Delays prior to arrival for treatment in the emergency department contribute to the decrease in successful emergency medical or surgical interventions and an increase in severity of illness.

A thorough understanding of the prehospital emergency services available in the community is necessary because of the widely varied local and state development of these systems. The ACEP's policy statement "Medical Direction of Pre-hospital Emergency Services"[7] suggests that all prehospital emergency services be managed by a physician who has authority over patient care and the responsibility to develop and implement medical policies and procedures, and is board certified in emergency medicine and experienced in emergency department management. Emergency medical technicians (EMTs) who respond by ambulance to crisis situations are required by the U.S. Department of Transportation to complete an 81-hour curriculum. Advanced levels of EMT training require from 280 to 1,000 hours. Some regions in the country are fortunate to have hospital-to-field communication systems that allow on-line medical direction in which physicians are directly responsible for orders given to field personnel regarding specific emergency conditions (see Box 23–1).

Box 23–1

Disputes and controversy arose when an oxygen tube was improperly inserted by an ambulance crew attending a collapsed fireman, causing brain damage, coma, and death. Volunteer ambulance workers allegedly refused to yield to emergency medical services paramedics and argued at the scene about which hospital to go to.[8]

Risk management concerns the field situation and approach to the medical emergency. Patients may be dead at the site or may arrive DOA (dead on arrival) at the emergency department. During transport to the hospital, the patient may experience cardiac and respiratory arrests, and there may be significant changes in prehospital diagnosis and emergency department diagnosis. Ambulances may be required to re-route to a hospital that is farther away than the one they originally set out for, due to overcrowding or understaffing at the original facility.

LEVELS OF SERVICE

Emergency departments are divided into categories based on the sophistication of the services provided. Established by the American Medical Association Commission on Emergency Medical Services,[9] these categories relate to availability of care, physician staffing, medical specialties required to be available in the hospital and on call, referral requirements, required biomedical equipment, medication availability, facility design, and support-department availability.

Patients often are not aware of the level of services available at the emergency department they choose to access, nor are they aware of the level of services that their medical condition requires. This lack of knowledge on the part of patients places the staff of the emergency department in a precarious position from a legal perspective. Hospitals can be successfully sued when they do not have the services, personnel, or facilities to render the care they have marketed to the community.

Many hospitals have established emergi-centers and/or urgi-centers in an attempt to access new markets within the community, provide additional services, and reduce the patient load on the hospital emergency department. Risk management concerns focus on the potential inappropriate public perception that urgi-centers are staffed and equipped to provide full emergency critical-care or trauma services.

Security issues are a major concern for emergency departments. Studies and media reports demonstrate that violence in emergency departments has escalated over the past 10 years.[10] During a 9-month period in just one emergency department, staff members were punched, kicked, grabbed, pushed, or spat on, 19 times.[11] Hospital workers may suffer psychological trauma and post-traumatic stress disorder because of the violent acts in emergency departments.[12] Ideally, security personnel should be in close proximity and availability to the emergency department 24 hours a day. Each institution should review the security risks and risk management issues and develop policies to minimize uncontrolled access into other sections of the hospital, to secure medications in controlled areas, and to deal with confiscated weapons.[13]

According to ACEP, emergency departments should be staffed by emergency-care physicians and other professionals, along with specialists on call, during all hours of operation, on the basis of the unique needs of the community and the level of emergency care offered.

Often, emergency departments are staffed by contract physicians or residents, who may be training or "moonlighting." Studies have shown that full-time attending physician coverage can result in a decrease in claims filed and claims paid out.[13] If residents are to be used, it is imperative that attending-physician supervision be available on-site.[14] A recent study found that "only about half of the nation's 25,000 jobs in

medicine are filled by doctors certified to provide emergency care."[15] It is important to realize that the attending physician is the primary physician responsible for the patient. Attending physicians who practice "long-distance" supervision of residents, and facilities that allow such practice, may experience greatly increased liability.

Contracted physicians, if used, should be board certified in emergency medicine, credentialed and privileged to practice in the department, and required to adhere to the policies and protocols of the hospital and to participate in quality-improvement activities.

In rural facilities, the number of physicians available may be limited, so the nursing staff needs to be able to stabilize the patient until the physician arrives or until adequate transfer conditions and plans have been met. Many hospitals have developed policies that require the on-call physician to be within 30 minutes of the hospital and that they provide guidance for the nursing staff regarding alternate physicians to be contacted. Frequently, the emergency department physician is required to cover in-house emergencies. From a risk management perspective, this responsibility must not compromise the availability of rapid medical or physician response to patients coming into the emergency department.

At a change in shift or change in professionals in the emergency department, each physician should be required to write a status note in the medical record regarding the patient, and the responsibility for patient care should be formally transferred.

Physicians in the emergency department should not practice outside their scope of training or expertise and are expected to contact the appropriate specialist, when needed, to reduce the potential for liability.

All physicians who provide care in the department are under the jurisdiction of the physician in charge, with whom final decisions concerning admission or patient discharge should rest. As soon as it is determined that a patient should be admitted, the attending physician should be notified. In most hospitals, emergency department physicians do not have admitting privileges. It is the attending physician's responsibility to admit the patient and assume further responsibility for the patient's care after discussing the situation with the emergency physician.

Liability increases when patients receive emergency care, are admitted or discharged, or leave without being evaluated by a physician. In addition, problems arise with unsigned and poorly documented medical records of services, consultations, and discussions between the emergency department physician and the attending physician.

TRIAGE

Once the patient arrives at the hospital, it is the responsibility of the staff to treat the patient as the medical situation dictates. Proper triage classifies patients by level of need.

Emergency Cases

Emergency cases require immediate medical attention, because delaying medical care would be harmful to the patient, as the disorder is acute and potentially threatens life or function. Examples include cardiac arrest, severe head injuries, chest pain with difficulty breathing, and a temperature greater than 105°F.

Urgent Cases

Urgent cases require medical attention within a few hours of arrival at the hospital because the patient is in danger of acute, but not life-threatening, problems. Examples include burns, back injuries, fractures, and persistent diarrhea.

Nonurgent Cases

Nonurgent cases do not require the resources of an emergency department, because the problem is minor or nonacute, or treatment

cannot affect outcome or suffering. Examples include nondebilitating headaches, minor fractures, or a case in which the patient is dead on arrival.

Risks most commonly related to triage include the failure to determine the existence of an emergency, improper categorization of the patient's status, improper diagnosis, and failure to communicate pertinent information. In addition to initial assessment, every patient should be reassessed prior to being discharged or transferred to another facility.

An advisory panel of the National Heart Attack Alert Program found that emergency departments could be doing more to quickly identify and treat patients with myocardial infarction.[14] During triage, opportunities also exist to identify battered women,[15] as well as cases of child abuse and neglect that require certain reporting and special social-service interventions (see Box 23–2).[16]

Managed-care insurance introduced the concepts of the physician gatekeeper, preauthorization of services, and limiting patients to the use of facilities approved by their insurance company. Decisions to assess and treat a patient should not be made on the basis of payment by managed-care organizations, Medicaid, or Medicare. Emergency care must be rendered as appropriate to the medical condition, regardless of the patient's ability to pay. Prior approval for payment purposes should not delay assessment or the provision of necessary emergency treatment.

Telephone advice also presents risk management concerns in the emergency department.

Box 23–2

The New York City Health Department criticized Woodhull Medical Center (Brooklyn, N.Y.) for failure to provide "considerate and respectful care" to a rape victim who was left unattended for 2 hours wearing only a hospital gown in an area where handcuffed male prisoners were also awaiting treatment.[17]

Frequently, patients and family members telephone the emergency department seeking advice on whether they should come to the emergency department or how they can treat an injury or illness at home. The ACEP position statement "Providing Telephone Advice from the Emergency Department" established some guidelines.[18] Some emergency departments provide this service; others do not.

Some hospitals respond to these calls with a set of physician-developed clinical algorithms designed to facilitate a telephone-triage process to determine whether the patient should be brought to the emergency department. If telephone calls are being responded to, a log should be maintained in the department containing details of the calls and any advice given.

PATIENT–PHYSICIAN RELATIONSHIP

One of the keys to a successful outcome of services is the rapport established by the healthcare professionals in the emergency department with the patient and the family. Physicians should inform patients of the treatment plan and the recognized accuracy of the diagnostic tests they are to receive, identify factors that pose special risks, and discuss the options. To the extent possible, the patient and/or family should be involved in decisions regarding care. Support staff should keep family members advised of the progress of the patient and how long they can expect to wait. Sometimes anger expressed by a patient is secondary to the clinical situation and can be appropriately evaluated and refocused. Other times, however, the anger results in a lawsuit. It is important that patients be made aware of the fact that, most often, emergency room physicians are not hospital employees.

Risk management should monitor emergency department visits and analyze the trends in specific situations, such as complaints and dissatisfaction about present or past treatment, patients seen for a complication resulting from a previous procedure, or patients who return within 72 hours of a previous admission. Some patients may try to establish disability as a result of the injury and treatment. Other patients may make repeated visits, demanding pain medication immediately upon arrival, and may cover their drug addiction with symptoms that mimic renal colic or cardiac pain.

DOCUMENTATION AND CONSENTS

Documentation is crucial to managing risk in the emergency department. From the point of entry into the system through triage, assessment, physicians' orders, testing, treatment, test results, and discharge, important pieces of communication need to be recorded. Some hospitals use voice-recognition programs for documentation;[19] others have instituted checklists to help ensure that a particular clinical path is followed. Software programs of emergency-care clinical-practice algorithms are available, as are computerized clinical protocols.

The time of the patient's arrival and departure and tests, as well as consent to procedures and tests, should be in the record, as should be evidence of patient education, transfer forms, and copies of discharge instructions.

Whenever possible, consent for examination, treatment, and invasive procedures or tests should be obtained from the patient or an authorized individual if the patient is unable to consent; however, whenever a life-threatening emergency exists and treatment is required to save a life, the presumption is that consent is implied by the patient's arrival at the emergency department. An additional presumption is that a delay in treatment would seriously increase the hazards to health by precipitating death or a serious impairment. When treating a minor, if an emergency condition exists and the parents of the minor cannot be located, the need for consent is generally obviated. Treatment should be limited to that which is necessary to cope with the emergency. Whenever a parent or guardian provides consent via the telephone, a second hospital representative should monitor the conversation as a witness and document his or her presence in the medical record. Subsequently, the parent or the guardian should be requested to sign the consent authorization.

A competent adult or emancipated minor who is deemed competent has the right to refuse medical and surgical treatment even if brought to an emergency department, unless the state can demonstrate a compelling, overriding interest. Usually, the patient's competency and strength of conviction are considered in such cases presented to the court.

SUPPORT SERVICES

Emergency department physicians are sometimes dependent on the analysis of tests performed outside the department to determine the diagnosis of the patient and how to proceed with the patient's treatment. For example, electrocardiograms reduce the number of missed diagnoses of heart attacks, when properly interpreted.

Accurate interpretation of X-rays is also critical for reliable diagnoses. Emergency physicians have limited training in radiology but may be required to perform an initial reading of the X-ray and prescribe treatment. The radiologist usually interprets the film on the following day or following week, especially in rural facilities. Teleradiology is quickly linking rural emergency departments for real-time radiographic interpretations. In this way, emergency departments without access to radiologists are linked to radiology departments in other hospitals. Missed readings or discrepancies in film interpretation need to be documented in the medical record and brought to the attention of the emergency physician immediately so that the patient can be notified and possible alterations in treatment advised.

Failure to communicate important medical information about a patient to the treating physician may be viewed as negligence, particularly if this information would have changed the physician's orders and assessment. Frequently, nurses contact physicians by telephone to discuss a patient presenting in the emergency department. Because of the recognized potential for information to be incomplete, not appropriately communicated, or misunderstood, risk managers recommend that the responsible physician personally evaluate the patient.

DEPARTURES, DISCHARGES, AND TRANSFERS

Patients who leave the emergency department against medical advice prior to medical evaluation pose special risks to the hospital. Some patients and their families tire of a lengthy wait and decide to leave before being seen by a physician. Other patients may not be pleased with the treatment they receive or may not agree with treatment plans suggested by the physician. Existing organizational protocols should delineate how to handle these patients to reduce the number who leave prematurely. Patients who voice their intent to leave should be advised of the possible medical and health consequences, and such conversations with the patient and the family members should be documented in the medical record. A patient's refusal to sign an AMA (discharge against medical advice) statement should also be noted.

For safe transfer of a patient to another hospital or facility from the emergency department, staff must ensure that the patient is approved and stable for transfer and that the mode of transfer selected is appropriate. A receiving facility must agree to the transfer in advance, and the original facility must provide the receiving hospital with medical records.[20] Many transferring patients (for example, newborns and cardiac or psychiatric patients) require attendance by specialty-trained professionals and high-tech group or air ambulances.

A statement authorizing the transfer should be signed by the physician and should

Box 23–3

A 32-year-old chronically homeless man verbally threatened to kill his treating psychologist. When brought to the hospital, he acted violently when told he would be committed to the county psychiatric hospital. Six police officers and additional hospital security personnel restrained the patient. He was involuntarily restrained to a gurney with four-point restraints. He was given a sedative, placed face-down on the gurney, and a backboard was placed over him in order to transfer him to the psychiatric hospital by ambulance. While being wheeled out of the emergency room he was found to not be breathing. Efforts to revive him failed.

The county coroner determined that the cause of death was positional asphyxia, and the death was a homicide. Negligence against the hospital, the emergency room physician, and the ambulance company was alleged. The verdict was a total of $2 million.[21]

detail the medical benefits anticipated at the receiving facility that outweigh the increased risks of transfer (see Box 23–3).

Patients discharged directly from the emergency department may require limited follow-up care. To reduce liability, it is recommended that written discharge instructions be given to the patient and family and that these instructions be available in all of the most commonly used foreign languages in the service community. Discharge instructions should be reviewed with the patient by a nurse[22] or the physician prior to the patient's discharge from the emergency department, and a copy should be filed in the medical record. Follow-up calls should be made to patients discharged with potentially high-risk problems, such as head injury, and such calls should also be documented.

RISK MANAGEMENT OPPORTUNITIES

Risk managers have several opportunities to monitor emergency department services:

from medical records, by specific notification by the department, or by complaints. All deaths in the emergency department, or within 24 hours of admission, should be investigated. Similarly, all adverse situations should be reviewed, such as transfer of a patient who requires CPR during the transfer, any DOA case, or a patient who dies within 24 hours of admission at the receiving facility.

Risk management should also monitor the emergency department records of patients who refuse hospitalization or treatment, patients who leave against medical advice, and family or patients who disappear from the waiting area. Patients should be seen within a reasonable waiting time to reduce complaints from the waiting area, so the time of arrival and time of treatment should be recorded. Useful information may also be gathered on patients who repeatedly use the emergency department for the same or similar diagnoses within a 7-day period.

OBSTETRICS AND NEONATOLOGY

Reviews of malpractice claims demonstrate that lawsuits related to obstetric and neonatal cases are frequently the most expensive in terms of claims settled and malpractice awards paid. With each birth it is hoped, and often expected, that the prenatal process, labor, and delivery will be uncomplicated and successful—the experience of a lifetime. Similar expectations hold true for the early hours and days of an infant's life. In large part because of these expectations and because of the belief that giving birth is typically a planned event, the physical and emotional impact can be severe when a maternal or neonatal complication or injury occurs. Clearly, this feeling is carried over into courtroom decisions that favor the plaintiff.

OBSTETRICS AND NEONATOLOGY LIABILITY RISKS

Multiple studies of obstetric claims have been performed. A study by the American College of Obstetricians and Gynecologists (ACOG) addressed the impact of professional-liability actions and costs on the practice of obstetrics and gynecology between 1990 and 1992, and again in 1999.[23] Of the physicians surveyed, approximately 79% had experienced at least one malpractice claim. This statistic represented an increase of more than 8% from information derived during the 1987 version of the same survey. Twenty-five percent of the physicians had been sued four or more times, an increase of more than 11% from the 1987 survey. More than 50% of the claims were carried through court or settlement. Of the claims not dropped or settled without payment, approximately 75% were settled with payment. In approximately 22% of the cases that went to court, the verdict favored the plaintiff. In terms of number of claims reported, the two most significant primary allegations for obstetric claims were neurological impairment to the infant and stillbirth or neonatal death. Additional allegations included maternal injuries, other infant injuries, failure to diagnose a problem, and maternal death. Labor/delivery and the nursery made up about 5.3% of all claims (9.6% of all losses in 2001), according to recent St. Paul Fire and Marine Insurance Company data. The average loss was a whopping $798,304.[1]

Primary allegations include for cesarean sections (C-sections): infant neuromuscular development problems, maternal hemorrhage, and maternal or infant death; for vaginal deliveries: infant neuromuscular development problems, Erb's palsy, retained vaginal sponge, intrauterine and ectopic pregnancies, and circumcision-related problems. Additional related allegations included delay in treatment of fetal distress and failure to obtain consent.[24]

While advanced medical technology has enabled physicians to save infants who may not otherwise have survived, it has simultaneously provided a larger base of complications on which lawsuits can be made. A recent study found that "infants weighing less than three

pounds are less likely to die or suffer serious problems if they are born in hospitals with neonatal intensive care units or transferred to such centers immediately after birth";[25] however, those infants who are "saved" are often medically compromised, increasing the likelihood of litigation in response to unsatisfactory results and poor long-term prognosis. School-age outcomes in children with birth weights under 750 grams were found to be at high risk for neurobehavioral dysfunction and poor school performance.[26]

Additional factors complicate litigation surrounding obstetrics. A *New York Times* investigative reporter discovered that a 1992 New York City report that was never published listed 64 lawsuits that were the direct result of brain damage to infants resulting from hospital negligence. Many of the worst cases involved obstetric residents in training who had little or no supervision from senior physicians.[27] A study of obstetric malpractice claims in Georgia found that 27% of the claims were indefensible because of breaches in the standard of care, problems with documentation, or a combination of both.[24]

Multiple surveys and studies of Florida obstetricians have examined the relationship between the mother's inclination to sue and the prior malpractice experience of the attending physician. A study of claims between 1977 and 1989 by mothers of infants who had incurred permanent injuries or had died identified numerous reasons for filing a malpractice claim: advice from knowledgeable acquaintances to file, recognition of a cover-up regarding the care of their infant, financial necessity, recognition that their child would have no future, lack of information as to why their child was injured or died, a desire to seek revenge, or desire to protect others from similar harm. This same study found two types of communication problems identified by the mothers: (1) their belief that some physicians had misled them, and (2) a failure on the part of the physician to provide sufficient information;[28] however, a second study found no relationship between prior malpractice claim experience and differences in objective or subjective measures of the quality of clinical care provided.[29]

An investigation of mothers who had not filed a malpractice claim but who had experienced viable infants, stillborn infants, or infant deaths found that "a consistent pattern of differences emerged when comparing women's perceptions of care received. Patients seeing physicians with the most frequent numbers of claims, but without high payments, were significantly more likely to complain that they felt abused, never received explanations for tests, or were ignored."[30]

These studies demonstrate the myriad factors that complicate the delivery process and increase a mother's inclination to sue. There are clinical issues, societal issues, communication problems, and administrative support issues that all may contribute in some manner to initiation of a lawsuit. While skilled caregivers are the most effective agents in managing the risk in obstetrics and neonatology, the physician–patient relationship is prominent. Informed consent and medical-record documentation must be actively monitored and maintained if litigation is to be successfully defended.

ETHICAL DILEMMAS

There are significant ethical and legal issues to be considered in the delivery and management of high-risk infants. Right to life, quality of life, wrongful life or birth, and right to die are issues that are personal to the parents of the infant and are also of concern to the medical profession. Do the parents have the right to know the status of their fetus, if compromised, and the possible resulting medical conditions in the newborn or as the child matures? To what degree and vigor should physicians prolong the life, with heroic treatments, of hopelessly ill newborns?

Members of the family should be involved in any ethical decision process. Risk managers agree that parents should be provided with all the available information regarding the condition of their fetus and the potential for development. All involved caregivers should be consulted and an attempt made to achieve consensus on the ultimate decision, if possible.

After an initial decision on care is reached, the matter may be revisited in the event of changes in the mother's or fetus/infant's condition or in response to the expressed desires of the family members. The American Academy of Pediatrics recommends ongoing evaluation of the infant's prognosis, with treatment decisions based strictly on what will benefit the newborn. Many facilities established ethics committees to assist in resolving conflicts in neonatal intensive care units.[31] All ethical discussions and decisions regarding care of the fetus or infant should be documented in the medical record.

STANDARDS AND GUIDELINES

Many professional organizations have developed clinical-practice guidelines in obstetrics and neonatology: American Academy of Family Physicians (AAFP), American Academy of Pediatrics (AAP), American Institute of Ultrasound and Medicine (AIUM), American College of Nurse-Midwives, American College of Obstetricians and Gynecologists (ACOG), American College of Radiology (ACR), American Pediatric Society (APS), Association of Women's Health, Obstetrics, and Neonatal Nurses, and National Association of Neonatal Nurses (NANN).

Hospital and department policies and procedures, revised annually and distributed widely, are essential in guiding healthcare providers in the management of obstetric and neonatal patients. Significant risk management problems can arise if practitioners are not fully aware of, and in agreement with, these policies and procedures.

Levels of Care: Institutional Capabilities

Obstetric- and neonatal-care services are provided in a wide range of hospital settings with varying capabilities throughout the United States. Both AAP and ACOG have established staffing, equipment, and support-service criteria that describe the classifications of the levels of care.[32]

Level-I facilities provide services that are the least intensive and designed to treat low-risk mothers and their infants. Even so, a level-I facility is required to provide the following:

- A protocol to identify and transfer high-risk patients to a higher-level facility
- The ability to perform a cesarean delivery within 30 minutes of determining the necessity
- The availability of blood and fresh frozen plasma
- Twenty-four-hour availability of anesthesia, radiology, ultrasound, electronic fetal heart rate (FHR) monitoring, and laboratory services
- Infant and maternal resuscitation capabilities at all deliveries
- The availability of blood typing, cross-matching, and Coombs' testing
- A qualified physician or nurse-midwife present at all deliveries

In addition to meeting level-I criteria, level-II facilities must be able to manage high-risk mothers, high-risk fetuses, and small, sick neonates. A decision to transfer a high-risk or critically ill neonate to a level-III facility rests with the referring physician, in consultation with the level-III neonatologist. Level-II-facility staff must be able to monitor and maintain critical functions, including cardiopulmonary, metabolic, and thermal status. Staffing requirements include: a board-certified obstetrician as chief of newborn services; a board-certified anesthesiologist supervising obstetric anesthesiology; 24-hour availability of a radiologist and clinical pathologist; support staff, including a medical social worker, a physical therapist, a dietitian or nutritionist, and a respiratory therapist; and nursing staff capable of identifying and responding to obstetric complications.

A level-III facility delivers more complex care. In addition to meeting all level-I and level-II criteria, level-III facilities must provide professional staffing with experience in neonatal medicine, maternal–fetal medicine, obstetric and neonatal diagnostic imaging, advanced nursing specialties, and pediatric subspecialties. In addition, the nurse-to-patient ratio of staff is more intensive than is required in level-I or level-II facilities.

Risk managers should periodically survey their facility to document the level classification and to determine compliance of the obstetric service to the staffing, equipment, and support-service requirements established by AAP and ACOG.

Except in emergency situations, and depending on the availability of healthcare providers, the family's wishes, and the condition of the mother and fetus, the prenatal care and delivery of the infant may be performed by an obstetrician, family practitioner, resident, or nurse-midwife. A report in the *New York Times* stated that nurse-midwives, who are responsible for delivering and caring for the babies of many of the lower-income women at New York City's public hospitals, "routinely exceed the limits of state law to handle high risk delivery cases . . . and that these cases are virtually impossible to defend."[33] Credentialing and privileging of these healthcare providers should be specific to the clinical tasks that they will be required to perform.

In some clinical situations, the family practitioner and nurse-midwife are required to consult with, or refer the case to, an obstetrician. Hospitals should have policies and procedures for required consultations and referrals, as well as for precipitous deliveries. Emergency departments should have delivery packs on hand and have staff available who are trained in emergency-delivery procedures and infant care.

PRENATAL AND PERINATAL CARE

Most physicians agree that prenatal care is paramount to ensuring the health and

> **Box 23–4**
>
> A baby was born with profound disabilities. Parents of the newborn alleged negligence in not being adequately informed of the results of a prenatal blood test. Their successful lawsuit claimed damages due to "wrongful birth" and "wrongful life."[34]

well-being of the newborn. Unfortunately, not all expectant mothers avail themselves of prenatal care, perhaps because of societal pressures, perceived lack of access, lack of money, or lack of knowledge. Regardless of the reason for foregoing prenatal care, it is imperative that physicians and hospital support staff document whatever steps are taken to ensure adequate prenatal care and record the actual extent of care received by the mother. During the prenatal period a multitude of clinical problems can develop, such as hypertension and diabetes, which may have a future negative impact on the mother and unborn child. Physician counseling of the patient should include a discussion of the level of accuracy of diagnostic procedures and the variability of test-result interpretations. Mothers should be informed as to realistic expectations regarding morbidity, mortality, tests, and procedure limitations (see Box 23–4).

An important step in determining the appropriate course of care for the expectant mother is an assessment of the gestational age of the fetus. Once pregnancy has been confirmed, the clinician should determine the appropriate plan for patient management on the basis of a thorough risk assessment, patient and family history, physical examination, environmental history, and findings that result from specialized diagnostic procedures and laboratory tests. One insurance study found that the cost of a claim rose 300% when these standards are not followed.[1]

Genetic Counseling and Testing

Genetic testing is available to determine the potential and/or occurrence of genetic prob-

lems during the perinatal period. The most commonly used tests are chorionic villus sampling, percutaneous umbilical blood sampling, and maternal serum alphafetoprotein testing.

Genetic testing is recommended where familial history or previous obstetric history provides an indication of the potential for a problem. In the general population, the risk of delivering an infant with a serious genetic birth defect has been found to be between 3% and 5%.

Each genetic test carries identified maternal and fetal risks. Prior to genetic testing, ultrasound studies should be performed to locate the placenta, confirm gestational age, determine fetal viability, and identify multiple fetuses if present. Maternal risks for select genetic tests include spontaneous abortion, abruptio placentae, penetration of the fetal vessels resulting in maternal hemorrhage or death, transient vaginal bleeding, and amniotic-fluid leakage. Fetal risks include fetal demise, limb and oromandibular defects, intrauterine growth retardation, premature birth, and Rh isoimmunization.

Genetically at-risk mothers and their families should be given information and advice about the possible consequences of inherited disorders that may or may not be detectable and the various options that are available for diagnosis, management, and prevention. A full and complete informed consent should be obtained from the mother prior to genetic testing acknowledging an understanding of the specific risks of the tests to both herself and the fetus. Infants born with unanticipated congenital abnormalities where there is no documented evidence of genetic counseling and/or testing continue to be a liability risk (see Box 23–5).

> **Box 23–5**
>
> Failure to diagnose a genetic disorder was the allegation in a Florida malpractice case that allowed recovery for all extraordinary expenses incurred during the child's life expectancy.[36]

Several hospital facilities, insurance companies, and health-maintenance organizations have developed perinatal case-management programs to decrease the number of preterm births.[35] Screening programs are utilized to identify at-risk patients. A perinatal case manager coordinates medical, social, and reimbursement resources, and enhances patient education and communication to facilitate an optimal outcome and to improve the quality of care received.

Antepartum Fetal Surveillance

The ability to monitor the clinical status of both the mother and fetus is an important step in preparing for a safe delivery and ensuring the well-being of the mother and unborn infant. Underlying medical disorders may contribute to a high-risk pregnancy. A host of clinical risks and complications can occur during the perinatal period. Adequate assessment of the mother and fetus requires that clinicians recognize which parameters require monitoring, the most effective techniques, and how to interpret normal, abnormal, and interference data. Appropriate equipment must be available and operating properly, and staff must be fully trained. Mothers should be informed of the importance and risks of monitoring and should provide their consent.

Physicians who conduct examinations and interpret tests utilizing sophisticated biomedical equipment should be specifically evaluated for those clinical privileges. Monitoring of the clinical parameters during the antepartum and perinatal periods offers clinicians the opportunity to recognize problems early and institute early intervention.

Establishment of the expected date of delivery (EDD) is of major importance in being able to determine the gestational age of the fetus, to evaluate fetal growth and maturity, and to plan for delivery. Additionally, medical care of ongoing medical problems or problems new to the pregnancy must be assessed through a review of the history, physical examination, and testing so that the impact on the pregnancy and the fetus is minimized.

Fetal surveillance through antepartum testing indicates the degree of fetal well-being. Results of FHR monitoring, nonstress testing, and visualization of the intrauterine contents through ultrasound/sonography studies provide the information needed for a "biophysical profile." A quantitative score to evaluate fetal oxygenation and the potential for fetal hypoxia is derived from the following five parameters with a possible total score of 10: (1) fetal breathing movement; (2) fetal body movement; (3) fetal tone, demonstrated by extension and reflexion of fetal limbs; (4) fetal heart rate, measured by a nonreactive stress test; and (5) quantitative amniotic-fluid volume. A cumulative score of 8–10 is interpreted as a normal infant at low risk for asphyxia. A score of 4 or less strongly suggests asphyxia. If asphyxia persists beyond 2 hours and is unexplained by other factors, immediate delivery is indicated.[37]

Ultrasound/sonography is a relatively noninvasive diagnostic procedure and one of the most widely used imaging and monitoring techniques during pregnancy. Ultrasound is performed by obstetricians, perinatologists, and radiologists, as well as by some family practitioners, to assist in determining the gestational age of the fetus at about the 18th week, to identify fetal anomalies, to view fetal activity, to aid in amniocentesis, and to evaluate fetal growth in high-risk or suspicious situations.

Standards for the use of ultrasound were developed by the American Institute of Ultrasound and Medicine, the American Academy of Pediatrics, and the American College of Radiology, but there is no mandatory training or certification for physicians who perform sonography. Past studies on the quality of ultrasound films revealed failure rates of 65%. Films evaluated were considered to be of poor or inadequate image quality and technique,[38] and such inadequate documentation poses risks if the films are needed for a defense.

The nonstress test is based on the assumption that the FHR will temporarily accelerate with fetal movement and be a good indicator of fetal autonomic function. Fetal heart rate is monitored externally, and the tracing is evaluated for accelerations. Occasionally, heart-rate accelerations may be induced by the use of a vibro-acoustic stimulator to waken the healthy but sleeping fetus. Actual strips and documentation of the professional interpretation are important parts of the medical record. Some loss of reactivity has been reported to be associated with central nervous system depression, ingestion of alcohol, and fetal acidosis.[39] There are no published contraindications for a nonstress test. By the use of low doses of intravenous oxytocin or nipple stimulation, the contraction stress test monitors the FHR response to induced uterine contractions. This test is rarely used at present but may appear in older medical records. Risks of this test, while rare, include preterm labor, induced fetal hypoxia, and perinatal death.

Blood-flow studies have been used to evaluate intrauterine fetal growth, low birth weight, placental insufficiency, and severe pregnancy-induced hypertension. In addition, blood-flow studies have been used to monitor Rh isoimmunization, fetal cardiac arrhythmias, and diabetes mellitus. When combined with Doppler techniques, ultrasound can measure the blood-flow patterns through the vessels of the umbilical cord or the maternal artery. The ACOG noted that there is insufficient evidence to support the use of Doppler velocimetry in reducing the risk of antepartum fetal demise or in improving neonatal outcomes.[37]

Uterine activity can be monitored in the home with a small, pressure-sensitive electronic device that is placed on the woman's abdomen. Movements associated with uterine contractions are converted into electronic signals for transmission over a telephone line to a computer for printout and evaluation. When the device was introduced to the marketplace, it was believed that it would aid clinicians in the early detection of preterm labor and thereby improve outcomes. In 1993, the Preventive Services Task Force of the U.S. Public Health Service found insufficient evidence of clinical effectiveness to recommend for or against home monitoring of uterine activity.[40,41] A recent study of 1,300 women also found that the monitor did not specifically aid in the identification of mothers at risk for preterm labor, nor did it improve pregnancy outcomes in terms of factors such as birth weight, gestational age at delivery, or infant complications.[42] Nurses, with or without the information from the uterine activity monitor, were equally as effective in managing preterm labor patients.

For all these surveillance techniques the documentation in the medical record becomes a major defensive tool when a breach of standard practice is alleged. Consent forms need to be present that document the what, when, and who of testing, the results of evaluation, and monitoring outputs. Of particular importance is the medical care responsiveness to tests and clinical evaluations indicating fetal distress and abnormalities and the interventions taken, if possible, to minimize poor outcomes of the pregnancy.

INTRAPARTUM PERIOD

Critical adverse events can occur in the intrapartum period, and the well-being of the mother or the newborn cannot be taken for granted. According to ACOG and AAP, 20% of perinatal morbidity and mortality occurs during the intrapartum period with mothers who have had no previous complications during their pregnancy.[43] In obstetric claims, ACOG reports that the most significant perinatal injury is acidosis leading to asphyxia at birth, or to death.[44] Usually, the allegation is that the fetus suffered hypoxia or anoxia for a period of time during the labor and delivery process sufficient to cause clinical injury to the brain, kidney, heart, or lung. Systemic symptoms may appear shortly after birth.

Labor can occur early in the pregnancy (preterm), amniotic membranes can rupture prematurely, the fetus may present in a difficult delivery position, or labor may not progress adequately or at all. Fetal heart rate monitoring and fetal blood sampling help determine the appropriate clinical approach.

Preterm Labor

Some mothers experience labor prior to 37 weeks of gestation, when the fetus has not had the opportunity to develop fully. In such cases, physicians must decide on the appropriate clinical course of treatment: either suppression of labor, or preterm delivery if it is neither desirable nor possible to suppress labor.

Risk management considerations include policies and procedures that require the physician to be present in the hospital during the administration of tocolytic (suppression) drugs, continuous monitoring of the mother and fetus, notification of the pediatrician or neonatologist of a potential preterm delivery, and the availability of resuscitation equipment.

Fetal Heart Rate Monitoring

Physicians evaluate the FHR to identify changes that may be associated with problems related to fetal oxygenation and placental perfusion, such as hypoxia, umbilical-cord compression, tachycardia, and acidosis. "The ability to interpret FHR patterns and understand their correlation with the fetus' condition allows the physician to institute management techniques including maternal oxygenation, amnioinfusion, and tocolytic therapy."[45]

Fetal heart rate can be evaluated effectively either by auscultation or by internal or external electronic monitoring. The ACOG has not been able to determine the most effective method of FHR monitoring, nor the specific frequency or duration of monitoring to ensure an optimal outcome; however, ACOG has established guidelines for monitoring, interpretation, and patient management, depending on various FHR patterns.

If patient-management interventions are not successful in improving fetal oxygenation and placental perfusion, ACOG recommends delivering the fetus by the most expeditious route, whether abdominal or vaginal. Multiple researchers and clinical practitioners have found that continuous FHR monitoring is associated with an increased rate of cesarean deliveries but a decrease in the incidence of intrapartum stillbirth.[42] Electronic FHR monitoring is presently used in 50–70 % of all U.S. births.[46]

Fetal Blood Sampling

The sampling of capillary blood from the fetal scalp and the evaluation of the fetal response to scalp stimulation have been found useful in intrapartum fetal monitoring for fetal hypoxia and abnormally high blood acidity.

Induction and Augmentation of Labor

The ACOG has established guidelines for the induction of labor prior to spontaneous onset and for augmentation of labor to improve the quality of contractions.[47] Prior to induction or augmentation of labor, it is important to determine fetal maturity and assess gestational age and the status of the cervix. The ACOG guidelines require that a physician who has C-section privileges be readily available and that trained personnel be in attendance to monitor the FHR and uterine contractions during the administration of the induction drug (oxytocin).

Surgical induction, such as rupturing or stripping the membranes, increases the risk of infection, bleeding, fetal dislodgement, and interference with cord presentation. Medical augmentation with intravenous drugs requires careful administration with an infusion pump or controller that permits precise flow-rate control. Hospital policies should address immediate availability of the delivering physician from the outset of induction or augmentation; protocols for use in fetal distress, uterine hyperstimulation, and infusion rates; and required documentation.

THE DELIVERY

Injuries or problems that develop during the perinatal period may be present at birth in addition to specific birth-related injuries or problems (see Box 23–6). Clinical injuries identified in malpractice claims as a result of vaginal delivery include newborn cardiopulmonary problems, neuromuscular developmental problems, shoulder dystocia, infant death, and Erb's palsy. Infants delivered by C-section may experience the same complications that are reported in vaginal deliveries. Additional maternal complications claimed include poor maternal outcomes, such as hemorrhage, perforation or laceration of tissue, coma, paralysis, and death.

Pain Management and Obstetric Anesthesia

Despite the current fad for natural childbirth, most women accept the concept of "natural childbirth without pain" and agree to epidural anesthesia during labor and delivery; however, there are deliveries in which the administration of other types of anesthesia becomes medically necessary. Anesthetic and analgesic agents act not only on the mother, but may affect the respiratory and cardiovascular status of the fetus as well.

Box 23–6

A series of articles in the New York Times on excessive maternal and neonatal morbidity and mortality among patients treated in municipal hospitals prompted the New York State health commissioner to order a review of all municipal obstetric wards and, if necessary, close them.[48]

Anesthesia and analgesics may be administered for pain management during either a vaginal delivery or a C-section. Options include intravenous analgesia and regional anesthesia, primarily epidural, for labor and vaginal delivery, and general anesthesia or spinal anesthesia for a C-section.

A study using the American Society of Anesthesiologists' Closed Claim Database reviewed malpractice claims filed against anesthesiologists in obstetric cases. The most common complications were, in order of severity: maternal death, newborn brain damage, and maternal headache. Minor complications included backache, pain during anesthesia, and emotional injury. Claims involving general anesthesia were frequently associated with severe injuries and resulted in higher payments than did claims involving regional anesthesia.[49]

The prime focus of anesthesia personnel is to cater to the mother and provide pain relief. Under extreme circumstances, they assist the neonatologist or pediatrician if their help is required or if the baby is compromised and other physicians are not available. Certain families and cultures prefer concentrated efforts on the newborn baby, especially male infants; however, in the United States there are professional and ethical questions regarding the primacy of either the mother or the fetus.

Obstetric anesthesia services should be supervised by an anesthetist with special training in obstetric anesthesia. Any hospital that provides obstetric services, at a minimum, should have a qualified physician or certified registered nurse anesthesiologist (CRNA) readily available, preferably within 15–30 minutes, in an emergency; however, it is generally recommended that 24-hour in-house anesthesia coverage be available. Qualifications include the ability of the professional to manage life-threatening respiratory and cardiovascular failure, toxemia, convulsions, and aspirations.

Pre- and postanesthesia evaluations that include both maternal and fetal status should be performed by anesthesia personnel. Decisions to use a particular type of pain relief and route of administration should be discussed with the mother by the professional intending to administer the anesthesia. That discussion should include the advantages, disadvantages, and risk implications to both the mother and fetus. Documentation of the discussion and the mother's consent to anesthesia should be reflected in the medical record.

Vaginal Delivery

Vaginal delivery is the most common route for births. Adequate staffing to care for both the newborn and the mother is required. It is preferred that a pediatrician be available for all deliveries and imperative that a pediatrician or neonatologist be present at all high-risk deliveries. C-section, infant resuscitation, and anesthesia services should also be available.

In some deliveries, labor will have to be interrupted and a C-section performed. Breech presentations are often delivered through C-section, although it has been shown that vaginal delivery may be attempted if certain obstetric criteria are met.[50]

Delivering babies underwater in so-called water births is now being offered as an option in about 200 hospitals in the United States. Proponents feel that the warm-water bathtub is more comfortable for the mother and less traumatic for the baby because it simulates the uterine environment. At the Oregon Health and Science University program, the neonatologist warns that the immersed baby should be removed from the water quickly to avoid near-drowning or death. Caution is advised in developing such new programs because of the high risk.[51]

Dystocia

A difficult birth caused by fetal or maternal abnormalities is known as dystocia. The most common causes of dystocia are cephalopelvic disproportion (the inability of the fetal head to pass through the maternal pelvis) and malpresentation (arrival of the fetus at the opening of the uterus in a position other than the normal head-first position). Each of these complications may indicate the need for a C-section delivery, use of tocolytic agents to relax the uterus, or fetal manipulation. If a vaginal delivery is to be attempted, it is recommended that a second physician be present to assist, anesthesia be readily available, and provision for emergency C-section be made.

Forceps and Vacuum Extraction

Obstetric forceps and vacuum extractors are designed to assist in removing the fetus from the birth canal at delivery when maternal contractions are insufficient. There is significant controversy in the medical literature regarding the use of these techniques. Maternal injuries associated with these adjunctive procedures include mild abrasions to severe lacerations of the vagina, cervix, and uterus. Fetal injuries include bruising; serious scalp, cranial, or brain injury; neurological damage; and eye injury. Litigation claims in neurologically impaired infants point to these techniques as the *prima facie* cause of permanent impairment, despite contrary research findings.

Cesarean Section

C-sections are performed in response to a variety of maternal and fetal indications, including previous cesarean delivery, dystocia, breech presentation, and fetal distress. Medical and legal literature suggests that the rate of C-sections performed is, in large part, dependent on a physician's concerns about malpractice litigation. Although the C-section includes inherent surgical risks, when elective it is a more rapid method of delivery. Studies indicate that the C-section rate has increased since 1997, reversing a former steady decline. A goal of having only 17% of births delivered via C-section has not been met, and the national average has risen to 22%.[51]

If the physician has decided to proceed with a C-section, it is generally recommended that the gestation be at term and that the mother be in active labor. An anesthesia consult should be obtained, blood should be typed and screened, fetal heart tones should be monitored immediately prior to preparation of the abdomen for surgery, infant resuscitation personnel should be in attendance, and a vaginal examination should be performed.[52]

Vaginal Birth After Cesarean

Many pregnant women and their physicians opt for a trial of labor and a vaginal delivery even after they have had as many as two C-section deliveries. With a vaginal birth after cesarean (VBAC), the medical profession recognizes that the need for anesthesia may decrease, some surgical risk is eliminated, and hospital stays are shorter. Documented risks include those associated with any vaginal delivery, as well as uterine rupture.[53] The ACOG has issued a press release regarding the potential risks of VBACs[54] and has developed guidelines for VBACs.[55] It is important that the physician carefully identify appropriate candidates on the basis of limiting maternal or fetal clinical criteria. Past obstetric complications and certain social and geographic issues may justify the patient's electing to have a repeat C-section. Should the patient elect to try a VBAC, however, personnel and facilities for an emergency C-section should be readily available.

INFANT RESUSCITATION AND MANAGEMENT

On occasion, newborns require resuscitation immediately following birth. These compromised infants may be apneic or gasping at delivery. In collaboration with the American Heart Association and the American Academy of Pediatrics, the National Resuscitation Program was implemented to create infant resuscitation guidelines and to provide certification for health professionals. Guidelines recommend that at least one person skilled in resuscitating infants be present at every delivery. It is imperative that prior to the delivery the team be aware of who is designated to be responsible for infant intubation and resuscitation.[56]

Documentation of resuscitation efforts, meconium status, Apgar scores, umbilical-cord blood-test results, and the placental examination are important risk management issues in cases of compromised neonates, which could lead to litigation.

Meconium Management

Heavy or thick meconium (the first stools of a newborn) can indicate past, recent, or ongoing fetal risk or distress. Meconium should be described in the medical record by color, amount, consistency, and amount of staining of the neonate or placenta. If meconium is observed in the amniotic fluid, a staff member trained in neonatal resuscitation should be present at the delivery.

Management of the newborn is aimed at preventing aspiration of the meconium and should include immediate suctioning, direct visualization of the trachea, and if necessary, suctioning using an endotracheal tube and meconium aspirator. During this procedure, the infant's heart rate should be monitored. If the heart rate falls, ventilation with 100% oxygen is recommended.[56]

Apgar Scoring

Apgar scoring is probably the most commonly used newborn-assessment tool. Derived from an assessment of select clinical parameters, the score assists the clinician in determining the degree of infant resuscitation required as well as the effectiveness, over time, of the resuscitation efforts. Many clinicians associate a low Apgar score with subsequent identification of neurological disorder, although AAP and ACOG have recommended against using the Apgar score alone as "evidence of or consequent to substantial asphyxia."[57] Additional factors that should be considered include central nervous system immaturity, maternal sedation, and congenital malformations.

Umbilical-Cord Blood Acid–Base Assessment

Both ACOG and AAP believe that umbilical-cord blood acid–base assessment is a more objective measure of the acid–base status of a newborn than is the Apgar score.[58] If there is a question of intrapartum asphyxia or a low Apgar score, the literature recommends performing cord blood sampling. In the depressed newborn, the assessment can exclude intrapartum hypoxia as the cause of the depression. Because the sample may be delayed for up to 60 minutes before testing, the 5-minute Apgar score should be determined prior to testing.

Placental Examination

An examination of the placenta can sometimes demonstrate whether an injury to the fetus, fetal maldevelopment, or birth trauma is responsible for asphyxia. It has been suggested that a placental examination "may reveal the cause of preterm labor, premature membrane rupture, fetal undergrowth, or antenatal hypoxia."[59] Several groups have examined the value of the placental examination. When based on specific clinical indicators and guidelines, this examination can prove beneficial as a risk management tool in the handling of claims related to fetal injury.[60]

Indications for pathological placental examinations are based on several maternal, fetal, and placental conditions.[61] Maternal conditions include severe preeclampsia, Rh isoimmunization, substance abuse, and insulin-dependent diabetes. Fetal conditions include fetal distress, meconium staining,

suspected sepsis, and seizures. Placental conditions include abruption, masses, and abnormal appearance of the placenta or cord. Physicians can protect themselves from being sued over neurologically impaired newborns by saving the placenta when they suspect something is wrong.[62]

If clinical conditions indicate that a placenta examination may help provide answers to clinical complications, the physician should examine the placenta, document any abnormalities, and forward the placenta to the pathology department for further examination. Placental specimens should be retained for subsequent examination by a placental specialist for possible trial testimony. "The placenta may well be the key to a solid defense for these cases in the courtroom."[63]

MATERNAL EXAMINATION AFTER DELIVERY

From a risk management perspective, it is important that following the delivery the uterus be checked for retained vaginal sponges and retained placental fragments. Some obstetricians choose not to explore the uterus following birth, for fear of causing pain or introducing infection, and may use ultrasound for the examination. A jury may find it difficult to understand why a physical examination was not performed.

With the trend toward shortened hospital stays following a normal delivery, mothers should be advised to call immediately if they experience excessive bleeding or discomfort when at home prior to their scheduled follow-up office visit.

FAMILY ATTENDANCE AND VIDEOTAPING OF BIRTH

Attendance of the father, significant others, and siblings has become so commonplace at births that many clinicians do not associate the act as potentially damaging in the event of a malpractice lawsuit. A videotape of the birth may prove to be even more harmful during court proceedings. Most hospitals have a policy that provides guidance for the physician or nurse to ask visitors attending the birth to leave the delivery room or to stop videotaping. This request may be viewed by the visitors as a sign that something has gone wrong or that the medical team is trying to cover up their actions. In one case, the father's videotape was used to support his contention that errors were made during the delivery.[64] But a jury may view a normal-delivery videotape and misinterpret what they see. If hospital staff is not simultaneously videotaping the medical team's actions during the delivery, the father's version of actions taped may be all that is presented in court. Lifesaving actions crucial to the case may not be captured on tape.

Standard practice seems to dictate that it would be impossible to bar visitors and videotaping during deliveries. Hospital policies and guidelines should be available to assist clinicians in directing visitors to turn off the camera and leave the delivery room when requested. Staff should be reminded that a videotape is a permanent record of what they say and do during the birth and that requests to cease filming without direction to leave may lead to covert filming of subsequent actions. If the staff is interviewed on camera after the event, they must understand that the words they say may be subject to misinterpretation and used against them in a court of law.

Some hospitals and physicians have considered videotaping deliveries as a permanent part of the medical record. This policy could be very expensive and may not be in the best interests of the hospital in the event of an error or deviation from standard practice by the medical team. Other facilities choose to tape selected parts of the delivery or take still photographs of the pathology. Whatever the decision, in the event that visitors and videotaping are permitted, information such as visitors' names and the fact that videotaping occurred should be entered into the medical record. If a visitor is asked to leave the room and/or stop videotaping, this request should also be entered into the medical record.

MEDICAL-RECORD DOCUMENTATION

Since legal action may be initiated as long as 21 years following the delivery in the case of an injured newborn, it is important that medical-record documentation be accurate, objective, and complete, and provide the rationale to support all patient-management decisions, including the decision not to intervene. A medical record should be created for all patients who present for care. Documentation should include the consent prior to all testing, the results of prenatal examinations and tests, and instructions given over the prenatal course. Testing or treatment refused by the mother, missed appointments, and attempts to contact the mother should also be recorded.

Physicians and risk managers alike have found that to ensure the best continuum of care, "copies of the initial history, physical findings, and laboratory data should be received by the hospital from the delivering physician or midwife soon after the first prenatal visit. At 36 weeks gestation, the patient's prenatal-care record at the hospital should be updated and the patient counseled by her physician or a designee with regard to labor instructions and warnings."[39] If there was no prenatal care and there are indications of complications or a possibly difficult pregnancy, case management and risk management personnel should be notified to monitor the outcome of the mother and infant, as well as to facilitate subsequent follow-up. It is important that all events during the labor process and delivery be recorded, even if the mother has signs of early labor and is sent home to await more active labor. This record should include the physician's orders and discharge instructions given to the patient.

Fetal heart monitor tracings are considered a part of the medical record and should be filed in a manner that allows them to be retrieved easily up to 21 years after the birth. Tracings and tracing segments should be marked so that the record clearly reflects the event sequence, physician's interpretations, and assessments. Documentation during the delivery should include the condition of the mother, fetal station, and fetal status. Detailed notes in the medical record should include the indications and rationale for the delivery method selected. All maneuvers used in vaginal delivery, including those related to breech presentation or dystocia, should be listed. A narrative labor and delivery summary note should be recorded for each delivery, especially if there are clinically significant FHR patterns, low Apgar scores, low cord pH values, dystocia, preterm deliveries, fetal demise, or a newborn with significant morbidity. All adverse events or poor outcomes should be reflected through documentation of relevant clinical facts; however, it is vitally important that the caregivers not speculate in the medical record regarding a poor outcome.

Postpartum documentation should include the postdelivery examination, and clinical indicators such as wound checks, bleeding, vital signs, and pain medications. With the shorter hospital stays for normal deliveries, there is less time for nursing interaction with the mother. Mothers at risk for infant care and self-care problems following discharge should be identified and referred to case management. Many facilities have introduced interactive video programs to facilitate the patient education and discharge process; however, an interactive video does not take the place of patient–nurse or patient–physician interaction. All discharge instructions, as well as planned follow-up for mothers with complications, should be documented in the medical record.

NEONATAL SERVICES

Following birth, infants are admitted to a nursery. The level of nursery service depends on the condition of the infant, the desires of the pediatrician or neonatologist, the availability of beds (for example, radiant warmers, incubators, bassinets), and staffing. In addition to the level I, II, and III nurseries, many hospitals divide their nurseries into well-baby and sick-baby nurseries. Neonatal intensive care units (NICUs) are reserved for infants who are medically compromised and in need of complex medical technology and specially trained medical professionals. While providing benefits to the infants, these technologies also pose significant risk due, in part, to the compromised condition of the infant, the invasive nature of some therapies, and the sometimes inherent risks of the medical devices.

For routine births, neonatal services pose few liability risks. With premature births, however, the expectation of malpractice claims is heightened. Infants with a low birth weight are biologically compromised and require time to mature and grow. Advances in science and technology have increased the ability of pediatricians and neonatologists to support tiny infants successfully for months with intensive care. During this time, diagnostic evaluation of the biological status of the infant is documented; congenital malformations are detected; corrective or emergency pediatric surgery may be performed; and general support of respiration, nutrition, fluid balance, and physiological functions is provided and monitored.

"Premature or otherwise compromised infants require a significant amount of clinical support during the first few weeks after birth."[64] Continuous observation in a therapeutic milieu with highly trained clinicians and nurses, high-tech equipment, and immediate attention to detectable alterations in status and adverse situations reduce the potential for liability in these units (see Box 23–7).

Risk management with these babies involves early detection and speedy intervention in identifying conditions. Transient hypoxic events and intraventricular hemorrhages, pneumonitis, sepsis, ABO blood

---

Box 23–7

Because her insurance company would not pay for a longer stay in the New Jersey Shore Medical Center (Neptune), Diane Weber and her newborn son left the hospital 36 hours after his birth. Her son became dehydrated, developed high bilirubin, and ended up in the neonatal ICU. A physician at the hospital said a longer stay would likely have meant that the conditions would have been spotted and treated before they became serious.[65]

Box 23–8

In a newspaper "debate over care of pre-emies," a mother said it had never occurred to her and her husband to limit treatment to their premature son, who weighed 2.5 pounds at birth. She said that miracles happen in NICUs regularly.[67]

---

incompatibility, and excess bilirubin may not be avoidable, but these conditions should be evaluated with a subsequent appropriate response. Individualized case management and an interdisciplinary team approach are essential to improving medical neurodevelopmental outcome while reducing overall hospital charges.[66]

Detailed documentation of the continuing care in regular nurseries and intensive care units is extremely important for defense in lawsuits. Daily status and changes, diagnoses, test results, consents from the parents, indicated medications and treatments, and periodic updated care plans are necessary parts of the infant's medical record.

Policies and procedures concerning the care of anencephalic infants and infants with multiple malformations, the use of universal precautions, the isolation of infected babies, routine screening tests, the involvement of parents in caring for the baby, and decision making are crucial.

Appropriate maintenance of equipment and training of staff in the use of, and response to, alarms and indicated infant problems help solidify the team approach to care. If used inappropriately or if malfunctioning, some equipment may cause unnecessary injury.

In comparison with the normal newborn nursery, where neonates stay only 2 days, ICU infants stay for months, and the staff may become emotionally attached, as well

as involved with family and visitors (see Box 23–8). Despite the best efforts and highest quality of care, deaths do occur. These serious events may be viewed by staff as personal failures and undermine confidence in their respective professional abilities. Group discussions and opportunities for venting feelings and attitudes should be promoted to reduce staff anxiety, stress, and potential loss of experienced staff to other professional activities.

The prolonged medical attention that babies who are born prematurely or with a very low weight require in order to survive to be discharged home raises issues concerning the quality of life.[68] Developmental delays, behavioral problems, neuromuscular deficits, mental retardation, cerebral palsy, and seizure disorders have been identified as unwanted sequelae and major contributions to the instigation of lawsuits.

When negligence claims are reviewed, it becomes difficult to distinguish among the various contributing factors: obstetric care versus anesthesia care versus neonatal care versus the risk itself of prematurity, which may be primary. Typically, in a scattershot approach, all parties are named in the suit: hospital, obstetrician, anesthesiologist, neonatologist, pediatrician, consultants, and other caregivers identified in the medical record. From the risk manager's point of view, every baby treated in the NICU is a potential liability action.

INFANT TRANSPORT

An infant's medical condition may require transport to a facility where a higher level of care is available. Level-II and level-III facilities treat not only the infants born at the respective facilities, but also infants transferred from lower level facilities. Infants being transported are typically medically compromised and in need of specialized support and equipment.

Before transfer can occur, the sending facility must contact the receiving facility to ensure acceptance of the infant. Both AAP and ACOG have outlined the components of infant transport between facilities, including requirements for communications, staffing, essential equipment, vehicles, patient care, and program evaluation.[32] The referring physician is responsible for providing the receiving physician with pertinent clinical information regarding the infant. Generally, it is preferred that the maternal patient be transferred with the fetus in utero, when possible. It is important to remember that sound clinical judgment, as well as the Emergency Medical Treatment and Active Labor Act (EMTALA), requires that a pregnant patient not be transferred until she has been examined, stabilized, and has provided consent. Transport should be ordered only if the risks of the transfer do not outweigh the risks of remaining at the original facility.

Copies of all records, tests, monitor tracings, and clinical-status details of the pregnancy, labor, and delivery, as well as information related to the infant's physical examination, diagnostic tests, and therapeutic interventions, should be sent along with the patient. Transport records should include the team names, mode of transport, time of arrival and departure from the sending hospital, and time of arrival at the receiving facility. Procedures performed en route, medication administered, and periodic vital signs should be documented, as well as the condition of the patient upon arrival at the new facility.

Risk management should review transport events and investigate any difficulties during transport or technical and professional problems en route to reduce inherent risks in these transfers.

INFANT ABDUCTION

The mass media has paid a significant amount of attention to infants kidnapped from hospitals. Ninety-seven cases of infants abducted from medical facilities were reported between 1983 and 1997. The number of infant abductions appears to be declining, however, in large part probably because of proactive security measures, educational efforts, and a shortened length of stay in the hospital. In an attempt to circumvent infant abductions, many hospitals have discontinued publishing the names of newborns in the local newspapers.

Abducted infants are typically between a few hours and a few days old. In all documented abductions, the abductor was a female with no past criminal record. Usually, the woman had convinced friends and family that she had been pregnant for the past 9 months.[69] The kidnapper typically posed as a medical caregiver and dressed in a hospital uniform. A majority of abductions occurred in the mother's room, followed by nursery, pediatrics, and other on-premise locations. Hospitals with delivery services, and thus an increased potential for infant abductions, should identify security-problem areas, design access-control systems, develop emergency procedures for responding to an abduction, and promote staff and patient education to reduce risks. Generally, security measures control entry into the nursery; secondarily, they supplement infection-control efforts by minimizing traffic into the nursery. Many nurseries are located behind electronically locked doors that have alarms. Only staff with a need to enter should be provided access to the codes and/or electronic keys. Some hospitals utilize closed-circuit television and electronic-alarm wrist bands. Other areas to consider securing include stairwell and exit doors to maternity, postpartum, and pediatric units.

Risk management guidelines suggest that all staff who have contact with infants wear a photograph identification badge at all times, which should be checked by other staff, and especially by the mother. Although a difficult public relations issue, visitor control is of paramount importance.

Infant identification plays an important role in decreasing the likelihood of abductions and minimizes the potential for giving the wrong infant to the wrong mother. This process should start in the delivery room and include duplicate banding of the infant, mother, and significant other, along with the footprint, blood typing, photograph, and written assessment noting birthmarks and identifying features. If there is a need to remove the infant's identification band, it should be replaced immediately and the incident should be documented in the medical record.

HOME APNEA MONITORING

A major risk management concern with home apnea monitoring is the documented rate of parental noncompliance. Between 1985 and 1993, the Medical Device Report File of the Food and Drug Administration (FDA) found that noncompliance or misuse of prescribed infant-apnea monitors in the home setting occurred more than 54% of the time.[70] Noncompliance or misuse was shown to be more prevalent in homes where there was a lack of food, lack of sufficient financial resources, prevalence of illicit drugs, involvement in gangs, and lack of extended family to assist in child care. Monitor-related problems include false alarms, interference, and power loss. Because of these problems, ideally the selected device should have a secondary monitoring modality, such as heart rate monitoring, electrodes that cannot be inadvertently connected into electrical outlets, power-loss alarms and/or low-battery alarms, and remote alarm capability.[71]

Identification of mothers at risk for noncompliance should prompt intense educational efforts and involvement of social services. Physician reaffirmation of the need for monitoring is imperative. Apnea moni-

tors are primarily a prescription item available through a durable or home-medical-equipment supplier whose only roles are to supply the equipment and provide preventive maintenance for it. It is the responsibility of the prescribing physician, and sometimes of case managers, to ascertain compliance, monitor progress, and discontinue use when indicated.

SURGERY AND ANESTHESIA

After ambulatory care in the office or clinic, the inpatient surgery department has the highest volume of claims (see Box 23–9). Approximately 24.2% of all claims are for inpatient surgery and 2.8% for outpatient surgery, according to the St. Paul's Fire and Marine Insurance Company. The average loss for surgery in the hospital was $115,405, and for the ambulatory care surgicenter it was $73,973.[1] The most frequent allegations related to surgery were:

- Postoperative complications
- Inadvertent acts
- Inappropriate procedures
- Postoperative death
- Unnecessary surgery

The most frequent allegations related specifically to inpatient surgery were:

- Treatment complications or bad results
- Injury adjacent to the treatment site
- Foreign body left in the patient
- Equipment malfunction or failure
- Infection, contamination, or exposure

Box 23–9

- A Philadelphia jury awarded $100 million to a plaintiff in a malpractice case involving surgeries and other care to an infant born after only 26 weeks of gestation.
- In West Virginia, a jury awarded $2 million (even though there was a $1 million cap) for a patient who died from complications after anti-reflux surgery.

Box 23–10

- In June 1995, the headline read "Physician Erred in Brain Surgery." A neurosurgeon at a world-renowned hospital specializing in the treatment of cancer operated on the wrong side of a patient's head. Mistakenly, the surgeon brought another patient's diagnostic films into the operating room, then opened the wrong side of the surgical field and probed the healthy side of her brain for the tumor.[72]
- In February of 2002, the recurring headline read "Florida Hospital Neurosurgeon Slices Wrong Side of Head."[73]

Box 23–11

- A review of 146 medical-malpractice cases involving surgery of the lumbar spine disclosed that unintended "incidental" durotomy (23 cases) occurred with perioperative morbidity and long-term sequelae.[75]
- For colon and rectal surgeons, causes of malpractice litigation in 98 cases from 103 allegations fell into five major categories: failure to diagnose colorectal cancer and appendicitis (43%), iatrogenic colon injury (24%), iatrogenic medical complications of diagnosis or treatment (15%), sphincter injury (10%), and lack of informed consent (8%).[76]
- Four-year-old Desiree Wade bled to death 4 days after undergoing a tonsillectomy. The New York State Health Department initiated a full-scale investigation into the death.[77]
- A District of Columbia ophthalmologist lost a malpractice lawsuit for allegedly failing to diagnose adenocarcinoma of the lacrimal duct.[78]

Of these allegations, the most common were injuries incurred adjacent to the treatment site, infections from orthopedic surgery, and burns during inpatient surgery as a result of laser or cautery equipment failure. In outpatient claims, most allegations fell into the category of treatment problems, complications, or bad results, or involved postoperative infections in orthopedics. Postoperative complications account for 50% of the claims and nearly 50% of the cost of claims involving surgical issues (see Box 23–10).

NEGLIGENCE AND MALPRACTICE

Surgery and accompanying sedation or anesthesia are, by nature, risky. For example, surgical risk includes the potential for inadvertent amputation of the wrong limb, accidental damage to an organ or artery, hemorrhage, infection, or unexpected death or brain damage. Except in elective procedures, the patient undergoing surgery with accompanying anesthesia is usually in a medically compromised condition; however, from a legal perspective, patients of higher medical risk, such as the elderly, do not represent the greatest liability risk. It is the young, otherwise healthy, patient having elective or semi-elective surgery for whom damages can be considerable.

There are a plethora of surgical specialties, each with inherent risks and specialized technologies. Many hospitals require mandatory consultation and referrals for each specialized area. Surgery may be performed in various clinical settings, including tertiary teaching hospitals, community hospitals, ambulatory surgery centers, and physicians' offices.

Liability in the ambulatory surgery center rests on many of the same legal principles that apply to the inpatient setting.[74] As a result, it is imperative that consents be documented, adequate and complete preoperative assessments be made, and diagnostic testing and discharge instructions be provided to the patient (see Box 23–11).

SURGICAL-SERVICES STAFF

Legally, the surgeon is considered the "captain of the ship" and works closely with teams to accomplish high-quality services. Surgical teams may consist of general surgeons, specialty surgeons, family-practice physicians, podiatrists, anesthesia personnel, nursing staff, surgical technicians and assistants, surgical and anesthesia residents, heart–lung pump technicians, and radiology technicians, to name a few. Each team member is trained to perform specific tasks. Their actions may or may not be regulated by national certification or state licensure. With the advent of new procedures and technologies, it is imperative that all members of the specific surgical team for the surgery contemplated have appropriate training. Team members should perform only those procedures for which they have clinical privileges as provided by the medical staff bylaws and department regulations. Risk managers recommend that surgical operating room scheduling managers be provided with the list of hospital surgeons and their approved privileges to ensure that inappropriate surgeries are not scheduled.

Sales representatives who promote new equipment and technology present a host of risk management concerns. Physicians recognize the wealth of specific technical knowledge that these sales representatives have gained in areas such as implantable cardiac pacemakers and balloon pumps; however, the sales representative should only provide technical advice and not be allowed to scrub or to operate any equipment in the operating suite.

A continuing risk management issue for rural hospitals concerns the credentialing of "outreach" surgeons. Guidelines for the use of outreach surgeons were developed by the American Hospital Association's Division of Medical Affairs.[79] These surgeons should be credentialed and privileged in the same manner as all other medical-staff members. Specific procedures appropriate for outreach surgery should be determined in advance by the medical staff, with approval by the hospital board of directors. Outreach surgeons should be included in the preoperative

assessment of the patient and should be instrumental in the decision to operate. Attending physicians should also be competent in the skills required for postoperative care.

PREOPERATIVE ASSESSMENT AND TREATMENT

Successful surgery requires quality clinical and technical skills of the surgical team and effective preoperative assessment, treatments, and diagnostic testing that prepare the patient for surgery. The Joint Commission on Accreditation of Healthcare Organizations (JCAHO) states that surgery can be performed only "after a history, physical examination, any indicated diagnostic tests, and the preoperative diagnosis have been completed and recorded in the patient's medical record."[80] Both aggressors and defense factors should be included in the assessment.[81] Aggressors include the type of surgical procedure and anesthesia, carcinoma, infection, medications, chemotherapeutic agents, and radiation. Defense factors include the immune system, nutritional condition, and physiological status.

Preoperative treatments may prepare the physiological state of the patient to deal with factors of aggression; yet, one study, based on a population of more than 2,500 patients in New York, found that nearly 40% of patients undergoing inpatient surgical procedures may not have received antibiotics in the proper time frame to be most effective. Medical literature indicates that 25% of all postoperative nosocomial infections occur at the site of the surgical incision.[82]

Risk managers must be concerned that often insufficient attention is paid to preoperative protocols. Patient education about what to expect as a result of the surgery, with an emphasis on what the patient's responsibilities are for care and monitoring, can improve the preoperative preparation of the patient.

INTRAOPERATIVE RISK ISSUES

Risk management should be notified of all unusual occurrences in surgical patients and the operating room, such as surgery on the wrong patient, performance of the wrong procedure, medication error, patient return to surgery for repair or removal of an organ or body part damaged in surgery or subsequently, and unexpected patient return to surgery or unplanned readmission to hospital (see Box 23–12). No operation or procedure should be performed for which the surgeon does not have clinical privileges.

Many intraoperative issues are of high risk and pervade several surgical specialties: anesthesia services, blood contact, implants, retained foreign bodies, and burns.

Sedation and Anesthesia

In their many forms, sedation and anesthesia remove the patient's ability to control his or her own actions—in some cases introducing paralysis of limbs, cessation of unassisted breathing, and inability to respond to pain. Responsibility for assuring quality of life, viability, and a minimum of pain remains with the surgeon, anesthesiologist, and surgical support team. Anesthesia services may be provided by anesthesiologists, certified registered nurse anesthetists (CRNAs), and in some rural facilities, by general surgeons and obstetricians.

Perioperative complications that result from anesthesia include hypertension; myocardial ischemia or infarction, and arrhythmias or cardiac arrest; oliguria; hypothermia; malignant hyperthermia; and respiratory arrest or anoxic episodes.[86] On the basis of more than 3,000 cases over a 9-year period (1986–1995), the American Society of Anesthesiologists Closed Claims Project indicated that the frequency of anesthesia-related claims for adverse respiratory events and the frequency of claims involving death and brain injury were both decreasing.[87]

Because of the complex and life support nature of anesthesia equipment, the FDA introduced recommendations for anesthesia apparatus checkout in 1986. In 1993, the use of a revised FDA checklist or a similar one was recommended to inspect the anesthesia system prior to each use.[88] The inspection checklist includes:

- Emergency backup equipment
- Anesthesia machine
- Waste-gas-scavenging system
- Oxygen supplies
- Oxygen-pressure-failure system
- Flow meters
- Warning systems
- Accessory equipment
- Machine or breathing-equipment leaks
- Ventilator
- Patient-suction apparatus
- Electronic monitors
- Airway-pressure alarms
- Volume-monitor alarms
- Central and cylinder supplies of nitrous oxide and other gases

A preanesthesia assessment should be based on the patient's medical, anesthesia, and medication history; an appropriate physical examination; a review of diagnostic data;

Box 23–12

- The wrong wrist of an 83-year-old woman with carpal tunnel syndrome was operated on.[83]
- Comedian Dana Carvey settled a $7.5 million lawsuit against New York Hospital and his cardiothoracic surgeon when coronary artery bypass graft surgery in 1998 bypassed the wrong artery. He had undergone three prior angioplasty surgeries and was subsequently successfully treated with another angioplasty in California.[84]
- An intravenous line was preoperatively inserted into the radial nerve of a 29-year-old woman admitted for outpatient, elective nose reconstruction. The arbitration award was $155,000.[85]

and the formulation and discussion of the anesthesia plan with the patient. Provision of detailed information about the risks of complications of general anesthesia on the eve of surgery generally does increase the patient's knowledge without increasing the patient's level of anxiety.[89] Patients must also be reevaluated immediately before the induction of anesthesia.

Noninvasive patient monitoring during anesthesia usually includes blood pressure, pulse, respiratory efforts, skin color, temperature, and electrocardiograms. Capnometry is used on expired gas to measure the concentration of end-tidal carbon dioxide as a reflection of patient oxygenation, whereas pulse oximetry can provide an indication of arterial oxygen saturation. Electro-encephalography (EEG) and evoked potentials, although not widely in use, have been used as indicators of unacceptable changes in brain activity as a measure of oxygen perfusion. Invasive monitoring, such as central venous pressure, continuous arterial blood pressure, or pulmonary artery monitoring, is typically used for critically ill patients and complex surgical procedures (for example, bypass surgery) that allow and require a more continuous method of monitoring.

If intravenous sedation, also called conscious sedation, is frequently administered to patients undergoing outpatient surgery, and there are no anesthesia staff present, there should be strict protocols in place regarding the types of cases and clinical parameters to be monitored by nurses, and steps to be taken in the event of complications.

Prevention of hypothermia is an important aspect of anesthesia management. Some methods used for its prevention, such as warmed intravenous fluid bags or bottles, cause cutaneous burns and are not recommended.[90] Adverse results of anesthesia can result from injury during intubation or extubation, allergic reaction to drugs or transfusions, and equipment failure. Death during surgery implicates surgeons and anesthesia personnel, as well as all other members of the team.

Perioperative Blood Contact

A major risk to surgical team members includes perioperative blood contact and sharps injuries. Blood exposure is associated with increased risk of infection from blood-borne pathogens, including hepatitis B, hepatitis C, HIV, and AIDS. Several authors believe that the incidence of blood exposure among surgical team members has been vastly underreported (see Box 23–13).[91]

A study of more than 8,500 surgical cases in nine hospitals showed that more than 10% of the cases resulted in one or more instances of blood contact. Of these contacts, 2% were the result of punctures. Other studies found percutaneous blood exposure of almost 5% and glove perforation as high as 50%, although the surgeons were only aware of 15% of the perforations.[93] Blood contact included blood soaking through surgical attire and onto the skin of the team member, mucous-membrane contact, blood spatter on the face or neck, and sharps lacerations or punctures. Blood exposure is a two-way street. Staff members need to protect themselves from the patient, but the patient also needs to be protected from staff (see Box 23–14).

Risk management should include careful attention to the requirements of universal

---

Box 23–13

A surgeon who put patients at risk by operating on them while knowing he was a hepatitis B carrier was sentenced to 1 year of imprisonment.[92]

Box 23–14

In *Faya v. Almaraz*, a Maryland appellate court ruled that a surgeon who was HIV-positive had an obligation to inform patients, thus suggesting the opportunity for recovery of damages by patients even if they had not been infected.[94]

precautions as recommended by the federal Centers for Disease Control and Prevention and mandated by the Occupational Safety and Health Administration (OSHA); however, reputable authorities have commented that careful adherence to the OSHA recommendations alone may not be effective in reducing exposure risks, since constant vigilance is not possible to maintain or expect. Many facilities are using fully fluid-resistant surgical gowns rather than gowns with fluid-resistant panels; double gloving, or replacement of surgical gloves at intervals throughout the surgery; protective eyewear such as face shields or splatter guards; "no-touch" instrument passing; blunted instruments; and careful attention to sharps management.

Whenever possible, needleless systems should be used.[95] Self-sheathing or blunting needles and appropriate sharps-waste-disposal units should be available. Vaccinations, such as for hepatitis B, should be encouraged for staff. Protocols for responding to an exposure should be in place and understood by everyone. In some types of surgery, it is important to understand the potential "sharpness" of patient anatomy. A fractured bone end poses a risk to a finger probing in an open fracture or surgical wounds.

Surgical teams must be vigilant and recognize and report risky events such as major breaches of sterile technique or blood contact with patients at high risk for blood-borne pathogens.

Biomedical Implants

Medical implants are a significant concern in surgical liability. Breast augmentation has become the most often-performed plastic surgery; conservative estimates are that 1 million procedures have been performed in the United States.[96] Implant materials, such as some polymers, have been alleged to contribute to systemic and local clinical complications that arise years after the implant surgery (see Box 23–1).

Box 23–15

Brenda Toole, a woman who had to undergo three operations to have silicone removed from her body after her breast implants ruptured, was awarded $6 million in her lawsuit against the implants' manufacturer, the Baxter Healthcare Corporation.[97]

Implants of all types may also wear excessively, break or fracture, and be useless years after the surgery. The question of whether to remove an implant is one of great concern to the medical community. Although there are potentially serious risks to allowing the defective implant to remain in situ, there are also serious concerns about the clinical hazards of removing the implant.

Mandates of the Safe Medical Devices Act (SMDA) require tracking of specific medical implants from point of purchase through the implant's end of life. Implants that require tracking are:[98]

- Replacement heart valve (mechanical only)
- Implantable cardiac pacemaker pulse generator
- Implanted diaphragmatic or phrenic nerve stimulator
- Implantable infusion pump
- Vascular graft prosthesis
- Implanted cerebellar stimulator
- Cardiovascular permanent cardiac pacemaker electrode
- Temporomandibular joint prosthesis
- Glenoid fossa prosthesis
- Mandibular condyle prosthesis
- Abdominal aortic aneurysm stent grafts
- Dura mater
- Automatic, implantable, cardioverter defibrillator

Because hospitals, licensed practitioners, and ambulatory surgical facilities are required to participate in this program, they should have policies that require tracking and that designate staff responsibility for tracking.

Information must be sent to the manufacturer about the implant, the physician, and the patient at the time of receipt, implantation, and the end of the implant's useful life. Failure of permanently implantable devices could have serious adverse health consequences.

Retained Foreign Bodies

Defense of cases involving a retained foreign body after surgery are very difficult. Courts expect surgeons to be aware of what they use on the patient in the operating room as well as what is removed from the patient. In an effort to minimize the risk of leaving these items in the surgical cavity, the American Association of Operating Room Nurses has developed recommended practices regarding sponge, sharps, and instrument-count procedures.[99] If the initial and final counts are not in agreement, an X-ray of the surgical field is recommended prior to the patient's leaving the surgical table. Incorrect instrument, sponge, or sharps counts may necessitate further exploration at the surgical site (see Box 23–16).

Claims of foreign objects or material found following surgery should initiate a thorough investigation by risk management of the medical record to identify lapses in procedure and to prevent further occurrences.

Patient Burns and Pressure Injuries

During surgery, a patient may experience what appears to be a chemical or thermal burn or a pressure injury. Chemical burns may result from the fluid used to clean the surgical site prior to the surgical procedure or the adhesive conductive gel used under the dispersive electrode of an electrosurgical unit (ESU). Thermal burns may result if the patient is placed too close to a surgical light, if an operating microscope is reassembled incorrectly, or if an ESU is used. Pressure injuries, which mimic the appearance of burns, may result from sustained normal pressure during surgery, from body weight, and from external objects that reduce or impede local circulation.[101] Vascular insufficiency may also contribute to pressure injuries. Incorrect positioning of the patient may lead to neural injuries or impairment. Additional risks are inherent in surgical patients who are elderly, malnourished or obese, or whose delicate skin is compromised by their basic medical status.

Because the majority of the patient's body is beneath surgical drapes and not visible to the surgical team, constant attention to placement of the patient's extremities is important. Meticulous attention to detail in positioning the patient, pressure-distribution devices, and padding, as well as careful clamping of towels, may help eliminate some pressure injuries. Inspection, maintenance, and appropriate placement of electrical accessories and use of devices will reduce unintended burns and future patient discomfort. Documentation of positioning and placement of electrodes protects staff from allegations of poor practices.

Any type of patient injury, reddening of the skin, or break in skin integrity not identified prior to surgery or noticed immediately after surgery or during postoperative recuperation should be examined, treated, and documented in the medical record, as well as thoroughly investigated and reported to risk management.

Laser Surgery

Laser surgery has introduced new and specialized risks to the surgical team and the

---

Box 23–16

- A blue towel and part of her colostomy bag were left behind in the body of a woman after two separate operations in a city-owned hospital. She was awarded a settlement of $125,000.[83]
- Eight surgical patients required second operations to retrieve sponges, cotton, or metal instruments left inside their bodies.[100]

patient. To ensure safe laser practices, guidelines were developed by the American National Standards Institute (ANSI) the Association of Operating Room Nurses (AORN), the American Society for Laser Medicine and Surgery (ASLMS), and the Laser Institute of America (LIA).

According to the ANSI, the most common accidents related to laser medicine are burns and eye injuries to the surgical team members, fires, patient burns, and accidental laser activation. The FDA reported that the most common cause of laser-related incidents was mechanical malfunction.[102] Malpractice claims associated with laser surgery have included allegations of lack of informed consent, improper usage, fire, explosion, nerve damage, scarring, disfigurement, and infection. Safety protocols typically include the use of nonflammable surgical drapes, nonreflective surgical instruments, skin preparation of the surgical site with nonflammable agents, endotracheal intubation with tubes made of nonflammable materials specific to laser type, and the use of nonflammable anesthetics.

Several recent newspaper series relative to elective plastic surgery in the *Sun Sentinel* (Florida),[103] the *Philadelphia Inquirer,*[100] and the *Boston Globe*[104] exposed the problems of unexpected deaths, scars, burns, and disfigurements from laser surgeries. Most of these procedures are done in outpatient offices in the community, but the patients are then seen in the hospital after trouble erupts. Some practitioners are unqualified for the procedures they perform.

Physicians should be credentialed and privileged prior to using lasers in surgery. Privileging should encompass specific laser types, as well as types of laser surgery to be performed. Access to the laser and the activation mechanisms should be controlled, and protective eyewear and/or in-line eye-protective measures should be provided to staff. Adequate smoke evacuation and filtering is important, as is the availability of a secondary means to control bleeding. Poten-

tially reflective surfaces should be identified and steps taken to minimize the risk. The availability and application of operational safety guidelines and manufacturer's protocols for staff will help reduce the risks inherent in this technology.[100]

POSTOPERATIVE RECOVERY CARE

Following surgery, patients are transported to the postanesthesia/recovery room or intensive care unit for monitoring and stabilization by specially trained physicians, nurses, and ancillary staff. The patient's postoperative status should be assessed on admission to the unit and reassessed prior to discharge. Monitoring should include the patient's physiological and mental status such as vital signs and level of consciousness; pathological findings; medication, fluid, blood, or blood-components administration; and unusual events or postoperative complications, as well as management of those complications.[90]

Postoperative risk management issues concern serious adverse clinical events during transfer to the recovery area, adverse results of anesthesia, medication or transfusion reactions, cardiac or respiratory arrest or death, and postoperative neurological deficits not present on admission (see Box 23–17).

It is usually the responsibility of the anesthesia personnel to discharge a patient from the recovery room, but some facilities permit

---

Box 23–17

Following 7 hours of surgery to correct a congenital heart condition in a 2.5-year-old, the girl was weaned from a respirator, developed difficulty breathing, turned blue, and was revived. The surgeon was sued for negligent postoperative care because the lack of oxygen left the child clinically blind and mentally retarded. Seventeen years later, the jury awarded $5 million to the girl's family.[106]

the nursing staff to use discharge-criteria protocols. Such protocols are developed through the joint efforts of anesthesia, surgical, and nursing staff, and should have the approval of the medical board.

INFORMED CONSENT

Consent is of particular importance when discussing risk management in surgery and anesthesia. Because of the significant potential for injury, the invasiveness of the procedures, and the medical alternatives sometimes available, there is general consensus that the patient and/or legal medical guardian is entitled to an understanding of the procedure, including risks and benefits, as well as alternatives to the procedure. Although requirements for the level of information to be afforded to the patient are highly dependent on state consent laws, there are universally accepted principles expected by risk management and the legal community.

Achieving an informed consent from the patient is primarily the responsibility of the healthcare practitioner delivering the service. While the surgeon is responsible for the consent discussion with the patient regarding the surgical procedure to be performed, it is the anesthesiologist's responsibility to discuss anesthesia risks and to obtain consent from the patient for anesthesia services. Consent forms are viewed by the court as administrative evidence that healthcare practitioners had a consent discussion with the patient, not that consent was fully achieved. A witness who signs the consent form is attesting to the signature of the patient, not to the patient's informed consent to proceed with the procedure.

Of particular interest to surgical and anesthesia personnel is the issue of advance directives and whether they are to be honored during surgical procedures or while the patient is under the influence of anesthesia. Many facilities have addressed this dilemma through their ethics committees.

MEDICAL-RECORD DOCUMENTATION

Medical-record documentation concordant with surgical procedures requires that documentation of the preoperative stage include diagnosis, review of the patient's history and physical status, preoperative nursing, review of diagnostic test results, assessment of the risks and benefits of the procedure, the need to administer blood or blood components, consent, and preanesthesia documentation. A plan of care should be generated to include the nursing care, the operative plan, the level of postsurgery care, and the need for additional diagnostic testing or monitoring. Documentation should also reflect the anesthesia process, as well as the nursing and medical course of the surgery.

Postoperative documentation must reflect the care delivered to the patient and the patient's condition in the recovery room and/or intensive care unit, as well as the clinical parameters monitored. Medical records must identify who provided direct patient-care nursing services and who supervised that care if provided by someone other than a qualified registered nurse. Daily charting of the physician's assessment of the patient's progress, monitoring and testing, dressing changes and medications, and plans for discharge are necessary. Medical records should also note the name of the licensed, independent practitioner responsible for the discharge, and record discharge instructions for care and follow-up services.

The JCAHO requires that the patient's medical record contain evidence of known advance directives, informed consent for procedures for which informed consent is required by hospital policy, and documentation of all operative procedures performed. The JCAHO also requires that the medical record of patients undergoing operative procedures and/or anesthesia include the following elements:[90]

- The name of the licensed, independent practitioner who is responsible for the patient, as well as the name of the primary surgeon and all assistants

- The preoperative diagnosis documented by the licensed, independent practitioner responsible for the patient
- Operative reports dictated or written in the medical record immediately following surgery
- The operative report that includes the findings, technical procedures used, specimens removed, and postoperative diagnosis
- Authentication of completed operative report by the surgeon as soon as possible
- An operative progress note in the event that there is a delay in placing the operative report in the medical record

IT'S A RISKY BUSINESS

All the contacts between a patient and the multiple professionals and ancillary personnel involved in the provision of healthcare services should be meticulously documented. This documentation is the major defense against allegations of medical negligence or incompetence when there has been no breach of community-accepted standards of care. Although accidents and misadventures are not entirely avoidable, the organization's and risk manager's objective is to provide high-quality services, prevent medical disasters, and limit damages resultant from, and incidental to, unintended adverse occurrences.

References

1. *Health care update.* (2002). Hospital issues. The St. Paul's Health Care Claims Analysis. St. Paul, MN: The St. Paul Companies.
2. Mayer, T.A. (1995, June 12). Emergency diagnoses are mostly accurate. *Wall Street Journal,* p. A13.
3. Rogers, J.T. (1985). *Risk management in emergency medicine* (pp. 1–36). Dallas: American College of Emergency Physicians.
4. St. Paul's Fire & Marine Insurance Co. (1993). Patient care area, emergency and inpatient surgery generate most hospital claims. *Hospital Update* annual report, St. Paul, Minnesota.
5. American Hospital Association, Special Member Briefing. (1992). *Emergency medical treatment and active Labor Act requirements and investigation* (pp. 1–12). Chicago: American Hospital Association.
6. Centers for Disease Control and Prevention. (2002). Emergency department statistics. Washington, DC: United States Department of Health and Human Services.
7. American College of Emergency Physicians. (1987). *Policy statement on medical control of pre-hospital emergency medical services.* Dallas: ACEP.
8. Sexton, J. (1995, March 8). Differing accounts of a firefighter's care. *New York Times,* p. B6.
9. American Medical Association Commission on Emergency Medical Services. (1989). *Guidelines for the categorization of hospital emergency capabilities* (pp. 7–29). Chicago: American Medical Association.
10. Reigner, W. (1993). Escalating risk: Violence in the ED. *QRC Advisor, 9*(8), 1–4.
11. Foust, D., & Rhee, K.J. (1993). The incidence of battery in an urban emergency department. *Annals of Emergency Medicine, 22*(3), 583–585.
12. Managing traumatic stress. (1994). *Occupational Hazard, 56*(10), 212.
13. Protection from physical violence in the emergency department. (2001). *Clinical policies.* Irving, TX: American College of Emergency Physicians.
14. Hobgood, C.D., John, O., et al. (2000). Emergency medicine resident errors: Identification and educational utilization. *Academic Emergency Medicine, 7*(11), 1317–1320.
15. ED doctors don't always have the right skills. (1994). *American Medical News, 37*(37), 11.
16. Reilly, B.M. (2002). Impact of a clinical decision rule on hospital triage of patients. *Journal of the American Medical Association, 288,* 342–350.
17. Hevesi, D. (1994, December 31). State assails mistreatment by hospital in rape case. *New York Times,* p. A29.

18. American College of Emergency Physicians, Professional Liability Committee. (1989). Providing telephone advice from the emergency department: Position statement. Dallas: American College of Emergency Physicians.

19. Clark, S. (1994). Implementation of voice recognition technology at Provenant Health Partners. *Journal of American Health Information Management Association, 65*(2), 34–37.

20. (1990). Principles of appropriate patient transfer. *Annals of Emergency Medicine, 19*(2), 337–338.

21. Healthcare Providers Service Organization. (2001). Case of the month, May. http://www .hpso.com/case/.

22. Mantel, D.L. (1995). The legal perils of patient discharge. *RN Journal, 58*(3), 49–51.

23. American College of Obstetrics and Gynecologists (ACOG). (2002, May 6). Nation's obstetrical care endangered by growing liability crisis. News release.

24. Ward, C.J. (1991). Analysis of 500 obstetric and gynecologic malpractice claims: Causes and prevention. *American Journal of Obstetrics & Gynecology, 165*(2), 298–303.

25. Bronstein, J.M., Capilouto, E., Carlo, W.A., et al. (1995). Access to neonatal intensive care for low-birthweight infants: The role of maternal characteristics. *American Journal of Public Health, 85*(3), 357–361.

26. Hack, M., Taylor, H.G., Klein, N., et al. (1994). School-age outcomes in children with birth weights under 750 grams. *New England Journal of Medicine, 331*(12), 753–759.

27. Failing our babies. (1995). *Neonatal Intensive Care, 8*(3), 11.

28. Hickson, G., Clayton, E.W., Githens, P.B., & Sloan, F.A. (1992). Factors that prompted families to file medical malpractice claims following perinatal injuries. *Journal of the American Medical Association, 268*(11), 1359–1363.

29. Entman, S.S., Glass, C.A., Hickson, G.B., et al. (1994). The relationship between malpractice claims history and subsequent obstetrical care. *Journal of the American Medical Association, 272*(20), 1588–1591.

30. Hickson, G.B., Clayton, E.W., Entman, S.S., et al. (1994). Obstetricians' prior malpractice experience and patients' satisfaction with care. *Journal of the American Medical Association, 272*(20), 1583–1587.

31. American College of Obstetricians and Gynecologists (ACOG). (2001). *Code of ethics.* Washington, DC: ACOG

32. Frigoletto, F.D., & Little, G.A. (1992). *Guidelines for perinatal care* (3rd ed., pp. 37–47). Elk Grove Village, IL: American Academy of Pediatrics and the American College of Obstetricians and Gynecologists.

33. Midwife care generates NY ruckus. (1995). *Medical Liability Monitor, 20*(5), 5, 8.

34. Capen, K. (1995). New prenatal screening procedures raise specter of more "wrongful-birth" claims. *Canadian Medical Association Journal, 152*(5), 734–737.

35. Kotula, C. (1994). High risk pregnancy. *Continuing Care, 13*(3), 16–19, 28.

36. Statute of repose runs from time of negligence. (1995). *American Medical News, 38*(11), 19.

37. American College of Obstetrics and Gynecology. (1994). Antepartum fetal surveillance. *Technical Bulletin, 188,* 3.

38. Evans, H. (1995, June 20). Technology: Doctors who perform fetal sonograms often lack sufficient training and skill. *Wall Street Journal,* p. 2.

39. Maley, R.A., & Epstein, A.L. (1993). *High technology in health care: Risk management perspectives* (pp. 235, 244). Chicago: American Hospital Publishing.

40. U.S. Department of Health and Human Services, Public Health Service, Preventive Services Task Force. (1993). Home uterine activity monitoring for preterm labor: Policy statement. *Journal of the American Medical Association, 270,*(3), 369–370.

41. McClinton, D.H. (1995). Monitoring devices are not essential for improving birth. *Continuing Care, 14*(2), 5.

42. Petrikovsky, B. (1993). Is fetal heart rate monitoring during labor and delivery justified? *Neonatal Intensive Care, 6*(4), 19–20, 48.

43. Catanzarite, V.A., Perkind, R.P., & Pernoll, M.L. (1987). Assessment of fetal well-being. In A.H. DeCherney, & M.L. Pernoll (Eds.), *Current obstetric & gynecologic diagnosis & treatment* (p. 286). Norwalk, CT: Appleton & Lange.

44. American College of Obstetrics and Gynecology. (1992). Fetal and neonatal neurologic injury. *Technical Bulletin, 163.*

45. American College of Obstetrics and Gynecology. (1995). Fetal heart rate patterns: Monitoring, interpretation and management. *Technical Bulletin, 207.*

46. Curran, C. (1993). The fetal monitoring position. Second source. *Biomedical Bulletin, 7*(3), 28.

47. American College of Obstetrics and Gynecology. (1991). Induction and augmentation of labor. *Technical Bulletin, 157,* 1–3.

48. Frankel, D.H. (1995). New York's obstetric mess. *Lancet, 345*(8951), 716.

49. Chadwick, H.S., Posner, K., Caplan, R.A., et al. (1991). A comparison of obstetric and nonobstetric anesthesia malpractice claims. *Anesthesiology, 74*(2), 242–249.

50. American College of Obstetrics and Gynecology. (1986). Management of breech presentation. *Technical Bulletin, 95.*

51. Report says water-birth may be risky. (2002, August 6). *Home News Tribune,* 7:1.

52. American College of Obstetrics and Gynecologists (ACOG). (2000). OB-Gyns issue recommendations on cesarean delivery rate. News release.

53. American College of Obstetrics and Gynecology, Committee on Obstetric Practice. (1991). Guidelines for vaginal delivery after a previous cesarean birth. *Committee Opinion,* no. 64.

54. American College of Obstetrics and Gynecologists (ACOG). (2001). ACOG addresses latest controversies in obstetrics: When planning for vaginal delivery may not be appropriate. News release.

55. Marta, M.R. (1994). Current topics in obstetrical risk management, part II. *Journal of Healthcare Quality, 6*(6), 6.

56. Osbourne, S.E., & Kassity, N.A. (1993). Neonatal resuscitation program update. *Neonatal Intensive Care, 6*(6), 32–33.

57. American College of Obstetrics and Gynecology, Committee on Obstetric Practice and American Academy of Pediatrics, Committee on Fetus and Newborn. (1991). *Use and misuse of the Apgar score.* ACOG/AAP committee opinion. Washington, DC: ACOG.

58. American College of Obstetrics and Gynecology, Committee on Obstetric Practice and American Academy of Pediatrics, Committee on Fetus and Newborn. (1994). *Utility of umbilical cord acid–base assessment.* ACOG/AAP committee opinion. Washington, DC: ACOG.

59. Marta, M.R. (1994). Current topics in obstetrical risk management, part I. *Journal of Healthcare Quarterly, 6*(5), 7.

60. Stoeckmann, A. (1994). Placental examination as a risk management tool. *Journal of Healthcare Risk Management, 14*(1), 9–14.

61. Arizona Medical Association. (1992). Placental project. *Enhancing placental examination: The vision and the professional opportunity.* Phoenix: Arizona Medical Association.

62. Clements, B. (1994). Don't get sued. *American Medical News, 37*(29), 15–17.

63. Schindler, N.R. (1991). Importance of the placenta and cord in the defense of neurologically impaired infant claims. *Archives of Pathology & Laboratory Medicine, 115*(7), 685–687.

64. OB/GYN claims: Analysis and advice. (1994). *Forum, 4*(5), 105.

65. Shaheen, J. (1995, March 5). Longer stay needed, a mother says. *New York Times,* p. 14.

66. Als, H., Lawhon, G., Duffy, F.H., et al. (1994). Individualized developmental care for the very low-birthweight preterm infant. *Journal of the American Medical Association, 272*(11), 853–858; Merenstein, G.B. (1994). Individualized developmental care: An emerging new standard for neonatal intensive care units? *Journal of the American Medical Association, 272*(11), 890–891.

67. Umansky, A.B. (1994, December 8). Parents thankful for tiny miracles. *Wall Street Journal,* p. A19.

68. Solomon, S.D. (1995). Suffer the little children. *Technology Review, 98*(3), 42–51.

69. Colling, R.L. (1994). Code pink—code pink. *Continental Rx, 6*(2), 4.

70. McIntyre, C.H. (1995). Monitoring compliance. *Home Health Care Dealer/Supplier, 6*(2), 51.

71. Picciano, L.D., & Keller, J.P. (1993). Hospital and home apnea documentation systems: Device acquisition and application. *Neonatal Intensive Care, 6*(4), 28–31.

72. McShane, L. (1995, June 23). Physician erred in brain surgery. *Philadelphia Inquirer,* p. A18.

73. *Naples Daily News.* (2002, February 27).

74. Quan, K.P., & Wieland, J.B. (1994). Medicolegal considerations for anesthesia in the ambulatory setting. *International Anesthesiology Clinics, 32*(3), 145–169.

75. Goodkin, R., & Laska, L.L. (1995). Unintended "incidental" durotomy during surgery of the lumbar spine: Medicolegal implications. *Surgical Neurology, 43*(1), 4–12.

76. Kern, K.A. (1993). Medical malpractice involving colon and rectal disease: A 20-year review of U.S. civil court litigation. *Diseases of the Colon & Rectum, 36*(6), 531–539.

77. Rosenthal, E. (1995, April 4). Full inquiry into death of girl, 4. *New York Times*, p. B3.

78. "Migraine sinus" was lacrimal gland cancer. (1995). *American Medical News, 38*(9), 19.

79. McCormick, B. (1989). Hospital policy on outreach surgery. *Trustee*, 17.

80. The Joint Commission on Accreditation of Healthcare Organizations (JCAHO). (1995). *Accreditation manual for hospitals: Standards* (Vol. 1, pp. 6–7, 16–17, 58–59). Oakbrook Terrace, IL: JCAHO.

81. Gagner, M. (1991). Value of pre-operative physiologic assessment in outcome of patients undergoing major surgical procedures. *Surgical Clinics of North America: Complications of General Surgery, 71*(6), 1141–1150.

82. Surgical patients in New York hospitals may not receive optimum antibiotic treatments. (1994). *Island Peer Review Organization Quality Initiatives*, 10.

83. Why it matters: The medical system is a leading killer. (2002). *Medical errors and malpractice*. Minneapolis: The Association of Health Care Journalists.

84. Falcon, M. (2001, November 5). Heart operation no laugh for Dana Carvey. *USA Today*, Health Spotlight.

85. Delegal, M.K. (2001, January). IV inserted to nerve results in radial nerve injury: $155,000 arbitration award. *Legal Review & Commentary Supplement, Healthcare Risk Management*.

86. Entrup, M.H., & Davis, F.G. (1991). Perioperative complications of anesthesia. *Surgical Clinics of North America: Complications of General Surgery, 71*(6), 1151–1174.

87. Saidman, L.J. (1995). Anesthesiology. *Journal of the American Medical Association, 273*(21), 1661.

88. U.S. Department of Health and Human Services, Food and Drug Administration. (1994). *Anesthesia apparatus checkout recommendations*. Rockville, MD: Food and Drug Administration.

89. Inglis, S., & Farnill, D. (1993). The effects of providing preoperative statistical anaesthetic-risk information. *Anaesthesia & Intensive Care, 21*(6), 799–805.

90. Cheney, F.W., Fosner, K.L., Caplan, R.A., & Gild, W.M. (1994). Burns from warming devices in anesthesia: A closed claims analysis. *Anesthesiology, 80*(4), 806–810.

91. Lynch, P., & White, M.C. (1993). Perioperative blood contact and exposures: A comparison of incident reports and focused studies. *American Journal of Infection Control, 21*(6), 357–363.

92. Choo, V. (1994). Jail for putting patients at risk of hepatitis B. *Lancet, 344*(8928), 1012.

93. Noera, G. (1994). Blood contact during open heart operations: Reducing the risk. *Annals of Thoracic Surgery, 57*(3), 785–786.

94. Patients can recover from HIV-positive doctor. (1995). *American Medical News, 38*(10), 19.

95. Needlestick Safety and Prevention Act (House of Representatives 5178) H.R. 5178. Passed November 6, 2000. Washington, DC: United States Congress.

96. Moran, T. (1995). Battle scars. For plastic surgeons, psychological effects linger from silicone breast implant controversy. *Texas Medicine, 91*(1), 30–34.

97. $6 million award in implant suit. (1995, February 5). *New York Times*, p. 18.

98. Low, N., & Wollerton, M.A. (1992). Food and Drug Administration user facility reporting. *FDA Medical Bulletin, 3*, 6.

99. Association of Operating Room Nurses, Recommended Practices Committee. (1995). *Proposed recommended practices for sponge, sharp and instrument counts*. Denver: AORN.

100. Gerlin, A. (1999, September 12). Medical mistakes. *Philadelphia Inquirer*.

101. Gendron, F.S. (1990). *Unexplained patient burns: Investigating iatrogenic injuries*. Brea, CA: Quest.

102. Carl, L. (1992). The health care team approach to laser medicine risk management. *Laser Nursing, 6*(1), 6–8.

103. Schulte, F., & Bergal, J. (1998, November 29). Plastic surgery: The risks you take. *Sun-Sentinel* (Florida).

104. Tye, L. (1999, March 14). Patients at risk. *Boston Globe*.

105. Harding, G.H. (1993). Laser surgery. In R.A. Maley, & A.L. Epstein (Eds.), *High technology in health care: Risk management perspectives* (pp. 149–150). Chicago: American Hospital Publishing.

106. Schwaneberg, R. (2001, April 20). $5 million award stands against MD. *Star-Ledger,* p. 53.

24

IMPROVING RISK MANAGER PERFORMANCE AND PROMOTING PATIENT SAFETY WITH HIGH-RELIABILITY PRINCIPLES

Stephen Pavkovic, JD, MPH, BSN
Kristopher Goetz, MA
Amit Prachand, MEng
Scott Stanley, JD, BSN

INTRODUCTION

While investigating a medication-administration event that reached the patient and resulted in temporary harm, an experienced risk manager recalls a series of factually similar medication events from the preceding months. Unable to recall the disposition of the similar cases, the risk manager reviews the files and discovers that there were four similar cases that reached the patient and resulted in temporary harm. Each case was investigated and "closed," with different levels of organizational response from the risk manager, clinical manager, and quality committee. After aggregating the four cases and reviewing common themes, as well as differences, along with the organizational responses, the risk manager, in a reflective moment, asks:

> Why did I investigate essentially the same case four different ways? Have I done this before with more serious events? If I handled these similar cases differently, would the other risk managers in my organization do the same? What were the lessons learned and how were they communicated to the front-line staff? Can I do better? Can our risk management department do better?

Historically, the role of the healthcare risk manager closely paralleled the retrospective view of an insurance-claims manager. For organizations that ardently work to ensure patient safety, the healthcare risk manager's role has evolved into one of a prospective patient safety champion. Healthcare risk managers are in a unique position to excel as patient safety champions, because their loss-control focus combines the operational realities of their organization with their regular contacts with front-line care staff. Despite this critical role in patient safety, many experienced risk managers recognize that far too often their event response is determined by an "I'll know it when I see it" approach.

When pressed to further define this type of risk-response criterion, descriptions emerge of ill-defined independent-triage processes enacted after *some* vulnerable internal-vigilance system determines that *some* action threshold has been met.

When internal individualized approaches are utilized as the primary risk management investigative response, the ability to reliably create loss-control opportunities from reported events is marginalized or completely lost, and the ability to replicate processes over time is impossible. Although each risk management investigation is distinct and some investigations involve scenarios only encountered once in a career, the majority of investigations involve recurring, common-place clinical facts and patterns of behaviors. Risk managers who investigate both common and rare events can support patient safety with reliable, predictable responses. Through such responses to recurring clinical events, risk managers can optimize their roles as patient safety champions by diligently investigating events and efficiently responding to the novel patient safety and loss threats.

This chapter provides an overview of the concepts of reliability as practiced in high-reliability organizations (HROs; see Chapter 22) and discusses how these concepts can create dependable patient safety event response for the individual risk manager and risk departments. Additionally, structured process-improvement methods, including lean-process-analysis concepts, are presented to demonstrate methods that can decrease individual risk manager performance variability, eliminate wasted risk department efforts and resources, and create sustainable change.

Through adopting the interrelated principles presented here, risk managers can begin to transform their activities from the individualized and intuitive to the routine and reliable. In this process risk managers can begin to reliably lead loss-control and patient safety activities and avoid the case-to-case discrepancies presented in the opening hypothetical scenario.

CONCEPT OF RELIABILITY

Reliability is one measure of a consistent, dependable performance within a system.[1] Embracing reliability to direct behavior can promote safety and prevent avoidable injury. This principle is the basis for safety engineering and error proofing of critical systems. Many patient-focused providers embrace these principles and design healthcare-delivery processes that create optimal care with predictable, reliable behaviors. Examples of engineered patient safety practices include:

- Requiring computerized physician order entry (CPOE) to limit prescriber ordering options and remove prescription-legibility errors
- Mandating pre-procedure "time-outs" and checklists to ensure that the appropriate patient, procedure, and supplies are in order[2]
- Communication tools, including SBAR (situation background-analysis recommendation), that create efficient predictable dialogues at critical transitions in patient care
- "Smart pump" technologies that create programmable medication-delivery systems with safety-focused lockouts and dosing parameters
- The use of approved and restricted abbreviation lists for clinical documentation

As with the aforementioned healthcare examples, predictable, coordinated risk management performance can also improve safety and support an organization's enterprise risk management objectives. Examples of an engineered risk department's response could include:

- Determining the appropriate types of matters for risk management intervention—for example, all anesthesia-related patient events involving dental injuries will be handled as a claim through the Department of Anesthesia with notice of matter disposition to the Risk Management Department—and determining with other organizational members an agreed-upon disposition for those matters outside the scope of risk management.

- Determining risk department best practice for conducting investigations including procedures for file opening and closing, utilization of medical record review templates, and handoff procedures to other organizational entities, such as quality committees, to appropriate sharing of the findings of risk management investigations with all necessary departments.
- Utilizing standardized, scripted risk management responses to common advice questions including medical records release issues, consent processes, and documentation practices for patients discharged against medical advice.
- Determining appropriate processes and taxonomy to ensure inter-rater agreement for the classification and severity rankings of reported events, and identifying a process to evaluate and record risk manager decisions.
- Conducting random and focused audits at fixed times to ensure compliance with established departmental processes.

RELIABILITY ALONE IS NOT ENOUGH

For healthcare providers and risk managers, creating an environment that solely supports reliable performance does not promote patient safety.[3] In *Critchfield v. McNamara*, hospital liability was determined based on the failure of the overnight neonatal intensive care unit (NICU) staff to report non-reassuring physical assessments to physicians. The NICU notes reliably documented the signs and symptoms of increasing respiratory decompensation and the evolving acute neurological injury, but there was no staff action on these findings.

Similarly for risk managers, performing accurate and reliable event investigations does not inherently promote patient safety, unless these findings are reliably applied to support a larger coordinated, patient-focused system-wide effort. For example, after an organization implemented a revised patient-identification process that required that both the patient and admitting staff initial armbands, the risk manager identified several incident reports where the patient was unable to initial. This possibility was not considered by the implementing committee. When the risk manager provided the committee with this crucial information, a revised process was enacted and the larger coordinated patient-identification goal supported.

HIGH-RELIABILITY ORGANIZATIONS COMBINE RELIABILITY WITH PERFORMANCE

Organizations that embrace reliability as an operating tenet are called high-reliability organizations (HROs). This operational method is adopted by industries involved in complex processes with the very real potential for catastrophic failures. Specific examples of HROs include nuclear power plants, commercial aviation, chemical manufacturing, and professional motor-sport teams. The HROs organize their activity around five reliability concepts, thereby creating a mindfulness regarding organizational actions, problem solving, and system functioning. Although the nature of defects in healthcare delivery do not always manifest as transparently as those in chemical manufacturing or in other HRO endeavors,[4] the HRO concepts create an excellent analytical framework by which to organize patient safety efforts and risk manager performance.

The five HRO concepts as described for healthcare leaders are:[4]

1. Sensitivity to operations. Preserving constant awareness by leaders and staff of the state of the systems and processes that affect patient care. This awareness is key to noting risks and preventing them.

2. Reluctance to simplify. Simple processes are good, but simplistic explanations for why things work or fail are risky. Avoiding overly simplistic explanations of failure (unqualified staff, inadequate training, communication failure, etc.) is essential in order to understand the true reasons that patients are placed at risk.

3. Preoccupation with failure. When near misses occur, these are viewed as evidence of systems that should be improved to reduce potential harm to patients. Rather than viewing near misses as proof that the system has effective safeguards, they are viewed as symptomatic of areas in need of more attention.

4. Deference to expertise. Allowing front-line staff—sharp-end healthcare providers—an opportunity to provide their insights in identifying patient safety threats and including them on developing patient safety improvement efforts.

5. Resilience. Leaders and staff need to be trained to know how to respond when system failures do occur.

In a healthcare setting, the HRO concepts facilitate a systems-oriented problem-solving focus and response. For example, when responding to a potential communicable-disease outbreak, an HRO-oriented organization may include both front-line housekeeping staff along with epidemiologists for their unique perspectives (deference to expertise). If an outbreak is not identified, HRO-oriented organizations will focus their efforts to capture potential lessons from the investigation (preoccupation with failure).

Similarly for the risk manager, the HRO concepts provide valuable guidelines to systematically construct investigations and identify loss-control opportunities. For example, using the opening scenario that involved five medication errors that reached the patient when conducting a risk investigation, the risk manager should engage the appropriate experts, which would include pharmacy leadership (deference to expertise). Pharmacy, through their own tracking systems, might have a better awareness of the scope of the issue (sensitivity to operations). In developing a plausible solution, the group should not only consider events that reached the patient, but also any near misses where staff may have actively prevented the event from reaching the patient (preoccupation with failure). Even if it is determined that there were appropriate system safeguards in place that should have prevented any of the five events, it is important to identify system weaknesses, opportunities (sensitivity to operations, reluctance to simplify), and a possible plan for responding to similar events in the future (resilience).

HRO FOR RISK MANAGERS

Healthcare risk managers maintain a series of formal responsive investigative tools and techniques, including root-cause analysis (RCA), failure-modes-and-effects analysis (FMEA), and human-factors analysis, to identify underlying causal factors that resulted in patient harm or threat; however, if the risk manager cannot reliably identify when to employ these techniques, important injury and loss-prevention opportunities are missed. The five HRO concepts provide the risk manager with a framework to reliably conduct individual investigations and reliably coordinate patient safety promotion with loss-control efforts.

When utilized by risk managers, the HRO concepts can control for individual variation and promote improved patient safety. As adopted here with specific risk management applications, the HRO concepts include the following:

1. Sensitivity to operations
   a. Knowing and practicing, through vetted risk department policies, the factors that support an organization's enterprise risk management goals including compliance with

non-negotiable legal, regulatory, and institutional demands, and an understanding of an organization's litigation posture

b. Determining a common patient-safety-focused taxonomy to prevent the misidentification of events and inappropriate responses

2. Reluctance to simplify
   a. Identifying the investigational standards required to complete an investigation
   b. Identifying the additional information sources available to a risk management department for investigations, and determining when this information should be consulted

3. Preoccupation with failure
   a. Establishing routine investigation processes and leading RCAs for near-miss events to learn from, and improve, faulty systems before they result in patient harm
   b. Establishing protocols for investigating all filed claims without prior notice to risk management to determine if the risk department should have known about them
   c. Trending all data, including near-miss data, by clinical department (e.g., emergency, surgery) and/or locations (e.g., radiology, sleep lab, electrophysiology studies [EPS] lab)

4. Deference to expertise
   a. Determining RCA participants based on their role in the presenting matter, rather than organizational title
   b. Identifying internal resources and external subject-matter experts available for conducting risk investigations

5. Resilience
   a. Conducting reliable disclosure discussions with patients after adverse events
   b. Developing predictable risk management responses when investigations fall outside of expected time frames for completion

ENGINEERING RELIABILITY WITH PROCESS IMPROVEMENT

The HRO concepts provide the individual risk manager and the risk management department with a proven framework for ensuring a more reliable risk response. Structured process-improvement approaches may provide risk managers with tools that can reliably lead to adoption of the HRO concepts and sustained change. In health care, popular approaches to systematic process improvement and patient safety promotion include six sigma, lean process analysis, and plan–do–check–act. The success of process-improvement techniques is maximized for organizations that have embraced an environment or culture of safety with internal and external transparency, clear lines of accountability, and engaged executive leadership.

Risk managers interested in engineering reliability into clinical and risk department performance should coordinate with quality improvement and patient safety practitioners, define systematic problems to understand and measure processes from a patient and provider's perspective, and implement solutions focused on sustainability. Once an organization has embraced this culture, the risk manager is ideally positioned to become a partner in quality improvement. For the purposes of discussion here, all process-improvement approaches contain foundational elements that guide change. As discussed below with risk management application, these elements include:

- Assessment of the current state. Once a problem is discovered, the existing process(es) should be defined and measured. This is achieved through collaboration with key stakeholders and often multidisciplinary teams to define the current state processes from their perspective. For example, from a risk perspective, quantifying the average number of days an investigation is open and the distribution of severity-score ranking per risk manager should be considered as the first steps for the risk department interested in creating a reliable risk department performance. It is important to note that even though there may be an agreed practice on average number of days an investigation is open, there may be external departmental factors that might impact the risk manager's ability to adhere to the agreed approach.

- Uncovering root causes. Experienced risk managers are well versed in the benefits of using RCA and FMEA to identify key drivers of clinical error. These same analytical tools provide the risk manager with a valuable approach to identify the causes of unreliable or variable risk manager performance. For example, did the prior clinical experiences of one risk manager create investigative assumptions that were not supported by the actual clinical practice in the presenting event while a second risk manager investigating the same event—and without that clinical experience—identified a more systemic breakdown in communications? The HRO concept of reluctance to simplify is critical for risk manager success at this stage.

- Implementing solutions. Developing and implementing new patient-centered processes can result in change when the solutions are generated as the product of the entire improvement team's cumulative efforts. Engagement of both frontline staff and executive leadership with improvement efforts is a critical requirement for successful implementation of clinical and risk department improvement efforts. Based on the frequently close collaborative relationship with clinicians, risk managers may possess firsthand knowledge of information that could impact the success of improvement efforts and data based on reported events to determine the effectiveness of those efforts.

- Ensuring sustainability. When implementing new patient safety improvements, process-improvement teams can ensure sustainability by embedding the solution into a revised, and when possible error-proofed, program of action. This is achieved when a new process is viewed and accepted as the new daily routine, rather than a temporary change in practice. Improvement teams should be skeptical of solutions that create additional work, extra processing, or require continued monitoring, because these steps will likely break down over time, once the novelty and the Hawthorne effect of the improvement activities have subsided.[5] Through error proofing of revised risk response processes, risk managers can obtain increased levels of reliability. For example, requiring a risk manager to complete a required field in an electronic form before closing an electronic investigation report will ensure that the field is complete.

Especially in larger healthcare organizations, many factors determine the role of the risk manager in formal process-improvement efforts; yet, with these approaches risk managers are particularly suited to adopt process-improvement efforts and engineer reliability for their own activities.

"LEAN" APPROACHES FOR RISK MANAGERS

The concept of "lean thinking" has rapidly permeated the healthcare landscape after initially starting as a manufacturing system designed to improve production efficiency.[6] Lean thinking has become more apparent in the healthcare industry because it provides a state of organizational mindfulness that increases performance efficiency with less human effort and resources while providing customers with exactly what they want.[7] Lean organizations see that every problem and cause of variation, whether a highly visible severe harm event or a seemingly minor precursor-type event, must be addressed to prevent the problem from becoming a severe event with harm.

Lean thinking links strongly with both the HRO concepts and the role of a proactive risk manager. In lean-thinking organizations, one focus is to review work and determine that the work is actually "value-added" in the eyes of the customer. For a lean-thinking risk manager, value-added activities include the prevention of avoidable injury to patients. Risk activities that do not support this goal are considered waste. For example, when a risk manager conducts an investigation, waste may present when phone calls are unanswered and when time and effort is spent searching for missing medical records. By adding a lean-thinking, value-maximizing, and waste-minimizing perspective to their investigations, risk managers can improve patient safety and capture loss-control opportunities.

The HRO concepts and lean thinking can promote reliable risk management event responses and reliable department performance. When risk managers work to create reliable performance with structured process-improvement techniques, sustainable change is achievable and increased patient safety is attainable.

References

1. Agency for Healthcare Research and Quality. (2008). *Becoming a high reliability organization. Operational advice for hospital leaders.* Executive summary. AHRQ publication no. 08-0022. http://www.ahrq.gov/qual/hroadvice/hroadvice.pdf/. Accessed April 20, 2010.

2. World Health Organization. (2008). *WHO surgical safety checklist and implementation manual.* http://www.who.int/patientsafety/safesurgery/ss_checklist/en/index.html/. Accessed April 20, 2010.

3. Critchfield v. McNamara. 1995. 532 N.W.2d 287.

4. Gibbs, V.C., & Auerbach, A.D. The retained surgical sponge (Chapter 22). In: *Retained surgical foreign body. Prevalence and severity of the target safety problem.* Agency for Healthcare Research and Quality. http://www.ahrq.gov/clinic/ptsafety/chap22.htm/. From the AHRQ publication "Making Health Care Safer: A Critical Analysis of Patient Safety Practices." Evidence Report/Technology Assessment, No. 43. Kaveh G. Shojania, Bradford W. Duncan, Kathryn M. McDonald, & Robert M. Wachter, Eds.

5. Leonard, K., & Melkiory, C. (2006) Outpatient process quality evaluation and the Hawthorne effect. *Social Science & Medicine, 63*(9), 2330–2340.

6. Graban, M. (2009). *Lean hospitals* (pp. 4–5). Boca Raton, FL: CRC Press.

7. Womack, J., & Jones, D. (1996). *Lean thinking* (p. 15). New York: Simon and Schuster.

25

THE BENEFITS OF USING SIMULATION IN RISK MANAGEMENT AND PATIENT SAFETY

Jeffrey F. Driver, JD, MBA
David M. Gaba, MD
Geoffrey K. Lighthall, MD, PhD

WHAT IS SIMULATION?

Simulation in health care is a set of techniques, often but not necessarily always involving technology, for replicating sufficient aspects of the clinical world for particular purposes of education, training, performance assessment, or research. Simulation can be used as a replacement for real-world clinical activities, or more commonly, as a supplement to them.

Why is simulation a useful and powerful technique? What makes it potentially worthwhile to "replicate reality" when we have reality all around us? Why have so many intrinsically hazardous endeavors (e.g., aviation, military, nuclear power production) relied so heavily on simulation, whereas health care has been relatively late to the party?

There are many reasons why simulations in health care, even if imperfect, are potentially valuable:

- Whatever the activity, there is no direct risk to real patients, unlike in real clinical situations. More and more clinicians in training are unable to experience the true nature of being fully responsible for their decisions, because they are always under supervision. In simulations, trainees can be "it"—they can make the decisions and implement treatments themselves.

- During simulation, instructors can allow errors to be made and to play out to their conclusion. If such errors were seen in real cases, the instructor would have to intervene to protect the patient.

- Simulations are controlled situations. Events can be created "on demand," especially those that are life critical or require highly invasive therapy. Clinicians do not have to learn only from the rare random occurrences of each of these situations.

- Simulation allows the use of teaching techniques that are not possible with real patients. One can pause the simulation to allow discussion; the simulation scenario can be rewound or fast-forwarded. One can let the simulated patient get very ill without having a cardiac arrest (like allowing pilots to fly underground and get back into the sky during aviation simulations). One can restart the simulation from the beginning or from a known situation. Furthermore, unlike in real clinical medicine, in simulation the instructors know what the underlying diseases and events are, and thus what the most relevant treatments should be.

- Simulation facilitates making detailed audio/video recordings of what happened for use in later debriefing; this is difficult in real cases.
- Simulation can be conducted in actual clinical work units ("in-situ" simulation) as well as in dedicated simulation centers. When conducted in-situ, the simulation exercises can probe the way the clinical system works, finding problems that can be fixed.

For all these reasons, those involved in simulation believe that, if done well, it can often be (with a nod to the rock band U2) "even better than the real thing."

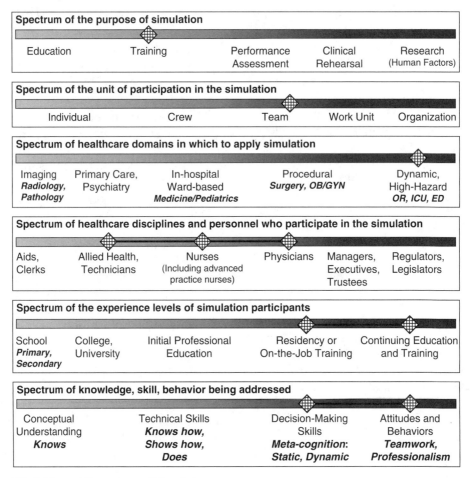

Figure 25–1 Eleven Dimensions of Simulation

There are many different uses and aspects of simulation, and this complexity can be broken down into at least 11 separate "dimensions" or factors.[1,2] Each dimension is a spectrum of choices; while these essentially form a continuum, they can be segmented into four to six choices per dimension. Any particular simulation activity can be classified by delineating the one or more characteristics in each of the 11 dimensions (see Figure 25–1). Of particular relevance are the goals and purposes of the simulation, the target population, the modalities of simulation, and the pedagogical approach that is used.

DIMENSIONS OF SIMULATION

Dimension 1: The Purpose and Aims of the Simulation Activity

The most obvious application of simulation is to improve the education and training of clinicians, but other purposes are also important. As used in this chapter, *education* emphasizes conceptual knowledge, basic skills, and an introduction to work practices. *Training* emphasizes the actual tasks and work to be performed. Simulation can be used to assess performance and competency of individual clinicians and teams, both for low-stakes or

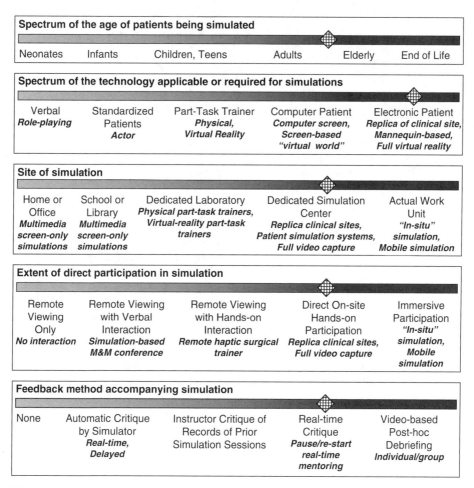

Figure 25–1 (Continued)

formative testing and (to a lesser degree as yet) for high-stakes certification testing. Simulation rehearsals are being explored as adjuncts to actual clinical practice, for example, where surgeons or an entire operative team can rehearse an unusually complex operation in advance using a simulation of the specific patient. Simulators can be tools for research and evaluation, concerning organizational practices (patient-care protocols) and for the investigation of human factors (for example, of performance-shaping factors, such as fatigue, or of the user interface and operation of medical equipment in high-hazard clinical settings). In fact, simulation-based empirical tests of the usability of clinical equipment have already been used in designing equipment that is currently on the market. Ultimately, such practices may be required by regulatory agencies before approval of new devices.

Simulation can be a "bottom-up" tool for changing the culture of health care concerning patient safety. Firstly, it allows hands-on training of both junior and senior clinicians about practices that enact the desired "culture of safety." Simulation can also be a rallying point about culture change and patient safety that can bring together experienced clinicians from various disciplines and domains along with healthcare administrators, risk managers, and experts on human factors, organizational behavior, or institutional change.

Dimension 2: The Unit of Participation in the Simulation

Many simulation applications are targeted at individuals. These applications may be especially useful for teaching knowledge and basic skills, or for practice on specific psychomotor tasks. Individual skill is a fundamental building block, but a considerable emphasis of simulation is applied at higher organizational levels in various forms of teamwork and interpersonal relations (often summarized under the rubric of crew-resource management, CRM, adapted from aviation).[3] Team training may thus be addressed first to crews (also known as single-discipline teams), consisting of multiple individuals from a single discipline, and then to teams (or multidisciplinary teams).[4] The advantages and disadvantages of each of these approaches are discussed later in this chapter.

Teams exist in actual work units in an organization, each of which is its own target for training. Going further, simulation can be applied to non-clinical personnel and work units in healthcare organizations (e.g., to managers or executives) and to organizations as a whole (e.g., entire hospitals or networks).

Dimension 3: The Experience Level of Simulation Participants

Simulation can be applied along the entire continuum of education of both clinical personnel and the public at large; however, for the purposes of risk management, simulation is aimed primarily at those who have a direct role in the care of patients. For the most part, this means either experienced personnel (staff) or those in advanced apprenticeship training (e.g., new-nurse orientation, interns, and residents).

Dimension 4: The Healthcare Domain in Which the Simulation Is Applied

Simulation techniques can be applied across nearly all healthcare domains. Much of the attention on simulation has focused on technical and procedural skills applicable in surgery, obstetrics, invasive cardiology, and other related fields, while another bastion of simulation has been recreating whole patients for dynamic domains that involve high-hazard and invasive intervention such as anesthesia, critical care, and emergency medicine. Immersive techniques can be used in imaging-intensive domains, such as radiology and pathology, and interactive simulations are relevant in the interventional sides of such arenas. In many domains, simulation techniques have been very useful for addressing non-technical skills (such as CRM) and professionalism or ethical issues, such as communicating with patients and coworkers, and in challenging situations such as end-of-life-care discussions or disclosure of bad news. There are now several textbooks that describe simulation in health care across all these domains.[5–7]

Dimension 5: The Healthcare Disciplines of Personnel Participating in the Simulation

Simulation is applicable to all disciplines of health care, not only to physicians; nor is simulation limited to clinical personnel. It may also be directed at managers, executives, hospital trustees, regulators, and legislators. For these groups, simulation can convey the complexities of clinical work, and it can be used to exercise and probe the organizational practices of clinical institutions at multiple levels.

Dimension 6: The Type of Knowledge, Skill, Attitudes, or Behavior Addressed in Simulation

In this way and others, simulation is applicable to clinicians throughout their careers to support lifelong learning. It can be used to refresh skills for procedures that are not performed often. Furthermore, knowledge, skills, and practices honed on the individual level must be woven into effective teamwork in diverse clinical teams, which in turn must operate safely in work units and larger organizations. Perpetual rehearsal of responses to challenging events is needed, because the team or organization must be practiced in handling them as a coherent unit. Because simulation recreates aspects of the real world, it provides a tool for probing or teaching about affective and emo-

tional issues of work that translate into attitudes and behaviors.

Dimension 7: The Age of the Patient Being Simulated

Simulation is applicable to nearly every type and age of patient, literally "from cradle to grave." Simulation may be particularly useful for pediatric patients and clinical activities, because neonates and babies have smaller physiological reserves than do most adults.

Dimension 8: The Technology Applicable or Required for Simulations

To accomplish these goals, a variety of technologies (including no technology) are relevant for simulation. The different modalities of simulation that are applicable for risk management purposes are discussed in more detail later in this chapter.

Dimension 9: The Site of Simulation Participation

Some types of simulation—those that use videos, computer programs, or the Web—can be conducted in the privacy of the learner's home or office using his or her own equipment. More advanced screen-based simulators might need more powerful computer facilities available in a medical library or learning center. Part-task trainers and virtual-reality (VR) simulators are usually fielded in a dedicated-skills laboratory. Mannequin-based simulation can also be used in a skills laboratory, although the more complex recreations of actual clinical tasks require either a dedicated patient-simulation center with fully equipped replicas of clinical spaces or the ability to bring the simulator into an actual work setting (in-situ simulation). The advantages and disadvantages to doing clinical simulations in situ versus in a dedicated center are discussed in detail later in this chapter.

Dimension 10: The Extent of Direct Participation in Simulation

Most simulations, even screen-based simulators or part-task trainers, were initially envisioned as highly interactive activities with significant direct "on-site" hands-on participation; however, not all learning requires direct participation. For example, some learning can take place merely by viewing a simulation involving others, as one can readily imagine being in the shoes of the participants. A further step is to involve the remote viewers either in the simulation itself or in debriefings about what transpired.[8] Because a simulation can be paused, restarted, or otherwise controlled, the remote audience can readily obtain more information from the on-site participants, debate the proper course of action, and discuss with those in the simulator how best to proceed.

Dimension 11: The Pedagogical Methods That Accompany Simulation

Much as in real life, one can learn a great deal just from simulation experiences themselves, without any additional feedback. For the most complex uses of simulation, especially when training relatively experienced personnel, the typical form of feedback is a detailed post-simulation debriefing session, often using audio/video recordings of the scenario.[9] Waiting until after the scenario is finished allows experienced personnel to apply their collective skills without interruption and also allows them to see and discuss the advantages and disadvantages of their behaviors, decisions, and actions.

SIMULATION AS A DATA SOURCE ABOUT CLINICAL PERFORMANCE

Simulation has another role to play in risk management: it provides a crucial window on clinical processes and clinician performance. In 1992, David M. Gaba described the complementarity of simulation with other methods of investigating performance, relating it to a jigsaw puzzle where each window on performance provides another piece of a larger puzzle.[10] Recently, McIntosh elaborated further on this model, terming it "Gaba's Jigsaw."[11] Simulation studies can add considerably to our knowledge of the issues and problems surrounding the way that patients are handled, because it allows the study of what people actually do (albeit in simulations) rather than what they think should be done, or what is reported in retrospect. Each method of assessment has strengths and weaknesses.

Prospective non-biased assessment of clinical process and clinician behavior in real-case situations would clearly be better. For some questions this can be accomplished by making recordings of data (through electronic medical records, the medical equivalent of aviation's "black box") or even sight and sound (through embedded microphones and cameras, the equivalent of the cockpit voice recorder) of many cases to capture those of interest for detailed study. Many clinical situations of relevance to the risk manager are, by definition, low-frequency events, so to really understand them, one would have to capture very many cases prospectively to get a fair sample of such situations (or else have either expert observers or a camera crew waiting patiently and immediately available for the few cases that come along). Even if this is warranted, the medicolegal, ethical, and logistical issues raised by filming in the clinical environment are daunting. Moreover, each such clinical situation is different, making it hard to see the spectrum of performance in responding to a "standardized" challenge. Case reports of real cases also offer a different window on performance. Such cases are actual clinical situations, and only salient ones would be brought to researchers' attention; however, the retrospective nature of these reports limits the information available, and memory recall of complicated cases is often faulty and subject to various hindsight biases. Moreover, there is likely to be a selection bias. Reporters are only likely to report cases in which there were significant problems, and not those for which care processes were faulty but whose results were unremarkable. Even without these limitations, there is still the problem that all the cases are different, making it hard to generalize from the reports.

Simulation therefore closes some of the holes left by the other techniques while possessing some of its own. Each case scenario is standardized, so all clinicians face the same challenges and conundrums; these can be as difficult as desired. Observation can be prospective and recorded in a non-biased fashion, typically using audio/video capture. Recordings allow for analysis by multiple observers or in multiple passes. Observers can be chosen with special expertise or training, if desired. The big limitation is that simulations are not real cases, and all participants know that this is true. This hole can either be closed or another piece of the puzzle if the simulations can be conducted such that the clinicians are unaware that it is not real. Such an approach is used when unannounced clinic visits by standardized patient actors are employed for quality assurance or research purposes in the outpatient clinic setting. For acute-care treatment situations, where actors cannot be used, such surreptitious simulations would require an "android" so good that it could be slipped into the clinical environment as if it were a real patient. This technology does not exist now and it may never be available; thus, a fundamental limitation of acute-care simulations for the foreseeable future is that clinicians know they are simulations. How is this likely to affect their performance? On the one hand, when they know that the "patient" is not a real patient, we can imagine that they will not take the situation seriously and will not perform all the actions as they would with a real patient. This can sometimes manifest as unusually sloppy or "cavalier" behavior, or clearly acting like it is all a game. Conversely, we sometimes see "hypervigilance" where participants later

admit to doing more than they usually would do, or to jumping too quickly on signs of possible trouble. Often this is because, knowing that it is a simulation, they were expecting problems to occur and acted on the first glimmer of abnormality. Other times they say that it is because they knew that they were being filmed and thus felt that they should do everything "by the book," even if the book is usually honored more "in the breach than the observance" (in the modern twist on Shakespeare's meaning).

Another thing that remains difficult in simulation is to reproduce the "motivational structure" of real work—that is, the incentives, disincentives, and culture of the workplace. This is a real problem for investigating performance in situations that depend on subtle judgments, negotiation between personnel, and the concerns for personal advancement, administrative discipline, or risk of litigation; nonetheless, despite its limitations, the window on performance offered by simulation is unique and may be of great utility in forward-thinking risk management approaches to quality management.

MODALITIES AND APPLICATIONS OF SIMULATION IN MORE DETAIL

As simulation is a technique that is conducted in many different ways that may or may not use various technologies, it is worthwhile to describe the different "modalities" of simulation in more detail.

Verbal Simulation and Storytelling

Human beings have long recreated experiences for others by telling or writing stories. Clinicians tell stories informally, or more formally as at morbidity and mortality conferences. These stories often are told in chunks, so that the outcome is unknown and the listeners or readers can simulate in their heads the decision-making processes that they would have used if faced with the same situation. Verbal simulations (i.e., "what if" exercises) can be specifically created for this purpose. The potential impact of this ultra-low technology can be seen when the mere act of reading or listening to a story brings tears to one's eyes.

Trigger Videos

Videos of salient cases are often used as "triggers" for reflection or for facilitated discussion, and are termed "trigger videos." While some trigger videos are created from footage of actual patient-care situations, they are frequently produced using simulation environments to present or recreate the intended set of clinical and behavioral challenges.

Role Playing

A step up from listening, reading, or viewing, with or without reflection or discussion, is acting out the situation by role playing. This allows participants to "walk the walk" rather than just "talk the talk." Such simulations are useful where thinking and communication skills need to be practiced, or where it is helpful to try to see a situation from another person's point of view. Role-playing techniques are often combined with technological simulation.

Standardized Actors

As long as one does not need to do anything to a patient (but only to talk with them or possibly examine them), the best simulator for a human being is another human being. Standardized patient (SP) actors are specially trained to consistently represent a patient with a particular medical history and chief complaint within a particular context. They understand enough about their condition to credibly improvise in response to any question of clinical staff. Standardized patients are used extensively for early learners (and they are also trained to rate their encounter with the trainee). They can also be used for advanced trainees or experienced staff, and some institutions use them surreptitiously to

probe the clinic's processes and quality. Standardized actors can also be used as family members for clinical encounters.

Computer-Screen Simulations (Screen-Only Simulators or Microsimulators)

One technique to represent the patient and the clinical environment is photos, videos, or animations with an interactive simulation that runs on a computer. Typically, the display is "on the screen" and choices of actions are made by clicking on menus, buttons, or sliders. To be considered a simulator, rather than just computer-assisted-instruction, the program must respond appropriately to a wide set of naturalistic interventions, rather than to a restricted set of choices. Such computer-screen simulations are aimed at a single user, who plays the role of the clinician(s) while the computer represents the patient. In non-medical settings, the prototypical simulator of this type would be the venerable Microsoft Flight Simulator (Microsoft, Redmond, Wash.).

Virtual Worlds

A virtual world is an on-screen environment that is shared with multiple participants, each of whom has a movable representation in the world (called an "avatar"). The participants are linked either by a local network, or over the Internet. The prototypical such non-medical world is the multiplayer on-line game World of Warcraft (Blizzard Entertainment, Irvine, Calif.), which has millions of participants enrolled worldwide. In medical virtual worlds, the role of the patient may be played by the computer, or it may in some cases be played by another participant. Similar to a computer-screen simulator, the clinical actions available to participants in the virtual world are often made by clicking on menus, buttons, or sliders, but in some cases the avatar's in-world actions may be needed. There is work ongoing to connect real-world actions to in-world actions. There is a popular generic virtual world called Second Life (Linden Research, San Francisco, Calif.), which anyone can join (for free) and allows participants to construct objects, facilitate virtual meetings, and offer services. There are already a small number of medical applications in Second Life.

Part-Task and Procedural Trainers

A set of simulation devices that target the learning of specific procedures or tasks are known as part-task trainers or surgical or procedural simulators. Such devices replicate the elements of the particular psychomotor task but may or may not include any elements of the rest of the patient or clinical care. Typical examples are simulators for laparoscopic surgery or endoscopy, or endovascular (catheter-based) procedures. The most complex of these procedural simulators presents a limited "virtual reality" in which the organs under manipulation exist only in a virtual computer world (and are represented on a two-dimensional screen). This is highly appropriate for clinical procedures such as minimally invasive surgery or interventional radiology/cardiology where the images used by clinicians in real practice are also two dimensional.

Very simple part-task trainers also exist, such as "IV arms" used to practice drawing blood or inserting IV catheters. Interestingly, food products are also used extensively as appropriate part-task trainers. For example, students may learn to suture wounds or incisions using pigs' feet, and cardiac surgeons practice coronary bypass grafts on cow hearts.

Mannequin-Based Simulation

A very common form of simulation uses computerized mannequins to take the place of the patient. The computer not only drives vital signs apparent in the mannequin, but also can present the data streams available from electronic monitors (e.g., the electro-cardiogram, pulse oximetry, invasive blood pressures). The computer integrates all mannequin-derived data with monitor findings such as a faint pulse occurring with the same timing as an ECG tracing showing damage to the heart. Depending on the particular device, the simulator's computer can be controlled either manually, semi-automatically (with the patients' vitals controlled by a pre-programmed script), or using mathematical models of physiology and pharmacology. The mannequin allows procedures such as intubation, pleural decompression, and cardiopulmonary resuscitation. Simulators must be used where the patient must have dynamically changing vital signs, where the patient has a lethal condition (e.g., cardiac arrest, severe anaphylaxis), and/or when significant interventions (medications or procedures) need to be administered. The mannequin may also provide a voice-link and speaker so that an instructor or actor can talk to clinical participants. It is thus common for the mannequin to also be a "standardized patient."

Complete Virtual Reality

The "holy grail" of simulation would be a complete VR that allows fully natural interaction of the participants with virtual environments so realistic that they could not be distinguished from the real world. The prototypical examples are the *Star Trek* Holodeck, or more chillingly, the world as depicted in the film *The Matrix*. Virtual-reality simulations are used in some non-medical environments (particularly the military and spaceflight), but there have been no complete VR applications yet in health care. A more limited variation, termed "mixed reality simulation," has been utilized. Here elements of the environment are represented virtually (and some participants may be virtual avatars) while other elements (typically the patient, some equipment, and some participants) are physically present. It is expected that eventually complete VR representations of the patient, of clinical equipment and supplies, and even of fully interactive computer-generated coworkers will be utilized in healthcare simulation. It is not known how far in the future this will occur.

Hybrid Simulations

It is noteworthy that the boundaries between these modalities are porous, and combinations and hybrids are possible. Actors are often mixed with part-task trainers or with mannequin-based simulators. Hybrid simulations aim to combine the best characteristics of each modality into a technique that is more than the sum of the parts.

APPLICATIONS OF SIMULATION TECHNIQUES IN HEALTH CARE

There are a large variety of simulation applications; as indicated in the section on the various dimensions of simulation, there are a variety of choices that define a given application. Rather than discuss each choice separately, we will discuss some of the most important high-level issues of simulation applications, largely assuming that the target population (for most risk management purposes) is at least one experienced clinician (house staff or above). In many cases the applications and choices are complementary—that is, we imagine that in a robust comprehensive simulation program many different types of simulation will be used, and that clinicians would cycle through different modalities and different applications throughout their careers, participating as individuals, in teams, and as entire work units.

Learning Objectives

Some simulations (especially computer-screen simulations) are aimed at helping to convey knowledge in a more interactive way. Psychomotor skills are addressed using part-task and procedural trainers, which have a role to play in risk management, because ensuring that all relevant clinicians have the appropriate knowledge and skills to do their jobs safely is a cornerstone of safe practice; however, much of the simulation that can help in risk management will address higher levels of cognitive performance, in particular abilities of dynamic decision making and management of a team in challenging situations. This involves the flexible use of "deployable knowledge" coupled with interpersonal and communication skills linked by team-oriented attitudes and an ability to stay calm and focused in a crisis. The prototypical approach to these issues adapts the crew-resource management (CRM) approach from aviation for use in health care. This was first accomplished at VA Palo Alto and Stanford for anesthesiology (where it was termed "anesthesia-crisis resource management," or ACRM).[12] The ACRM-like approach in health care spread extensively from anesthesiology to many other domains, especially those that involve dynamic management of patients over seconds to hours, rather than over days to months. There are a number of different formulations of the key principles of ACRM.

Figure 25–2 and Table 25–1 show one such formulation and distinguishes the CRM principles from the medical and technical skills that can also be addressed using simulation.

In the ACRM-like approach, simulations are conducted to present challenging clinical situations to individuals working in teams either with confederates or with real coworkers from other disciplines and domains (see below on "single-discipline" vs. "combined-team" training). Scenarios are chosen that stress both the individual's diagnostic and problem-solving abilities and the core aspects of CRM.[4] Typically, approximately 60% of the emphasis of simulations is on CRM or systems-thinking issues, and 40% or less is on disease-specific knowledge and treatment issues. ACRM-like courses, especially with participants having the experience of interns, or more, typically allow participants to manage the situation without pause and without help or advice from an all-knowing instructor.

Medical/Technical Skills	Non-technical Skills (Key Points of CRM)	
Medical knowledge and its application	Decision-making and cognition	Team and resource management
Physical examination	Knowledge of the team and environment	Taking a leadership role
Data evaluation	Anticipation and planning	Calling for help early
Differential diagnosis	Wise allocation of attention	Communicating effectively
Knowledge of therapeutic plans and pathways	Use of all available information and confirmation of key data streams	Distributing the workload
Hands-on skills	Use of cognitive aids (e.g., checklists, reference materials)	Mobilization and utilization of all available resources

Figure 25–2 Skill Sets Historically Targeted by Simulation-Based Training

Table 25–1 Use of Patient Crisis Simulation to Address CRM Concepts

CRM Point	Scenario or Condition	Rationale
Situational awareness	• Sepsis, obstetric disaster, bleeder, MI. Have arriving participant ask what's going on. • Diseases with secondary findings (i.e., tachycardia in hemorrhage)	• Assesses ability to understand and verbalize nature of situation • Assesses whether team maintains focus on primary abnormality
Leadership	• High complexity cases with shifting needs (mechanical ventilation, procedures, CPR, etc.) • Send in senior physician when junior physician (current leader) is doing an adequate job.	• Assesses ability to focus on priorities while maintaining view of larger problems • Set up for power struggle—does leader support or take over? What is best for patient?
Use of cognitive aids	• Malignant hyperthermia • Pulseless electrical activity	• Forces use of MHAUS* direction sheet • Forces one to find list of "five Ts and five Hs"**
Anticipation/acquiring help	• Hemorrhage, myocardial infarction, increased intracranial pressure • Any rapidly deteriorating patient	• Requires engagement of others for definitive control of time-sensitive disease processes • Is patient receiving more attention or monitoring? • Are junior-level trainees in over their heads?

(continues)

Table 25–1 (Continued)

CRM Point	Scenario or Condition	Rationale
Checking of all data streams	• Pulseless arrest; equipment disruptions • Pneumothorax, hypopnea, bronchospasm, heart murmur	• Requires examination of all sources confirming pulsatile blood flow • Is a team member actually examining the patient?
Distribution of the workload	• Sepsis or hemorrhage with several tasks to attend to—send in someone asking if they can help. • Send in ECG tech or X-ray tech (radiographer) who asks trainees to move away. Patient has PVCs (ventricular ectopic beats).	• Assesses leader's monitoring of workload and task pairing • Assesses if anyone is watching patient
Prevention of fixation errors	• Equipment malfunctions, pulseless patient • Novel, rare, or other problems with poor outcomes (malignant hyperthermia, machine malfunction, tamponade)	• Assesses whether finding is related to overall situation, and whether new information changes plans or there are overriding beliefs that all is fine • Can the team accept compelling information establishing a diagnosis?
Communication	• Data probes (information passed on to a single group member) • Send in extra people, create noise	• Assesses presence of healthy two-way communication, willingness of junior members to contribute information • Forces use of techniques such as readback that assure requests are properly received
Wise allocation of attention	• Pneumothorax, shock, tamponade, hemorrhage	• Cases requiring high-level of technical skill that may force senior leader to perform procedure (assesses whether leader gets other to do the procedure, watch patient, lead team)

* Malignant Hyperthermia Association of the United States
** American Heart Association Advanced Life Support algorithm

Where possible, the simulation is followed by a detailed debriefing, often using strategically chosen snippets of video from the simulation scenario. Teaching via debriefing is a powerful technique that requires special aptitude and training for optimal results.

Unlike seminar types of CRM-oriented training in which personnel may discuss how CRM principles apply to their work or to specific situations, simulation-based CRM-oriented training makes them actually put these principles into practice while engaged in the medical/technical problem solving and interventions. The integrated application of medical knowledge and skill with behavioral aspects of management lies at the heart of expert clinical care in dynamic environments. It is widely believed that problems in CRM are a major root cause of adverse outcomes, because retrospective analysis often reveals that a clinical problem was, in theory, treatable, but that adequate coordination of all decisions and therapies was not made sufficiently well or in time to make a difference.

Table 25–2 Individual Versus Team Simulations

	Pros	Cons
Individual	Targets specific needs of the individual	Much clinical care is rendered in teams, not just by individuals
	Allows practice at own pace	Richer discussion with more than one participant and more than one view
	Formative evaluation unique to individual performance	Hard to achieve high throughput of learners with 1:1 sessions
	Learner is safe from scrutiny by supervisors, peers, or subordinates	Some participants enjoy the support of peers during experiential learning
	Ideal for focused psychomotor simulations or for development of individual knowledge or skill	
Group or Team	Can address and practice issues of team management and behaviors	Hard to schedule multiple learners at one time
	Increased efficiency of sessions (>1 learner per session/instructor)	Often limited to addressing issues of "lowest common denominator" of group
	Take advantage of team cohesion and spirit; peers reinforce learning	Sub-optimal group dynamics can sabotage learning of some individuals

With regard to unit of participation—i.e., individual vs. team (see Table 25–2) and single discipline vs. combined team (see Table 25–3)—some modalities of simulation are, by their nature, targeted at individuals. This is true of part-task and procedural trainers used to learn the specific psychomotor skills of a given manual procedure. The typical use of such a device is aimed at an individual, although they might be incorporated into hybrid simulations that involve a team. Other forms of simulation (e.g., mannequin based) might well be equally targeted at an individual learner, or at a team, or even a whole work unit; thus, there is a choice of the unit of participation. If the choice is for a team or group, there is also a choice of whether to target a single discipline (e.g., anesthesiologists) as the learner population, or to make the target a multidisciplinary team or group (e.g., the staff of the ICU, including doctors, nurses, allied health personnel, and adjunctive unit personnel). There are pros and cons to each type of unit of participation.

Dedicated Simulation Center Versus In-Situ Simulations

As described in dimension 9 (site of simulation participation), a given activity can be carried out in different sites (dedicated center vs. in situ). An obvious difference is the need in a dedicated center for space, utilities, and fixed infrastructure, all of which are a significant expense especially for a smaller institution. In-situ simulation, while not inexpensive (the simulator is only a tiny fraction of the aggregate cost of running simulations), is within the reach of nearly every hospital. Our group has recently completed an AHRQ-funded study in which we taught a diverse set of client hospitals to do multidisciplinary simulation (AHRQ U18 HS16630-02, "Preparing rural and urban hospitals to improve safety culture using simulation").

Table 25–3 Single-Discipline Versus Combined-Team Simulations

Single-Discipline Group	Can address issues of particular interest to that discipline without boring other discipline personnel	Does not train real teams to work as teams
	Sometimes easier to assemble group from single discipline only	
	Can present full spectrum of behavior or performance of other team members (using "confederates") rather than being limited to behavior of real team members from other disciplines	Difficult to represent real motivational structure and group dynamics of a real team
	Not always possible to provide credible (simulated) work for every team member from every discipline	
Combined Team	Trains real team to work as a team	Limited to behaviors of actual team members in that session
	Facilitates cross-discipline understanding and cross-training	Often logistically difficult to assemble all team members
		Hard to provide credible (simulated) work for all team members depending on their discipline (e.g., simulations only available for certain kinds of surgery)

One client hospital was a 25-bed critical-access hospital in a rural part of a small state. They have successfully launched simulation programs both in situ and with a small center built in an unused ward room. If such an institution can conduct meaningful simulation, we believe that it can be done almost anywhere. Clearly, techniques of in-situ simulation and the use of a dedicated center are complementary (see Table 25–4).

Scheduled Versus Unannounced Simulated Events (or In-Situ Simulations)

In-situ simulations can be conducted as scheduled exercises either for personnel in their regular-duty roles or for personnel on their off-duty or education days. Alternatively, in-situ simulations may be "unannounced mock events" that are "sprung" on unsuspecting personnel. Again, these are complementary approaches, each with its own pros and cons (see Table 25–5).

APPLICABILITY TO RISK MANAGEMENT

From a risk management standpoint, simulation has a number of potential ways in which it might prevent claims or mitigate losses: (1) prevent adverse events or mitigate the outcome of evolving events when they do occur; (2) reduce the likelihood of a claim; and (3) enhance the chances of a favorable settlement or decision on a claim.

Prevention or Mitigation of Adverse Events

There are two ways that simulation may be useful to prevent or mitigate events; one is training and the other is systems probing. Like all training paradigms, simulation can be used

Table 25–4 Dedicated Simulation Center Versus In-Situ Simulation

	Pros	Cons
Dedicated	High level of control and infrastructure (e.g., AV system)	Not a good replica of every clinical setting; Does not probe actual clinical system.
	Easy to schedule	Remote from site of clinical work
	Setup time is minimized	Creating and maintaining dedicated center is expensive.
	Protects personnel from being pulled into real clinical work	
	Facilitates conduct of detailed debriefing of simulation, often involving video review	
In Situ	Probes actual clinical site(s) and system(s)	Vacant clinical space is not always available.
	Can involve personnel near their site of clinical work	Personnel are vulnerable to being pulled away to real clinical work; distraction from onlookers is hard to control.
	Less expensive than operating dedicated simulation center	Setup and cleanup takes more time.
		Debriefing usually limited, brief, or absent; Less AV recording capability

Table 25–5 Scheduled Versus Unannounced In-Situ Simulation

(In Situ)	Pros	Cons
Scheduled	Desired participants can be targeted.	Participants know session is coming; may prepare work unit for simulation (may lose some systems probing ability)
	Protected time for exercise	
	Pre-work/reading can be assigned; simulations can be coordinated with existing lecture program.	Scheduled sessions may have to be in addition to participants' standard tour of duty and may require extra/overtime pay.
Unannounced	Probes individuals, team(s), and system as they actually are.	Pulls personnel from actual patient care work
	Personnel participate as part of their regular duties (no extra pay).	Only minimal setup is feasible for unannounced mock events.
		Whoever is on duty participates, but some may have participated before.

to improve the knowledge, skills, and performance of individual clinicians, teams, and systems by regular practice. There is now a growing body of evidence that simulation can improve technical skill on procedures, especially for those relatively new to the procedure. This makes simulation applicable to help ensure the ability (and the documentation of ability) of house-staff physicians and also in nursing personnel on relevant procedures. Training is typically only one component of comprehensive quality-improvement plans, and in fact, it is a truism of human-factors engineering that "design" of devices or work processes "trumps training." It requires an enormous amount of training to overcome device design or work processes that tend to lead people to do the wrong thing; nonetheless, continuous and intensive training of individuals and teams is a key tenet of high-reliability-organization theory, and it is a cornerstone of safety management in nearly all industries with intrinsically high hazard.

Currently, procedural training is being used to reduce the rate of iatrogenic injury for central venous cannulation and for thoracentesis.[13–15] It is also being used to improve the performance of novices on laparoscopic surgery before they actively engage in surgery under supervision.[16,17] The principle of having early learners climb large parts of the learning curve with simulation before they begin apprenticeship practice is growing.

Beyond invasive procedures, simulation may also be an adjunct to process change in fostering the adoption of evidence-based best practices such as "bundles" aimed at reducing ventilator-associated pneumonia, improving sepsis management, or reducing central-line-complication rates.

Another important target of training is teamwork skills and CRM. While there is not level-1a evidence to prove that adverse events and outcomes are due to CRM failures that can be remedied by CRM training, there is a widespread belief that this is true. It may never be possible to prove this connection with level-1a certainty, or not for all potential applications. It is expected that a comprehensive and sustained program of CRM-oriented training in the domains that most need it will, over time (possibly a long time), lead to better overall clinical performance and thus to better clinical outcome. This may not always be true, of course, especially for patients whose prognosis is already dire. Probably most patients who have an in-hospital cardiac arrest will have a poor prognosis even if the technical and team resuscitation efforts are perfect; however, no one signs up for suboptimal hospital care, even if their prospects are poor.

In determining which clinical arenas would most benefit from simulation-based training, there may be different priorities for education and training between the needs of house-staff programs, quality management, and risk management. Areas of keen interest for one may not be of immediate interest for another. Not all quality issues end up as risk management issues (although eventually they probably do), and certainly many issues of professional education do not directly affect quality, risk, or patient safety.

Examples of clinical areas that have chosen to address known risks include, but are not limited to, the following:

- Radiology. Training radiologists, nurses, and technicians to respond to catastrophic medical events in the radiology suite, including allergy to radiocontrast injection
- Neonatology. Training personnel to conduct extracorporeal membrane oxygenation
- Anesthesiology. Training anesthesiologists and/or operating room teams to manage catastrophic events such as malignant hyperthermia
- Internal Medicine. Training leaders and combined teams for cardiac-arrest resuscitation ("code teams") or rapid response
- Critical Care. Training combined teams to manage serious manifestations of respiratory failure, circulatory failure, or sepsis

- Emergency Medicine or Trauma. Training team leaders and/or teams to handle extreme events including massive hemorrhage, multiple injuries, multiple simultaneous patients, and disaster triage

Training on How to Perform the Non-clinical Response to a Serious Adverse Event

Another training paradigm of high salience for risk management is to use simulation techniques to allow clinicians (along with appropriate risk management personnel) to prepare for, or practice how to respond to, a serious adverse clinical event. This training can include simulations for practice in talking with patients or families and disclosing bad news. It can also include in the clinical simulations practice in securing the workspace, ensuring proper acquisition and safeguarding of key clinical data, and inclusion of risk management as a partner in these activities. Although typically we use standardized patient actors to play the role of family members, we have also on occasion used risk management personnel to play this role. Although they are not trained actors (and thus may not be able to portray as skillfully as broad a spectrum of family response as can the actors), playing this role can give risk management personnel a better appreciation for the family's side of the disclosure of an adverse event.

Systems Probing Using In-Situ Simulation

There are few quality-improvement tools that prospectively identify sources of patient risk. Sentinel-event reporting and root-cause-analysis (RCA) investigations—processes for discovering operator error and latent conditions following adverse events—address adverse events *after* adverse events or near misses occur. Although necessary and effective, RCAs cannot be thought of as a wholly preventive method of error avoidance.

A prospective method for error prevention is the healthcare failure-mode-and-effects analysis (HFMEA), a methodology adapted from other industries (especially nuclear power) to health care in the early 2000s.[18] Investigators conduct HFMEA by generating a list of potential but theoretical hazards (i.e., failure modes) through creative thinking about work-flow processes. Although prospective in nature, HFMEA methodology is limited by human inability to imagine all of the potential directions an emergency response can take, and by the limitless varieties of human behavior in emergencies. We have found that in real patient-care scenarios, a complex mixture of individual and social behaviors evolves in response to challenging situations, and that they lead to sources of errors that are difficult to predict. Patient simulation, and in particular in-situ simulation, can therefore be viewed as a powerful adjunct to the prospective identification of failure modes.

Even simulations in a dedicated center provide good triggers for discussing systemic problems in particular clinical settings. When the simulator is taken to the actual workplace, such probing becomes far more powerful. People and systems are challenged to respond where and how they actually would be challenged. Whole work units can be involved along with ancillary systems throughout the institution. Even small things can go wrong, but, in the proverbial "for want of a nail the shoe was lost" cascade, finding those small things that make a big difference can be very important, especially because they can be fixed systematically.

With in-situ simulation, the "patient" resides within a real workplace, and event management depends upon mastering the immediate environment in addition to diagnosing and providing therapy for the patient's problem. To increase the "yield of discovery" we find it important to require interaction with the unit's real resources and conditions—such as actual equipment, supplies, and people—to the greatest extent possible. That way, if, for example, key materials are not properly stocked, if the system of obtaining help does not work, if modes of communication are not reliable, or if training programs do not prepare providers for real conditions, these facts can be discovered and documented in a simulated event. Both hospital-wide and unit-specific responses to emergency situations can be assessed. Researchers have reported on the use of these techniques to assess the management of pediatric trauma, rescue from sedative overdosing, and management of adult cardiopulmonary arrests.[18-22]

In-situ simulation has also proven worthy in discovering and troubleshooting problems and response systems prior to the use of new patient-care facilities, and may become the standard for assessing the readiness of a new work unit, clinical program, or entire facility prior to its first use for patient care.[20,23-25]

Stanford Experience in Simulation for Systems Probing: The "Hemorrhage Project"

An example of systems probing with in-situ simulation was a series of exercises at our hospital aimed at understanding the factors that impact on the care of patients with life-threatening hemorrhage. Stanford's captive insurance company identified hemorrhage situations as worthy of investigation. Simulation was helpful because the patient outcome in such events is dependent upon a complex set of activities including timely diagnosis of the problem, followed by institution of stabilizing therapy to maintain life-critical hemodynamic functions (e.g., administration of banked blood and products, rapid-response or code teams), controlling the source of bleeding (e.g., interventional radiology, gastroenterology, and surgery), and transfer of care for definitive therapy and follow-up (OR, ICU, etc.). Management of hemorrhage emergencies thus requires high-level skills in communication and leadership, teamwork, and medical decision making.

We hypothesized that there might be some issues unique to specific work areas, and others that would pertain throughout the hospital. To properly understand these differences, we conducted surprise simulations of critical events—usually, but not always, of life-threatening hemorrhage—at a variety of plausible locations throughout the hospital. We allowed all relevant patient-care and support services to be engaged in their usual fashion. For example, if the cardiac-arrest team was requested, it was called without being told that it was a simulation. The team was expected to perform as usual using the same equipment and supplies it would use in a real cardiac arrest. At the outset, we secured support from the leadership of many departments including medicine, surgery, critical care, nursing, patient safety, transfusion medicine, and quality management. Support from the top was an absolute necessity for unannounced mock events to run smoothly without resistance from front-line staff. Our in-situ simulations were organized with assistance from unit managers who chose a staff nurse to be the initial point of contact for the simulated patient. We did provide a very short briefing to the initial nurse as to the capabilities of the simulator and the "rules of the game," but we did not indicate the nature of the upcoming problem. All other personnel were mobilized naturally by the system, and then undertook their usual duties. Using a small camcorder and video cart, we acquired video recordings of the simulations, supplemented by direct observation by project staff. After each simulation, there was a short debriefing in the workplace with those personnel who could stay.

In the case of the hemorrhage project, our results suggested (among other things) the need to standardize the content and methods of communicating with the transfusion department (in one case a doctor phoned the blood bank only to discover that the phone would not ring; the doctor wisely sent a runner), and the lack of widely known standardized protocols for rare but catastrophic problems such as blood loss or allergic reactions.

We conduct unannounced in-situ simulations on a regular basis in different locales throughout the medical centers for code teams and rapid-response teams. They serve a dual role of training for the members of these teams and for continuous system probing.

POTENTIAL APPLICATIONS OF SIMULATION SPECIFIC TO RISK MANAGEMENT'S OWN ACTIVITIES

There are also several possible applications of simulation that specifically target the activities performed by, are under the aegis of, or are directly relevant to risk management itself. To date, there are only a handful of examples, and few have been published; nonetheless, it is worth describing these applications so that, where appropriate, they might be tried.

With regard to case reconstruction, during the investigation or analysis of an actual adverse event it can sometimes be useful to perform a simulation that attempts to reconstruct the details of the event. If simulation models were perfect representations of actual human beings, it would be possible to recreate the physiologic situation to determine quantitatively whether one treatment or another would have been more successful, or the effect of different timing of a treatment. Currently, simulator models are not robust enough to do this, except on a very qualitative basis, with only certain variables, and generally only at the extremes. For example, a simulator model could predict the likely decrease due to apnea of arterial $p_{art}O_2$ (or S_aO_2) in a patient of known size, pulmonary status, body temperature, effort level, and starting alveolar FiO_2.

For full physical recreations of an event, in some cases it can be done with the actual personnel involved, because it may jog their memory for key details that may not come out during interviews; however, their responses in the simulation may be prone strongly to hindsight bias about what "must have happened" or "should have happened." Sometimes a reconstruction is attempted with completely naïve participants (perhaps more than one set) to determine if the behavior of the actual individuals or team was typical or highly aberrant. Any of these techniques may also be used to enhance the individual and organizational learning resulting from the event, such as during a morbidity and mortality conference, in addition to its analytical role in an RCA.

Simulation can be used as an aid in the defense of a malpractice claim. First is the analytical role in helping to understand what may have occurred (whether quantitatively or qualitatively). As suggested previously, in some cases (perhaps not many) simulations can rule in or rule out particular theories or hypotheses about what happened. Simulation can also play a role—often via video recordings—in explaining to a jury the clinical-care processes involved in the case and some of the issues under dispute in the litigation.[26] Such a simulation can illustrate the equipment and procedures involved and demonstrate a typical sequence of events. A more ambitious role, which is alluded to in the previous section, is that simulations with naïve participants may demonstrate that a particular response to a set of occurrences is, in fact, common among reasonable and prudent clinicians trying to solve the problem. Such an undertaking would require a scope of simulation and number of subjects that is typically beyond that which risk management would sponsor, but it could be attempted.

It has also been suggested that, because simulation is still relatively novel for use in hospitals and with experienced personnel, institutions that have regular programs of simulation for training or for systems probing could promote this as a signal of their commitment to patient safety by providing state-of-the-art training and systems assessment for its staff and clinical procedures. To our knowledge, no one has attempted this process. Moreover, as simulation becomes more widely utilized, the relative value of this argument will be undermined.

THEORETICAL LEGAL RISKS OF CONDUCTING SIMULATION TRAINING OR PERFORMANCE ASSESSMENT

In theory, and based on analogy with some other industries, there are potential legal risks involved in conducting simulation training or performance assessment. Where litigation involves a clinician who has undergone simulation training, there are several possibilities. A plaintiff's attorney might allege that the training was faulty ("negative training"), leading the clinician to perform improperly (this might also be argued by the defendant clinician against the provider of the training). Or a plaintiff's attorney might argue that the clinician's performance in the simulation was poor, and that the simulation instructor should have recognized the erroneous performance and intervened administratively with the participant's department or practice group. To the best of our knowledge, neither kind of legal action has yet been attempted in healthcare litigation.

There are programs underway in which simulation is used as an adjunct to evaluate or remediate clinicians whose skills are in question.[27,28] Some of these programs operate under the aegis of a state medical board or equivalent. We do believe that because of the unique window on performance that simulation can give, it can be a useful component of the evaluation and retraining of the marginal clinician; however, a set of simulation exercises by themselves should not be the sole basis of decision about a clinician, and the simulation providers are unlikely to declare a clinician safe vs. unsafe, or competent vs. incompetent. At the most, they would provide data and interpretation about the performance in the simulations that can be used by a duly constituted credentialing or review panel in making their determination. In the long run, it will be beneficial to establish empirical benchmarks of performance by known competent clinicians on challenging scenarios in order to compare the performance of those being scrutinized.

When used as a part of credentialing, there is also a theoretical risk of legal action by the clinician if their privileges are suspended or terminated. Again, we are not aware of any such litigation as yet; nonetheless, the fear of such risks has been a barrier to the widespread use of simulation for remedial assessment and training. Any simulation center that initiates a remedial evaluation and training program is advised to clarify the potential legal risks and the potential need for targeted insurance to cover them.

THE POWER AND THE PROMISE OF SIMULATION IN MANAGING HEALTHCARE RISK

Simulation is a very powerful technique that has multiple applications in healthcare risk management. Although some forms of simulation are inexpensive, many require investment in both hardware and "people-ware." It is not simple to conduct good simulations, and they are only as good as the skill of the instructors who run them. We believe that these investments will pay off over the long run, through enhanced clinician skill, smoother-functioning clinical systems, and smarter risk management. The ultimate goal is to make patient care safer and more effective for everyone. Risk management cannot get any better than that.

We started this chapter asking, "Why have so many intrinsically hazardous endeavors relied so heavily on simulation, whereas health care has been relatively late to the party?" Indeed, it is a very important and provocative question. Undoubtedly, the inherent appeal of simulation, as far as risk management applications are concerned, is that it is intuitive. So many of the benefits from education, training, rehearsals of complicated procedures, performance and competency assessment, human-factors investigations, and exploration of team behaviors and safety culture (single discipline and multidisciplinary) are, in a word, "obvious"; yet, health care lags significantly behind other high-risk industries such as aviation, military, and nuclear power production. Why is that the case?

There may be several reasons for this lag, but from a risk management perspective, the authors of this chapter believe strongly that the risk management profession has the potential to lead the way with others in the vigorous adoption of simulation throughout the healthcare sector. Healthcare risk management has been on a journey since its wide adoption in the midst of the medical-malpractice crisis decades ago to the modern patient safety movement in the wake of the Institute of Medicine report on medical error and injury in health care.[29] The modern trend in healthcare risk management is transitioning from heavy reliance on retrospective analysis of accidents (e.g., RCA, claims analysis, peer review) to incorporate, and even shift, emphasis to the prospective analysis of risk using analytical tools such as such as FMEA and the triangulation of risk information generated from traditional sources of risk information such as incident reports, patient-complaint systems, and sophisticated claim-information systems that utilize rich accident-causation taxonomies to identify the genesis of accidents (e.g., strategies from CRICO/RMF [Controlled Risk Insurance Company of Vermont/Risk Management Foundation], a risk retention group belonging to the Harvard Medical Institutions).

The ultimate "BHAG" (big-hairy-audacious-goal) in healthcare risk management is to identify and prevent accidents waiting to happen, or, in terms of James Reason's model of accident causation, to close as many "Swiss cheese holes" (latent errors) as possible in order to prevent accidents and harm to patients.[30] At Stanford, simulation is embraced by its captive insurance company because this has been proven to be an effective risk management technique. For exam-

ple, in-situ simulation is readily sponsored and funded in an open offer to all of its insured hospitals and faculty physicians, because it is recognized as an effective—if not the most effective—and efficient prospective method for identification of failure points in medical care so that they can be quickly corrected before they lead to accidents and harm to patients. We think of in-situ simulation as FMEA on steroids in real time! Simulation also has proven intrinsic value, because it prepares care providers for low-frequency/high-severity events (e.g., massive hemorrhage protocols) by stress testing and probing for systemic errors while simultaneously teaching clinicians the principles of crisis resource management, teamwork, and understanding deep-rooted cultural behaviors in the context of health-care delivery. Provoking accidents and mistakes in the simulated environment for the purpose of individual and team learning, as well as accident prevention, has inherent worth; yet, widespread adoption and integration of simulation application in health-care risk management has not occurred at a pace that is commensurate with other high-risk industry sectors.

The promise of simulation in risk management is bright. A crucial issue to the further spread of simulation for risk management applications is the funding of simulation ventures. We believe that managers of risk stand in an excellent position to influence simulation funding either through reinvestment of self-insured gains, calling upon their insurance companies, partnering with hospital administration and medical group leadership, or seeking public or private grants such as those funded by organizations such as the American Society for Health Care Risk Management. The future is now, and the present authors look to the risk management community to help advance the risk management applications of simulation with sincere optimism—one that matches the intense passion that drives the profession toward its vision of safe and trusted health care.

References

1. Gaba, D.M. (2007). The future vision of simulation in healthcare. *Simulation in Healthcare, 2,* 126–135.

2. Rall, M., & Gaba, D. (2010). Patient simulation. In R. Miller (Ed.), *Anesthesia* (pp. 151–192). Philadelphia: Churchill Livingstone.

3. Helmreich, R., & Foushee, H. (1993). Why crew resource management? In E. Weiner, B. Kanki, & R. Helmreich (Eds.), *Cockpit resource management* (pp. 3–46). San Diego: Academic Press.

4. Gaba, D., Howard, S., Fish, K., Smith, B.E., & Sowb, Y.A. (2001). Simulation-based training in anesthesia crisis resource management (ACRM): A decade of experience. *Simulation & Gaming, 32,* 175–193.

5. Riley, R.H. (2008). *A manual of simulation in healthcare.* Oxford: Oxford University Press.

6. Kyle, R., & Murray, W.B. (2008). *Clinical simulation: Operations, engineering and management.* Burlington, MA: Academic Press.

7. Gallagher, C.J., & Issenberg, S.B. (2006). *Simulation in anesthesia.* Philadelphia: Saunders.

8. Cooper, J.B., Barron, D., Blum, R., Davison, J.K., Feinstein, D., Halasz, J., et al. (2000). Video teleconferencing with realistic simulation for medical education. *Journal of Clinical Anesthesiology,* 12:256–261.

9. Fanning, R.M., & Gaba, D.M. (2007). The role of debriefing in simulation-based learning. *Simulation & Healthcare, 2,* 115–125.

10. Gaba, D. (1992). Improving anesthesiologists' performance by simulating reality (editorial). *Anesthesiology, 76,* 491–494.

11. Mcintosh, C. (2009). Lake Wobegone for anesthesia. Where everyone is above average except those who aren't: Variability in the management of simulated intraoperative critical incidents (editorial). *Anesthesia & Analgesia, 108,* 6–9.

12. Howard, S., Gaba, D., Fish, K., Yang, G., & Sarnquist, F.H. (1992). Anesthesia crisis resource management training: Teaching anesthesiologists to handle critical incidents. *Aviation Space & Environmental Medicine, 63,* 763–770.

13. Wayne, D.B., Barsuk, J.H., O'Leary, K.J., Fudala, M., & McGaghie, W. (2008). Mastery learning of thoracentesis skills by internal medicine residents using simulation technology and deliberate practice. *Journal of Hospital Medicine, 3,* 48–54.

14. Duncan, D.R., Morgenthaler, T.I., Ryu, J.H., & Daniels, C.E. (2009). Reducing iatrogenic risk in thoracentesis: Establishing best practice via experiential training in a zero-risk environment. *Chest, 135,* 1315–1320.

15. Gaba, D.M., & Dunn, W.F. (2009). Procedural risks in thoracentesis: Process, progress, and proficiency (editorial). *Chest, 135,* 1120–1123.

16. Seymour, N.E., Gallagher, A.G., Roman, S.A., O'Brien, M., Bansal, V.K., & Andersen, D.K., et al. (2002). Virtual reality training improves operating room performance: Results of a randomized, double-blinded study. *Annals of Surgery, 236,* 458–463.

17. Grantcharov, T.P., Kristiansen, V.B., Bendix, J., Bardram, L., Rosenberg, J., & Funch-Jensen, P. (2004). Randomized clinical trial of virtual reality simulation for laparoscopic skills training. *British Journal of Surgery, 91,* 146–150.

18. De Rosier, J., Stalhandske, E., Bagian, J.P., & Nudell, T. (2002). Using health care failure mode and effect analysis: The VA National Center for Patient Safety's Prospective Risk Analysis System. *Joint Commission Journal of Quality Improvement, 27*(5), 248–267.

19. Blike, G.T., Christoffersen, K., Cravero, J.P., Andeweg, S.K., & Jensen, J. (2005). A method for measuring system safety and latent errors associated with pediatric procedural sedation. *Anesthesia & Analgesia, 101,* 48–58.

20. Kobayashi, L., Shapiro, M.J., Sucov, A., Woolard, R., Boss III, R.M, & Dunbar, J., et al. (2006). Portable advanced medical simulation for new emergency department testing and orientation. *Academic Emergency Medicine, 13*(6), 691–695.

21. Hunt, E., Walker, A.R., Shaffner, D.H., Miller, M.R., & Pronovost, P.J. (2008). Simulation of in-hospital pediatric medical emergencies and cardiopulmonary arrests. *Pediatrics, 121,* e34–e43.

22. Marsch, S.C.U., Franziska, T., Semmer, N., Spychiger, M., Breuer, M., & Hunziker, P.R.. (2005). Performance of first responders in simulated cardiac arrests. *Critical Care Medicine, 33*(5), 963–967.

23. Villamaria, F.J., Pliego, J.F., Wehbe-Janek, H., Coker, N., Rajab, M.H., & Sibbitt, S., et al. (2008). Using simulation to orient code blue teams to a new hospital facility. *Simulation & Healthcare, 3,* 209–216.

24. Rodriguez-Paz, J.M., Mark, L.J., Herzer, K.R., Michelson, J.D., Grogan, K.L., & Herman, J. et al. (2009). A novel process for introducing a new intraoperative program: A multidisciplinary paradigm for mitigating hazards and improving patient safety. *Anesthesia & Analgesia, 108,* 202–210.

25. Nunnink, L., Welsh, A.M., Abbey, M., & Buschel, C. (2009). In situ simulation-based team training for post-cardiac surgical emergency chest reopen in the intensive care unit. *Anaesthesia and Intensive Care, 37,* 74–78.

26. Kofke, W.A., Rie, M.A., & Rosen, K. (2001). Acute care crisis simulation for jury education. *Medical Law, 20,* 79–83.

27. Rosenblatt, M.A., & Abrams, K.J. (2002). The use of a human patient simulator in the evaluation of and development of a remedial prescription for an anesthesiologist with lapsed medical skills. *Anesthesia & Analgesia, 94,* 149–153.

28. Levine, A.I., & Bryson, E.O. (2008). The use of multimodality simulation in the evaluation of physicians with suspected lapsed competence. *Journal of Critical Care, 23,* 197–202.

29. Kohn, L., Corrigan, J., & Donaldson, M. (Eds.). (2000). *To err is human: Building a safer health care system.* Committee on Quality of Health Care in America, Institute of Medicine. Washington, DC: National Academy Press.

30. Reason, J. (1990). *Human error.* Cambridge: Cambridge University Press.

26

CREATING A MINDFULNESS OF PATIENT SAFETY AMONG PHYSICIANS THROUGH EDUCATION

Barbara A. Connelly, RN, MJ
Mahendr S. Kochar, MD, MS, MBA, MACP, FACC, FRCP (London)

INTRODUCTION

Although much has been achieved in patient safety over the past decade, medical education rarely includes patient safety and quality-improvement education in medical school or residency training. The physicians lead the healthcare team but fall behind when it comes to patient safety. Today, there are few physicians who have the knowledge and experience to teach it. This chapter examines the barriers to patient safety education in medicine and identifies how the healthcare risk management professional is uniquely qualified to teach physicians about patient safety and quality improvement. The chapter provides an outline of a comprehensive patient safety and quality-improvement curriculum and discusses how integrating patient safety and quality improvement into clinical practice is necessary to create a culture of safety.

While there were many studies available in the 1980s and early 1990s that described the breadth of medical errors in health care, two things captured the attention of the media and created a lasting focus on the need to avoid patient injuries; the first was a series of reported tragic injuries and deaths due to medical errors (see Table 26–1),[1] and the second was the release of the Institute of Medicine's (IOM) report titled, "To Err Is Human: Building a Safer Health System."[2] The IOM report stated that most medical errors are system based, and most patient safety activity should be driven from a system perspective rather than blaming individuals for errors.[2] Over the past decade there has been an explosion of information on patient safety. The number of patient safety initiatives and the number of required hospital-quality reports have increased markedly. Although physicians drive the majority of health care in the United States, little has been done to require their participation in patient-safety-improvement activities.[3] Physicians admit patients to hospitals, discharge them, diagnose, develop plans of care, order

Table 26–1 Selected Medical Errors That Garnered Extensive Media Attention in the United States Accreditation Council for Graduate Medical Education (ACGME)

Error	Institution	Year	Impact
An 18-year-old woman, Libby Zion, daughter of a prominent reporter, dies of a medical mistake, partly due to lax resident supervision	Cornell's New York Hospital	1984	Public discussion regarding resident training, supervision, and work hours; led to New York law regarding supervision and work hours, ultimately culminating in ACGME duty-hour regulations
Betsy Lehman, a Boston Globe healthcare reporter, dies of a chemotherapy overdose	Harvard's Dana Farber Cancer Institute	1994	New focus on medication errors, role of ambiguity in prescriptions and possible role of computerized prescribing and decision support
Willie King, a 51-year-old diabetic, has the wrong leg amputated	University Community Hospital Tampa, Florida	1995	New focus on wrong-site surgery, ultimately leading to The Joint Commission's Universal Protocols to prevent these errors
Two healthy young volunteers (Jesse Gelsinger and Ellen Roche) die while participating in research studies	University of Pennsylvania (J.G.); Johns Hopkins Hospital (E.R.)	1999 and 2001, respectively	New focus on protecting research subjects from harm
18-month-old Josie King dies of dehydration	Johns Hopkins Hospital	2001	Josie's parents form an alliance with Johns Hopkins leadership (leading to the Josie King Foundation and catalyzing Hopkins' safety initiatives), demonstrating the power of institutional and patient collaboration
Jesica Santillan, a 17-year-old girl from Mexico, dies after receiving a heart–lung transplant of the wrong blood type	Duke University Medical Center	2003	New focus on errors in transplantation, and on enforcing strict, high-reliability protocols for communication of crucial data

diagnostic tests, and determine which treatments are needed and what medications should be ordered. They manage and control 70–80 % of all healthcare dollars spent.[4]

Throughout medical school and residency training, physicians are taught to be autonomous and not taught to view medical errors from a system perspective.[5,6] Is it any wonder that there is a disjointedness between most patient safety initiatives, which take a systems approach, and engaging physicians in quality and safety?

Physician participation in patient safety is imperative for health care to achieve a substantial and lasting improvement in patient safety. Physicians need education about patient safety, quality improvement, and system-related causes of error throughout their training and professional career. This will prepare them to create an awareness of safety at the worksite and lead efforts to improve patient care.

BARRIERS TO PHYSICIAN INVOLVEMENT IN PATIENT SAFETY

Most physicians have a strong allegiance to their patients and strive to provide the best possible care. Physicians do not want to see their patients injured by a medical error, yet the literature is full of comments about the lack of physician involvement in the patient safety and quality-improvement initiatives. Brennan reported that physicians actually impede efforts to improve quality.[3] The IOM reports, "To Err Is Human"[2] and "Crossing the Chasm,"[7] were aimed at the public, instead of the medical community, to avoid physicians' "inertia" when it comes to quality improvement.[3] Lucian Leape, an early investigator of medical errors and a physician expert on patient safety, remarked that most physicians do not contemplate patient safety and are apathetic about it.[8] It is important to understand the barriers to physician involvement in patient safety when designing a patient safety and quality-improvement curriculum (see Table 26–2).

CULTURE OF MEDICINE

While the lack of active physician involvement in patient safety efforts frustrates those in health care who are charged with moving the patient safety agenda forward, it can be linked to how physicians are educated and

Table 26–2 Barriers to Physician Involvement in Patient Safety

Culture of Medicine	Medical Education	Practice	Limited Patient Safety Measures
Autonomy	Limited education on quality, patient safety	Small group or solo practices	Lack of comparative data
Personal responsibility	Lack of interdisciplinary training	Recent changes in healthcare business practices	Quality of data dependent on voluntary reporting
Hierarchical authority	Crowded medical-school curriculums	Increasing demands created by complex system	Limited expertise in research in safety
	Service needs in residency and on-call demands	Financial disincentives	
	Duty-hour restrictions		

the culture within the medical profession that forms the beliefs, norms, and values that are the foundation of physician behavior. During their medical education, and throughout residency and fellowship training, physicians are taught to be autonomous and to have a deep sense of personal responsibility for their individual patients. [9]

The National Patient Safety Foundation conducted a needs-assessment survey on patient safety among physicians and nurses and reported that 78% of physicians agreed that health care has a collective responsibility for errors, yet only 49% felt that errors were best addressed at the system level. Consistent with the profession's belief in personal responsibility, physicians asserted that errors are an individual's issue.[6] This focus on individual responsibility contradicts the current emphasis placed on system improvements by patient safety leaders who purport that most medical errors are made by competent providers who work in complex environments.[1]

Although breakdown in communication frequently contributes to, or causes, medical errors and patient injuries, there is an intrinsic hierarchical authority in health care that creates a steep power gradient that stifles communication. There is a clear order of authority with all other disciplines being subordinate to the attending physician. This hierarchical authority often leads to communication barriers between physicians, nurses, pharmacists, etc., and impedes the safety of patients. Medical students and residents learn early in their training that silence as a situational response can serve them well, rather than drawing the attention and criticism of their supervising physicians when they identify an error.[10] Errors that result in near-miss situations are often ignored because no actual harm was done. Research and surveys have identified that nurses and other healthcare providers perceive communication with physicians to be problematic; however, physicians rarely share this perception.[11]

Medical Education

As noted previously, the culture of medicine often limits physician involvement in patient safety. The foundation of this culture is built in medical school and residency training with a science-based curriculum that emphasizes memorization and acquisition of technical skills. The beliefs, norms, and values of the medical community are assimilated by medical students and residents through socialization resulting in the physician's intense sense of responsibility for patients and a strong reliance on self and other physicians. Medical students and residents are provided little, if any, education about quality improvement, patient safety, communication skills, or how healthcare systems or technical design can influence patient outcomes.[12] They are also not educated about the dynamics of teamwork, even though most health care is delivered by interdisciplinary teams.

In a review of recently published medical textbooks and the curricula of 125 medical schools, it was evident that little has been done to integrate patient safety into medical education since the publication of the IOM report "To Err Is Human." In 2007 and 2008, only 10% of the 125 U.S. medical schools reported having patient safety content in required or elective courses.[13] A significant roadblock to incorporating patient safety into a medical-school curriculum is the strong competition for time in an already full curriculum.

Instruction in patient safety should begin early in medical school and continue to be integrated into clinical course work and rotations. It is important that this instruction continue throughout graduate medical education training as a physician's pattern of clinical practice and professional behavior is established during residency training.[10] During their busy days and nights of on-call duty, residents often witness, or are involved in, errors, but it is unlikely that they have the skill set needed to effectively manage harm-producing errors or near-miss situations, or to critically examine them to study their prevention.

Graduate medical education, in certain ways, is an apprenticeship. The less-experienced physician learns from the more experienced, including how to deal with errors.[12] They also learn by doing. Unless an attending physician has developed an interest in patient safety, it is unlikely that it would be taught to medical students and residents. So while medical and hospital-accreditation organizations have recognized the need for medical education on patient safety and quality improvement, few physicians and program directors are prepared to provide that education.[14]

Practice Structure

The practice of medicine takes place in very complex and structured healthcare systems that consume physicians' time and attention, thereby creating a barrier for their involvement in patient safety. While the modern patient safety movement looks to other complex, highly reliable industries that rely on technology for their improvements to find examples of how to eliminate error, the provision of health care is unique in that it is dependent on human relationships between all members of the interdisciplinary team.[5] Frequently, the physician specialist and providers from other disciplines have overlapping patient-care responsibilities. The rapid advancement in technology and pharmaceuticals, and increased service demands, add to this complexity.[15] To successfully provide patient care in this work environment, providers must spend valuable time to increase their verbal- and written-communication skills. It is difficult to keep up with the workload and get through each day.[16] Physicians are frustrated with the escalating demands, which leave little time to focus on improvements.

Various business structures in which physicians practice result in a self-focus that also contributes to limited participation

in safety and quality. Today, many physicians still practice solo or in small groups,[17] and their practices are the focal point of their professional and business interests. Quality issues that arise in a physician's practice are often not in sync with those of the hospital. In addition, many physicians believe that most patient safety issues arise in hospitals and see few opportunities for improvement in their own practices. Similarly, physicians who are employed by healthcare systems or who practice in academic medical centers have other factors such as productivity demands, organizational expectations, bureaucracy, and hierarchy that they perceive as barriers to engaging in patient safety and quality. Often, today's physicians are members of multiple hospital medical staffs and can be in competition with each other or the hospital(s) for revenue.[9]

Perhaps the most insidious barrier to engaging physicians in patient safety and quality-improvement strategies may be the financial disincentives to do so. In the past, neither physicians nor hospitals that improve their patients' outcomes were financially rewarded for their efforts. Physician reimbursement has been based on a fee-for-service payment and hospital reimbursement has been based on a prospective payment system for most payors regardless of the quality of care provided or the clinical outcome. Until recently, providers have received higher reimbursement for patients that have complications. The Center for Medicare and Medicaid Services (CMS) has now begun to apply strategies for pay-for-performance and non-reimbursement for hospital-acquired conditions to physicians.[18]

Limited Patient Safety Data

It can be difficult to engage physicians' interest in patient safety without research and reports that accurately measure an organization's errors and injuries. Information and data on patient safety has been limited until recently because the science of patient safety is new. Furthermore, measurements of errors can be difficult to obtain when the errors do not result in an injury, and reporting of errors is often voluntary and sometimes anonymous (to encourage reporting). In his book *Understanding Patient Safety*, Wachter outlines the difficulty in obtaining reliable measurements related to patient safety.[1] Although written or electronic incident reports, the primary mode of reporting errors or injuries, are useful for gathering information to manage individual occurrences, they do not necessarily provide a true picture of the number, types, or trends of errors. As noted previously, incident reporting is voluntary and it is widely acknowledged that few physicians complete an incident report. A remarkable feature of incident reporting is that an increase in the reporting rate often represents increased voluntary reporting rather than an actual increase in the number of errors or patient injuries. Unfortunately, because of concerns about medical-malpractice lawsuits and patient-privacy rights, the data and contributing factors about medical errors are rarely shared with physicians and staff, thus creating missed opportunities for them to learn and improve.

HEALTHCARE RISK MANAGEMENT PROFESSIONALS AS TEACHERS OF PATIENT SAFETY

Risk management professionals are uniquely qualified to develop and deliver education on patient safety for physicians. They understand the quality-improvement principles that underpin patient safety initiatives. They possess finely honed skills in identifying risks that can lead to medical errors, and they work with and manage system-based issues on a daily basis. Additionally, they intimately know the downstream results of patient injury and are familiar with the tenets of medical malpractice. Risk management professionals are not only able to develop and teach a patient safety curriculum to physi-

cians, they are in a unique position to provide a framework for the applied learning of safety principles by consulting with and coaching physicians when medical errors occur.

Healthcare risk management professionals have worked with medical errors and patient injuries since the early 1970s when their role in health care arose to address rapidly escalating professional-liability insurance costs.[19] The risk management process in health care extends beyond a focus on economic losses by including prevention, early identification, and the management of risks related to patients, visitors, and staff. The risk management process also includes analysis of the specific behaviors and practices that result in injury and litigation.[20] Although the role and responsibility of the healthcare risk professional varies depending on the size and needs of the organization, and how the organization finances its losses, all healthcare risk management programs include functions aimed at preventing or reducing loss and managing claims and lawsuits. Such duties include thorough investigations and management of serious adverse events, the development of strategies to prevent injuries, education for providers at all levels within the organization, and responsibility for risk-related policies and procedures such as incident reporting, informed consent, sentinel-event management, and confidentiality.[20]

Healthcare risk management professionals are an excellent choice to teach or facilitate the instruction of patient safety to physicians, because they have a working knowledge of patient safety theory and the necessary skill set to do so. Healthcare risk management professionals are able to identify contributing factors and underlying causes of medical errors. They understand system theories, human-factors engineering, environmental factors, and the concepts of blame and accountability. Additionally, they have access to a great deal of information regarding potential loss from administrative sources as well as from data collected about patient injuries through incident reports and claims and lawsuits. They are familiar with and use quality-improvement principles to bring about change to reduce risk exposures.[21] More recently, healthcare risk management professionals have utilized modern patient safety theories to enhance their effectiveness and to help create a culture of safety in the healthcare environment. Successful healthcare risk professionals have a core skill set that enables them to manage, consult, lead, teach, and move their agenda forward. In a national survey of healthcare risk managers reported in 2006, 35% of all respondents said that they spend at least 50% of their time doing patient safety work. Only 3% reported that they do not do patient safety work.[22]

When adverse events occur, risk management professionals have the unique opportunity to reinforce patient safety and risk-reduction concepts through their consultative services to physicians and other healthcare providers. Adverse events create teachable moments at the bedside, because the provider is emotionally engaged in firsthand experience and is motivated for change. Teachable moments help providers learn patient safety and apply improvement concepts in a powerful way.

BUILDING A PATIENT SAFETY CURRICULUM FOR PHYSICIANS

An effective patient safety curriculum for physicians must include several elements. Firstly, the curriculum must be meaningful to physicians and it should complement the existing curriculum used in medical schools and graduate medical education.[15] Secondly, it should utilize multiple teaching techniques to engage physicians' interests. Thirdly, the curriculum should be flexible so that it can be taught in one course or across time. Fourthly, and most importantly, the curriculum should cultivate a mindfulness of patient safety at the worksite. The curriculum must

also demonstrate how each module and topic is relevant to the six general competencies for physicians. In 1999, the Accreditation Council for Graduate Medical Education (ACGME), the organization that accredits graduate medical education (GME), established a requirement that all resident physicians must be competent in six areas of practice.[23] These six competencies have been widely accepted by other physician organizations (see Table 26–3).

Instructors

As mentioned previously, healthcare risk management professionals are well qualified to teach a patient safety curriculum. There may be other clinicians, non-clinicians, educators, managers, or other health professionals within a medical school or organization who can be called upon to teach a patient safety curriculum.[15] In addition to being knowledgeable about the science of patient safety and quality improvement, the qualifications needed to teach a curriculum include strong interpersonal, analytical, and teaching skills.[21] Ideally, content experts from across the medical school or organization would teach sections of the curriculum that are related to their respective fields of expertise.

Teaching Methods and Learning Environment

The objectives of a patient safety curriculum for physicians are to engage them in patient safety, have them identify with the concepts, and, ultimately, have them apply the acquired knowledge in their practice. The teaching methods and case examples must capture their attention and interest and be seen as being applicable to real patient care. A study by Kolb and Kolb about the use of experiential learning in higher education demonstrated that when learners actively participate in the learning process, they have better retention of the material and a greater ability to transfer the

Table 26–3 Accreditation Council for Graduate Medical Education Core Competencies

Patient Care	Residents must be able to provide patient care that is compassionate, appropriate, and effective for the treatment of health problems and the promotion of health.
Medical Knowledge	Residents must demonstrate knowledge of established and evolving biomedical, clinical, epidemiological, and social–behavioral sciences, as well as the application of this knowledge to patient care.
Practice-Based Learning and Improvement	Residents must demonstrate the ability to investigate and evaluate their care of patients, to appraise and assimilate scientific evidence, and to continuously improve patient care based on constant self-evaluation and lifelong learning. Residents are expected to develop skills and habits to be able to meet the following goals: • Identify strengths, deficiencies, and limits in one's knowledge and expertise • Set learning and improvement goals • Identify and perform appropriate learning activities • Systematically analyze practice using quality-improvement methods, and implement changes with the goal of practice improvement • Incorporate formative evaluation feedback into daily practice; locate, appraise, and assimilate evidence from scientific studies related to their patients' health problems • Use information technology to optimize learning • Participate in the education of patients, families, students, residents, and other health professionals
Interpersonal and Communication Skills	Residents must demonstrate interpersonal and communication skills that result in the effective exchange of information and collaboration with patients, their families, and health professionals. Residents are expected to: • Communicate effectively with patients, families, and the public, as appropriate, across a broad range of socioeconomic and cultural backgrounds • Communicate effectively with physicians, other health professionals, and health-related agencies • Work effectively as a member or leader of a healthcare team or other professional group • Act in a consultative role to other physicians and health professionals • Maintain comprehensive, timely, and legible medical records, if applicable
Professionalism	Residents must demonstrate a commitment to carrying out professional responsibilities and an adherence to ethical principles. Residents are expected to demonstrate: • Compassion, integrity, and respect for others • Responsiveness to patient needs that supersedes self-interest • Respect for patient privacy and autonomy • Accountability to patients, society, and the profession • Sensitivity and responsiveness to a diverse patient population including, but not limited to, diversity in gender, age, culture, race, religion, disabilities, and sexual orientation

Table 26–3 (Continued)

System-Based Practice	Residents must demonstrate an awareness of, and responsiveness to, the larger context and system of health care, as well as the ability to effectively call on other resources in the system to provide optimal health care. Residents are expected to: • Work effectively in various healthcare-delivery settings and systems relevant to their clinical specialty • Coordinate patient care within the healthcare system relevant to their clinical specialty • Incorporate considerations of cost awareness and risk–benefit analysis in patient- and/or population-based care as appropriate • Advocate for quality patient care and optimal patient-care systems • Work in inter-professional teams to enhance patient safety and improve patient-care quality • Participate in identifying system errors and implementing potential system solutions

Accreditation Council for Graduate Medical Education. 2007 *ACGME Institutional Requirements*. Chicago, Illinois, Accreditation Council for Graduate Medical Education; July 2007. http://www.acgme.org/acWebsite/irc/irc_IRCpr07012007.pdf. Accessed March 28, 2009.

newly acquired information to different situations.[24] It is equally necessary to engage the learner emotionally. Experiential learning and emotion activation together allow the learning experience to be as realistic as possible. This allows the learner to assimilate the patient safety and quality-improvement concepts and apply them to clinical practice.[25] Accordingly, multiple teaching methods should be utilized whenever possible to enhance learning.[15] The examples include lectures, self-study, interactive group discussions, patient-based case scenarios, healthcare simulations, objective structured clinical examinations (OSCE), and clinical observations.

If physicians are expected to actively participate in learning, the environment should be stimulating yet safe. The instructor must create and control the learning environment so that physicians enrolled in the curriculum are comfortable participating, discussing, and reflecting without concern about being humiliated or ridiculed.

With regard to curriculum modules and topics, a patient safety and quality-improvement curriculum should not only *inform* physicians, but should also prepare them to lead (see Table 26–4). Accordingly, in addition to core topics, a comprehensive curriculum should explore the unique position physicians hold in health care and the barriers that exist to assimilating patient safety in both healthcare systems and medicine.[6] To effectively understand and manage medical errors and contribute to the improvement of healthcare delivery systems, a patient safety curriculum for physicians should include:

- The history and background of patient safety
- The culture of medicine and medical education
- System-based theories
- Quality improvement
- Communication
- Interdisciplinary teamwork
- Organizational and community demand for safer patient care
- Application of patient safety and quality-improvement theory, tools, and initiatives in clinical practice
- Liability exposure and legal actions that may arise from patient injuries

Table 26–4 Outline of a Patient Safety Curriculum for Physicians

Modules and Related Physician Competencies	Synopsis of Topics

Patient Safety
    Professionalism
    Systems-Based Practice
	History: an overview of the modern patient safety movement from the early 1990s work identifying serious concerns about patient safety to the present day.

	Culture of Medicine: a review of the physician's role in patient safety and quality improvement and the culture of medicine with a focus on tradition, medical education, and medical-practice structures.
	To Err Is Human: the IOM report published in 1999, which reported that up to 98,000 people die each year as a result of medical errors. This report garnered the public's interest in patient safety.
	Crossing the Chasm: the IOM report that suggested that there are large gaps in health care between the care patients receive and the care that is available.
	Definitions: the definitions of terms commonly used in discussions of, and study of, patient safety.
	Government and Private-Sector Response: see Table 26–5 for a list of many organizations that are active in patient safety. Often these organizations have initiatives that require hospital compliance.

Systems
    Practice-Based Learning
        and Improvement
    Systems-Based Practice
	Errors: a review of the different types of errors and learning how understanding errors can lead to improved health care.

	Swiss Cheese Model: the system model of active and latent failures as described by James Reason.
	Blunt-End and Sharp-End Model: the system model by David Wood that considers how the decisions made at the administrative level impact the delivery of patient care.
	Hindsight-Bias Theory: the theory by Richard Cook that investigations into errors often stop with the individuals involved in making the error without looking for causative or contributing factors.
	Root-Cause Analysis (RCA): the analytical method for identifying causative factors that lead to an error or potential harm. The Joint Commission requires all accredited hospitals to conduct an RCA when a sentinel event occurs.
	Failure-Mode-and-Effect Analysis: the prospective analysis of design processes to identify the potential for error.
	Utilizing a Defect Tool: utilizing a tool to analyze adverse events in a structured method to identify system failures.
	Just Culture: the theory by David Marx that encourages organizations to adopt a non-punitive philosophy while at the same time aligning the concept of personal responsibility for reckless or willful misconduct.

Table 26–4 (Continued)

Modules and Related Physician Competencies	Synopsis of Topics
	Human-Factors Engineering: the study of the interface between humans and machines or work-flow designs to prevent or minimize the potential for medical errors and patient injury.
Communication Professionalism Patient Care Medical Knowledge	Physician–Patient Communication: the basis that forms the relationship with the patient that takes into account the patient's level of health literacy.
	Informed Consent: the process of informing patients about their health status and proposed plans of treatment so that they understand the associated risks, benefits of treatment, and alternative treatment options so that they can make an informed decision about their health care.
	Disclosure: the discussion with patients about unanticipated outcomes as the result of care and treatment.
	Handoffs: the interactive process of passing patient information from one caregiver to another to assure the continuity of care and the safety of the patient.
	Team Training: the training needed to assure effective communication and work flow among all healthcare team workers to improve the safe delivery of care.
Quality Improvement Practice-Based Learning and Improvement Professionalism	Measurement of Quality: the measurement of structure, process, and outcome to effectively evaluate quality in health care as described by Avedis Donabedian.
	Identifying and Defining Quality Issues: the use of quality-improvement principles to identify and define problems.
	Quality-Improvement Tools: the use of quality-improvement tools to identify sources of unwanted variation in a process and the use of tools to introduce and evaluate interventions.
	Understanding and Using Data Effectively: the review of multiple databases reporting data on quality and patient safety.
	Leading a Team to Improve Quality: the selection of team members and the teamwork needed to lead quality-improvement efforts.
Risk Management Systems-Based Practice Professionalism	Incident Reporting: the reports used to document and manage adverse events and to capture related data for analysis.
	Investigation of Adverse Event: the process of collecting and analyzing information about adverse events and utilizing that information to prevent future occurrences.
	Patient Complaints: the management of individual complaints. Complaints are often a predictor of liability. Data from patient complaints should be collected and analyzed to avoid potential losses.

(continues)

Table 26–4 (Continued)

Modules and Related Physician Competencies	Synopsis of Topics
	Standard of Care: the standard of care is established by expert witnesses from the same field of medicine or health care.
	Medical Malpractice: the legal process in civil court to determine whether the defendant was negligent and, if so, provide compensation to plaintiffs.
	Documentation: the elements of good medical-record documentation that facilitate communication among providers and that gives evidence that the standard of care was met.

Clinical Patient Safety Initiatives
  Medical Knowledge
  Systems-Based Practice
  Practice-Based Learning
    and Improvement
	The Joint Commission National Patient Safety Goals: a list of problems that impact patient safety and recommended solutions that accredited hospitals and other providers are expected to implement.

	The Joint Commission Sentinel Alerts: the publication of The Joint Commission specifically identifying sentinel events and their underlying causes so that steps can be taken to avoid such events.
	Institute for Healthcare Improvement: strategies, including multidisciplinary rounds, rapid-response teams, and interventions to improve care of patients on ventilator support, aimed at reducing death and poor outcomes for hospital patients.
	Surgical Care Improvement Project: a partnership of public and private organizations focused on reducing surgical complications through the implementation of evidence-based measures.
	Infection-Control Practices: the implementation of proven measures that prevent infections especially when used for invasive procedures.
	Medication Safety: the review of errors and adverse events associated with medications and practice strategies that can make the use of medications safer.
	Evidence-Based Practice: the utilization of research results (evidence) when making decisions about health care.

A comprehensive patient safety curriculum is outlined in Table 26–4. The modules and topics can be taught in serial order or each can be taught as a stand-alone unit. For example, the modules could be taught across 4 years of medical school, integrated into a residency training program's core curriculum over the length of training, or a single topic could be presented for a continuing medical education (CME) offering to practicing physicians. Several modules are broad concepts that are central to multiple topics in the curriculum. For example, Informed Consent is a topic under the Communication Module; however, it could also be listed under the Clinical Risk Management Module because informed consent is commonly a cause of action against physicians in lawsuits.

An important part of the curriculum is to familiarize physicians with the demands by the community, government, and healthcare organizations for safer patient care. There are many organizations that are devoted to patient safety, quality improvement, and risk management, and most have initiatives (see Table 26–5). Many of the improvements in patient safety that have been made thus far have been achieved through these initiatives. This is true largely because hospitals have been required to comply with most of these initiatives through regulations, accreditation standards, healthcare payer requirements, or market pressure.

Assessment and Evaluation

An important part of any curriculum is the assessment of the student's learning and an evaluation of the curriculum. Tools that can effectively be used to evaluate learning include multiple-choice questions, short answer and essay questions, written reports, portfolios, presentation of a project or case, and structured oral exams. In addition to assessing student learning, it is equally important to evaluate the curriculum itself to determine its quality and effectiveness. Curriculum evaluation(s) should be developed based on the purpose of the evaluation. For instance, measuring the impact of a patient safety curriculum on patient perception of safety would be much different than evaluating the curriculum content. One method of evaluation is to employ surveys to gather student and faculty impressions on whether the curriculum goals and objectives have been met.[15]

APPLIED LEARNING OF PATIENT SAFETY THEORIES

Safer patient care should be achieved when patient safety theories and measures are applied in clinical practice, in management of an adverse event, and throughout the process of making systematic quality improvements. Patient care should be safer when all healthcare providers, including physicians, incorporate into their clinical practice patient safety measures such as the national patient safety goals, universal protocols, procedural check-

lists, safe medication practices, infection-control practices, better communication, and evidence-based medicine.

Both patients and physicians will be better off if adverse events are immediately reported, properly investigated, and fully disclosed to patients. As noted previously, patient safety concepts are best learned through real experience. Whenever adverse events occur, healthcare risk management professionals should use the moment to educate physicians. They should assist the physician to ascertain what happened, uncover what led to the adverse event, and help learn from the experience by identifying what could have been done differently. Finally, risk management professionals should offer physicians guidance and emotional support.

Physician leadership and perspective is critical to achieving lasting changes within healthcare organizations. For example, participation by physicians who know and understand system-based theories add an additional dimension to quality reviews, such as a root-cause analysis or a peer review. They can help identify system-based causes and develop real quality-improvement strategies. Likewise, involvement by more physicians trained in patient safety and quality improvement can lead to improved patient outcomes across the organization. Such participation should also strengthen physicians' professional satisfaction.

There are two significant changes in medical education that require physician training in patient safety and quality improvement. The first change came from the ACGME, which now mandates that the sponsoring institution demonstrate how residents participate in education on patient safety and quality improvement.[26] In addition, the ACGME also requires all residents to work in interprofessional teams to enhance patient safety and improve patient-care quality in order to meet its system-based competency requirements (see Table 26–3).[27] The second change came from the American Board of Medical Specialties (ABMS), the body that assists

Table 26–5 Selected National Patient Safety, Quality Improvement, and Risk Management Organizations

Organization	Sample Initiative(s)
American Board of Medical Specialties (ABMS) assists 24 approved medical-specialty boards in the development and use of standards in the ongoing evaluation and certification of physicians. http://abms.org/	Requires ongoing measurement of the six core competencies for recertification
Accreditation Council for Graduate Medical Education (ACGME) is responsible for the accreditation of residency and fellowship medical training programs in the United States. http://www.acgme.org/	Requires compliance with: • The number of duty hours that medical trainees may work • Practice-Based Learning and Improvement Core Competency requirement • System-Based Core Competency requirement
Agency for Healthcare Research and Quality (AHRQ) is an agency of the U.S. Department of Health and Human Services. Its mission is to improve the quality, safety, efficiency, and effectiveness of health care for all Americans. Information from AHRQ's research helps people make more informed decisions and improve the quality of healthcare services. AHRQ was formerly known as the Agency for Health Care Policy and Research. http://www.ahrq.gov/	The federal agency that: • Funds research projects on patient safety • Promotes evidence-based practice by funding Evidence-Based Practice Centers (EPC) that develop evidence-based reports and technology assessments on topics relevant to clinical, social science/behavioral, economic, and other healthcare-organization and healthcare-delivery issues—expensive and/or significant for the Medicare and Medicaid populations • Sets Quality Indicators, which are measures of healthcare quality that make use of readily available hospital inpatient administrative data; include prevention, inpatient, patient safety, and pediatric indicators • Administers CAHPS to collect data from standardized patient surveys • Administers the provisions of the Patient Safety Act dealing with Patient Safety Organizations • Administers Patient Safety Network (PSNet), is a national Web-based resource that features the latest news and essential resources on patient safety • Administers WebM&M (Morbidity and Mortality Rounds on the Web), is the online journal and forum on patient safety and healthcare quality. This site features expert analysis of medical errors reported anonymously by our readers, interactive learning modules on patient safety ("Spotlight Cases"), and Perspectives on Safety. Continuing Medical Education (CME) and Continuing Education Unit (CEU) available.

Table 26–5 (Continued)

Organization	Sample Initiative(s)
American Society for Healthcare Risk Management (ASHRM) is a personal-membership group of the American Hospital Association with more than 5,200 members representing health care, insurance, law, and other related professions. ASHRM initiatives focus on developing and implementing safe and effective patient-care practices, the preservation of financial resources, and the maintenance of safe working environments. http://www.ashrm.org/	Has patient safety curriculum for professional healthcare risk managers

Centers for Medicare and Medicare Services (CMS) is an agency of the U.S. Department of Health and Human Services that extends health coverage to almost all Americans aged 65 years or older and to low-income families and individuals with disabilities. http://www.cms.hhs.gov/	Links reimbursement to quality and patient safety by its:
	• Hospital-quality initiative (started in 2001)
	  – Submission of quality data on predefined measures
	  – Reimbursement strategies linked to data
	  – Patient satisfaction
	• Non-payment strategy for certain hospital-acquired conditions (started in 2008)

ECRI Institute is an independent non-profit organization dedicated to applying scientific research to discover which medical procedures, devices, drugs, and processes are best, all to enable one to improve patient care. ECRI Institute plays a major role in technology planning, procurement and management, patient safety, quality and risk management, healthcare policy and research, and healthcare environmental management. It is designated as both a Collaborating Center of the World Health Organization and an Evidence-Based Practice Center by the U.S. Agency for Healthcare Research and Quality. https://www.ecri.org/	Offers the following: • Accident investigation, facilitation of a statewide event-reporting system, and the expertise of a staff of clinical, legal, and quality-management professionals • Comprehensive membership programs, publications, and resources to supplement your patient safety efforts • Resources for tracking medical-device hazards and recalls, viewing problem reports, and reducing medication errors • Tools to address healthcare environmental and occupational safety issues, such as infection control, ergonomics, OSHA compliance, and emergency preparedness • Medical-device-related incident or deficiency reporting to its problem-reporting database • Onsite consulting and customizable programs and solutions to organization-specific challenges
Institute for Healthcare Improvement (IHI) is an independent not-for-profit organization helping to lead the improvement of health care throughout the world. Founded in 1991 and based in Cambridge, Massachusetts, IHI works to accelerate improvement by building the will for change, cultivating promising concepts for improving patient care, and helping healthcare systems put those ideas into action. http://www.ihi.org/IHI/	Develops initiatives for healthcare providers including, but not limited to, the following: • 100,000 Lives Campaign • 5 Million Lives Campaign • Surgical Safety Checklist • Model for Improvement

(continues)

Table 26–5 (Continued)

Organization	Sample Initiative(s)
Institute for Safe Medication Practices (ISMP) is a non-profit organization devoted entirely to medication-error prevention and safe medication use. ISMP started a voluntary practitioner error-reporting program to learn about errors happening across the nation, understand their causes, and share "lessons learned" with the healthcare community. Each year, the national Medication Errors Reporting Program (MERP), operated by the United States Pharmacopeia (USP) in cooperation with ISMP, receives hundreds of error reports from healthcare professionals. http://www.ismp.org/	Develops: • Medication safety tools and resources • Educational programs Has a program, ISMP Medication Errors Reporting Program (MERP), for reporting medication errors
The Joint Commission is an independent not-for-profit organization that accredits and certifies more than 15,000 healthcare organizations and programs in the United States. The Joint Commission accreditation and certification is recognized nationwide as a symbol of quality that reflects an organization's commitment to meeting certain performance standards. Its mission is to continuously improve the safety and quality of care provided to the public through the provision of healthcare accreditation and related services that support performance improvement in healthcare organizations. http://www.jointcommission.org/	Requires its accredited hospitals to comply with its: • Accreditation standards related to patient safety (50% of standards) • Sentinel Event Policy requiring investigations of sentinel events • Universal Protocol on site marking • Speak Up Initiative to educate the public • Quality Check and Quality Reports • Sentinel Event Alert publication to inform hospitals about high-risk situations
Leapfrog Group is a voluntary program aimed at mobilizing employer purchasing power to alert America's health industry that big leaps in healthcare safety, quality, and customer value will be recognized and rewarded. Among other initiatives, Leapfrog works with its employer members to encourage transparency and easy access to healthcare information as well as rewards for hospitals that have a proven record of high-quality care. http://www.leapfroggroup.org/	Rates hospitals on four identified practices: • Computer physician order entry • Evidence-based hospital referral • Intensive care unit staffing by physicians experienced in critical-care medicine • The Leapfrog Safe Practices Score
National Committee for Quality Assurance (NCQA) is a private not-for-profit organization dedicated to improving healthcare quality. Since its founding in 1990, NCQA has been a central figure in driving improvement throughout the healthcare system, helping to elevate the issue of healthcare quality to the top of the national agenda. http://www.ncqa.org/	Gathers statistics that track the quality of care delivered by the nation's health plans

Table 26–5 (Continued)

Organization	Sample Initiative(s)
National Patient Safety Foundation (NPSF) is an independent not-for-profit organization that has one mission: to improve the safety of patients. NPSF fosters collaboration on the issue of patient safety. Its founding sponsors include the American Medical Association, CNA/ HealthPro, 3M, and major benefactor Schering-Plough Corporation. http://www.npsf.org/	Sponsors Stand Up for Patient Safety Program for NPSF members. The program provides information on patient safety implementation strategies, along with practical tools to facilitate the incorporation of patient safety into the hospital culture and enhance existing safety and quality programs.
National Quality Forum is a not-for-profit membership organization created to develop and implement a national strategy for healthcare quality measurement and reporting. A shared sense of urgency about the impact of healthcare quality on patient outcomes, workforce productivity, and healthcare costs prompted leaders in the public and private sectors to create the NQF as a mechanism to bring about national change. Established as a public–private partnership, the NQF has broad participation from all parts of the healthcare system, including national, state, regional, and local groups representing consumers, public and private purchasers, employers, healthcare professionals, provider organizations, health plans, accrediting bodies, labor unions, supporting industries, and organizations involved in healthcare research or quality improvement. http://www.qualityforum.org/	The NQF publication, *Safe Practices for Better Health Care—2009*, presents 34 practices that have been demonstrated to be effective in reducing the occurrence of adverse healthcare events, better known as "never events."
Risk Management Foundation Center for Patient Safety (CRICO/RMF). Its mission is to design models and systems by which the delivery of patient care is made safer. The Center supports ongoing patient safety and medical-error-prevention efforts across the Harvard/CRICO healthcare system and serves as a resource in the rapid dissemination of learning from the data, including analysis, reports, education, publications, and other media. http://www.rmf.harvard.edu/patientsafety/index.html/	Online education on risk reduction and patient safety education
National Coordinating Council for Medication Error Reporting and Prevention (NCC MERP), founded by the US Pharmacopoeia (USP), is an independent body that comprises 24 national healthcare organizations, which are collaborating to address the interdisciplinary causes of errors and to promote the safe use of medications. http://www.nccmerp.org/	Develops recommendations to reduce medication errors

(continues)

Table 26–5 (Continued)

Organization	Sample Initiative(s)
National Center for Patient Safety of the U.S. Department of Veterans Affairs was established in 1999 to develop and nurture a culture of safety throughout the Veterans Health Administration. Its goal is the nationwide reduction and prevention of inadvertent harm to patients as a result of their care. http://www.patientsafety.gov/	Online resources: • NCPS handbook • Cognitive aids on root-cause analysis, fall prevention, escape and elopement, and health Care Failure-Mode-and-effect analysis
National Surgical Quality Improvement Program (NSQIP) by the U.S. Department of Veterans Affairs was implemented in 1994 to provide reliable, valid, and comparative information about surgical outcomes) morbidity and mortality rates) among the 123 Veterans Administration medical centers that perform major surgery. This information enables researchers, clinicians, and managers to identify factors that contribute to high-quality surgical care, as well as those factors that result in less-than-optimal care, and to identify best practices that will improve care. The American College of Surgeons now operates and administers a parallel NSQIP program for the private sector. https://acsnsqip.org/login/default.aspx/	This program develops performance measures that will result in better practices that improve the quality of surgical care. The program: • Provides patient risk-adjusted surgical outcomes to surgical programs to permit valid comparisons with other programs • Provides reliable, believable data • Empowers surgeons to review their quality and make quality improvements (not intended to point out "bad apples") • Emphasizes that quality resides primarily in systems, at program level
The World Alliance for Patient Safety was launched in October 2004 by the World Health Organization (WHO). The Alliance raises awareness and political commitment to improve the safety of care and facilitates the development of patient safety policy and practice in all WHO member states. http://www.who.int /patientsafety/en/	The Alliance delivers a number of programs that cover systemic and technical aspects to improve patient safety around the world. Examples include: • Safe Surgery Saves Lives • Clean Care is Safer Care • Patient Safety Curriculum Guide for Medical Schools

medical-specialty boards in the development and use of standards in the ongoing evaluation and certification of physicians. It now requires physicians to demonstrate professional development through continuous learning and ongoing measurement of the six core competencies in order to maintain their board certification.[28]

These two changes will accelerate the need for physicians to develop their knowledge about system-based errors and actively participate in system-based analysis to identify contributing factors. It is likely that the medical profession will utilize patient rounds, grand rounds, morbidity and mortality (M&M) conferences, and peer review to provide structure to teach and learn analytical and improvement processes. Some academic medical centers have already utilized M&M conferences to incorporate the ACGME core competencies of "System-Based Practice" and "Practice-Based Learning and Improvement" into that activity.[29,30] Berenholtz, Hartsell, and Pronovost have described how fellows in Johns Hopkins Multispecialty Surgical Critical Care Program incorporate what they have learned from system analysis of adverse events into their presentations at M&M conferences. This addition enhances the learning experience and meets the ACGME competencies.[31]

Finally, outcome data from studies and improvement initiatives will help incentivize physicians' involvement in patient safety. The Agency for Healthcare Research and Quality (AHRQ), which is part of the Department of Health and Human Services, has led the way in research studies on patient safety and quality. It has funded over 100 studies on patient safety to uncover the causes of injuries. One example of an AHRQ-funded research study that is having significant impact was the study conducted by Pronovost. It demonstrated that catheter-related bloodstream infections can be reduced to near zero in the ICU setting.[32] Another example comes from an estimated 123,000 patients' lives saved through the Institute for Healthcare Improvement initiative titled "100,000 Lives Campaign," which ran from December 2006 through December 2008. This initiative focused on reducing mortality through use of proven best practices in hospitals across the country.[33]

CONCLUSION

It is imperative to involve physicians so that a lasting culture of safety is achieved. Although few physicians today have sufficient education and training in patient safety, physicians at all levels of training and practice can be educated with a curriculum that incorporates concepts from patient safety, quality improvement, and risk management to create a solid foundation. Such a curriculum should be meaningful for physicians and designed so that it can be utilized at all levels of physician training. It should be flexible so that it can be used for lifelong learning and utilize a variety of teaching methods, including experiential learning, to engage physicians as active participants. Ultimately, patients will be best served if physicians are mindful of patient safety when they are practicing and use their knowledge to lead other physicians and healthcare providers in creating a safer healthcare system.

References

1. Wachter, R.M. (2008). *Understanding patient safety*. New York: McGraw-Hill.
2. Kohn, L., Corrigan, J., & Donaldson, M. (Eds.). (2000). *To err is human: Building a safer health care system*. Committee on Quality of Health Care in America, Institute of Medicine. Washington, DC: National Academy Press.
3. Brennan, T.A., Horwitz, R.I., & Duffy, F.D. (2004). The role of physician specialty board certification status in the quality movement. *Journal of the American Medical Association, 292*(9), 1038–1043.
4. Bain, K.T. (2007). Barriers and strategies to influencing physician behavior (editorial). *American Journal of Medical Quality, 22*(1), 5–7.
5. Leape, L.L., & Berwick, D.M. (2005). Five years after "To err is human": What have we learned? *Journal of the American Medical Association, 293*(19), 2384–2390.
6. VanGeest, J.B., & Cummins, D.S. (2003). *An educational needs assessment for improving patient safety: Results of a national study of physicians and nurses*. National Patient Safety Foundation. http://www.npsf.org/download/EdNeedsAssess.pdf/. Accessed January 31, 2009.
7. Institute of Medicine. (2001). *Crossing the quality chasm: A new health system for the twenty-first century*. Washington, DC: National Academy Press.
8. Buerhaus, P. (2007). Interview: Is hospital patient care becoming safer? A conversation with Lucian Leape. *Health Affairs, 26*(6), w687–w696. http://content.healthaffairs.org/cgi/content/full/hlthaff.26.6.w687/DC1/. Accessed April 3, 2009.
9. Reinertsen, J.L., Gosfield, A.G., Rupp, W., & Whittington, J.W. (2007). Engaging physicians

in a shared quality agenda. Institute for Healthcare Improvement Innovation Series, white paper. http://www.ihi.org/IHI/Results/WhitePapers/EngagingPhysiciansWhitePaper.htm. Accessed February 1, 2009.

10. Hoff, T., Pohl, H., & Bartfield, J. (2005). Implementing safety cultures in medicine: What we can learn by watching physicians. In *Advances in patient safety: From research to implementation* (Vol. 1, pp. 15–38). Agency for Healthcare Research and Quality, publication no. 050021 (1–4). http://ahrq.gov/qual/advances/. Accessed January 21, 2009.

11. Burke, M., Boal, J., & Mitchell, R. (2004). Communicating for better care. *American Journal of Nursing, 104*(12), 40–47.

12. Aron, D.C., & Headrick, L.A. (2002). Educating physicians prepared to improve care and safety is no accident: It requires a systematic approach. *Quality and Safety in Health Care, 11*, 168–173.

13. Kane, J.M., Brannen, M., & Kern, E. (2008). Impact of patient safety mandates on medical education in the United States. *Journal of Patient Safety, 4*(2), 93–97.

14. Thompson, D.A., Cowan, J., Holzmueller, C.,Wu, A.W., Bass, E., & Pronovost, P. (2008). Planning and implementing a systems-based patient safety curriculum in medical education. *American Journal of Medical Quality, 23,* 271–278.

15. World Health Organization. (2008). *WHO patient safety curriculum guide for medical schools* (1st ed.). World Alliance for Patient Safety. http://www.who.int/patientsafety/en/. Accessed February 20, 2009.

16. Veltman, L. (2007). Getting to Havarti: Moving toward patient safety in obstetrics. *Obstetrics and Gynecology, 110*(5), 1146–1149.

17. Shields, M.C., Sacks, L.B., & Patel, P.H. (2008). Clinical integration provides the key to quality improvement: Structures for change (editorial). *American Journal of Medical Quality, 23,* 161–164.

18. Centers for Medicare and Medicaid Services. (n.d.). Hospital-acquired conditions (present on admission indicator). http://www.cms.gov/HospitalAcqCond/. Accessed February 1, 2009.

19. Murphy, D.M., Shannon, K., & Puglise, G. (2006). Patient safety and the risk management professional: New challenges and opportunities. In R.C. Carroll & S.M. Brown (Eds.), *Risk management handbook for health care organizations* (Vol. 2, 5th ed., pp. 1–21). San Francisco: Jossey-Bass.

20. Sedwick, J. (2006). The health care risk management professional. In R.C. Carroll & S.M. Brown (Eds.), *Risk management handbook for health care organizations* (Vol. 1, 5th ed., pp. 115–153). San Francisco: Jossey-Bass.

21. American Society of Healthcare Risk Management, American Hospital Association. (2004). *The growing role of the patient safety officer: Implications for risk managers.* Chicago: American Hospital Association.

22. Gallagher, T.H., Brundage, G., Bommarito, K.M., Summy, E., A., Ebers, E.A., & Waterman, A.D., et al. (2006). *Journal of Healthcare Risk Management, 26*(3), 11–16.

23. Accreditation Council for Graduate Medical Education. (n.d.). *ACGME outcome projects.* http://www.acgme.org/outcome/comp/compMin.asp/. Accessed April 27, 2009.

24. Kolb, A., & Kolb, D. (2006). Learning styles and learning spaces: A review of the multidisciplinary application of experiential learning theory in higher education. In R. Sims & S. Sims (Eds.), *Learning styles and learning: A key to meeting the accountability demands in education.* Hauppauge, NY: Nova Publishers.

25. Rudolph, J.W., Simon, R., & Raemer, D.B. (2007). Which reality matters? Questions on the path to high engagement in healthcare simulation (editorial). *Simulation in Healthcare, 2*(3), 161–163.

26. Accreditation Council for Graduate Medical Education. (2007). *ACGME institutional requirements.* http://www.acgme.org/acWebsite/irc/irc_IRCpr07012007.pdf/. Accessed March 28, 2009.

27. Accreditation Council for Graduate Medical Education. (2007). *Common program requirements.* http://www.acgme.org/acWebsite/dutyHours/dh_dutyhoursCommonPR07012007.pdf/. Accessed March 28, 2009.

28. American Board of Medical Specialties. (2000). *ABMS maintenance of certification.* http://abms.org/Maintenance_of_Certification/ABMS_MOC.aspx/. Accessed March 28, 2009.

29. Kravet, S.J., Howell, E., & Wright, S. (2006). Morbidity and mortality conference, Grand Rounds, and the ACGME's core competencies. *Journal of General Internal Medicine, 21,* 1192–1194.

30. Bechtold, M.L., Scott, S., Dellsperger, K.C., Nelson, K., Cox, K.R., & Hall, L.W. (2008). Educational quality improvement report: Outcomes from a revised morbidity and mortality format that emphasized patient safety. *Postgraduate Medical Journal, 84,* 211–216.

31. Berenholtz, S.M., Hartsell, T.L., & Pronovost, P.J. (2009). Learning from defects to enhance morbidity and mortality conferences. (Published on March 3, 2009 as doi:10.1177/1062860609332370). *American Journal of Medical Quality OnlineFirst.* 2009. http://ajm.sagepub.com/cgi/rapidpdf/1062860609332370v1. Accessed April 3, 2009.

32. Clancy, C.M. (2005). Training health care professionals for patient safety (commentary). *American Journal of Medical Quality, 20*(5), 277–279.

33. Institute for Healthcare Improvement. (2006). *Protecting 5 million lives from harm.* http://www.ihi.org/IHI/Programs/Campaign/Campaign.htm?TabId = 6#LivesSavedCalculation/. Accessed April 28, 2009.

27

MANAGING PATIENT EXPECTATIONS THROUGH INFORMED CONSENT

S. Joseph Austin, JD, LLM

INTRODUCTION

Informed consent consists of more than having a patient sign a document granting permission for, or submitting to, a treatment or procedure. It is a process that involves dialogue, or exchange of information, between the treating physician and the patient, which results in the patient's comprehension of the proposed treatment and a mutual understanding between the patient and the treating physician. A valid informed-consent process culminates with the patient being knowledgeable about the nature of the proposed procedure, including the possible risks, benefits, complications, and alternative treatments. Only when this level of understanding is reached can the patient provide truly informed consent.

At a minimum, the treating physician should expect to provide the patient with information regarding the proposed treatment, including an explanation of what the treatment involves along with known significant risks, anticipated possible complications, and any expected temporary pain or discomfort. This disclosure should also incorporate the benefits of the proposed treatment and the alternative treatments or procedures that are available to the patient. Additionally, the treating physician should provide the patient with information regarding any likely permanent results from the proposed treatment (e.g., disability, scarring) and the projected outcome should the patient not consent to treatment.

It is noteworthy that some risks do not necessarily need to be disclosed to the patient; these include remote risks (unless it should be reasonably expected that such a risk carries a significance with the individual patient) and commonly known risks. Commonly known risks are defined either as those risks the existence of which a person of average experience would be aware, or those risks that an individual patient would be aware of based on previous experience.

INFORMED-CONSENT BACKGROUND

Consent Theory

There are two primary legal theories regarding informed consent in the healthcare industry. These two theories are premised on the torts of battery and negligence. The first theory, battery, has historically developed as a result of the high value placed on individual autonomy. The second theory, negligence, has developed more recently and tends to be associated with the recovery of monetary compensation for injuries.

Battery

According to common law, battery is defined as any intentional touching of, or use of force against, another person without that person's consent. The theory of battery, as applied to informed-consent matters, emerged in a concrete formulation under a 1914 case decided by the New York Court of Appeals (that state's highest court). The case, *Schloendorff v. Society of New York Hospital,* 211 N.Y. 125, 105 N.E. 92 (1914), is still presently cited by courts as persuasive law when reviewing informed-consent issues. Therein, Justice Cardozo stated, "Every human being of adult years and sound mind has a right to determine what shall be done with his own body: and a surgeon who performs an operation without his patient's consent commits an assault, for which he is liable in damage."

In application to the healthcare industry, the definition of battery has been expanded to include practices and procedures that are performed without the patient's consent, even when the practice or procedure does not necessarily implicate hands-on contact, such as the taking of radiographs. Similarly, liability for battery may be found in situations where the patient has consented to a proposed treatment to be performed by a given doctor and the procedure is subsequently performed by a second, unnamed physician. Under such circumstances, the consent may be considered to have been granted solely to the named treating physician and not to the unnamed practitioner; as a result, both physicians could be subject to liability.

Negligence

The emergence and utilization of allegations of negligence in association with informed-consent issues have resulted primarily because of compensation arrangements. Basically, a person is limited in battery litigation to recuperation for only actual damages or injuries that are sustained. Under negligence, however, a person is capable of receiving monetary compensation for actual, non-economic, and punitive damages. This broader scope of recoverable losses allows for patients to include claims of pain and suffering, loss of companionship, loss of consortium, etc.

Types of Consent

There are two principal types of consent that are generally acknowledged as valid in the medical and legal fields; these are implied consent and expressed consent. The former type relies upon the perception by the treating physician that the patient, through his or her actions, has consented to receive a proposed treatment. The latter type of consent, express consent, is premised on either verbal or written expression from the patient that a proposed course of treatment is acceptable. Additionally, in some circumstances, a patient may opt to waive his or her right to receive information regarding the risks, benefits, and alternatives of the proposed treatment.

Implied Consent

Implied consent is premised on an unspoken understanding between the treating physician and the patient that a proposed method of treatment is advisable and suitable to both parties. The landmark case regarding the acceptability of this type of consent is *O'Brien v. Cunard S. S. Co.,* 154 Mass. 272, 28

N.E. 266 (1891). Therein, the Supreme Judicial Court of Massachusetts was asked to determine whether there was adequate evidence to justify a jury finding that the defendant, through its agents, had committed an assault against the plaintiff.

The facts of that case indicate that the plaintiff, O'Brien, was a passenger onboard a Cunard Steam-Ship Company vessel bound for Boston, Massachusetts. At that time, Boston had implemented "strict quarantine regulations in regard to the examination of emigrants, to see that they [were] protected from small-pox by vaccination." Only those persons who had received a certification from the medical officer on board the ship confirming that the individual was so protected would be allowed to disembark without being subject to quarantine detention.

Notice of the quarantine regulations were posted throughout the ship in various languages, along with information stating that the ship's medical officer would be available to administer the requisite vaccination. Accordingly, the court there determined that it was justifiable for the administering physician to assume that the plaintiff understood the importance and the purpose of the vaccination.

O'Brien was vaccinated by the physician at the same time as approximately 200 other passengers. According to O'Brien's own testimony, she understood from conversations with the other passengers that the purpose of the gathering was to receive the vaccination. Additionally, O'Brien acknowledged that she stood alongside fellow passengers while the physician examined their arms and vaccinated those persons who did not visibly show signs of prior vaccination.

When the physician examined O'Brien, he found no visible indication that O'Brien had previously been vaccinated. O'Brien then stated that she had in fact received the small-pox vaccination in the past, but that it had not left a mark. The physician then advised that O'Brien should be vaccinated again, and O'Brien responded by baring her arm.

O'Brien did not indicate or verbalize that she did not desire to be vaccinated, or that she had already received the vaccination. She then accepted the certification that she was vaccinated and used that certification to avoid quarantine.

Based on these circumstances, and the fact that O'Brien did not indicate through conduct or word that she did not want to receive the small-pox vaccination, the court found that the actions of the physician were lawful. It was determined that O'Brien was aware of the procedure to be performed and that her actions indicated a willingness to participate in the vaccination procedure. This complacency, combined with her own testimony that she did not refuse the treatment, led the court to its finding that the physician had acted lawfully; thus, the physician was not guilty of assault against O'Brien.

As this case demonstrates, there are certain situations wherein a patient may submit voluntarily to a course of treatment under circumstances that tend to indicate that he or she is aware of the proposed treatment plan and has implicitly consented to it. When considering the validity of implied consent, courts will primarily look for two factors: firstly, the patient must comprehend the nature of the proposed treatment and be aware of the common risks that are associated with it; and, secondly, the patient must be provided with an opportunity to refuse or withdraw from the proposed treatment.

Physician reliance on implied consent remains, however, a risky enterprise. Courts give strong deference to the theory of individual autonomy and, therefore, the right of the patient to determine the course of acceptable treatment; thus, acceptance of implied consent should be utilized only for simple and routine matters or, as discussed in more detail below, emergency situations.

Express Consent

For procedures that are more than minimally invasive or possess more than minor risk, the treating physician should generally not rely on implied consent in order to proceed; instead, the treating physician should obtain express consent from the patient or from the patient's authorized representative (discussed below), before proceeding.

Express consent is premised on a verbalized understanding between the treating physician and the patient that a proposed method of treatment is both advisable and suitable to the parties. It is a grant of permission given by the patient to the treating physician that acknowledges that a proposed treatment or procedure is acceptable by the patient and that the patient desires the treating physician to so proceed. This agreement may be either written or verbal, but a written agreement may prove beneficial in the event of litigation.

Generally, express consent should be obtained prior to the performance of any of the following types of procedures:

- Surgery, including both major and minor surgical operations
- Anesthesia, whenever the proposed procedure requires the utilization of anesthesia
- Non-surgical procedures, when the procedures involve more than minimal risk
- Radiographic imaging and similar procedures
- Blood or blood-product transfusions
- Biopsies
- Experimental procedures, including the utilization of experimental drugs or devices
- Electroconvulsive therapy
- Sterilization

Individual institutions may also require that express consent be obtained prior to the performance of certain treatments. Physicians and medical practitioners should be aware of their institution's specific practices. Should the treating physician be uncertain as to whether a procedure necessitates expressed consent, it would be advisable to err in favor of obtaining it.

As noted previously, express consent may be either verbal or written. In the event of subsequent litigation, however, a written agreement acknowledging the consent of the patient provides a strong evidentiary basis. It is noteworthy, however, that even a signed "Informed Consent" form may not be sufficient in order to establish the validity of the consent or that the consent was truly informed. As discussed at the beginning of this chapter, informed consent requires a dialogue between the treating physician and the patient, and an understanding by the patient of the proposed treatment and its risks, benefits, and alternatives. It is a process that must be fully completed in order for consent to be truly informed.

Physicians would be advised to preserve the contents of such a dialogue through documentation. Such documentation does not necessarily need to be greatly detailed; rather, it should concisely address the matters discussed during the counseling session. For example, the physician should specify the procedure to be performed and include information regarding the capacity of the patient to consent, what possible risks and complications were disclosed, and the discussion related to alternative treatment options. Importantly, the physician should be sure to provide time to answer questions posed by the patient regarding the proposed treatment and would be advised to document the specifics of such an exchange of information. This documentation may prove invaluable should subsequent litigation ensue.

Waiver

Occasionally, a patient may choose to waive the disclosure of information, preferring instead to remain ignorant of the risks, complications, benefits, or alternative treatments associated with a proposed treatment. When such a situation arises, the treating physician would be advised to thoroughly document the patient's request to not receive the information. Additionally, if possible, it would be desirable to have the patient sign a statement verifying the request.

STANDARD OF EVALUATION

Historically, courts applied a "reasonable physician" standard when reviewing the sufficiency of disclosure by physicians to patients in informed-consent matters. Under that criterion, physicians were expected to provide information in accordance with what a similar physician in a similar community would have disclosed. Essentially, the sufficiency of disclosure was judged comparatively with the practices of similarly situated physicians.

In more recent years, however, courts have tended to shift analysis in favor of a "reasonable-patient" standard. Under this framework, the sufficiency of disclosure is judged primarily on what information a patient would reasonably expect to receive from a physician in order to make an informed decision. This patient-oriented approach requires that the information provided by a treating physician be tailored to the proposed treatment and that the disclosure incorporate the information that an average, or reasonable, person would want to know before agreeing to that treatment.

In informed-consent litigation, the primary question will most typically be whether the treating physician provided sufficient and appropriate information in order for a reasonable patient to make a well-reasoned decision on how to proceed. This tends to indicate that the "reasonable-patient" standard is the principal measure of evaluation employed by the courts. Failure on the part of the treating physician to provide the patient with sufficient information in order for the patient to make a rational and reasoned decision may be construed as a deviation from the appropriate standard of care. Such a deviation, in turn, may result in physician liability for battery, negligence, or both.

OBTAINING INFORMED CONSENT

Capacity

In order for a patient to validly consent to a proposed treatment, he or she must be an adult and able to make informed and reasoned decisions. This means that the patient must be able to fully understand the nature and extent of the proposed treatment, in addition to the associated risks, benefits, and alternatives. Capacity to consent may be adversely affected temporarily or permanently by any number of factors, such as inebriation, unconsciousness, disability, or the law (for example, minors).

Adult

An adult is commonly defined as a person 18 years of age or older. An adult patient is generally presumed to be competent enough to consent to his or her own medical treatment. This presumption assumes that the adult patient is capable of understanding the following four factors:

- The nature and severity of his or her condition
- The nature and severity of the proposed treatment
- The risks associated with the proposed treatment
- The risks involved should the patient refuse the proposed treatment

All four of these factors must be met in order for the patient to be considered competent enough to consent. If the patient comprehends these four elements but refuses to consent to the proposed procedure, the treating physician should not proceed with the treatment without a court order. This stands true even in situations where the proposed treatment is considered to be medically advisable. When presented with the refusal of a patient, the physician would be advised to thoroughly document that the patient was fully apprised of the expected risks and benefits of the proposed treatment, that the patient understood the risks involved in refusing consent to the treatment, and that the patient continued to refuse authorization.

In situations where the adult patient does not fully understand any of the above factors, the treating physician may make a determination that the patient is incapable of giving informed consent. Incompetence may be either temporary or permanent, and may be the result of a natural occurrence, age, shock, illness, injury, intoxication, inebriation, or any other form of incapacitation. When such a determination is made, the physician may then seek authorization from a surrogate decision maker (discussed later).

Minor

Consent issues that involve minors continue to create confusion as a result of the wide variation among state laws. Commonly, a minor is defined as a person less than 18 years of age. The general rule involving minors is that approval for the performance of medical treatments or procedures requires the consent of the minor patient's parent or other legal guardian. From a legal perspective, a person's status as a minor may be construed as a form of temporary incompetence, and the standard procedures utilized when obtaining consent from an incompetent patient should typically be followed (see discussion below about the appointment of a surrogate). In a limited number of circumstances, however, a minor patient may be authorized under the law to consent to a proposed treatment or procedure. The most common situations where the consent of a parent or other legal guardian is neither required nor valid may include the following:

- The minor is married at the time of treatment.
- The minor is pregnant or suspected of being pregnant at the time of treatment.
- The minor is emancipated.

Individual states may make further provisions that allow for a minor patient to consent to treatment for venereal diseases, alcohol abuse, drug abuse, or psychotherapy, or to receive birth-control services. Additionally, a minor patient who is the victim of sexual assault or sexual abuse may be permitted to give valid consent for counseling, diagnosis, or treatment of any related injuries or diseases.

Lastly, most states recognize an exception to the general rule, that a minor patient is incapable of consenting to a proposed treatment, for the "mature minor." The mature-minor doctrine is commonly defined as a minor who possesses the cognitive faculties to articulate reasoned decisions regarding his or her health and welfare. Application of the mature-minor doctrine is discretionary and dependent on the subjective evaluation of the treating physician. Should a physician opt to utilize this doctrine, the physician would be advised to document the minor patient's maturity and decision-making capacity, and any supporting information pertinent to making the determination. Because of the subjective nature of the evaluation, physicians should be cautious in reliance on the mature-minor doctrine.

Ultimately, due to the substantial variation among state laws regarding obtaining consent from, and on behalf of, minor patients, it is virtually impossible to assert any authoritative conclusions on the subject. Physicians and other medical personnel should consult the statutes of their home state and the policies of their practicing institutions for further guidance concerning such practices.

Surrogate

An adult patient who has the capacity to make reasoned decisions regarding proposed treatments has the right to give, withdraw, or refuse consent. In certain situations, however, the adult patient may be incapable of making informed and rational decisions. Determinations regarding such capacity may be decided either by the treating physician or through court adjudication.

In situations where the adult patient is determined to be incapable of giving consent based on physician determination, consent may be obtained instead from the patient's next of kin. State law generally establishes the order of lineage from which consent can be obtained. Typically, the order is as follows:

- Guardian
- Spouse
- Adult child
- Parent
- Adult sibling
- Adult grandchildren
- Grandparent

Some states have enacted provisions that enumerate additional surrogate decision makers including close friends of the patient, persons standing in *loco parentis* of the patient, or guardians of the patient's estate. Physicians and other medical-staff members should be aware of the laws and regulations of the state in which they practice, as well as the policies and guidelines of their medical institution.

In limited situations, when the patient is too incompetent to give consent, merely obtaining the consent of a family member or other surrogate may not be adequate. Individual states have enacted mandates that in certain non-emergency situations, due to their extreme nature, only a court-appointed guardian can consent on behalf of the incapacitated patient. For example, such procedures may include the following: sterilization, electroconvulsive therapy, or psycho-surgery. Additionally, when one family member consents to a proposed treatment and an equally close relative refuses consent, and the parties are unable to come to a consensus, the determination should be submitted to court adjudication for resolution.

Court adjudication may be initiated by any interested party. If the treating physician, or another member of the medical staff, is aware of the existence of relatives or friends who are interested in the patient's welfare, effort should be made to encourage those relatives or friends to initiate guardianship proceedings.

From the perspective of the healthcare provider, court adjudication should be commenced only where the patient is incapable of giving his or her own consent, there is no available next of kin to serve as a surrogate decision maker, and the treating physician has determined that the proposed treatment is medically necessary. Under such circumstances, a reviewing court will likely appoint a guardian or conservator to serve on behalf of the incapacitated patient.

DISCLOSURE

Responsibility

When attempting to obtain the consent of a patient, the treating physician should generally be forthcoming in the disclosure of possible risks, complications, benefits, and alternatives of the proposed treatment. This standard relates to the founding premise of informed consent, which was established in *Schloendorff v. the Society of the New York Hospital* and holds that "every adult of sound mind has the fundamental right to control decisions relating to his or her own medical care, including the withholding or withdrawal of medical or surgical treatment. As the probability or severity of risk to the patient increases, the physician's duty to inform also increases."

Importantly, the treating physician should be mindful that obtaining informed consent is a process that involves a dialogue between the physician and the patient. The nature of the disclosure for a given procedure may vary from patient to patient. In making the requisite disclosure, the physician should be mindful of the individual needs and expectations of the patient and take into consideration those factors that may personally affect the patient.

Additionally, physicians should be mindful of the fact that courts generally find that the duty of obtaining informed consent is an obligation of the treating physician. This result stems from the premise that the physician is more qualified to discuss such matters than a certified nurse practitioner, physician assistant, registered nurse, or other healthcare provider. It is noteworthy that although the treating physician may delegate the actual function of obtaining consent, the responsibility for ensuring valid informed consent cannot be delegated.

Scope

The treating physician should give particular attention to the scope of disclosure that is given to a patient regarding a proposed treatment. Disclosure needs to be tailored to the treatment under consideration and should include information regarding possible risks and benefits of the treatment, available alternatives, and the projected results from the treatment. Additionally, in ensuring valid consent from the patient, the treating physician will need to specify the nature and extent of the proposed treatment, and identify himself or herself as the treating physician. Notably, it is not sufficient to incorporate a "catch-all" provision allowing the treating physician to perform any necessary medical procedures that may be indicated.

Generally, a physician may be held liable if he or she exceeds the scope of the patient's consent. Since informed consent should be tailored to the proposed treatment, a physician may be held liable if he or she performs the wrong procedure or a procedure that has not been authorized by the patient. Courts have upheld such rules even when the erroneous or unauthorized procedure is performed flawlessly and benefits the patient.

An exception does exist, however, for situations wherein the treating physician discovers an unanticipated condition during an operation which, if not rectified, could endanger the life and health of the patient. Under such circumstances, the treating physician may justifiably extend or expand the authorized

operation without the patient's consent in order to remove, repair, or palliate the discovered medical condition. The breadth of this exception is narrow, however, and should only be utilized in order to treat conditions in immediate need of attention; non-emergency situations should be delayed until appropriate consent can be obtained.

State Mandates

Some states have enacted statutory provisions requiring the disclosure of certain risks for specific procedures. Physicians and healthcare institutions should consult the laws of their home state for such measures and ensure compliance with the provisions therein. Importantly, from the perspective of the healthcare provider, compliance with such statutes generally establishes a presumption that the healthcare provider adequately disclosed the risks associated with the given procedure.

SITUATIONAL CONSIDERATIONS

Therapeutic Privilege

Under limited circumstances, a physician may legitimately exercise "therapeutic privilege" in order to knowingly withhold information from a patient. This privilege is intended as a means to allow a physician, in his or her judgment, to withhold information when disclosure of such information is likely to adversely impact the patient's health. Although the privilege is considered to be discretionary, it should only be exercised in the most extreme situations and not utilized as a means of gaining consent for a proposed treatment, even if the treating physician believes that the proposed treatment is in the best interest of the patient.

Revocation and Refusal of Consent

Just as an adult patient who is of sound mind and capable of making intelligent decisions has the right to give consent for a proposed treatment, he or she also has the exclusive right to revoke consent or refuse treatment. A competent adult patient may revoke or withdraw a previously granted consent at any time prior to the initiation of the proposed treatment. Similarly, a competent adult patient may refuse medical treatment. The ability to revoke or refuse a proposed medical treatment is a right that may not be superseded, unless through court adjudication, even if the proposed treatment is medically advisable or medically necessary.

In either situation, whether a patient revokes a previously granted consent or refuses to provide consent, the treating physician would be advised to document the circumstances of the situation. In doing so, particular attention should be given to ensuring that the patient understands that risks, benefits, and alternatives to his or her decision, and that such information is included in the physician's documentation.

Non-Consensual Situations

Emergency

A medical emergency can commonly be defined as existing when a patient's life, health, or safety is in jeopardy, or when the patient may suffer disfigurement or loss of limb if the performance of a diagnostic or therapeutic procedure is delayed in order to contact the authorized or surrogate decision maker. Determination of the existence of a medical emergency relies upon the discretionary evaluation of the treating physician. Even when such an emergency exists, however, a competent adult patient retains the right to grant, revoke, or refuse consent.

Most states have enacted legislation that addresses the provision of health care and treatment during a medical emergency. In these states, consent to medical intervention may be implied when, in the opinion of the treating physician, a medical emergency exists and all of the following factors are satisfied:

- The patient is temporarily or permanently incapable of giving or refusing consent
- The patient has not previously refused consent for the proposed treatment
- The patient has no known advance directive or living will that is instructive on how to proceed
- There has not been a previous refusal of consent for the proposed treatment from an authorized or surrogate decision maker
- There is no authorized or surrogate decision maker immediately available

The implied consent of an emergency situation does not give carte blanche to the treating physician, however. Generally, when presented with such circumstances, the physician can only provide the reasonable care and treatment that is necessary in order to alleviate or eliminate the medical emergency. Once the patient is stabilized, additional medical care can only be provided after obtaining the consent of the patient or, if the patient remains either temporarily or permanently incapable of providing consent, by the patient's authorized or surrogate decision maker.

Importantly, reliance on implied consent in emergency situations should only occur when the desires or directives of the patient are unknown. Emergency consent should not be utilized as a tool to override the previously expressed wishes of the patient, whether those wishes have been conveyed verbally or in writing.

Court Orders

There are several scenarios under which a physician or healthcare institution may be presented with a court order on behalf of a patient. Such orders may be issued in order to mandate that a patient receive a proposed treatment; appoint a guardian, conservator, or other decision maker; or declare a minor capable of providing valid consent. As discussed previously, a court order may also be necessary when two equally close next of kin disagree over consent for an incompetent patient.

When a surrogate decision maker is appointed or otherwise acknowledged, that person is granted the right to consent on behalf of a patient. This authority also means that he or she holds the right to revoke or refuse consent for treatment on behalf of the patient. In the majority of states, however, courts have restricted this latter right to cases where the revocation or refusal is reasonable. If the treating physician or medical institution determines that the surrogate decision maker has acted unreasonably, the physician or medical institution can petition a court for an order authorizing the proposed treatment.

In order for a court to consider a request of this type, the petitioner must establish two factors: firstly, there must be a demonstrable need for the treating physician to proceed with the proposed treatment before the patient would be capable of considering the matter; and, secondly, the proposed treatment must be appropriate for the patient's condition. If the petitioner is able to satisfy both of these factors, the court will be more inclined to issue the requested order.

Lastly, a court order may be desirable in situations where the patient, although incompetent legally to make decisions regarding care and consent, takes a position in opposition to that of his or her guardian, conservator, or other surrogate decision maker. Some courts have indicated that the wishes of the incompetent patient should be taken into consideration in resolving the matter. Given this disposition, it may be advisable for a physician or medical institution facing a similar scenario to submit the matter to a court for resolution and thereby limit exposure to liability.

Law-Enforcement-Officer Orders

It is not uncommon for law-enforcement officers to bring persons to a physician or healthcare institution for examination or medical testing. Law-enforcement officers are not, however, authorized to provide consent on behalf of a patient; this rule holds true whether the law-enforcement officer is employed at the federal, state, or local level. Valid consent in such situations can only be provided by the patient, or by the patient's authorized or surrogate decision maker as determined through the appropriate procedures.

28

Improving Health Literacy to Advance Patient Safety

Caroline Chapman, JD

INTRODUCTION

Over 300 studies have shown that health information cannot be understood by most of the people for whom it was intended, suggesting that the assumptions made by the creators of this information, regarding the recipient's level of health literacy, are often incorrect.[1]

Almost 83 million adults in the United States struggle to understand basic information about their health and medical care. According to the 2003 National Assessment of Adult Literacy, conducted by the U.S. Department of Education, 36% of adults have below basic or only basic health literacy.[2] This means that over a third of adults in the United States cannot read a prescription drug label well enough to determine what time to take the medication with regard to eating. Over one third of adults in the United States cannot find the age range, using a table, in which a child should receive a vaccine, or understand a body-mass-index chart. Over one third of adults cannot read an over-the-counter drug label well enough to identify substances that may interact badly with the drug.[2] Perhaps an even more disturbing trend revealed by the study are the populations for whom health-literacy limits are endemic: elderly patients, non-native English speakers, and the poor. For these patients, many of whom already face barriers to getting medical care, limited health literacy places yet another obstacle in the way of accessing meaningful, appropriate, and safe care.

On the other side of the equation, only about 12% of adults in this country are proficient with health information.[2] In other words, just over 1 in 10 adult patients possess the reading and quantitative skills needed to process the full range of information about their health. Lest we feel confident with this 12%, even these numbers may deceive, because study participants answered questions under optimal conditions, with none experiencing the stress of acute illness or the fear that accompanies a life-threatening diagnosis. Physicians, nurses, pharmaceutical companies, and public health agencies are all talking to Americans, but the data show that we are simply not being understood.

That we concern ourselves at all with patients' health literacy is in large part a reflection of the changing role of patients in recent decades. Our current healthcare system is undergoing a revolution in perspective, challenging itself to become patient centered and asking individuals to take an active role in medical decision making, choosing quality providers, disease self-management, and safety efforts.[1] The simultaneous proliferation of pharmaceuticals and the increasingly complex web of health insurance have significantly complicated patients' roles in their own care. The degree to which patients have the capacity to obtain, process, and understand the information required for good medical decision making in all these arenas will directly affect how safe and effective their health care is. Never before have successful outcomes depended so directly on the skills not just of caregivers but of patients themselves. Upon this schematic, we must now impose the stark National Assessment of Adult Literacy (NAAL) data demonstrating that only about 1 in 10 patients has the skills for the task.

Even this brief introduction to the concept of health literacy evokes the obvious practical link between the ability of patients to understand and process health information and patient safety. When communication between patients and providers is derailed by patients' inability to meaningfully comprehend what they are reading or being told, opportunities for adverse events abound. After analyzing its extensive data on sentinel events, The Joint Commission concluded that the failures of communication are the root cause of nearly every reported unexpected death and catastrophic injury.[3] Similarly, studies reviewed by the Institute of Medicine (IOM) in its landmark report, "To Err Is Human," reveal that as many as 10% of adverse drug events arise from communication errors.[4] Patients who cannot accurately identify their medications or fill out medical-history forms, or who nod yes to any question asked because of limited English, are at risk for a panoply of errors with each and every medical encounter. To make sure that those encounters are safe, providers must make meaningful reciprocal communication of health information one of their highest priorities.

HEALTH-LITERACY DEFINITION

The definition of health literacy proposed by the National Library of Medicine and used in "Healthy People 2010"[5] has been adopted by the IOM in its recently published seminal report on health literacy titled, "Health Literacy: A Prescription to End Confusion" and has since become widely used.[1] Under this definition, health literacy is, at its most basic, "the degree to which individuals have the capacity to obtain, process, and understand basic health information and services needed to make appropriate health decisions."[1]

Beyond its most basic definition, health literacy has also been defined in more functional terms. Functional health literacy has been noted to include "the ability to understand instructions on prescription drug bottles, appointment slips, medical education brochures, doctor's directions and consent forms, and the ability to negotiate complex health care systems."[6] To be fully functional, health literacy also requires oral-communication skills such as being able to articulate symptoms, to formulate relevant questions, and to convey health history and current treatment.[1] In addition, health literacy in the information age requires quantitative literacy, or numeracy: the ability to perform computations and reason numerically. Health-literate patients thus need to be able to calculate dosages, interpret test results, weigh risks and benefits, and evaluate health information for quality and accuracy.[1] Notably, patients need to implement their health-literacy skills under less-than-ideal circumstances, generally, when they are sick or under the stress of discovering that they or a loved one have an illness.

These definitions of health literacy are multifaceted, and providers may see themselves as ill-equipped to improve the demonstrably poor skills of so many U.S. patients. This has led to a number of efforts to incorporate health-literacy building into the U.S. education system and even to a legislative proposal to fund the development of curricula for health literacy to be implemented in schools, colleges, and through agencies such as Centers for Medicare and Medicaid Services (CMS) and other public health departments;[7] however, a shift in perspective from the needs of the patients to what might be called the health-literacy quotient of providers shows what the latter group can do to ensure meaningful communication of health information. When seen from the perspective of providers, health literacy means the ability to speak and write clearly when addressing patients. Later in this chapter the components of clear communication are discussed in detail, but to begin, they include the ability to speak and write plainly about health information; to effectively use visual aids, pictograms, and videos; to implement teach-back techniques in which patients' true comprehension is tested; to provide interpreter services when required; and to provide culturally competent care to all patients. Providers have available to them a variety of fairly simple tools that can be universally applied that will facilitate a meaningful exchange with patients seeking care.

HEALTH LITERACY AND PATIENT SAFETY

The literature is replete with anecdotal evidence of a strong link between health literacy and patient safety. From the illiterate patient who nearly bleeds out after misunderstanding his doctor's instructions about taking a blood thinner, to the mother who pours an oral antibiotic into her child's infected ear, to the Spanish-speaking patient who receives another man's medication because he incorrectly nods in response to an identification question asked in English, these stories illustrate the concrete and commonplace medical errors that result from a failure to implement health-literacy initiatives.[1,3] There is also a strong logical connection between a patient with limited health literacy, or limited English proficiency, and an increased risk that a communication error with this patient will cause harm.

With this logical starting point, providers have gone to their own data for an evidence-based confirmation of their concerns. One hospital reported to The Joint Commission that they categorized their adverse events by native language of the patient and found "clusters of adverse events in patients with English as a second language."[3] According to the Center for Health Care Strategies, low-literacy patients at 659 public hospitals were five times more likely to misinterpret prescription information.[8] Low literacy also affected the proper use of a metered-dose asthma inhaler and medication compliance among HIV-positive adults.[8] As the field of health literacy has grown over the past decade, so have efforts to study and quantify this link on a broader scale. As the IOM report "Health Literacy: A Prescription to End Confusion" noted, limited health literacy has already been linked to problems with chronic-illness management, patient involvement in decision making about treatment, lower adherence to certain therapy regimes, and lower self-reported health status.[1]

The AHRQ also recently undertook a literature review regarding existing studies of the nexus between health literacy and health outcomes. The authors concluded that poor reading skills and poor health were demonstrably related. Additionally, the review confirmed anecdotal evidence that low health literacy does correlate with "a range of adverse health outcomes."[9] Low numeracy has also been linked to poor outcomes. One study linked low numeracy with poorer anti-coagulation control among patients taking warfarin to reduce stroke risk.[10] Another study found that less-numerate women aged 40–49 years could not accurately assess the risks and benefits of screening for breast cancer, although the National Institutes of Health (NIH) advises women in this age group to decide whether or not to have mammography based on a discussion of the risks and benefits with their physicians.[10] Although the IOM and the AHRQ have both noted that the causal connection between low health literacy and adverse events requires additional study, they concur that existing studies and clinical experience demonstrate a strong connection between the two.

A link has also been demonstrated between low-literacy patients and increased medical expense. Although it is hardly surprising that poor management of chronic illness or failure to adhere to therapy plans creates additional expense for the healthcare system, the IOM report and others have suggested that low-literacy patients have higher hospital-utilization rates, higher use of emergency services, and higher inpatient-spending rates.[1] The National Academy on an Aging Society estimates that the additional healthcare expenditures due to low health literacy were approximately $73 billion in 1998 healthcare dollars.[11] Money spent to address poor outcomes, increased emergency department use, and longer inpatient stays could be redirected to health-literacy programs and education for providers, and has the potential to improve outcomes and reduce communication-related errors for patients.

HEALTH-LITERACY DATA

It is not always easy to determine which patient has low literacy. These patients may have spent years developing sophisticated masking and coping strategies. These patients may be articulate and present well. One study of low-literacy patients suggested that low-literacy patients are not likely to front this information with healthcare providers.[12] The study revealed that 85% of them had not revealed their limited literacy to coworkers and 67% had not even told their spouse. Fifteen percent of these people had told no one. Another study revealed that clinic physicians accurately identified only 20% of their low-literacy patients.[8] Patients themselves may think that their health-literacy skills are adequate, but they may simply not be.

The lesson from these studies is twofold. Firstly, health-literacy efforts must be implemented universally and contain behavioral and communication changes that improve clarity of communication regardless of the literacy level of the patient or the accuracy of the perceptions of the provider. Secondly, specific data about populations that may be particularly vulnerable to low health literacy can help providers focus their self-assessment of patient safety issues on those patients at highest risk for communications-related errors.

From where might these data come? Providers now have an up-to-date and comprehensive resource in the 2003 NAAL. The NAAL was administered to more than 19,000 adults and, for the first time, contained a specific health-literacy component.[13] The assessment measured literacy by asking participants to complete literacy tasks, as opposed to self-reporting literacy, drawn from actual health-related materials. The assessment was thus designed to capture the true functional literacy of participants in real-life contexts. The assessment was also designed to measure different types of literacy, each of which reflected skills required to comprehend and properly process health information. The assessment measured prose literacy (basic reading and comprehension), document literacy (the ability to search and read through longer, non-continuous text), and quantitative literacy (the ability to perform computations using numbers embedded in print materials). The specific tasks focused on three areas of health information: clinical, preventative, and navigation of the healthcare system. None of the tasks required special knowledge of health-related vocabulary.

The assessment defined the following four categories of health literacy:

- "Below Basic" represents those individuals who range from non-literate in English to those able to locate easily identifiable information in a short prose text, to locate easily identifiable information and follow simple instructions in charts or forms, and to perform simple computations (such as addition) with concrete and familiar numerical information. Fourteen percent of U.S. adults' health literacy is limited to this level.
- "Basic" represents those individuals who could read and understand short prose text and simple documents and who could locate numerical information and use it to solve simple, one-step arithmetic operations. Twenty-two percent of adults have only basic health literacy.[13]
- "Intermediate" represents the individuals who could read and comprehend moderately complex prose and make simple inferences from it, locate information in dense documents and make simple inferences from it, and locate less-familiar quantitative information and use it to solve arithmetic operations not previously specified. Just over 50% of adults have an intermediate health-literacy level.
- "Proficient" included individuals who could read and comprehend lengthy and abstract prose, integrate and synthesize multiple pieces of information, and locate abstract numerical information and solve multi-step problems. Twelve percent of adults are proficient.[13]

Certainly, these numbers are not all discouraging. About two thirds of adults have intermediate health literacy or higher.[13] Although the skills required for intermediate health literacy may not include the full panoply of skills necessary to reliably navigate all medical encounters, there does appear to be a reasonable cohort of adults who have a degree of competency with medical information; however, a word of caution must be noted regarding this group: health literacy is contextual. The NAAL did mot measure the literacy skills of these individuals under the extreme stress of a health crisis. As the U.S. Department of Health and Human Services has aptly noted: "the health literacy of a 50-ish English speaking woman with two years of college and a head cold who is buying a familiar over-the-counter medicine are *different in that moment* from the capacities of that same woman when she undergoes diagnostic tests, learns that she has breast cancer, and has two different treatment options, neither of which she understands."[14] It is important to remember that although demographic information is unquestionably useful to providers, the benefit of applying health-literacy principles universally is the benefit to anyone whose literacy skills may be affected by external factors such as extreme stress or physical illness.

Not all of the news from the study was good. Just over one third of adults in the study had only Basic or Below Basic literacy skills.[13] These individuals cannot consistently read and follow directions on prescription bottles and may have difficulty reading and completing a medical-history form or reporting what medications they are currently taking.[13] Although this news is disturbing, the good news is that as a result of the NAAL study, we are now armed with the relevant data to begin addressing the problem. Although many of the programs discussed in the latter part of this chapter would be appropriate to implement for all patients, knowing the depth and breadth of the literacy crisis and knowing that sub-populations may face the greatest health-literacy challenges allow providers to target those groups whose literacy limitations may place them at the greatest risk for communication-related adverse events.

On average, women were more health literate than men, with men representing a higher percentage of the Below Basic population (4% more).[13] Breakdowns by race and ethnicity were even more marked. Although only 9% of Caucasians had Below Basic health literacy, and only another 19% had basic health literacy, 24% of African American adults had Below Basic health literacy and an additional 34% had Basic health literacy.[13] In total, over 50% of African American adults had not more than Basic health literacy. The study also revealed that 41% of Hispanic adults had Below Basic health literacy in English.[13] This means that almost 50% of the adult Hispanic population in this country is trying to navigate medical encounters with a very limited English literacy skill set. Another 25% of Hispanic adults had only Basic health literacy. When totaled, two thirds of Hispanic adults have health-literacy limitations.[13] The implications for providers from the race and ethnicity data in the study are profound. Depending on the racial and ethnic makeup of an institution's patient population, significant numbers of patients may need health-literacy assistance to ensure safe and appropriate care.

Disparities extended beyond race and ethnicity. Adults 65 years and older had the lowest average health-literacy score of any other adult age group. Twenty-nine percent of older adults had Below Basic skills and another 30% had only Basic skills.[13] Among seniors, 59% had no more than Basic skills.[13] The implications of this statistic are significant. We are an aging society, and older adults consume more health services and products than any other single group.[8] As of the year the NAAL was conducted, 78% of the Medicare population (people over 65 years and some disabled individuals under 65 years) "suffer from one or more chronic conditions that require ongoing medical management."[15] Strikingly, 20% of the older adult Medicare population have at least five chronic conditions.[15]

The NAAL did not measure the objective health condition of its participants; however, self-reports were taken from participants. Notably, of people who reported their health condition as poor, 42% had Below Basic health literacy and another 27% had only Basic health literacy. Of people who consider themselves to be in excellent health, 57% had intermediate health literacy and 19% had Proficient health literacy.[15] Although some consideration must be made for personal perception of health, the numbers strongly suggest that poor health and poor literacy are at least coincident, if not causally related.

Finally, the NAAL established that economic status had an effect on a group's health literacy. Adults living in poverty had a lower health-literacy score than non-poor adults. Thirty-five percent of this group had Below Basic literacy skills and another 27% had only Basic skills.[15] Critical to providers serving a poor patient population is the knowledge that well over 50% of these patients have very limited skills for comprehending medical information.

The NAAL data have obvious relevance in several areas. Firstly, the data highlight that those populations already at risk for disparities in healthcare provision (i.e., people of color and the poor) are also burdened by more limited skills for obtaining meaningful information about that care. To ensure that these patients get safe care and can participate in medical decision making, providers must evaluate the way that health information is provided. As the U.S. Department of Health and Human Services has noted: "Closing the gap in health literacy is an issue of fundamental fairness and equity and is essential to reduce health disparities."[5] Secondly, the data indicate that a substantial percentage of the adult population has health-literacy limitations. Implementing system-wide health-literacy measures has the potential to aid a significant portion of the patient population. Finally, providers now have the basic data needed to conduct analysis of their adverse-event data with an eye toward populations known to have health-literacy issues. If these populations are demonstrably more vulnerable to error than others, then health-literacy-oriented responses may lead to a more targeted error-reduction response.

SAFE CARE FOR NON-ENGLISH SPEAKERS: LIMITED ENGLISH PROFICIENCY, A CRITICAL COMPONENT OF HEALTH-LITERACY WORK

According to a national survey conducted by the Health Research and Educational Trust, 63% of hospitals treat Limited English Proficiency (LEP) patients either daily or weekly.[16] In analyzing its data on adverse events, The Joint Commission found that although only about 30% of English speakers suffered physical harm from reported adverse events, almost 50% of LEP patients were harmed by the adverse events they suffered.[3] As the NAAL study profoundly highlighted, the English health-literacy skills of the Hispanic population, many of whom are not native English speakers, is an area that merits significant attention from providers. The NAAL study reveals that 67% of them have only Basic health literacy, or lower, in English.[2] These statistics starkly indicate how critical health-literacy efforts targeted at LEP patients are to addressing potential safety issues.

Although a fundamental concern for the safety of all patients undoubtedly underlies providers' interest in tackling the health-literacy obstacles for LEP patients, Title VI of the federal Civil Rights Act also mandates that providers take action. Under Title VI, providers must provide interpretation services to their LEP patients. Title VI has also been interpreted by the Office of Civil Rights to demand that all vital written materials be translated, including consent and complaint forms; information about free translation programs; notices of eligibility criteria, rights, denial, loss, or decreases in benefits or ser-

vices; and intake forms.[17] In addition, a presidential executive order issued in 2000 mandates that all recipients of federal financial assistance (in other words, providers who receive Medicare or Medicaid funds) provide "meaningful access" to services to their LEP beneficiaries.[18] Under this mandate, the Centers for Medicare and Medicaid Services (CMS) have taken an aggressive position on LEP, mandating that all of its beneficiaries have access to interpreters. All of these legal requirements, however, beg the question of what exactly these translation and interpreter services will be at any given institution.

Interpreters

Who will be the interpreters that a medical institution provides? At what kind of encounter will those services be available? What, if any, training will be provided to these interpreters? Although the ease of using family members or friends as interpreters for LEP patients is undeniable, reliance on these individuals creates risks for the institution. A 2003 study on the error rates of medical interpretation provides a cautionary tale for the safety-minded health-literacy advocate. The study found an error rate of 31 interpretation errors per medical encounter.[3] The interpreters in the study included hospital-provided interpreters and ad-hoc interpreters, with the latter making significantly more errors than the former. Generally, the errors ranged from omissions, substitutions, editorializing, and additions, and included instructing a parent to put an oral antibiotic in a child's ear. The results of this study highlight two important points. Firstly, that the use of family members, friends, and other ad-hoc interpreters risks the miscommunication of vital health information. Because federal law mandates the provision of interpretation services, an error of this kind not only puts patients at risk but creates potential liability for hospitals. Whenever a provider is attempting to convey to, or obtain from, an LEP patient meaningful medical information, an ad-hoc interpreter is a poor choice. Secondly, even using institution staff as interpreters can present risks if that staff has not been trained as medical interpreters. Again, relying on the accuracy of interpretation by a fluent bilingual staff member may not shield an institution from liability if that interpreter was not qualified for the task. The Joint Commission recommends that providers evaluate the proficiency of their interpreters with regard to communicating medical information, guidance for which is available through the National Council on Interpreting in Healthcare.[17]

Translation

In addition to using appropriately trained medical interpreters and weaning providers off the use of ad-hoc interpreters, the provision of translated written materials can reinforce the communication of vital medical information. Translated written materials may be critical in informed-consent contexts and may provide a critical backup for oral communication under certain circumstances. Direct translation must be avoided because it is likely to produce materials that are confusing or even nonsensical in the second language. As the U.S. Department of Health and Human Services found when translating its "Five Steps to Safer Health Care," the metaphor of stairs evoking progression had to be entirely reworked because it had no meaning in Spanish.[19] Providers also need to be reviewing translated documents to check their clinical and cultural accuracy, and can use focus groups, translation services, or their own trained medical interpreters for this review. The Joint Commission recommends that providers consider pooling resources for translating critical and broadly used written materials.[3] Also important to the creation of appropriately translated materials is the health-literacy level of LEP patients in their native language. As CMS discovered when

surveying Medicare beneficiaries, Spanish-dominant persons were unfamiliar with terms such as ibuprofen or heart bypass surgery in either language.[19] Although providing translation services for these individuals is crucial, those written materials must be written in appropriately plain language that will communicate effectively to those at even the lowest literacy levels.

Cultural Competency

Another critical component to providing safe care to non-English or limited English speakers involves the concept of cultural competency. The Joint Commission defines cultural competency as "the ability of health care providers and organizations to understand and respond effectively to the cultural and language needs brought by the patient to the health care encounter."[20] Cultural competency requires organizations and their personnel to: (1) value diversity; (2) assess themselves; (3) manage the dynamics of difference; (4) acquire and institutionalize cultural knowledge; and (5) adapt to diversity and the cultural contexts of individuals and communities served.[17] Just as important as making your words understood is the concept of communicating with patients in the way that is most likely to achieve their desired outcome.

If, as did a provider in one well-documented case, you explain to a family that their child is dying and that family is from a culture that interprets this as threatening and offensive, the family might remove that child from your care in a way that puts the family and the child in unnecessary peril.[3] The chances of non-compliance, treatment refusal, and withholding of crucial information all arise when the provider is unaware of the cultural forces shaping patients' decisions. As the IOM has stated, "A principle of patient safety is to include patients in safety designs and the processes of care."[1] To do so, it is essential to understand cultural nuances of what patient safety means to different people and what beliefs, values, and actions that inform people's understanding of safe care come into play."[1]

The Joint Commission has issued two reports that directly confront cultural-competency issues for medical-care providers.[17,20] These reports outline best practices for dealing with LEP patients and cultural-competency issues, and highlight the current work being done by specific institutions to address these issues. The reports also indicate the emphasis that The Joint Commission, as an accrediting body, is placing on monitoring institutions' efforts in these areas. Also in recognition of the importance of cultural competency, the Department of Health and Human Services (HHS) created National Standards for Culturally and Linguistically Appropriate Services (CLAS) in Health Care. The CLAS dictates not only that "health care organizations must make available easily understood patient-related materials . . . in the languages of commonly encountered groups" but that these materials must be culturally responsive as well.[3] The Joint Commission's accreditation standards mirror the CLAS dictates, and that body has published a self-assessment tool for institutions to evaluate their cultural competence.

To better understand the potential health-literacy obstacles that your LEP patient population faces, the National Patient Safety Foundation (NPSF) recommends conducting an audit of all written, visual, and verbal patient points of contact.[21] Ask questions about the accessibility of written materials, the ability to navigate the physical layout of the hospital, the reading level of items such as medication instructions, and responses to patient questions. Understanding and responding to patient needs in this way not only can improve patient safety but can also help keep the institution from facing unfortunate legal consequences.

THE LAW AND HEALTH LITERACY

Informed Consent

The safety implications for effective communication between providers and patients is unquestionably a key force driving the health-literacy movement. There are, however, important liability issues that underlie the question of whether patients understand information presented to them concerning their medical care. First and foremost is the issue of informed consent. While specific laws vary from state to state, according to the American Medical Association's (AMA) general principles, in order to give informed consent to medical care, patients should be informed of their diagnosis, if known; the nature and purpose of a proposed treatment or procedure; the benefits, and particularly the risks, of a proposed treatment or procedure; alternatives and their risks and benefits; and the risks and benefits of undergoing no treatment.[22] The adequacy of the communication is judged by what a reasonable person would need to know to make an informed choice about the proposed treatment. Failure to obtain informed consent before treating a patient opens a provider to a malpractice claim. In obtaining a meaningful informed consent from patients, understanding that for every institution significant numbers of those patients have limited health literacy presents its own challenges.

Anecdotal evidence about the cryptic nature of informed-consent forms abounds, and the literature is replete with quotes from these forms that are unreadable by anyone who does not possess both a medical and legal education. A brief literature review conducted by the Agency for Healthcare Research and Quality (AHRQ) revealed the incompleteness and inadequacies of the majority of the informed-consent interactions studied.[23] From omissions of central aspects of the informed-consent components to level of satisfaction by patients with the amount of information they had prior to undergoing a treatment, to the readability of written consent forms, the studies all highlighted the health-literacy challenges presented by typical informed-consent procedures.

This literature review also included studies of the effectiveness of several different approaches to improving the communication effort in informed-consent processes. Although the AHRQ authors concluded that additional study is needed regarding the most effective means for conveying the information required for a truly informed consent, they recommended several evidence-based steps that providers can take to improve their informed-consent process. Firstly, consent forms should be revised for increased readability and written at a reading level that more accurately reflects the skills of a provider's average patients. Secondly, informed-consent discussions should be highly structured teaching sessions rather than ad-hoc discussions between providers and patients. Thirdly, the teach-back method significantly improved patient recall of risks. Finally, the use of visual or auditory learning aids assisted patients in recalling information about the proposed treatment. With these relatively simple steps, the AHRQ authors concluded that institutions could communicate far more effectively with not only low-health-literacy patients but with the general patient population as well.

An important subset of the informed consent dialog is providing patients information about the risks of the treatment of procedure. Because risk information is generally gathered in the aggregate, understanding risk and applying that information to oneself as an individual patient requires numeracy or quantitative literacy. Understanding risk requires weighing benefits and interpreting percentages, ratios, risk magnitude, and statistical information. The NAAL study revealed that a substantial percentage of patients have limited quantitative literacy, with many able to do no more than simple arithmetic compu-

tations when identified for them. It is critical, therefore, that institutions meet their obligation to inform patients about risks and benefits by finding effective ways to communicate quantitative risk information. Suggestions for communicating quantitative information effectively include providing smaller amounts of data at any given interaction, reducing the calculations and inferences from data required by the patient by providing more analysis and conclusions within the communication, and using visual displays.

LEP and Cultural Competency

The previous discussion of the challenges and requirements of providing information to LEP patients maps equally well onto the process of obtaining informed consent from these patients. Again, a successful approach must be comprehensive and unified. Translating an informed-consent form into another language has limited value without an interpreter to facilitate questions and answers between providers and patients, and almost no value if the patient has limited literacy in their native language. Likewise, issues of cultural competency do arise in the informed-consent context. As The Joint Commission has noted, a patient's cultural belief may have an impact on their decisions about care.[17] "Cultural brokers" can help providers communicate the importance of care that may be the subject of a cultural barrier with a patient by creating an environment of trust that allows the wishes of the patient and the provider to be more likely to align.

Advance Directives

A corollary to the issue of informed consent is the advance-directives issue. Advance directive can be a powerful tool in helping providers act on the wishes of their patients, but the forms used for these directives may be unreadable and not comprehensible for low-literacy patients. Considering that the NAAL census found consistently lower health-literacy rates among the elderly, critical advance-directive users, this area requires additional focus by providers. As the IOM noted in its report, one institutional provider developed a form written at the fifth-grade reading level that gave step-by-step, simple instructions for completing it and included text-enhancing graphics for low-literacy users. Because the provider had a significant Spanish-speaking patient cohort, the form was also translated into Spanish.

Accreditation

In addition to federal requirements, accreditation bodies, such as The Joint Commission, are becoming increasingly focused on health-literacy efforts at accredited institutions. The Joint Commission has directed a number of their National Patient Safety Goals to health-literacy-related subjects.[3] Institutions that seek to obtain or retain accreditation from The Joint Commission are expected to be in compliance with these goals. Similarly, the AHRQ is developing a new module for their Consumer Assessment of Healthcare Providers and Systems (CAHPS) survey that will measure patients' satisfaction with communication by providers.[9] The module will assess the clarity of communications concerning treatment, test results, and medications, among others.

HEALTH-LITERACY PRINCIPLES AND PROGRAMS

As the previous section stressed, adopting an institution-wide health-literacy program is a promising option for staying in compliance with the many legal and regulatory requirements that dot the current healthcare landscape. This is particularly true in light of the evidence that one cannot assess a patient's health literacy "just by looking." Making providers aware of the problem of low health literacy is only one part of the solution. Institution-wide health-literacy best practices can provide an important degree of protection against provider–patient miscommunication-based adverse events and, unlike the literacy level the average patient presents with, is under providers' control.

Although a number of programs now exist, one of the most important steps providers can take is to analyze their own patient population and keep current with the demographics of the people they serve. Staying aware of the number of non-native English speakers, the languages they speak, and the cultural issues that they bring with them when seeking care are vital to addressing the health-literacy issues that they may have. Maintaining current data on the number of senior patients at the institution will assist in addressing the particular health-literacy needs of this population. Institutions that serve a large number of patients at or below federal poverty levels will need to carefully examine their patient communications as well. Having staff who reflect the population that the institution serves is another technique to address health literacy at an organic level. Staff members that speak patients' native tongues, understand their cultural preferences, and are familiar with the obstacles that certain influences, such as poverty and age, have on literacy can help integrate an institution's efforts to ensure that literacy limitations do not lead to adverse events.[17]

Institutions are also their own best repositories for their particular risks related to health literacy. Examining adverse events and near misses for any components that can be attributed to patients' abilities to understand and communicate health-related information provides a starting place for an institution to identify and address the particular needs that its patient population faces. As an example, a hospital that serves a large population of Navajos with limited English proficiency had concerns about the safety of its medication self-administration program.[17] The hospital used sun and moon stickers to help patients understand when to take the medicines and dots to indicate how much medication to take. Implementing such an idea and then gathering data about adverse events in the medication self-administration program could provide an institution with specific patient safety initiatives tailored to that institution's particular needs.

Health-Literacy Programs

Although relying on their own data to pinpoint problems and test solutions is critical for institutions trying to eliminate health-literacy-related adverse events, there will also be efficiencies in adopting programs created by the many groups that have been studying health literacy over the past decade. The AMA, the NPSF, and even the federal government have also created health-literacy programs for healthcare providers.

The NPSF's "Ask Me 3" program centers around encouraging patients to understand three questions:[24]

1. What is my main problem?
2. What do I need to do?
3. Why is it important for me to do this?

The "Ask Me 3" program provides posters and brochures aimed at both, patients and providers. Providers are encouraged to understand the demographics and potential health-literacy issues of their patients, to use the program's tools to conduct in-service trainings for practitioners, and to audit their points of contact with patients for clarity and opportunities to assess patients' true understanding of what they are being told. Additionally, the AMA offers providers a "Health Literacy Kit," a clinician-oriented program designed to "define the scope of the health literacy problem; recognize health system barriers faced by patients with low health literacy; implement improved methods of verbal and written communication; and incorporate practical strategies to create a shame-free environment."[25] Also available are videos for clinicians showing patients describing barriers to their understanding of medical information.

While much attention has been paid to the oral communication between providers and patients, and the opportunity these moments create for providers to tailor their words to the specific skills of a specific patient, attention must also be paid to written communication. The federal government has initiated a "Plain Language" strategy to improve the clarity of written communication.[14] The strategy proposes techniques for plain writing, including putting the most important information first, breaking information into accessible chunks, using simple language and defining important technical terms, and providing enough white space to make pages easy to read. Plain language strategies also include speaking tips, including the "teach-back" method under which patients restate the information that they have gotten from providers in their own words so that providers can assess their comprehension. The information is repeated until the patient comprehends it well enough to restate it accurately. Demonstration techniques also assist with oral communication: showing a patient how to do something and then watching the patient do it.

As important as knowing the capabilities of your patient base is, it is also important to know the readability of your own materials. Several basic principles of clear writing have been generally adopted. Using common words and eliminating jargon help to clarify text for limited-literacy readers. Several different groups have created thesauri translating complex words and medical terms into plain language that is accessible to more readers. Other tips include writing in conversational sentences, limiting one idea to each paragraph, leaving white space on the page, emphasizing desired behaviors instead of medical facts, using headers and bullets as road signs for readers, and using only short sentences. Field testing materials and then revising based on comments can also help ensure that the materials accomplish their goals. Even providing surrogate readers may help some patients whose skills are the most limited.

The Group Health Research Institute provides a readability toolkit to help providers evaluate their written materials.[26] Also available is the Simple Measure of Gobbledygook tool that estimates the reading level required to understand a given text.[27] Similarly, the Maximus Center for Health Literacy is an online service that provides style manuals, translation services, and other readability services to state governments and other organizations.[28] Finally, Harvard University's School of Public Health, Health Literacy Studies Department, provides a variety of Web-based resources for organizations that seek to provide readable materials and to address other health-literacy challenges that their organizations face.[29]

Health-Literacy Case Study

Recent efforts by the Iowa Health System (IHS) provide an example of an institution using many of these resources to address health literacy head on. After assessing its own patient population and recognizing that half of its patients were at risk for low health literacy, the IHS created a Health Literacy Collaborative to coordinate a literacy initiative.[30] The collaborative conducted staff workshops, implemented the AMA's health-literacy toolkit, the Ask Me 3 program, and evaluated their efforts based on patient feedback. The collaborative had as its goals improving communication between providers and patients, using specific tools to help ensure patients' comprehension of health information, and simplifying paperwork, materials, referrals, and check-in. After implementing the program, the IHS saw an increase in the comprehension and retention of information by patients, and although the study did not specifically examine adverse events, the system met its primary goal of facilitating better-informed patients.

Health-Literacy Tests

Several tests have been developed for measuring an individual's health literacy. The most widely known tests are the Rapid Estimate of Adult Literacy in Medicine (REALM) and the Test of Functional Health Literacy in Adults (TOFHLA). The REALM assessment takes about 3 minutes and tests a person's ability to recognize and pronounce medical words.[9] The TOFHLA tests numerical ability and reading comprehension and takes about 20 minutes.[9] Both tests have proved highly valuable to people who conduct research in specific areas of health literacy; however, the formality of both tests and the limitations in what they can tell providers about a patient's true ability to process and evaluate medical information in the actual moment of treatment make them cumbersome and of limited value to providers on a day-to-day basis. These limitations indicate that the health-literacy techniques discussed herein, and those that will be coming out of ongoing research, should be applied as universally as possible. Using simple language, teach-backs, visual aids, trained interpreters, and culturally competent communication methods should become the best practice for all institutions and providers.

CONCLUSION

Although this book examines patient safety from the perspective of its myriad components, the nexus between good communication and safety resounds in each chapter. For over a decade, increasing attention has been paid to the provider–patient communication dyad and the concept of health literacy, and the role that the latter plays in patient safety has been developed. Although the starting point may appear to be the capabilities of patients to comprehend medical information, the IOM has recognized that "[e]qually important are the communication and assessment skills of the people with whom individuals interact regarding health."[1] Although the issues that underlie patients' limited literacy reach well beyond the control of providers, providers can take a lead role in combating the effects of limited health literacy on patient outcomes. As the "Healthy People 2010" authors note, "[[d]iagnoses and treatments require doctors to negotiate a common understanding with patients about what is to be done. The quality of provider–patient communication can affect numerous outcomes [and] [a]ppropriate information and communication with a provider not only can relieve patients' anxieties but also can help patients understand their choices, allow them to participate in informed decision making and better manage their own health concerns."[5]

In the final chapter of its report, the IOM has articulated the following 12 principles of health literacy that sum up the vision for the future of patient–provider communication:

1. Everyone has the opportunity to improve their health literacy.
2. Everyone has the opportunity to use reliable, understandable information that could make a difference in their overall well-being, including everyday behaviors such as how they eat, whether they exercise, and whether they get checkups.
3. Health and science content would be basic parts of K-12 curricula.
4. People are able to accurately assess the credibility of health information presented by health advocate, commercial, and news-media sources.

5. There is monitoring and accountability for health-literacy policies and practices.
6. Public-health alerts, vital to the health of the nation, are presented in everyday terms so that people can take necessary action.
7. The cultural contexts of diverse peoples, including those from various cultural groups and non-English-speaking peoples, are integrated into all health information.
8. Health practitioners communicate clearly during all interactions with their patients, using everyday vocabulary.
9. There is ample time for discussions between patients and healthcare providers.
10. Patients feel free and comfortable to ask questions as part of the healing relationship.
11. Rights and responsibilities in relation to health and health care are presented or written in clear, everyday terms so that people can take necessary action.
12. Informed-consent documents used in health care are developed so that all people can give or withhold consent based on information that they need and understand.[1]

References

1. Nielsen-Bohlman, L., Panzer, A.M., & Kindig, D.A. (Eds.). (2004). *Health literacy: A prescription to end confusion*. Institute of Medicine, Committee on Health Literacy. Washington, DC: National Academy Press.
2. National Center for Education Statistics, U.S. Department of Education. (2006). *The health literacy of America's adults: Results from the 2003 National Assessment of Adult Literacy*. http://nces.ed.gov/naal/. Accessed December 2, 2008.
3. The Joint Commission. (2007). *"What did the doctor say?": Improving health literacy to protect patient safety*. http://www.jointcommission.org/. Accessed December 2, 2008.

4. Kohn, L., Corrigan, J., & Donaldson, M. (Eds.). (2000). *To err is human: Building a safer health care system*. Committee on Quality of Health Care in America, Institute of Medicine. Washington, DC: National Academy Press.
5. Office of Disease Prevention and Control, U.S. Department of Health and Human Services. (2010). *Healthy people 2010* (Chap. 11: Health Communication). http://www.healthypeople.gov/document/pdf/Volume1/11HealthCom.pdf. Accessed 5/3/2010.
6. Glassman, P. (n.d.). *Health literacy*. National Network of Libraries of Medicine. http://nnlm.gov/outreach/consumer/hlthlit.html/. Accessed December 2, 2008.

7. The National Literacy Act of 2007, The 110th Congress S. 2424, introduced December 6, 2007. http://frwebgate.access.gpo.gov/cgi-bin/getdoc.cgi?dbname=110_cong_bills&docid=f:s2424is.txt.pdf. Accessed May 5, 2010.

8. Center for Health Care Strategies. (2005). *Health literacy fact sheets.* http://www.chcs.org/. Accessed December 2, 2008.

9. Agency for Healthcare Research and Quality. (2004). *Literacy and health outcomes.* Evidence report/technology assessment (No. 87). http://www.ahrq.gov/clinic/epcsums/litsum.htm/. Accessed December 2, 2008.

10. Peters, E., Hibbard, J., Slovic, P., & Diekmann, N. (2007). Numeracy skill and the communication, comprehension, and use of risk–benefit information. *Health Affairs, 26*(3), 741–748.

11. National Academy on an Aging Society. (n.d.). Fact sheet: Low health literary skills increase annual health care expenditures by $73 billion. http://www.agingsociety.org/agingsociety/publications/fact/fact_low.html/. Accessed December 2, 2008.

12. Parikh, N.S., Parker, R.M., Nurss, J.R., Baker D.W., & Williams, M.V. (1996, January). Shame and health literacy: The unspoken connection. *Patient Education and Counseling 27*(1), 33–39.

13. National Center for Education Statistics, U.S. Department of Education. (2006). *The health literacy of America's adults: Results from the 2003 National Assessment of Adult Literacy.* http://nces.ed.gov/naal/. Accessed December 2, 2008.

14. Office of Disease Prevention and Health Promotion, U.S. Department of Health and Human Services. (n.d.). *Plain language: A promising strategy for clearly communicating health information and improving health literacy.* http://www.health.gov/communication/literacy/plainlanguage/PlainLanguage.htm. Accessed May 5, 2010.

15. Medicare Rights Center. (2005). *Medicare statistics: The Medicare population, 2005.* http://www.medicarerights.org/maincontentstatsdemographics.html/. Accessed December 2, 2008.

16. The Commonwealth Fund. (2006). Quality matters: Health literacy (Vol. 21). http://www.commonwealthfund.org/publications/. Accessed December 2, 2008.

17. Wilson-Stronks, A., Lee, K.K., Cordero, C.L., Kopp, A.L., & Galvez, E. (2008). *One size does not fit all: Meeting the health care needs of diverse populations.* The Joint Commission.http://www.jointcommission.org/PatientSafety/HLC/. Accessed December 2, 2008.

18. U.S. Department of Justice, Civil Rights Division. (2000). *Improving access to services for persons with limited English proficiency.* Presidential executive order 13166. http://www.usdoj.gov/crt/cor/Pubs/eolep.php/. Accessed December 2, 2008.

19. Miranda, D., Zeller, P.K., Lee, R., Koepke, C.P., Holland, H.E., Englert, F., & Swift, E.K. (n.d.). *Speaking plainly: Communicating the patient's role in health care safety.* Advances in Patient Safety (Vol. 4). Agency for Healthcare Research and Quality. http://www.ahrq.gov/downloads/pub/advances/vol4/Miranda.pdf/. Accessed December 2, 2008.

20. Wilson-Stronks, A., & Galvez, E. (2008). *Exploring cultural and linguistic services in the nation's hospitals: A report of findings.* http://www.jointcommission.org/PatientSafety/HLC/. Accessed December 2, 2008.

21. National Patient Safety Foundation, Partnership for Clear Health Communication. (n.d.). *Ask Me 3: Program implementations guide for health care and information providers.* http://www.npsf.org/askme3/. Accessed December 2, 2008.

22. American Medical Association. (n.d.). *Informed consent.* Patient–physician relationship topics. http://www.ama-assn.org/ama/pub/category/4608.html/. Accessed December 2, 2008.

23. Pizzi, L.T., Goldfarb, N.I., & Nash D.B. (n.d.). *Procedures for obtaining informed consent.* Making health care safer: A critical analysis of patient safety practices. Agency for Healthcare Research and Quality. http://ahrq.gov/clinic/ptsafety/chap48.htm/. Accessed December 2, 2008.

24. Ask me 3. http://www.npsf.org/askme3/. Accessed December 2, 3008.

25. http://www.ama-assn.org/ama/pub/category/9913.html/. Accessed December 2, 2008.

26. Group Health Research Institute. (n.d.). *Our capabilities.* http://www.centerforhealthstudies.org/capabilities/capabilities.html/. Accessed December 2, 2008.

27. McLaughlin, G.H. (n.d.). *SMOG: Simple measure of gobbledygook.* http://www.harrymclaughlin.com/SMOG.htm/. Accessed December 2, 2008.

28. http://www.maximus.com/services/health/health-literacy/. Accessed May 5, 2010.

29. Harvard School of Public Health. (n.d.). Health literacy studies. http://www.hsph.harvard.edu/healthliteracy/. Accessed December 2, 2008.

30. The Commonwealth Fund. (2006). *Health policy, health reform and performance improvement.* Quality matters: Health literacy (Vol. 21). http://www.commonwealthfund.org/publications/. Accessed December 2, 2008.

29

THE IMPACT OF FATIGUE ON ERROR AND PATIENT SAFETY

Diana L. Alvarez, MT, (ASCP)CM
Barbara J. Youngberg, JD, MSW, BSN, FASHRM

INTRODUCTION

The effects of fatigue and sleep deprivation have been directly linked to increases in the occurrence of human error. The Exxon Valdez incident as well as the disasters at Three Mile Island, Bhopal, and Chernobyl each lists fatigue as a root cause.[1] In response to these incidents and to prevent these types of occurrences in the future, the aviation, mining, nuclear power, transport, and military industries have invested heavily in research to study fatigue and its effects on workers. The results of this research have been used to direct solutions that help prevent and mitigate the effects of fatigue, and thereby decrease the potential risk of associated error.

Certain occupations, such as airline pilot and truck driver, have had their work hours restricted by the Occupational Safety and Health Agency (OSHA) for a long time. Airline pilots are not permitted to work for more than 8 hours. On international flights that last more than 8 hours, there are two sets of crews. The second set of crew takes over in mid-air after the first set has worked their shift. Truck drivers have to take an 8-hour break after a 12-hour shift. Health care, which constantly involves performing critical tasks and is also at risk for errors due to worker fatigue, has only recently been added to this list of highly hazardous industries.[2]

Among industries, considerable research has been conducted to study fatigue and how it affects the human being. This chapter explains fatigue and its effects, and describes why healthcare providers are at increased risk for developing it. The chapter highlights research specifically focused on the effects of fatigue in the healthcare setting and its impact on healthcare providers and the patients they serve. Recommendations directed at improving provider and patient safety, and reducing the overall risks identified by this research, are discussed along with the reasons that many of these recommendations are met with resistance from some healthcare educators and professionals. Finally, a few practical solutions and proactive strategies aimed at raising awareness of the problem among healthcare workers are offered.

WHAT IS FATIGUE?

Fatigue is not easily defined, and people experience different and varying degrees of symptoms.[3] Generally, fatigue can be described as feelings of extreme tiredness, lack of energy, or exhaustion to the point that the ability to function and respond normally decreases.[3,4] Fatigue usually presents when a person is suffering from a lack of quality sleep that, over time, can adversely affect performance. Chronic sleep deprivation can result in a lack of vigilance and attention as well as short-term memory lapses, cognitive diminution and frontal-lobe-function deficits, and rapid and involuntary sleep onsets during waking hours.[5] Moodiness, emotional instability, clumsiness, lack of motivation, and even loss of appetite and digestive problems can also result when a person is chronically fatigued.[3] It becomes apparent that these effects can present a multitude of problems for the individual suffering from them, but when that individual is a healthcare provider, the risk for potentially adverse outcomes to not only the provider but also the patient increases dramatically.

WHY ARE HEALTHCARE PROVIDERS SUSCEPTIBLE?

As mentioned previously, many entities in the healthcare sector operate around the clock and must be staffed to provide adequate coverage at all times. In addition, many healthcare providers, particularly interns, residents, and attending physicians, are forced to either work long hours as part of their training or return to the hospital after hours to handle emergencies. In addition, providers work schedules that include various non-traditional types of shifts: evening, night, rotating, shifts of various lengths, and on-call. According to The Joint Commission Resources publication, "Strategies for Addressing Health Care Worker Fatigue," approximately 30% of nurses employed full time in health care participate in shift work.[6] Expanding this number to include the many other positions necessary to keep the entity functioning around the clock, it becomes apparent that the number of persons involved in shift work is significant and the problems associated with fatigue are common.

The effects of fatigue are exacerbated in those individuals who work night shifts. A primary reason that fatigue is common in night-shift workers is that they are awake and active at night, when the body expects to be sleeping. This causes disruption of circadian rhythms, which cycle on a 24-hour clock, are entrained by light, and regulate many important bodily functions including secretion of melatonin and cortisol.[3,5] These disruptions can negatively affect both the ability to stay awake during work hours as well as the ability to sleep during the day, and fatigue may ensue.[5] Another reason that off-shift work may contribute to fatigue involves the motivation of the employee and why they chose to work an undesirable shift. If an individual is under financial constraints, he or she may choose to work an evening or night shift to take advantage of the differential paid to employees who cover those hours. In addition, working an irregular shift allows the opportunity to moonlight or take a second job. Because these individuals are not using their time away from work to get adequate sleep, they may suffer more severe symptoms of fatigue.[7]

In addition to working different shifts, the length of shifts worked by healthcare providers must also be addressed. Many healthcare professionals routinely work 12-hour shifts and are often required to work longer due to staffing issues. One study gathered data on critical-care nurses' work hours and found, over a 28-day reporting period, that only 1 in 502 respondents reported leaving work at the end of their scheduled shift.[8] Long duty hours are infamously associated with residents in training who, until regulations were enforced by the Accreditation Council for Graduate Medical Education (ACGME) in 2003, sometimes worked more than 100 hours per week and shifts that lasted 36 hours or longer with little time for on-duty sleep.[3,7] Because residents in training are fulfilling an educational obligation, this was not viewed as excessive by some standards; however, research illustrates that both patient and provider safety are at risk when providers are forced to work extended shifts.

CORRELATING FATIGUE TO MEDICAL ERRORS

Research has demonstrated a definitive link between fatigue and a decrease in cognitive function. Caldwell et al. list the following skills/functions that are impaired by fatigue: accuracy and timing degrade, multi-tasking becomes difficult, ability to integrate information is lost, performance becomes inconsistent, and well-practiced activities become increasingly difficult.[5] Compound these conditions with a decrease in the ability to reason, waning attention, attitude/mood deterioration, and involuntary lapses into sleep,[5] and it is evident that when healthcare providers are suffering from these effects, there is a very high potential for medical error to occur.

A study by Barger et al. concluded that interns across the United States who worked extended-duration work shifts (more than 24 hours) "were associated with an increased risk of significant medical errors, adverse events, and attentional failures."[9] The study, conducted over a 10-month period, required participating interns to complete monthly surveys regarding work and sleep hours, number of days off, monthly activities, and number of shifts requiring extended duration. The surveys also required the interns to report signifi-

cant medical errors that they made and whether or not they felt the error was fatigue related. The results of this study demonstrated a correlation in the increase in the number of significant fatigue-related errors, including those that resulted in a fatality, as the number of extended-duration shifts increased. The occurrence of an intern suffering from an attentional failure, such as dozing during surgery or during an examination, also demonstrated a positive correlation with the number of extended-duration shifts worked.[9]

There have likewise been studies conducted that associate the effects of fatigue experienced by nurses and how these effects compromise patient care and safety. Due to a nationwide shortage of registered nurses, these professionals may be especially vulnerable to the effects of fatigue. They are often required to work longer than a regularly scheduled shift (which may be 12 hours to begin with), work through break periods, pick up extra shifts, and take call during their time away from work. A study by Rogers et al. analyzed the work patterns of nurses and found that the likelihood of a nurse making an error increased with increased work duration, overtime, and number of hours worked per week. Of 5,312 shifts worked, there were 199 errors and 213 near errors made by nurses, more than half of which were medication errors.[10] Another study, by Scott et al. that focused on critical-care nurses reported similar results, with 86% of shifts extending longer than scheduled by almost an hour, and 27% of nurses reported making at least one error and 38% reported making at least one near error.[8] Many of the errors reported were again medication errors, and other sources of error were in performing procedures, charting, and transcription;[8] thus, research demonstrates that fatigue does negatively affect the healthcare professional's ability to perform tasks and puts the patient on the receiving end of this care at risk.

PIVOTAL MOMENTS

In 1984, Libby Zion, an 18-year-old, died at New York Hospital within a few hours of admission.[11] Although her death was the result of a culmination of mishaps, contributing factors included that Libby was being cared for only by residents, who routinely worked 36 hours at a time with minimal to no sleep, and that these residents were undersupervised.[4,11] Libby's father turned the tragedy of losing his daughter into a mission aimed at limiting resident work hours and increasing their supervision.[11] As a result of his crusade, limitations on resident work hours were recommended by a New York State commission in 1987.[4] Although this was a step in the right direction, this effort met with little success and no other states followed in instituting work-duty limits; however, following the 1999 publication of the Institute of Medicine (IOM) report, "To Err Is Human: Building a Safer Health System," which brought public attention to the frequency of medical errors and the acute need to improve patient safety, it became apparent that duty-hour reform was necessary. In 2003 the Accreditation Council for Graduate Medical Education (ACGME) instituted duty-hour regulations that limit resident duty hours to an average of 80 hours/week, applicable to all ACGME-accredited programs throughout the United States, although there are exemptions for a few specialties.[4] Similarly, the Association of periOperative Registered Nurses (AORN) and the American Association of Nurse Anesthetists (AANA) have made recommendations intended to limit fatigue in nursing professions and thereby improve patient and provider safety.[12]

ACGME REGULATIONS: OPPOSING VIEWS

Although the primary purpose of the ACGME institution of resident duty-hour limits was to promote patient and provider safety as well as resident well-being, these new regulations met with some opposition. Many physician educators believe that the extremely long hours incurred in resident education are necessary to expose residents to the rigors of real-world practice, and that reducing them will leave the resident ill-prepared for life after residency;[13] others feel that regulations imposed by an outside agency result in a loss of autonomy by physician training programs.[13] A third argument against shorter duty hours is that decreased work hours will result in more frequent patient handoffs, which has a negative effect on continuity of care for the patient.[13] Costs associated with implementation of shorter duty hours will require additional staff, and this is also a concern to the institutions that sponsor resident training programs.[14] Many of these issues present valid reasons for arguments against implementing the 2003 ACGME regulations. The recent IOM recommendations offered in response to the 2003 ACGME regulations address many of these issues.

In response to the ACGME guidelines, Congress and the Agency for Healthcare Research and Quality (AHRQ) requested that the IOM form a committee to focus on resident schedules relative to healthcare safety and develop strategies to improve safety in health care by optimizing these schedules.[4] This committee, the IOM's Committee on Optimizing Graduate Medical Trainee (Resident) Hours and Work Schedules to Improve Patient Safety, recently published their findings and recommendations in "Resident Duty Hours: Enhancing Sleep, Supervision, and Safety," which supplements the ACGME regulations by focusing not just on reducing work hours but on increasing opportunities for sleep during resident training to prevent chronic sleep deprivation and thus decrease the occurrence of fatigue-related errors.[4] The IOM committee concentrated on a few pertinent factors, including resident educational requirements, resident safety and well-being, patient safety, as well as the economic implications of instituting recommended changes, in developing their recommendations.[4] The IOM committee makes the following general recommendations: [4]

1. The ACGME should adopt and enforce requirements of resident training such that:
   a. They limit duty hours and develop schedules that allow for prevention of sleep loss and fatigue.
   b. When fatigue is unavoidable, additional measures are taken to mitigate the effects.
   c. Schedules provide predictable, protected, and sufficient recovery sleep to relieve acute and chronic sleep loss.
   d. They promote resident well-being.
   e. They ensure that learning requirements are met.
2. The ACGME should amend its current requirements on moonlighting to require that all moonlighting be included in the duty-hour limits, that residents get approval for these activities from their program director, and that their performance be monitored to ensure adequate resident performance.
3. The ACGME and residency programs should strengthen monitoring practices, and the Centers for Medicare and Medicaid Services (CMS), as well as The Joint Commission, should oversee these activities.
4. Those institutions with residency programs provide safe alternate transportation options for any resident who is too tired to safely drive home.
5. The ACGME should require residency-training institutions to adjust resident workload by limiting tasks that provide little or no educational value and provide adequate time for the resident to perform patient evaluations and reflective learning to ensure that the resident fulfills all core educational requirements.
6. The ACGME should ensure that there is adequate, direct, onsite supervision of residents.

7. Teaching hospitals should institutionalize structured handover processes to ensure continuity of care and patient safety.
8. Residents should be fully involved in reporting, learning, and quality-improvement systems at their respective institutions, and this should be included as part of the educational experience.
9. All recommendations should be supported by financial stakeholders, e.g., CMS, Department of Veterans Affairs (DVA), Department of Defense (DOD), Health Resources and Services Administration, state and local governments, private insurers, and sponsoring institutions, to ensure promotion of patient and resident safety and education.
10. ACGME should gather data and monitor implementation of these recommendations as well as plan for revision to achieve the desired result. The CMS, AHRQ, National Institutes of Health, DOD, DVA, and others should financially support this effort.

This information and set of recommendations are very specific to resident training. Because the healthcare industry is comprised of many different allied health professionals, alternative recommendations are discussed in the next section, which can apply to anyone who may be at risk of suffering from fatigue and its effects. Table 29–1 provides a comparison of the 2003 ACGME Duty Hour Limits and the 2008 Institute of Medicine Recommendations.

ALTERNATIVE RECOMMENDATIONS AND SOLUTIONS

Much has been learned about fatigue from the research conducted across different industries that can be used to develop solutions for combating it and its effects. Traditionally, working more and sleeping less was considered by some to be an indication of a

Table 29–1 Comparison of the 2003 Accreditation Council for Graduate Medical Education (ACGME) Duty Hour Limits with the 2008 Institute of Medicine Recommendations

Variables	2003 ACGME Duty Hour Limits	2008 Institute of Medicine Recommendations
Maximum hours of work per week	80 hours, averaged over 4 weeks	No change
Maximum shift length	30 hours (admitting patients up to 24 hours, then 6 additional hours for transitional and educational activities)	30 hours (admitting patients for up to 16 hours, plus 5-hour protected sleep period between 10 p.m. and 8 a.m. with the remaining hours for transition and educational activities) 16 hours with no protected sleep period
Maximum in-hospital on-call frequency	Every third night, on average	Every third night, no averaging
Minimum time off between scheduled shifts	10 hours after shift length	10 hours after day shift 12 hours after night shift 14 hours after any extended duty period of 30 hours and not return until 6 a.m. the next day
Maximum frequency of in-hospital night shifts	Not addressed	Four nights maximum; 48 hours off after three or four nights of consecutive duty
Mandatory time-off duty	4 days off per month; 1 day (24 hours) off per week, averaged over 4 weeks	5 days off per month 1 day (24 hours) off per week, no averaging One 48-hour period off per month
Moonlighting	Internal moonlighting is counted against 80-hour weekly limit	Internal and external moonlighting is counted against 80-hour weekly limit All other duty-hour limits apply to moonlighting in combination with scheduled work
Limit on hours for exceptions	88 hours for select programs with a sound educational rationale	No change
Emergency room limits	12-hour shift limit, at least an equivalent period of time off between shifts; 60-hour work week with an additional 12 hours for education	No change

person's motivation, training, or professionalism;[5] however, research has demonstrated that it is impossible for a person to adapt to inadequate sleep.[5] The Joint Commission Resources recently published "Strategies for Addressing Health Care Worker Fatigue" and names education as the foundation of raising awareness and thereby reducing fatigue in the workplace.[3] Education should include basic information about how sleep works, sleep deprivation and identifying symptoms of fatigue, good sleep hygiene, identifying sleep disorders, effects of caffeine, exercise, and prescription drugs on sleep, as well as environmental conditions that improve alertness, including lighting and ventilation, and taking short breaks from tasks.[3] Other solutions to help prevent worker fatigue include improving work/rest schedules, optimizing sleep, and faster circadian entrainment.[5]

Many solutions are relatively easy to implement, and the cost of start-up and maintenance may prove to be considerably less than the cost of the medical error that it may prevent. It is imperative, for these solutions to be successful, that the institution place value on and support efforts toward preventing worker fatigue at every level. Examining and adjusting work schedules, taking into consideration shift length, number of consecutive days, start and end times, on-call or overtime, and allowance for adequate recovery time after each worked shift can be very effective in reducing worker fatigue and burnout.[3] If a person is required to work rotating shifts, ensure that shifts rotate forward to facilitate circadian entrainment.[5] Schedulers may benefit from using FAST (Fatigue Avoidance Scheduling Tool), a software program initially developed for the U.S. Air Force and Army that is used in other industries as well. It allows a user to enter a potential or actual work schedule to determine if the schedule allows for adequate rest based on the SAFTE model (Sleep, Activity, Fatigue, and Task Effectiveness).[3]

Enhancing the ideas of teamwork and effective communication among providers can help alleviate the issue of more frequent patient handoffs and disruptions in continuity of patient care resulting from staff changes. Fostering teamwork in the healthcare setting is critical to improving communication and thereby providing patient care in a safe and effective manner.[3] According to The Joint Commission Resources, to improve teamwork and communication an organization should:[3]

- Eliminate the hierarchy, which may be difficult for some physicians. Everyone needs to work as a team and communicate effectively and respectfully with one another.
- Define each team member's role and responsibilities.
- Provide training on teamwork and how to communicate effectively.
- Have and enforce a zero-tolerance policy for abusive behavior.
- Have a means of measuring team performance.

These solutions are relatively easy to implement and can prove very effective in preventing fatigue and associated medical errors, if they are supported by every person at every level of the institution.

CONCLUSION

Many unfortunate events have spurred research on fatigue and its effects on the human being. Although fatigue and its effects have been realized in the aviation, mining, nuclear power, transport, and military industries, health care has just recently been identified as one of these high-risk industries due to the around-the-clock nature of the business. As a result, there has been increasingly more research performed that addresses specifically the effects of fatigue on healthcare workers. Born from this research are a multitude of regulations and recommendations that are all aimed at preventing fatigue and thereby improving patient safety by decreasing the number of associated medical errors. Many cost-effective and easily implemented solutions are available for organizations to increase the awareness of fatigue and learn ways to prevent it and/or mitigate its effects when working fatigued is unavoidable due to circumstances. Working together to raise awareness of fatigue, this often-ignored but very real consequence of working in an industry "that never sleeps" can help create a safer environment not only for the patient but for the provider as well.

References

1. Griffith, C., Hallbert, B., & Mahadevan, S. *Inclusion of fatigue effects in human reliability analysis.* Department of Civil and Environmental Engineering, Vanderbilt University. http://www.reliability-studies.vanderbilt .edu/projects/briefs/griffith_c.htm. Accessed May 5, 2010.
2. Dinges, D.F. (1995). An overview of sleepiness and accidents. *Journal of Sleep Research, 4*(Suppl 2), 4–14.
3. The Joint Commission Resources. (2008). *Strategies for addressing health care worker fatigue.* Oakbrook Terrace, IL: The Joint Commission on Accreditation of Health Care Organizations.
4. Institute of Medicine. (2009). *Resident duty hours: Enhancing sleep, supervision, and safety.* Washington, DC: The National Academies Press.
5. Caldwell, J.A., Caldwell, J.L., & Schmidt, R. (2008). Alertness management strategies for operational contexts. *Sleep Medicine Reviews, 12,* 257–273.
6. Blachowicz, E., & Letizia, M. (2006). The challenges of shift work. *Medsurg Nursing, 15*(5), 274–280.
7. Clancy, C. (2009). *Navigating the health care system.* How Tired is Your Doctor. Agency for Healthcare Research and Quality. http://www .ahrq.gov/consumer/cc/cc030309.html/. Accessed May 7, 2010.
8. Scott, L.D., Rogers, A.E., Hwang, W.T. & Zhang,Y. (2006). Effects of critical care nurses' work hours on vigilance and patients' safety. *American Journal of Critical Care, 15,* 30–37.

9. Barger, L.,Ayas, N.T., Cade. B. E., Cronin, J.W., Rosner, B., & Speizer, F. (2006). Impact of extended-duration shifts on medical errors, adverse events, and attentional failures. *PLoS Medicine, 3*(12), 2440–2448. http://www .plosmedicine.org/article/info:doi/10.1371/ journal.pmed.0030487. Accessed May 6, 2010.
10. Rogers, A.E., Hwang, W.T., Scott, L.D., Aiken, L.H., & Dinges, D.F., (2004). The working hours of hospital staff nurses and patient safety. *Health Affairs,* 202–212. http://content .healthaffairs.org/cgi/reprint/23/4/202. Accessed May 6, 2010.
11. Lerner, B.H. (2009, March). A life-changing case for doctors in training. *The New York Times,* p. 3., http://www.nytimes.com/2009/ 03/03/health/03zion.html?_r=1&partner =rss&emc=rss. Accessed May 5, 2010.
12. Association of periOperative Registered Nurses. (2005). AORN position statement on safe-work/on-call practices. http://www.aorn.org/ PracticeResources/AORNPositionStatements/ Position/. Accessed May 7, 2010.
13. Cherr, G.S. (2004). The origins of regulated resident work hours: New York and beyond. *Bulletin of the American College of Surgeons, 87*(11), 23–27.
14. Medline Plus. (2009). *Limiting work hours for medical residents could be costly.* http://health .usnews.com/health-news/managing-your -healthcare/healthcare/articles/2009/05/20/ limiting-work-hours-for-medical-residents -could.html. Accessed May 7, 2010.

30

MANAGING THE FAILURES OF COMMUNICATION IN HEALTHCARE SETTINGS

Sherri DeVito, JD, BA

INTRODUCTION

Medical errors are an unfortunate aspect of modern health care. Despite the best intentions and efforts of healthcare practitioners, errors occur and patient injury results. Although most people think of medical errors as individually caused (e.g., the doctor operated on the wrong leg, the nurse gave the wrong medication), the reality is that medical errors often have system-level causes that set up doctors and nurses to fail and ultimately harm patients. Communication, or the lack thereof, is one such system-level cause of medical errors. The failure of communication, especially during handoffs (the transfer of patients between healthcare practitioners), is a widespread problem that results in confusion, frustration, near misses, and adverse events. How could a highly trained industry be plagued by such a simple human problem? This chapter discusses the impact that poor communication has on healthcare providers and their patients. Firstly, the chap-ter explains what is "good communication" versus "bad communication" and why the distinction matters. Next, it analyzes the common reasons behind communication breakdowns and why the problems persist. Lastly, the chapter explores possible ways to fix this situation and discusses settings where such remedies have already been successfully implemented.

EFFECTIVE COMMUNICATION VERSUS POOR COMMUNICATION: WHY DOES IT MATTER?

Communication, commonly seen as an innocuous component of healthcare delivery, is a real and dangerous threat to patient safety if handled poorly.[1] Effective communication is clear, complete, detailed, and thorough. Poor communication takes various forms and can be divided into the following categories: failures of occasion, content, purpose, audience, and process. Communication failures due to occasion occur where the timing of an information exchange was requested or provided too late to be useful.[2] Content failures happen when critical information needed to care for a patient is not communicated, either verbally or in writing, or is inaccurate.[2] Failures of communication purpose take place where the issues were not resolved.[2] Exclusion of key individuals from the communication constitutes a failure of audience.[2] Lastly, the process itself can cause communication failures in various ways, such as through the lack of face-to-face communication, use of unclear or illegible handwritten notes, and as a result of the use of night-float residents.[3] Night-float residents are second covering resident physicians, who generally care for patients between midnight and 7 a.m.

As a consequence of communication failures through the multiple types listed previously, various negative results can occur. For instance, in a study by Awad et al., 36% of communication failures were found to result in visible effects on system processes including inefficiency, team tension, resource waste, work-around, delay, and patient inconvenience.[4] Additionally, there is the chance of severe patient injury or mortality as a result of the failure to effectively communicate important information. As seen in other industries, simple errors of communication have the ability to cause deadly catastrophes.[5] Well-known examples of disasters that resulted from communication errors are the explosion of the space shuttle Challenger and the release of methocyanate in Bhophal, India.

Despite recognition of the various ways in which communication errors manifest, the multiple consequences that result, and the presentation of best-practice solutions, the issue still persists. This is quite troubling, particularly because those who work in the healthcare industry are generally well educated, well trained, and committed to patient care. Why, therefore, is something so basic as communication so difficult to achieve? Surprisingly, the answer has much

more to do with system-level factors than it has to do with individual failures. Seven such system-level factors that contribute to communication failures are hierarchies, healthcare culture, education/training, insufficient staffing, poor team integration, lack of standardization, and decreased work weeks.

PRESENCE OF HIERARCHIES

The presence of hierarchies in medicine is perhaps one of the biggest contributors to communication problems. In most industries there is a clear chain of superiority, running from the lowest link, such as interns, to the highest link, such as the chief executive officer, with intermediate-level supervisors and managers in between. Ideally, the lower links would feel free to go to their superiors with problems and concerns, whether those issues be about their work or about the superior's work. In medicine, however, the opposite is true: there is a widespread feeling that those who are superior cannot and should not be bothered by an inferior. This mentality can be seen in four types of specific, problematic relationships that exist in healthcare settings: residents/attending physicians, hospital residents/community physicians, internal-medicine residents/specialists, and residents/nurses.[6]

Communication problems typically arise between residents and the attending physician who has a supervisory role over the resident.[7] Sutcliffe et al. found that while the attending physician is a teacher and the resident performs the bulk of the decision making and patient care, the residents are hesitant to appear incompetent by communicating information that might be unfavorable to them.[7] This is a particularly odd feature of the resident/attending-physician relationship, because by definition, a resident is a student and therefore mistakes occur because they simply do not have the knowledge that the attending physician possesses. In addition to residents' hesitancy to communicate information where they might appear incompetent, residents are also hesitant to offend those in power.[7] This manifests particularly when residents debate calling an attending physician in the middle of the night; thus, residents feel tension between wanting to be sure that they are taking the correct course of action and wanting to possess enough knowledge to not have to contact the attending physician.[8] Sutcliffe et al. also found that residents are further discouraged from disagreeing with a superior because of pervasive perceptions that those in power would not listen to them or hear their point of view.[9] Additionally, residents are frequently given too little information by their attending physician, and for all the previous reasons, residents do not feel that they can contact the attending physician for further details, thereby jeopardizing patient care on account of pride.[10]

Faulty communication also frequently occurs between hospital residents and community physicians, most often where the hospital resident admits a patient who was previously under the care of a community physician to the care of a team of staff physicians.[11] When that care transfer occurs, information about the patient is often lacking, sometimes completely, because of role conflict and ambiguity.[11] The community physician may desire to maintain some role in the patient's care, and as a result of convoluted communication links between the large team of healthcare providers now involved, miscommunication and disagreements over patient care are common.[11]

Internal-medicine residents and specialists also suffer from communication problems, the most common of which is the lack of timely and effective exchange of pertinent information.[11] Concerns about offending or being ignored by the superior party, as seen in the relationship between residents and their attending physician, are present in situations where residents must interact with other attending physicians in specialty departments.[12] In particular, internal residents often find themselves admitting

patients sent to them by emergency room attending personnel, and may find it difficult to disagree with the specialty attending physician because of the hierarchy in place.[12] Exacerbating the problem is the lack of face-to-face communication between the internal-medicine residents and specialty consultants and communication through patient charts, which often are incomplete or illegible.

Lastly, residents and nurses also experience failures in communication, despite the fact that they work together closely in managing patient care. Part of the problem can be attributed to written orders. Although writing or typing orders in a patient's medical record allows for better documentation, such orders are impersonal and cannot appropriately address certain situations, such as where action must be taken quickly.[12] In those circumstances, oral communication would be superior, because it would allow the resident to convey the urgency and afford the nurse the chance to ask any questions regarding further treatment. Additionally, the personal characteristics of the communicator can also contribute to communication failures.[12] Besides perceptions that a superior is, or is not, receptive to receiving information, non-verbal information displayed by the parties also plays an important role. Eye gaze, posture, facial expression, and voice tone can cause a party to look nice or aggressive, thereby influencing how others respond to that person's concerns regarding a patient.[12]

Problematic hierarchies are not limited to coworkers, however, and commonly exist between providers and patients. Part of the problem is the historical, paternalistic treatment of patients whereby firm, professional decisions are taken on a patient's behalf with a minimum of discussion.[13] As a result, patients can feel powerless and that the choices for their care and treatment are not theirs to make. Furthermore, the large education gap that often exists between providers and patients further exacerbates the inequality between the two groups. The use of medical terminology, although appropriate between colleagues, confuses most patients and prevents full understanding of their medical conditions. Without such knowledge, patients cannot effectively participate in their care and make well-informed decisions with their healthcare provider; therefore, many patients retreat from active involvement, leading practitioners to behave in a paternalistic manner.

THE IMPACT OF CULTURE

Medical culture also plays a significant role in communication problems. For instance, professional autonomy has long been cherished by the medical community.[14] Many healthcare practitioners feel that they should be able to manage patient care without outside influence or the need to go to another for assistance. Additionally, individual accountability is valued, meaning that if an error occurs, it can and should be directly attributed to the patient's caregiver or the one who "caused" the error, with little to no focus on outside, system-level factors.[14] Deeply embedded in the culture is also the idea that error-free performances and quality care are the result of being well trained and trying hard.[15] When mistakes inevitably occur, they are viewed as a result of the personal failure of the healthcare practitioner who simply did not try hard enough.[16]

EDUCATION AND TRAINING

The education and training of healthcare practitioners is a third factor that contributes to errors in communication. Nurses and doctors receive different training in communication, and that discrepancy leads to problems in practice.[16] Doctors are taught to be concise and get to the "headlines" without haste, while nurses learn to be broad, narrative, "paint the big picture," and not make diagnoses when providing clinical descriptions.[16] As a result, nurses may feel that they get inadequate information from doctors, while doctors feel nurses waste their time with

extraneous information. Additionally, many healthcare practitioners do not even know how to communicate errors once they have occurred because of a lack of training on the hospital's error-reporting system;[17] thus, personal and system-level factors can combine to prevent effective disclosure.

STAFFING PROCEDURES

A fourth factor in communication problems is that of staffing procedures. Numerous hospitals experience budgetary shortfalls, and as a solution to save money, the hospital staff is limited to a minimum. Although such cutback may help the hospital's bottom line, it leads to stress for the rest of the staff because there are fewer people to handle the same amount of work. Additionally, such a lack of redundancy means that there is less time for practitioners to communicate properly, either through team meetings or otherwise.[18] As a result, there is decreased understanding about the goals for that patient's care, which could possibly lead to an adverse event.

TEAM INTEGRATION

Team integration also plays a role in faulty communication. Team instability, such as a circulating group of scrub nurses, can lead to inferior outcomes because team members simply do not know each other and their work styles.[18] As discussed previously, hierarchies and interpersonal dynamics can also contribute to a lack of team integration.[19] Additionally, role conflict and ambiguities, as seen in the previous discussion of hospital residents and community physicians, often cause communication difficulties.[20]

LACK OF STANDARDIZATION

The lack of standardized instruction regarding communication is a sixth factor that contributes to errors in communication.[4] Although the inevitable daily changes in a patient's hospitalization make[21] the task of communicating an important one, few medical trainees receive formal instruction, supervision, or feedback in the handoff process. Part of the problem is that communication skills are underemphasized in residency programs, and the formal teaching programs that are available, such as medical-team training, are not entirely effective.[22]

LIMITS IN DUTY HOURS

A seventh system-based factor that causes communication problems is the shift to the 80-hour work week. In 2003, the Accreditation Council for Graduate Medical Education implemented duty-hour limits for resident education and related patient care.[23] Currently, residents are limited to 80-hour weeks, averaged over 4 weeks.[23] The duty-hour standards were adopted out of concern that fatigue resulting from excessive hours for residents jeopardized the quality of care and subjected them to working environments that were not conducive to learning.[23] However, there is a downside to the limit on hours: there is an increased volume of transfers of patient care as a result;[22] therefore, there is an increased chance for communication errors because there are increased patient handoffs as a result of the new standard.

Although system-based factors overwhelmingly contribute to communication problems, particularly when there is a change in personnel managing a patient's care, individual-level factors also play a role. Perhaps most basic is the fact that many practitioners are tired at the end of their shift and therefore either forget to mention all pertinent aspects of a patient's care or are simply too fatigued to provide a thorough recap.[20] Practitioners' interpersonal skills also play an important role in communication mishaps.[7] An introverted practitioner may find it exceedingly difficult to speak up, whereas an extroverted one may provide too much information, causing others to tune out his or her words.[18] Along the same lines,

supervisor hostility is another individual-level factor that would negatively affect communication, regardless of the interpersonal skills of the supervisor's subordinate.[7]

THE RESULTS OF INEFFECTIVE COMMUNICATION

What results from all of these various factors is that there is a pervasive breakdown in quality, elementary communication where it is most needed. Although communication difficulties may occur at anytime, it is particularly problematic in the context of patient handoffs where many of these factors combine and render highly educated and well-trained persons incapable of effectuating the simple human task of talking.

The impact of such a breakdown affects not only healthcare practitioners and their ability to perform at optimal levels but patients as well. Communication problems are one of the most frequent contributing causes of adverse outcomes, occurring in 30% of cases.[24] Even where the error does not rise to the level of an adverse outcome, errors in communication may cause frustration and confusion to the patient over his or her medical condition, because the patient could be told different things by different healthcare providers. Additionally, patient distrust of the medical system is likely to arise, because obvious errors in a relatively simple task can indicate latent errors elsewhere in the healthcare system; therefore, it is paramount that the medical community take seriously the problem of communication and implement solutions so as to change the way healthcare practitioners interact and also to serve patients better.

SUGGESTIONS ON HOW TO AMELIORATE THE CURRENT SITUATION

Communication problems, unlike errors of machinery, are difficult to fix because there is no simple repair or recall to effectuate an improvement; instead, remedying errors in communication necessitates a modification in the personal behavior of a large number of people, something that is quite challenging to do. Although such a change will be difficult to implement system-wide, it is necessary and possible through the following eight methods: standardized training/education, change in culture, elimination of hierarchies, use of technology, face-to-face communication/required debriefings, personality awareness in healthcare settings, redundancy, and critical-language use.

Although effective verbal communication is important to ensure proper transmission of information, standardized methods of doing so are largely absent from the medical community.[25] This is particularly problematic at the time of handoffs, where proper information exchange is imperative. Because proper verbal communication during sign-out is important for safe patient care, standard educational programs should be considered to train healthcare practitioners to communicate effectively at the time of handoff.[25] One such standardized program is the Situational Debriefing Model, also known as "SBAR," which stands for situation, background, assessment, and recommendation.[25] This model originated in the U.S. Navy but can be applied in healthcare settings to improve communication of critical information in a timely and orderly fashion.[25] A second standardized program that could be utilized by the healthcare community is a five-part briefing protocol, currently used by the U.S. Forest Service, known as STICC (situation, task, intent, concern, calibrate).[25] Under STICC, communicators describe the circumstances, what they think they should do, the reasons why, and what they should keep their eye on, and they discuss the situation with others for deeper understanding.[25]

A third program, known as the situational awareness (SA) model, is essentially a shared understanding of what is going on and what is likely to happen next.[26] This model is particularly useful because it recognizes the coexisting roles of systems and cognitive errors and helps to minimize hindsight bias in understanding clinical decision making.[27] Although SA is used primarily in aviation, it can be applied to health care because it takes into account a person's perception, comprehension, projection, and resolution, which are factors that correspond closely to the steps in making a clinical decision.[28]

A second way to improve the communication problems is to implement a change in the medical culture. The current culture expects error-free practice, emphasizes individual accountability, and blames the individual when he or she fails to perform.[29] In order to change this mentality, it is best to target the group as a whole, rather than simply changing one's individual-level actions.[20] This is because the community must know that the change is being implemented system-wide, and that compliance is mandatory. On the other hand, targeting individuals would yield less-desirable results because they might feel that changing their actions alone is not enough to make a significant difference in the culture.

In addition to the change in group mentality, a change in culture requires an increase in strong leadership.[30] This is different from strong senior leaders, such as attending physicians, who are already respected by their peers and subordinates. Strong leadership requires all levels of practitioners to come forward, stand up for the right thing to do, openly support it, and encourage others to do the same.[30] When healthcare professionals stand up for what they believe in and exhibit positive, effective communication, others will follow. In the context of communication, that means vocalizing concerns in a concise and respectful manner despite pressure to do the opposite. At the same time, the healthcare environment must become more cooperative so as to encourage physicians to be leaders instead of chastising them for going against the system.[31]

Additionally, medical culture should be approached from a bottoms-up perspective, not the traditional top-down perspective currently in use.[31] The top-down approach blames the individual and says "you have a problem that needs to be corrected";[31] instead, there needs to be a shift from "who did it" to "what happened."[32] Human-performance factors should be dissociated from issues of clinical competency, because more often than not it is bad systems that set up good people to fail.[15]

Closely related to the problem of medical-culture change is the issue of hierarchies. To truly effectuate a change in culture and improve communication, elimination of medical hierarchies is necessary. Although hierarchies are seemingly innocuous, they have a real, negative effect on communication. Such power relationships serve only to crystallize the difference in status between groups and add nothing to proper patient care.[18] Because such hierarchies are a barrier to effective communication, active steps must be taken to equalize healthcare practitioners and do away with status differentiation. One way to do so is to have a penalty-free culture that allows for physicians to speak up, particularly when they disagree with a supervisor.[33] Additionally, senior practitioners should report or act on errors, regardless of whose error it is.[34] A senior healthcare provider who not only encourages others to speak up but admits when he or she makes a mistake will undoubtedly demonstrate to others that hierarchies are a thing of the past.

A fourth way to achieve culture change is through the use of technology. Computerized physician order entry can reduce the rates of medication-related errors and improve other processes, because the order will be clear and much easier to read than a handwritten order in illegible scrawl.[35] Additionally, a computer-based system can potentially reduce content omissions through the use of standard fields.[25] A less-expensive method would be to use standardized written sign-out forms. Such forms should include required fields for necessary content, such as code status and active/anticipated medical problems, to prevent omissions.[1,25] More attention must be paid to writing legibly, however.[1]

Conversely, face-to-face communication plays a paramount role in decreasing errors during an information exchange, particularly during patient handoffs. Arora et al. found that the most frequent suggestion to improve handoff procedures was to verbally communicate any anticipated problems and review face-to-face any relevant medical issues that might affect patient care.[21] In an ideal situation, physician orders should not only be entered by computer, but should also be communicated orally during handoff procedures, allowing the incoming practitioner a clear record of the patient's treatment and a personal appraisal of what might come; therefore, formal debriefings should be required for all handoffs. Such a briefing promotes people-to-people transfer of information in real time, establishes a platform for common understanding, gives people permission to be frank and honest, puts members of the team on the same page, and provides a structure for collaborative planning.[36] The briefings should involve not only physicians but nurses as well, because they are essential to patient care and require accurate information just as much as the doctors do.[37]

A sixth method for reducing communication errors is to increase awareness of the various personalities present in the healthcare system.[18] Whereas introverts may need training to help them make necessary and clear communications, extroverts may require help reducing their communications to only pertinent information.[18] Assertiveness training is one possible helpful method for introverts, whereby a supervisor announces that he or she will intentionally make an error that day and expects the medical or nursing staff to speak up when that happens.[34] By understanding the different personalities of the medical staff and training them on a regular basis, proper communication techniques will become familiar and will equalize the various personalities present on the staff.

Redundancy is the seventh way by which communication can be improved. Healthcare settings that have more than minimal staffing allow people the time to communicate properly.[18] Having adequate numbers of staff members means communications are less rushed and the communicators can be thorough in their relaying of information. In the context of patient handoffs, communicators are better able to give complete information because they are not as stressed and also not responsible for an overly large number of patients.

Given that medicine is hierarchical, culturally stagnant, and suffers from the same budgetary concerns that affect numerous industries at this time, changing basic features is admittedly quite difficult. Even if none of the other suggestions are put into place, the following proposition is perhaps the most important: the development of critical language. Healthcare facilities can decide for themselves what the exact language should be, but each should adopt language that essentially translates to "we have a serious problem, stop and listen to me."[37] This decreases the threshold to get help and creates a clearly agreed-upon communication model that helps avoid the tendency to speak indirectly and differentially.[37] The idea behind this is similar to language used for codes: people understand that something bad is happening and that action must be taken. Thus, if healthcare practitioners are armed with a critical-language phrase, they may feel more comfortable eliciting help despite an environment that can discourage such behavior.

These suggestions demonstrate that change is indeed possible, and that expensive or unduly burdensome programs are not required to effectuate a change. It costs nothing to tell residents to speak up, or require face-to-face communication during handoffs, or do away with hierarchies, and such inexpensive steps may prevent costly errors that would have continued to occur but for the intervention.

EXAMPLES OF SUCCESSFUL CHANGE

Although changing the behaviors of an entire system is admittedly difficult, it is imperative that appropriate actions be taken to do just that. Although there are various alterations that can be made to technical elements of patient care, such as electronic charting instead of handwritten charts and altering staffing procedures, the majority of proposed reforms target human behaviors. Modifying the day-to-day practices will take time and dedicated effort by everyone involved, but eventual change is possible. Kaiser Permanente, Orange County Kaiser, and Veterans Affairs Medical Center are just three examples of large health entities that implemented successful measures to improve communication problems that were plaguing the institutions.

Kaiser Permanente is one of the largest non-profit health systems in the United States, employing more than 11,000 physicians and caring for over 8.3 million patients.[37] In response to communication problems, Kaiser Permanente standardized communication at shift changes using the SBAR method, requiring both physicians and nurses to participate.[37] Additionally, the health system instituted critical-language phraseology between subordinates and superiors, and when a subordinate says "I need you now," the superior attends to the issue 100% of the time.[37]

Surgical teams at Orange County Kaiser implemented formalized briefings into their surgical-care process with great success.[37] The supervisor begins by telling the others what he or she thinks they need to know in a given case, and afterward the other team members are allowed to tell the supervisor what they need to know.[37] All team members are required to be present for such briefings, which have specified meeting times.[37] As a result, errors decreased, nursing turnover decreased by 16%, employee satisfaction increased by 19%, and perceptions of the safety climate improved from "good" to "outstanding."[37] The formalized briefing process has since been expanded to the departments of radiology, and labor and delivery, in the hospital.[37]

Successful communication-improvement measures have been implemented at the Veterans Affairs Medical Center in Houston, Texas, as well. After noting that poor communication among surgeons, anesthesiologists, and nurses may lead to adverse events that can compromise patient safety, Awad et al. looked at their own institution and found low communication ratings from staff members.[38] To determine if communication in the operating room could be improved through medical-team training, Awad et al. had study participants attend a dedicated training session, which involved didactic instruction, interactive participation, role playing, training films, and clinical vignettes, using crew-resource-management principles.[38] At the end of the session, a change team, composed of representatives from general surgery, anesthesiology, and nursing, was created to drive the implementation of the principles discussed in the training session through the development of a preoperative briefing system.[39] The team held weekly meetings and made adjustments to the briefings based on team feedback.

The results were inspiring: after the implementation of the team training, preoperative briefings increased from 64% at the first month after implementation to 100% by the end of the fourth month.[40] Additionally, the communication scores for the anesthesiologists and surgeons increased significantly by 4 months after implementation of the training sessions.[40] Furthermore, there was a substantial increase in the number of patients who received prophylactic treatments where such actions were appropriate.[40] Lastly, preoperative briefings led to a decrease in dangerous surgeries, because they identified patients before induction who were high-risk candidates for surgery.[40] Thus, Awad et al. found that by using crew-resource-management techniques along with the use of a change-implementing team, communication can be

dramatically improved through the use of preoperative briefings.[4]

Although the situations described do not specifically address the issue of communication in handoff procedures, the examples are still valid. They are illustrative of the idea that simple changes can be made in a hospital setting that can improve communication between staff members and thereby improve patient care. The methods used and the successes achieved in the examples can be extrapolated to the issue of patient handoffs because there are substantial similarities: Kaiser Permanente addressed problems that occur at shift changes, which is when patient handoffs typically take place. Additionally, Orange County Kaiser and Veterans Affairs Medical Center dealt with communication practices occurring between physicians and nurses, superiors and subordinates. This directly translates to patient handoffs, because such transfers of care do not merely occur between peers but between various groups of healthcare practitioners with a range of statuses; therefore, the examples of Kaiser Permanente, Orange County Kaiser, and Veterans Affairs Medical Center all demonstrate that it is possible to ameliorate poor communication practices, which are endemic to patient handoffs, through uncomplicated initiatives.

CONCLUSION

The phrase "good people are set up to fail in bad systems"[15] perhaps has no truer application than in the context of communication. For the most part, healthcare practitioners do not come to work with the intent to purposely leave out information pertinent to a patient's care or to make others feel as though they cannot go to that person with critical information because of that healthcare practitioner's personality; however, that is exactly what happens on a daily basis in hospitals around the country because of pervasive system problems that allow such actions to occur. Although people may not go to the hospital with bad intentions, years of poor habits and lack of attention have effectively indicated that such behavior will be tolerated, in some cases at the expense of the patient.

Regardless of what the situation is currently, change is possible. Through the use of training, culture change, dismantling of hierarchies, improved forms, mandatory debriefing, personality awareness, redundancy, or critical language, communications that occur at the time of patient handoffs can be improved. Kaiser Permanente, Orange County Kaiser, and Veterans Affairs Medical Center each stand out as examples of the successes that can be achieved through the implementation of one or more of the suggested methods.

Hospitals should take it upon themselves to speak out against the problem, set out a solution, and require that all of its physicians and nurses comply with the proposal. Once armed with the knowledge that communication errors at the time of patient handoffs do occur, are a multi-faceted problem, and have a large number of available solutions, there is no reason why such bad systems should continue to exist.

References

1. Arora, V., Johnson, J., Lovinger, D., Humphrey, H.J., & Melyzer, D.O. (2005). Communication failures in patient sign-out and suggestions for improvement: A critical incident analysis. *Quality Safety Health Care, 14,* 401.
2. Awad, S.S., Fagan, S.P., Bellows, C., Albo, D., Green-Rashad, B., & DeLa Garza, M. (2005, Nov.). Bridging the communication gap in the operating room with medical team training. *American Journal of Surgery, 190,* 770, 773.
3. Supra note 1, p. 402.
4. Supra note 2, p. 773.
5. Sutcliffe, K.M., Lewton, E., & Rosenthal, M.M. (2004). Communication failures: An insidious contributor to medical mishaps. *Academic Medicine, 79*(2), 186, 187.
6. Ibid, pp. 188–192.
7. Ibid, p. 188.
8. Ibid, pp. 188–189.
9. Supra note 5, p. 189.
10. Supra note 5, pp. 189–190.
11. Supra note 5, p. 190.
12. Supra note 5, p. 191.
13. Brewin, T.B. (1984, March). Who should decide? Paternalism in health care. *Journal of Medical Ethics, 10*(1,) 51–52.
14. Garbutt, J., Brownstein, D.R., Klein, E.J., Waterman, A, Krauss, M.J., Marcuse, E.K., et al. (2007). Reporting and disclosing medical errors. *Archives of Pediatric Adolescent Medicine, 161* (2), 179.
15. Leonard, M. (2004). The human factor: The critical importance of effective teamwork and communication in providing safe care. *Quality Safety Health Care, 13,* i85, i86.
16. Ibid, p. i86.
17. Supra note 14, p. 181.
18. Firth-Cozens, J. (2004). Why communication fails in the operating room. *Quality Safety Health Care, 13,* 327.
19. Singh, H., Thomas, E.J., Petersen, L.A., & Studdert, D.M. (2007). Medical errors involving trainees. *Archives of Internal Medicine, 167*(10), 2030, 2034.
20. Supra note 5, p. 193.
21. Supra note 1, p. 404.
22. Supra note 19, p. 2034.
23. Accreditation Council for Graduate Medical Education. (n.d.). *ACGME duty hour standards.* Fact sheet 1. http://www.acgme.org/acWebsite/newsRoom/ACGMEdutyHoursfactsheet.pdf/.
24. White, A.A., Wright, S.W., Blanco, R., Lemonds, B., Sisco, J., Bledsoe, S., et al. (2004). Cause-and-effect analysis of risk management files to assess patient care in the emergency department. *Academy Emergency Medicine, 11,* 1035.
25. Supra note 1, p. 405.
26. Singh, H., et al. (2006). Understanding diagnostic errors in medicine: A lesson from aviation. *Quality Safety Health Care, 15,* 159.
27. Ibid, p. 162.
28. Ibid, p. 163.
29. Supra note 14, p. 183.
30. Supra note 15, p. i89.
31. Supra note 24, p. 1040.

32. Walton, M.M. (2006). Hierarchies: The Berlin Wall of patient safety. *Quality Safety Health Care, 15,* 229, 230.
33. Jain, M., Miller, L., Belt, D., & Berwick, D.M. (2006). Decline in ICU adverse events, nosocomial infections and cost through a quality improvement initiative focusing on teamwork and culture change. *Quality Safety Health Care, 15,* 235, 239.
34. Supra note 32, p. 230.
35. Supra note 24, p. 1039.
36. Supra note 2, pp. 771–772.
37. Supra note 15, p. i87.
38. Supra note 2, p. 770.
39. Ibid, p. 771.
40. Ibid, p. 772.

31

IMPROVING HANDOFF PROCEDURES IN HEALTH CARE TO REDUCE RISK AND PROMOTE SAFETY

Jayne Westendorp-Holland, JD, BA
Barbara J. Youngberg, JD, MSW, BSN, FASHRM

INTRODUCTION

The purpose of this chapter is to explore the risk and patient safety concerns associated with handoff communications. A look at current research on the impact of poor communication between and among healthcare providers, its impact on patient safety, and current strategies to reduce this system-level factor that contributes to error are discussed.

DEFINITION OF A HANDOFF

Handoffs are broadly defined by The Joint Commission on Accreditation of Healthcare Organizations as the "transfer of information, responsibility, and authority regarding a patient's care from one caregiver to another."[1] There are many variations in how handoffs are defined. The British National Safety Agency defines handoff as "the transfer of professional responsibility and accountability for some or all aspects of care for a patient, or group of patients, to another person or professional group on a temporary or permanent basis."[2] Ideally, handoff communication is "the contemporaneous, interactive process of passing patient specific information from one caregiver to another or from one team of caregivers to another for the purpose of ensuring the continuity and safety of the patient's care" (R. Crouteau, commenting at the 2006 National Patient Safety Goals, The Joint Commission International Center for Patient Safety Teleconference, July 8, 2005). Most definitions in the literature seem to look at a transfer that involves two factors, information and responsibility. The complexity of conditions that many patients present with often require that their care is managed by many different professionals and specialists. These care transitions can lead to errors caused by failed coordination or failed communication during the handoff process. At first glance the definition implies a fairly simple interaction between the off-going and oncoming caregiver(s), which usually takes place at change of shift in the hospital setting. The process, however, has a much broader scope of application. There are multiple times in the course of a hospital stay when care must be handed off to another caregiver of equal or varied training and background, which compounds the opportunity for failed or missed communication in the continuum of care for the given patient.

The Joint Commission has studied the problem of handoff communication through review of sentinel events, which they receive from healthcare providers across the country, and reports that "communication issues were a root cause of approximately 65% of the 2,966 sentinel events reported to them from 1995 to 2004 and nearly 70% of the 582 sentinel events reported for 2005."[3] In the Institute of Medicine report, "Crossing the Quality Chasm: A New Health System for the 21st Century," it is noted that patient handoffs increase the possibility for error. The report notes that in a safe system, information is not lost, inaccessible, or forgotten in transitions.[4] In 2006, The Joint Commission added handoff communication to their list of National Patient Safety Goals. Goal number two is to improve the effectiveness of communication among caregivers (NPSG.02). Listed under this goal is NPSG.02.05.01, which applies specifically to handoff communications. NPSG 2 states that the "primary objective of a handoff is to provide accurate information about a [patient]'s care, treatment and services; current conditions; and any recent or anticipated changes." Also included are five elements that should be included in each handoff. These elements include:

1. Interactive communication that allows for the opportunity for questioning between the giver and receiver of patient information.
2. Up-to-date information regarding the patient's condition, care, treatment, medications, services, and any recent or anticipated changes.

3. A method to verify the received information, including repeat-back or read-back techniques.
4. An opportunity for the receiver of the handoff information to review relevant patient historical data, which may include previous care, treatment, and services.
5. Interruptions during handoffs are limited to minimize the possibility that information fails to be conveyed or is forgotten.

The Joint Commission's 2010 Safety Goals have been released. Handoff communication has been changed from a requirement to a standard. This means that there is "less of a need to spotlight the issue and less emphasis will be placed on it during survey."[6] This in no way should diminish the importance of handoff communications. The Joint Commission "spotlighted" the issue and the healthcare industry has begun the process of researching the best way to most effectively carry out the handoff process in a wide variety of circumstances.

CREATING A CULTURE OF COMMUNICATION

The Birmingham VA Medical Center participated in a program initiated by the National Center for Patient Safety.[7] It is a 12-month program that builds on each session presented. The program's ultimate goal is to protect patients from harmful errors. The program was designed to improve communications among healthcare workers by making them more aware of the way they presently communicate and possibilities for improvement. The program used role playing to get the staff to act out situations, and by slowing down, stepping back, and looking at what was occurring, they could see missed opportunities for communication. Once identified, they were taught how to communicate in the most effective manner.

To create a culture of communication it is important that everyone, at every level, not be intimidated to speak up when they see something that could endanger a person. The understanding is that everyone working in patient care is there for the good of the patient, and the better the medical professionals communicate the better it will be for the patient. Ultimately, one wants to develop "enhanced levels of communications throughout the hospital, with all players participating."[7] The VA stated that "Between receiving handoffs and giving handoffs a medical resident may be doing 50–60 handoffs a day, [and] it is hard to keep up a high standard of communication."[7] Awareness of the communication process is needed to assist in maintaining a consistent and necessary high standard of communication.

STANDARDIZED HANDOFFS IN A MULTIFACETED SYSTEM

Ross D. Silverman's book-review essay on Robert M. Wachter's book, *Understanding Patient Safety*, states that "communication among care providers is at the core of many safety challenges."[8] Wachter compares other high-hazard fields and describes how they have dealt with improving teamwork communication. He speaks of the airline industry being able to reduce communication errors with an adoption of training programs; however, in the medical field, communication among team members "will be confounded by the presence of a wider variety in personnel education and experience, steeper authority gradients, more deeply entrenched hierarchies, and dramatically different professional cultures, perspectives, and use of language."[8] Considering these variables, one can see how easily errors can occur even when all participants have the best of intentions concerning the well-being of the patient.

In the healthcare system there is a greater variance in circumstances as well. A standardized checklist that works well in getting a plane off the ground, flying it, and landing safely has fewer variations than that of an individual patient with any number of diag-

nosed or possibly undiagnosed variables. The concern with the standardized process is that one wants to ensure that enough information is being passed to ensure the safety of the patient, but not so much that the "receiver of the information is overwhelmed with unnecessary information."[5] Another concern is that with a reliance on a standardized form, a false sense of security may occur and important information that is not on the form may be overlooked.

HANDOFF STANDARDIZATION

The Quarterly Journal for Health Care Practice and Risk Management's "Infocus" divides handoff standardization into three levels. The first level of standardization is a simple cross-unit transport form used in cross-unit handoffs. The checklist covers basic information concerning the patient such as identification, medications, vitals, infections, etc.[9]

Johns Hopkins has taken the checklist to a higher level. In a recent "Johns Hopkins Medicine Quality Update," they highlight just what can be done with a simple, carefully constructed checklist. They developed a one-page checklist that concerns steps for use of a central catheter from cleaning to insertion. It is widely used at other facilities, even in the United Kingdom. The use of the checklist has greatly reduced bloodstream-infection rates. A point emphasized is that it is not enough to develop a new tool, but the staff that utilizes it needs to be educated as to how to use it and the rationale behind its use. Equally important is keeping the staff updated on how the tool has impacted the targeted use.[10]

Johns Hopkins took the same approach with improving postsurgical handoffs. They looked at where the breakdowns were occurring. They recognized that the handoffs were far more complex than a change of shift, in that information and technology were being transferred. It was typically a confusing time that lacked sequential steps. They broke it down and created a postoperative handoff process that involved a gathering of core team providers at the bedside immediately after surgery. It is a focused time with a postoperative checklist that ensures that all aspects of a report are covered.[10]

Standardized Methods for Improving Handoffs

The second level that "Infocus" lists are "more ambitious methods, such as SBAR, teamSTEPPS, and ANTIC-ipate." The most widely known and utilized method is SBAR.

SBAR

SBAR stands for:

- Situation: brief patient information (vitals, code status)
- Background: context, brief history, relevant condition
- Assessment: problem and conclusions
- Recommendation: action that needs to be taken, follow-up actions, and time frame

SBAR-R tracks and adds one more step to the process:

- Repeat back: handoff team verbally confirms information

The SBAR system was not originally designed for the healthcare system. It was designed for use in change of command on nuclear submarines.[11] The system is helpful but does not always meet the criteria needed for a complete and safe handoff. Many facilities have customized SBAR to meet their needs. Some personnel need more details, and some less, depending on the departments that are doing the handoff.

In the "Hospital Peer Review" July 2009 edition, Amber Cocks, the senior quality- and process-improvement consultant, and Christiane Levine, patient safety program manager at Children's Healthcare of Atlanta, teamed up, strengthened the SBAR

system, and utilized it to raise patient awareness of patient deterioration and shock. Their hospital system saw a drop of preventable codes by 70%.[12] They started by looking at what was missing in their system. They worked with the clinicians to gather input as to what and how transfers were occurring. "The two assembled 'transfer of care champions' in each area and identified the nurse-to-nurse; shift to shift transfer as the greatest area for evaluation." Their goal was to isolate the minimum set of information and to identify the most important things that needed to be communicated during patient transfers of care. Each department, with their assistance, was able to modify the list as needed and post it. They also put the elements into the electronic health system and were able to put it up on the screen.[13]

In implementing their plan they utilized the same techniques as those discussed in the section on creating a culture of communication. Rather than just sending out a memo, they educated with simulation. They programmed a shock patient into the computer system. The staff "walked through the scenarios and made decisions or recommendations on what they saw." They learned the list of essential elements to communicate and were told to speak up if these issues were not communicated. They were given the scripted communications for situations that required that they speak up. Cocks and Levine feel that what made their endeavor successful was building a program based on their failures. They "built a team on [their] failure points," not on what other hospitals were utilizing.[14]

Another element key to their success was incorporating PEWS into their program. PEWS is an early-warning score system that was developed by a U.K. hospital. Through a series of quick, second assessments, done every 4 hours, the pediatric patient receives a score.[14] This score is used by nurses, but doctors are educated so that when a nurse calls with a score they understand the predictor value for deterioration.[14]

I PASS the BATON

In contrast to the simpler SBAR tool, I PASS the BATON is a more detailed mnemonic tool, created by the U.S. Department of Defense Patient Safety Program, that is also frequently referenced in healthcare literature as an effective handoff communication tool. This tool is a more extensive template developed to cover key areas of both simple and complex patient handoffs.

Simply explained, the acronym stands for:

- Introduction: introduce yourself, your role, and patient name.
- Patient: name, identifiers, age, gender, location.
- Assessment: presenting chief complaint, vital signs, symptoms, and diagnosis.
- Situation: current status, medications, circumstances, code status, recent changes, response to treatment.
- Safety concerns: critical lab values/reports, socio-economic factors, allergies, alerts (falls, isolation, etc.).

[the]

- Background: comorbidities, previous episodes, past/home medications, family history.
- Actions: what actions were taken or are required *and* provide brief rationale.
- Timing: level of urgency and explicit timing, prioritization of actions.
- Ownership: who is responsible (nurse/doctor/team) including patient/family responsibilities.
- Next: What will happen next? Anticipated changes? What is the plan?

Contingency Plan

A more detailed explanation of the Contingency Plan tool is given on the Web site of the U.S. Department of Defense Patient Safety Program (http://dodpatientsafety.usuhs.mil/).

TeamSTEPPS: A Military Solution

TeamSTEPPS was developed by the U.S. military to increase the "precision of care provided both on the battlefield and in the combat support hospitals in Iraq and Afghanistan." The military agreed to collaborate with the Department of Health and Human Services Agency for Healthcare Research and Quality (AHRQ) and the Health Care Team Coordination Program (HCTCP) to integrate the TeamSTEPPS program into health care. The collaborative goal was "to help doctors and hospitals integrate teamwork principles into their daily activities as a way to reduce clinical error and to improve patient outcomes, patient satisfaction and hospital staff satisfaction."[16] This approach has been used with great success in high-risk settings, such as the emergency department and labor and delivery, and now is moving into medical–surgical settings and to perioperative patient care.[11,17]

TeamSTEPPS provides tools to help develop a cohesive team. The core framework has four key principles/skills that are integrated to foster delivery of safe, quality care as a cohesive patient care team, which includes the patient, direct caregivers, and those who play a supportive role in the healthcare-delivery system. The four key skill areas are:

1. Leadership. The ability to coordinate activities. Changes in information are shared and team members are given the necessary resources. These short planning sessions involve problem-solving huddles and process improvement through debriefing.
2. Situation monitoring. The process in which the individual actively scans the behavior and actions of those around him or her to assess the situation or environment. Situation monitoring fosters mutual respect and team accountability, and provides a safety net for the team and the patient.

3. Mutual support. The ability to anticipate and support other team members' needs through accurate knowledge about their responsibilities and workload. Mutual support protects team members from work-overload situations.
4. Communication. The process by which information is clearly and accurately exchanged among team members. Here the program integrates SBAR.[18]

"The tools found in TeamSTEPPS can advance culture change by providing the health care workforce with a shared simple set of words to describe critical communication behaviors. Effective teamwork and communication are vital to the success" of the program.[19] The Association of periOperative Registered Nurses (AORN) and the U.S. Department of Defense Patient Safety Program (DoD PSP) developed a Web-based, Perioperative Patient Handoff Tool Kit[20] with extensive resources to help caregivers standardize handoff communications in perioperative settings. The kit is based on TeamSTEPPS.

Blount Memorial Hospital in Tennessee created its own four-step handoff system, Just Go NUTS. (The process is unique to issues regarding tubes safety.) This system puts in additional information concerning tubing and safety issues in their handoff.[11]

ANTIC-ipate

Another tool that is being used successfully to minimize errors in handoff communication, especially by physicians, is a written "sign out" using the mnemonic "ANTICipate."

ANTIC-ipate was developed at the University of San Francisco and University of Chicago. It stands for:

- Administrative information that focuses on accuracy in patient identification and location.
- New information (clinical update) that includes diagnosis and a brief history, updated medications, problem lists, baseline status, recent procedures, and significant events.

- Tasks in an if/then format. Tasks are the "to do" list, the things that must be done during the cross-coverage period.
- Illness is the primary provider's subjective assessment of severity of illness.
- Contingency planning ("what if" scenarios), which includes information that assists the covering physician in anticipating the "what ifs" by talking through past successful therapeutic interventions for the particular patient in the event of the same or a similar presentation.

Anticipation is the key, and communicating necessary information is vital as recognized by this tool.

Ticket to Ride

To minimize error when handoff is taking place between professional and nonprofessional caregivers, many facilities have developed a "ticket to ride" or similar tool, as recommended by The Joint Commission. The need for a "ticket to ride" arises when a patient is leaving the unit temporarily for diagnostic testing or therapy in another department and is not going to be accompanied by his primary professional caregiver.

The tool, a "ticket," must be a short document that can be easily completed by the professional handing off care to the nonprofessional, usually an interdepartmental transporter, whenever the patient leaves the home unit. It is a fill-in-the-blank document that requires completion of all essential information necessary for safe continuum of care of the patient while away from the home unit. Prior to return to the home unit, the "return ticket to ride," usually the back of the document, is completed and updated with any changes that did not require a direct conversation between the professional caregivers.

These are the most frequently referenced tools in the current literature. Medical-care facilities are encouraged to use the given models to guide handoff communication.

Synopsis

The final level that "Infocus" listed for standardized handoffs is a technology-based approach. Synopsis is a technology-based program that assists in safe handoffs. It allows one to enter pertinent patient data, such as lab results, code status, administrative information, vitals, diagnosis, etc. The program can create printed handouts to be used with the handoff process.[11] The Nurse Knowledge Exchange (NKE) system "combines a software handoff template with face-to-face exchange and overlapping rounds to improve sign-outs for nursing shifts."[11] Electronic health records (EHR) are part of the HITECH Act (Health Information Technology for Economic and Clinical Health Act), which is part of the 2009 American Recovery and Reinvestment Act. The Act has allocated money for the development of EHR systems that support a nationwide exchange of patient information in a secure and accurate manner. This will expedite the technology-based options for handoff communications.

TYPES OF HANDOFFS

Handoffs in Large Medical Groups in the Ambulatory-Care Setting

In 2002, the *Journal of Health Politics, Policy and Law* published a special issue on Managed Care Redux. In the article "Efforts to Improve Patient Safety in Large, Capitated Medical Groups: Description and Conceptual Model," the authors saw a large gap in the amount of energy going into inpatient problems and solutions in terms of safety but felt that the large physician groups were being overlooked.[21] The ambulatory-care processes "tend to consist of numerous, small, interrelated, and often sequential transactions that occur over time in multiple locations and organizations (or organizational units) and can involve multiple people, including patients."[22] Their study sought to identify the key determinants concerning patient safety

and evolving methods to reduce patient injuries. They found that the participants who had some type of electronic technology with which to work were able to better identify where their problem areas were and to deal with them. In terms of handoffs, any system that could "increase the information flow" to clinicians as well as staff were key. The ideal was electronic systems that could interface with each other so that lab results, medication lists, and diagnoses could be accessed in "result-viewing systems." The most advanced systems had reminder systems built into them to help track results, reminders for screenings, and drug-interaction alerts.[23] This is the direction the HITECH Act hopes to facilitate in the ambulatory setting as well as the inpatient setting.

If the organization can reduce the number of steps required in a handoff, they can reduce the possibilities for errors. The authors highlight a group who were dissatisfied with the "proportion of breast cancers that went undetected until an advanced stage." They relocated to a space where the specialist and technicians could move into one building. Routine mammograms were only scheduled in the morning so that if any were abnormal, a radiologist was available to discuss the case with the patient and, if necessary, pathologists were available for needle biopsies in the afternoon. The new system eliminated the delay in diagnosis and reduced stress on the patients and their families.[24]

Handoffs in the Hospital

"Modern Healthcare" did an interview with the outgoing president of The Joint Commission, Dennis O'Leary. He stated that he would not want to be admitted to a hospital as a patient without having someone along with him to monitor his care: "I would bring someone with me and have them stay the night, and I would always be asking questions. I think caregivers find that helpful, and it prevents them from making human errors. If I go in a hospital, I know I'm vulnerable, and I will do what I can to protect caregivers from unintentionally harming me."[25] The same article quotes a story from the *Wall Street Journal* (November 14, 2006) concerning a collaboration between Great Ormond Street Hospital, the largest children's hospital in Britain, and Italy's Formula One Ferrari racing team. The hospital asked Ferrari to look at the hospital's handoff process and assist them by sharing their strategies in terms of leadership, specific roles, contingency planning, and addressing small problems before they became big ones. They combined Ferrari's strategies with a human-factors analysis to develop handoff procedures. A 2-year follow-up found that they had reduced their information omissions by 50% and technical errors by 42%.[11]

In "Deconstructing Negligence: The Role of Individual and System Factors in Causing Medical Injuries," the authors define "system" as "a set of independent elements, both human and non-human, interacting to achieve a common aim."[26]

The authors further state:

> The concept refers to the interrelationships among health care providers, the tools they use, and the environment in which they carry out their work. The system view of accident causation asserts that it is misguided to prioritize, and dead wrong to focus exclusively on, lapses by individual health care providers because most medical outcomes, including those that flow from errors, are essentially the product of organizational structures and processes. The relationship between individual and systems factors in the production of medical injury has been little studied until recently.[26]

In their empirical results, the authors list 18 variables as factors that contribute to harmful errors. Three of the factors have a communication element: teamwork and communica-

tion, 40% of all error-related injuries; handoffs, 15%; and other communication problems, 13%. In total, 68% of all error-related injuries had a communication issue of some kind.[26]

An article titled "The Bermuda Triangle of Healthcare" examines the OSF Medical group, which owns and operates a variety of healthcare facilities including seven acute-care facilities.[27] OSF was already using the GE Centricity Enterprise clinical information system but needed to find a way to integrate the handoff process into their system. Their goal was to find a way to put all of the information needed into a one-page-per-person format with the ability to access additional information online if needed. SBAR was used as a framework for their project. The multi-disciplinary team was willing to work with various prototypes to refine the form. The team was able to get the 12-step process down to 8 steps by using a new electronic report. An application was designed to pull data from their clinical system and place it into the SBAR handoff format. The report could be utilized online or in print. Prior to this format, it took the facilities an average of 8.7 minutes to complete a handoff; after, the average was 4.1 minutes. By the end of 2007, six OSF facilities were "creating an average of more than 66,000 handoff reports per month. By the end of March 2008 . . . more than 85,000 a month." They attribute their success to two key elements, the support of the corporation as well as the individual facilities, and that nursing drove the format and content due to the fact that they would be the primary users.[28]

Sealing the Cracks, Not Falling Through: Using Handoffs to Improve Patient Care

The report, "Sealing the Cracks, Not Falling Through: Using Handoffs to Improve Patient Care," states that "the ideal handoff takes place face to face between the two parties, at the bedside, with the patient's chart or electronic medical record in front of them."[5] Whether high tech or low tech, one of the key elements to the handoff is that it is a structured communication process with an opportunity for the receiving party to ask questions and clarify information.[5] Handoffs should be regarded as a time to see the patient with new eyes, a chance for redundancy, a chance to prevent errors, and a time to catch possible errors.

Handoffs Involving Residents

There is a lot of literature concerning fatigue-related errors as they pertain to residents. The Institute of Medicine (IOM) released a report in December 2008 proposing revisions in residents' hours and workloads to decrease the chance of fatigue-related errors. The report recommends that there be overlapping schedules for residents, because patient handoffs have been identified as the likeliest time for errors to occur. Communication deteriorates with fatigue. With overlapping shifts, communication could be optimized.[29]

Managed Care Weekly Digest reported that with the increased restrictions on resident hours, handoffs increased in frequency. In looking more closely at the resident handoffs, they were shown to be problematic. In surveys sent out to residents, over 50% of the respondents reported that although handoffs were done face to face, they were not done in quiet or private settings and typically had frequent interruptions. Studies are being funded to work on minimizing the issues concerning the problematic handoffs.[30]

Handoffs with Language Barriers

"Infocus" addressed the issue of limited English proficient (LEP) patients in their November 2007 issue. The statistics show that many LEP patients receive substandard care due to miscommunication. There are resources available to help set up a language-access strategy. They suggest looking at the compo-

sition of your patient cohort. Know which languages for which you need to be prepared. Hire bilingual staff when possible, hire interpreters, train staff, and have policies in place. There are agency and contract interpreters if you do not have them on staff.[32]

Nursing Handoffs

In the hospital setting most handoff communication policies for nurses include the following:

- Handoffs must be interactive so that the nurse receiving the patient has the opportunity to question and confirm what is reported.
- There should be minimal interruptions. The content of the report should be objective, concise, and related to the patient's care.
- Nurses are responsible for all handoff communications to contain specific information such as age, gender, diagnosis, allergies, medications, and code status.

Each clinical area is responsible for developing guidelines pertinent to their clinical area.[32] Change-of-shift report is an extremely important handoff in terms of patient safety. A lot of information must be transferred to the oncoming shift. One of the methods utilized is the nurse-to-nurse bedside report.[33] Shift report among nurses has been defined as "a system of nurse-to-nurse communication between shift changes intended to transfer essential information for safe, holistic care of patients."[33]

Caruso recounts the experience of changing from a standard unit report in a medical/surgical cardiology unit to a bedside report.[33] The initial interest arose out of Caruso attending a seminar where there was a presentation on bedside report. The next step was to review the literature. The institution was motivated with The Joint Commission's Safety Goals and felt that a bedside report assisted in the recommendation for two means of identification as well as improving the effectiveness of communication. After educating the nursing staff, the plan was implemented. After 1 month, a meeting was held to discuss the pros and cons of the system. Nurses reported an uneasiness in discussing the patient in front of the patient and felt that they were interrupting at times. They had a difficult time including the patient and the report took longer. They reported that they often found that it was a time, they had realized, that IVs needed adjusting, chest tubes needed draining, etc. They did feel better starting their shift after having viewed their patients, and they were able to establish a brief assessment of each patient.

Overall, the feedback from the patients and their families was favorable. They liked knowing who their nurse was at the beginning of the shift and what the plan was for their care. Caruso stated that they were continuing with the bedside report with adjustments, because overall they felt that it gave the patient a better sense of security and also enhanced patient safety.

Handoffs of Critical Test Results, Medications, and Discharges

Handoffs of critical test results, medications, and discharges are some of the additional handoffs that occur in the healthcare setting. These categories, as well as others not mentioned, involved the same processes discussed previously and, just like those processes, con-

tain elements that are specific to their discipline. Therefore there is a need to take systems that are already in place and tailor them to their particular discipline.

CONCLUSION

Having a system in place that allows for clinical data to go into a system designed for handoffs, necessary information that is accurate and condensed, with additional information available online if needed, is the ideal system to strive for and utilize. A major challenge ahead is in the area of information technology. With the HITECH Act and major advances in technology, there will be many glitches to deal with, but whether the process involves high or low technology, the goal remains the same: to keep the patient safe and give him or her the best care possible.

As Silverman states:

> While we gain knowledge about how and why errors and adverse events occur in our health system, perhaps what has become most clear about patient safety can be found in the words of Lao-tzu: we are finding that there are no one-size-fits all means of identifying, categorizing, or addressing health care quality and safety concerns . . . the complex problems raised in health care delivery largely defy straightforward solutions.[34]

References

1. ECRI Institute. (March 2007). *Ensure that handoff process is standardized, interactive.* Operating Room Risk Management, pp. 7–12. Available at https://www.ecri.org/Documents/OROM_Newsletter_0307.pdf. Accessed May 8, 2010.
2. British Medical Association. (2005). *Safe handover: Safe patients.* London: British Medical Association.
3. Gregory, B.C. (2006). Standardizing handoff processes. *AORN Journal, 84*(6), 1059–1061.
4. Groah, L. (2006). Handoffs: A link to improving patient safety. *AORN Journal, 83*(1), 227–230.
5. Paine, L.A., & Millman, A. (2009). *Sealing the cracks, not falling through: Using handoffs to improve patient care.* Westlaw News Room 6176696, pp. 1–2.

6. Comak, H. (2009, October 1). The Joint Commission's 2010 Patient Safety Goals reduce requirements. *HealthLeaders Media,* pp. 1–2.

7. Gordon, T. (2008, November 24). Westlaw News Room 22538671, *Birmingham News,* p. 3.

8. Silverman, R.D. (2008). Book Review Essay: Understanding Patient Safety by Robert M. Wachter. *Journal of Legal Medicine, 29*(561).

9. FOJP Service Corporation. (2007, September). The ethics of conscience. *Infocus Journal,* Vol. 4. http://www.fojp.com/inFocusSept07.pdf/. Accessed May 8, 2010.

10. Points from Pronovst "Are Their Hearts In It?" (2009). *Johns Hopkins Medicine Quality Update, 5*(1). http://www.hopkinsmedicine.org/bin/s/i/Quality_Update_Spring_2009_final.pdf. Accessed May 7, 2010.

11. FOJP Service Corporation. (2007, November). *Handoff communications: Heeding the call to change. Infocus Journal.* http://www.fojp.com/inFocusNov07.pdf/. Accessed May 9, 2010.

12. Hospital peer review. (2009). *Raising staff awareness of patient deterioration, shock.* Westlaw News Room 12712901, p. 1.

13. Westlaw News Room 12712901. (2009). pp. 1–2.

14. Westlaw News Room 12712901. (2009). p. 3.

15. Ferguson, S.L. (2008). *TeamSTEPPS: Integrating teamwork principles into adult health/medical–surgical practice.* Westlaw News Room 25511106, p. 2.

16. Westlaw News Room 27125118. (2008), p. 1.

17. Ferguson, S.L. (2008). *TeamSTEPPS: Integrating teamwork principles into adult health/medical–surgical practice.* Westlaw News Room 25511106, p. 1.

18. Splete, H. (2008). *Teamwork training may help improve inpatient safety: Good communication can prevent errors.* Westlaw News Room 25511106, pp. 4–5.

19. Ibid, p. 3.

20. AORN. (n.d.). Perioperative Patient Handoff Toolkit, available at http://www.aorn.org/ PracticeResources/ToolKits/PatientHandOff ToolKit/. Accessed May 8, 2010.

21. Miller, R.H., & Bovbjerg, R.R. (2002). Efforts to improve patient safety in large, capitated medical groups: Description and conceptual model. *Journal of Health Politics, Policy and Law, 27*(3), 401.

22. Ibid, p. 404.

23. Ibid, pp. 407–408.

24. Ibid, p. 408.

25. Westlaw News Room 26202126. (2007). p. 1.

26. Mello, M.M., & Studdert, D.M. (2008). Deconstructing negligence: The role of individual and system factors in causing medical injuries. *Georgetown Law Journal, 96*(599), 3.

27. White, R.S., & Hall, D.M. (2008). *The Bermuda Triangle of healthcare.* Westlaw News Room 12792977, p. 1.

28. Ibid, pp. 2–3.

29. Feder, H.H. (2009). Work hours for residents need to be limited and monitored. *Journal of Health Care Compliance, 11*(1).

30. *Managed Care Weekly Digest.* (2008). Hospital residents report patient-handoff problems common, can lead to patient harm adverse drug reactions. Westlaw News Room 18756631, pp. 1–2.

31. FOJP Service Corporation. (2007, November). Improving communications with better interpretation choices. *Infocus Journal.* http://www.fojp.com/inFocusNov07.pdf/. Accessed June 6, 2010.

32. Brigham and Women's Hospital. (2009, October 6). *BWH nurse.* http://www.brighamandwomens.org/. Accessed June 6, 2010.

33. Caruso, E.M. (2007). The evolution of nurse-to-nurse bedside report on a medical–surgical cardiology unit. *MedSurg Nursing, 16*(1), 17–22.

34. Silverman, R.D. (2008). Book Review Essay: Understanding Patient Safety by Robert M. Wachter. *Journal of Legal Medicine, 29*(561).

32

THE RISKS AND BENEFITS OF USING E-MAIL TO FACILITATE COMMUNICATION BETWEEN PROVIDERS AND PATIENTS

Sara Greening Truss, MBA

INTRODUCTION

Chapters 30 and 31 addressed the importance of communication as a strategy to reduce risk and advance patient safety. This chapter speaks to a specific trend that many providers believe will enhance communication, but only if the risks are correctly understood and managed.

There is a lot of discussion about the use of technology in health care today. The Obama Administration has stated that information technology (IT) is expected to play a large role in the way healthcare services are delivered, backing that up with federal funding. Medicare participants will be required to have electronic medical records in the next few years, and many insurance companies now require that claims and payments be transmitted electronically. The use of IT reduces costs, allows patient information to be immediately available to clinicians, and reduces the overall risk to patient safety; however, the percentage of clinicians and

healthcare organizations that use IT systems is very small in comparison with the percentage of people in the United States who use electronic devices as a way to communicate on a daily basis. One of the most popular electronic methods of communicating today is through the use of electronic mail (E-mail).

In 1999, it was estimated that by 2001, more than 50% of the U.S. population would be using E-mail.[1] It is safe to assume that the number has increased even more since then, with the use of hand-held devices such as cell phones and personal digital assistants (PDAs), and with the increase in computer availability. In today's business world, to ask someone for their phone number is almost inappropriate. E-mail is the primary way that most professionals interact with each other. With more and more people using E-mail as their primary contact information, there is more of a consumer demand for healthcare professionals to be accessible to their patients by way of E-mail, which provides "speed, convenience, utility for managing simple problems, efficiency, improved documentation, and avoidance of telephone tag."[2]

Although healthcare facilities and providers incorporate IT systems into daily use, physician–patient E-mail is still new and creates some concerns for healthcare providers. Patient–physician or patient–provider E-mail is defined as "computer-based communication between clinicians and patients within a contractual relationship in which the health care provider has taken on an explicit measure of responsibility for the client's care."[2]

There can also be communication between doctors and "consumers" who are seeking medical advice but are not patients of the doctor. This chapter makes reference to that scenario but focuses on provider–patient E-mail.

The following scenario is used to demonstrate the safety and liability concerns expressed by many healthcare professionals with using E-mail. The risks in using E-mail and how to limit liability with regard to this scenario will also be addressed in this chapter.

SCENARIO

One of your physicians, Dr. Smith, comes to you and tells you that he has been giving out his home E-mail address as a way of communicating with his patients. He told his patients that he is more accessible via E-mail and they should feel free to contact him at any time if they have a problem. The physician went on vacation, and when he returned, he read an E-mail that was 5 days old from one of his patients. The patient wrote that he needed assistance in managing what he thought was a severe allergic reaction. At the end of the E-mail, the patient wrote "I will await your response prior to taking any action."

The following is an example of a response from the risk manager to Dr. Smith detailing advice on the subject of E-mail communication with patients:

Dear Dr. Smith,

This letter is in response to the scenario you presented to me the other day. After we had determined that the patient was fine, we discussed some of the risks involved in using E-mail. In addition to our discussion, I thought it would be important to provide you with the same information in writing. I have also included company policies, which have been approved by the board. These policies will go into effect immediately.

First, I would like to acknowledge your dedication to communicating with your patients. Some physicians are hesitant to use E-mail, as they feel it would create more work for them for which they do not get reimbursed. Other doctors, such as Dr. Daniel Z. Sands at Harvard Medical School, who uses E-mail with his patients, reports that he views E-mailing patients as the same as calling them.[3] Our physicians do not get paid for phone calls, but it is expected that they will respond to their patients' needs in a timely manner.

I am in agreement that E-mail is useful. There are patient non-emergencies that come up but still need a provider's attention. Patients with a multi-disciplinary team of providers benefit from having the clinicians exchange information amongst themselves and the patient. The E-mail message should be saved either electronically in the patient's electronic medical record, or a hard copy printed and entered into the paper chart.[4] E-mail can also reduce manual work, administration time, and minimize human errors that come with written messages (incorrect spelling, illegible handwriting, losing a paper message, etc.). E-mail may also allow patients to feel more at ease and willing to discuss things with their physician.[1] And another benefit of E-mail is the prevention of "phone tag."[2] Unlike leaving voice messages with the fear that a person other than the patient overhears the message, a provider can respond to a patient's inquiry in writing, as long as it is within the company's guidelines. Finally, with more patients demanding E-mail ability with their provider, E-mail could soon be a market differentiator.[2] With all of the above being said, I must make one thing very clear. The American Medical Association emphasizes that E-mail should not replace face-to-face time with patients.[3] Our organization fully supports the AMA's recommendation and expects the same from our staff.

Though I believe you had good intentions, your use of E-mail has created risk for your patient, yourself, and this organization. Another one of the main reasons why many providers are hesitant to use E-mail, which can be seen in your situation, is the concern about patients sending medical emergency E-mails, and not receiving a response in a timely manner. This is a patient safety issue and could create a liability for both the doctor and organization.

Patient safety is our primary concern with using provider–patient E-mail. You can put patients at risk by not providing them with guidelines of how to communicate with you appropriately via E-mail. Knowing that your patients communicate with you via E-mail, you had the responsibility to inform your patients that you would not be available via E-mail for the time that you were on vacation.

In the future if you have any questions about potential liability regarding E-mail use or how to assure that your practice staff are all aware of our policy concerning it, please contact me.

Sincerely,
Sara Truss
Risk Manager

LEGAL ISSUES

The U.S. healthcare system has laws with regard to patient health information and the provider's responsibility to uphold patient confidentiality. These laws include:[1]

- Provider's duty to maintain confidentiality (see *Alberts v. Devine*, 395 Mass. 59, cert. denied, 474 U.S. 1014 [1985])
- Patient privacy; Massachusetts Privacy Act (M.G.L. c. 214, 1B)
- HIPAA: Health Insurance Portability and Accountability Act of 1996 (PL 104-191, 110) Stat. 1988 (1996) (codified in portions of 29 U.S.C., 42 U.S.C. and 18 U.S.C.)
- Federal Privacy Act of 1974 (5 U.S.C. 552a)
- Federal Electronic Communications Privacy Act of 1986 (18 U.S.C. 2510)
- Massachusetts Patients' Bill of Rights, 1979 (M.G.L. c.111, 70E)

When providers are transmitting patient health information, they must meet the standards that these laws require. Patient confidentiality must not be broken when using E-mail. Some important questions that a provider must ask him- or herself are given by Morlang as follows:[4]

- Are the networks secured?
- Are you encrypting your messages?
- Do you have password-protected computers and screen savers?
- Who can access your computer other than yourself?
- Have you ever sent a mass E-mail from your address book to all your patients, thereby providing each with a list of all your other patients?
- Do you know that the person sending you a message is indeed who she or he reports to be?
- When you reply to an E-mail, do you know who in that household has access to your response? Have you ever forwarded an E-mail to a third party without obtaining prior consent from the patient to divulge the information contained therein?

Another legal issue and patient safety issue is the content of what providers provide to their patient via E-mail. The Texas State Board of Medical Examiners has specific rules for what a physician cannot do via E-mail. Some of the rules may seem to be obvious, such as not prescribing controlled substances without establishing a physician–patient relationship, but other areas of concern may not be so obvious. A physician must verify that the person sending the E-mail is truly the patient.[4] There are stories on the news of minors purchasing drugs over the Internet claiming to be of the legal age, and identity theft creates concern. This is again another reason why physicians should use E-mail to exchange information with "minimal privacy-related consequences such as appointments or flu shot reminders."[5]

Two other legal issues to take into consideration are (1) what the state rules are for a provider to practice medicine (diagnose, treat, or offer to treat) via E-mail to a patient out of the state (i.e., on vacation), and (2) that the information that the patient provides to the doctor may not be considered "medically relevant material" and may be legally used in litigation such as child-custody hearings or divorce.[4] Once again, this supports the recommendation from many healthcare providers to limit information in E-mails exchanged with patients.

GENERAL E-MAIL POLICIES

The only circumstances in which an E-mail should be used to share identifying and confidential patient information is when both parties use secure E-mail encryption software. If an encrypted E-mail is opened by someone other than the intended person, the text is encoded so that it does not make sense to the reader.[6] Larger healthcare institutions may have a secure system set up that requires patients to sign into their system to send an E-mail to the physician, ensuring that the E-mail is secure. This does require a complex server as well as people to monitor and update it, which a smaller company might not be able to afford; however, there is software that can be used that allows for the same securities that larger facilities have.[7]

Using a personal E-mail address and accessing it away from the office should be against an organization's policy. As previously stated, E-mail correspondence between a provider and a patient is considered to be a part of the patient's medical record.[4] In accordance with HIPAA guidelines, a patient's medical record cannot leave the office and must be kept in a securely locked place or a secured electronic-medical-record (EMR) system. A healthcare professional's personal E-mail is not a secure E-mail, and therefore that professional would be putting the patient's confidentiality at risk. Not only is such an E-mail not secure, but one does not know if the person to whom one is writing has a secure E-mail. Both the professional and the patient must have their computers set up to send and receive encrypted E-mail to ensure total security.[8] By using personal E-mail, the professional is creating a liability for him- or herself; thus, no healthcare professional should ever use personal E-mail to communicate any information related to their patients.

HAND-HELD AND WIRELESS DEVICES

Due to the vulnerability of hand-held and wireless devices, provider–patient E-mails cannot be exchanged using these tools. The only exception to this is if the hand-held device is provided by the organization and has E-mail encryption abilities. This is not a preferred way to communicate with patients and should not be the primary form of communication.

COMPANY POLICIES AND PROCEDURES TO MINIMIZE LIABILITY

The present author's institution is called Vital Rehabilitation (Chicago, Illinois). If Vital Rehabilitation's providers intend to use E-mail with their patients, her role as risk manager is to minimize risk. Company policies are implemented to train Vital Rehabilitation's providers on how to use E-mail with their patients. Every organization and every state may have different laws that dictate company policies. Vital Rehabilitation's E-mail policies are meant to be used by its providers and patients, and do not represent any other facility. Vital Rehabilitation's policies may also change as new laws and guidelines are developed by state healthcare organizations (e.g., Centers for Medicare and Medicaid Services, Healthcare and Family Services) or federal organizations.

Based on the research done for this chapter, the present author has developed a proposal for a provider–patient E-mail policy for Vital Rehabilitation. She obtained written consent from the director of business to use the company's name and descriptive information. Any information herein about the company is not confidential information or company trade secrets.

Vital Rehabilitation is a therapist-owned, private rehabilitation outpatient clinic that provides physical, occupational, speech, and developmental therapy and counseling services. There are five locations in the greater Chicago area. The therapists provide therapy at the clinic or in the patient's home. Many therapists are contracted therapists who see patients in the home, and rarely come to the office; therefore, the main way of communicating with patients is via phone, fax, and E-mail. Vital Rehabilitation's referral sources also use E-mail to obtain information about a therapist's availability at present, not much patient information is shared, but that may change soon. Currently, Vital Rehabilitation's population of patients, the elderly and children, do not use E-mail very often; however, as the company grows and provides services to different populations of patients, management wants to ensure that an E-mail policy is in place to decrease the risk of using E-mail with the patients. These policies are meant for all company staff, not just the therapists.

Specific E-mail Policy

All E-mail correspondences must be done via the company's E-mail system, which has the E-mail address format of: (person's name) @vitalrehabilitation.com. E-mail cannot be used to share or exchange medical information about the patient. E-mail can be used to remind the patient of an appointment, allow the patient to cancel or reschedule an appointment, or provide the patient with basic information about services from other providers to whom the patient was referred.[9] E-mail cannot be used for marketing purposes, and in no event should a mass E-mail be sent to Vital Rehabilitation's patients. This would violate patient confidentiality, because the recipients could see the other patients' E-mail addresses. (Although E-mail does provide a BCC option to prevent others from seeing who received the E-mail, to ensure the safety and privacy of patients, mass E-mailing is strictly prohibited at Vital Rehabilitation.)

A disclosure statement must be included with every E-mail sent with patient information. Vital Rehabilitation's current company disclosure statement, which the company uses for faxes, will be modified for E-mail use. That statement is the following:

> This facsimile transmission— EMAIL—contains confidential information, some or all of which may be protected health information as defined by the federal Health Insurance Portability & Accountability Act (HIPAA) Privacy Rule. This transmission is intended for the exclusive use of the Individual or entity to whom it is addressed and may contain information that is propriety, privileged, confidential and/or exempt from disclosure under applicable law.

> If you are not the intended recipient (or an employee or agent responsible for delivering this facsimile transmission to the intended recipient), you are hereby notified that any disclosure, dissemination, distribution, or copying of this information is strictly prohibited and may be subject to legal restriction or

sanction. Please notify the sender by telephone (773-685-XXXX) to arrange the return or destruction of the information and all copies.

If a patient contacts a provider via the company's E-mail from his or her own E-mail, and it contains confidential information, the patient is not breaking any HIPAA laws. However, if the provider responds with confidential information, HIPAA laws are being violated;[8] therefore, we request that all providers respond to such E-mails with the following statement:

> I have received your email. Due to patient confidentiality, I will contact you directly at the phone number listed in your medical record. Please allow me 24 hours to contact you. Thank you for your understanding.

If the patient continues to contact the provider via unsecured E-mail, Vital Rehabilitation requests that the provider speak to the patient directly and remind him or her of the E-mail policy. Although providers do not often report patients harassing them, or writing lengthy E-mails, if there is a problem with a specific patient, the provider must discuss that with his or her immediate supervisor to determine if he or she should no longer accept E-mails from that patient. According to Sands, a good rule of thumb for E-mail use is: "any message that takes more than two volleys back and forth should not be done by email."[3]

If a provider is contacted by someone seeking medical advice, other than his or her patient, the provider is not to respond. Vital Rehabilitation's system generates an automatic response, which must be used:

> Unsolicited patient email seeking medical advice will not be answered. If you have a medical emergency, dial 911 for police, fire, and ambulance.

Finally, under no circumstance can instant messaging be used to relay patient information.[5] Such programs cannot be uploaded to any of Vital Rehabilitation's computers. If an instant-messaging program is found, it will be deleted, and the person who installed it will be issued a written warning.

Vital Rehabilitation also recommends the assignment of staff to monitor E-mails from its patients. Although this process is still new, having someone assigned to check E-mails from patients would minimize the risk of ignoring an E-mail. Vital Rehabilitation's policy states that the company is not obligated to respond to any E-mail, but to provide good customer service, all E-mails should be reviewed. Another recommendation is to have one inbox, or one E-mail address per clinic, which is given to patients instead of an individual therapist's E-mail address. This would allow one person to be designated and responsible for reviewing all E-mail. A back-up person must also be identified in the event that the regular person is not in the office. The designated person should be a full-time person who agrees to check E-mail first thing in the morning, and then throughout the day at his or her discretion. For the weekend, when no one is checking the inbox, an automatic response should be used stating the following:

> We are not in the office at this time and no one can respond to your email at this time. We will check email the following business day and respond in the order received. You may also call on the next business day to speak to one of our staff. If this is an emergency, please dial 911.

Patient Consent

Once the patient has been informed of the risks of using unsecured E-mail, the patient must give consent to exchange information that is allowed by company policy. The patient consent form must include the following statements:[5,9]

- Vital Rehabilitation does not guarantee the confidentiality of any E-mail message.

- Please provide your full name in the *Subject* line of the E-mail. In addition, please leave a phone number in the message for where we can call you. If we have patients with the same name, we will contact you by phone, and not respond to your E-mail.
- E-mail is not to be used for medical emergencies.
- If you require immediate attention during business hours, please call the office.
- All E-mails will be printed and kept in the patient's record.
- Our therapists will not initiate E-mail and only respond to those that we deem to be appropriate. We will contact you directly to share medical information.
- Our therapists are not obligated to respond to any E-mail.
- Vital Rehabilitation is not liable for any patient sending E-mails via a secured computer over an encrypted network.
- Therapists may not respond immediately— please allow 24 hours for a response.
- If an E-mail is returned to us with a "bad address" message, Vital Rehabilitation will not attempt to contact you again via E-mail without directly speaking with you first.
- Our policies are subject to change at any time. You will be informed of such changes in writing.

Once the patient agrees to and signs the consent, a copy will be given to the patient and a copy will be kept in the patient's file.

EDUCATING PATIENTS

The best way to minimize patient risk is to educate patients about the risk of using E-mail.

They must be informed of the risk of using unsecured E-mail, and how their medical information can be mistakenly or intentionally seen by unintended parties. Patients must also be made aware of the risk of sending E-mail messages from their own company's E-mail system, because many employers have the ability to monitor employee E-mail transmissions.[2]

Vital Rehabilitation's patients must also be informed of the company's E-mail policies (above) and must abide by them if they want to communicate with the staff via E-mail. Some providers have developed a system in which the patient must agree, verbally and in writing, to the company's policies before an E-mail address is even provided to the patient. After that, the patient is given a card with the E-mail address and the E-mail policy.[1] Vital Rehabilitation is strongly urged to consider incorporating this policy.

CONCLUSION

Doctor Tom Delbanco, of Beth Israel Medical Center (New York, N.Y.), who uses E-mail with his patients says: "Medicine is very conservative. It changes slowly." For example, when telephones became widely available in the late 1800s, doctors were concerned that they would be swamped with phone calls. Delbanco continues to say that he also believes that technology will become a routine part of medicine; it is just a matter of time.[3] With appropriate training of clinicians and educating the patients, the use of E-mail between the two can work while reducing physician and patient risk.

References

1. Sands, D.Z. (2003). Sharing electronic medical record information with patients via the Internet. http://www.mahealthdata.org. Accessed May 10, 2010.

2. Kane, B., & Sands, D.Z. (1998). Guidelines for the clinical use of electronic mail with patients. *Journal of the American Medical Informatics Association* 5(1), 1204–1211.

3. Associated Press. (2008, April 22). Only 1 in 3 doctors use e-mail with patients. http://www .msnbc.msn.com/id/24260074/. Accessed May 10, 2010.

4. Morlang, H. (2002). *Talking to your patients by e-mail? What physicians should know about electronic relationships.* http://www.law.uh.edu/ healthlaw/perspectives/Internet/020430 Talking.html. Accessed May 10, 2010.

5. Yale University. (n.d.). Guidance on the use of email containing PHI. http://hipaa.yale.edu/ guidance/emailconfidentiality.html/. Accessed May 10, 2010.

6. E-mail as a provider-patient electronic communication medium and its impact on the electronic health record (AHIMA Practice Brief). (2003). Available at http://library.ahima.org/xpedio/ groups/public/documents/ahima/bok1_021588 .hcsp?dDocName=bok1_021588. Accessed May 10, 2010.

7. Veniegas, M. (n.d.). http://ezinearticles.com/ ?HIPAA-and-Email—How-Does-Your-Practice -Deal-with-Compliance-in-a-Digital -Age?&id=123458/. Accessed May 10, 2010.

8. Clinical Lawyer. (2007). *Those confidentiality disclaimers at the end of your email.* http:// clinicallawyer.com/2007/07/those -confidentiality-disclaimers-at-the-end-of -your-email%e2%80%a6%e2%80%a6/. Accessed May 10, 2010.

9. Kaiser Permanente Northern California e-mail policy. (n.d.) Available at http://134.174.100 .34/. Accessed May 10, 2010.

Internet Resources

http://www.cwclaw.com/publications/article Detail.aspx?id=161/

http://www.ericgoldman.org/Articles/emailtricks article.htm/

http://healthcare.zdnet.com/?p=228/

http://134.174.100.34/

http://www.healthyemail.org/

http://www.informatics-review.com/thoughts/ pat-email.html/

http://www.1800calldoc.com/articles/patient_email .htm/

http://134.174.100.34/NEJM/Delbanco-Sands _NEJM.pdf/

http://www.annals.org/cgi/content/full/129/6/495/

http://www.fergusonreport.com/articles/tfr07-01.htm/

http://www.ihealthbeat.org/Data-Points/ 2009/How-Important-Is-It-for-Health-Care -Providers-To-Use-Electronic-Health-Records .aspx/

http://www.pediatrichealthcare.com/about/email .htm/

http://med.stanford.edu/shs/smg/email.html/

https://www.relayhealth.com/

http://www.castleconnolly.com/healthcare/advocate .cfm?id=31&keyword/

http://www.hschange.com/content/875/

http://e-patients.net/archives/2008/04/why-doesnt -my-doctor-answer-my-email.html/

http://www.nytimes.com/2008/07/15/health/views/ 15mind.html?ex=1373774400&en=a13c40e 0a6956439&ei=5124&partner=digg&exprod =digg/

http://www.nytimes.com/2004/04/27/health/take -two-aspirin-e-mail-me-tomorrow.html?scp =1&sq=Take%20Two%20Aspirin,%20email %20me%20tomorrow&st=cse/

http://hosted.ap.org/specials/interactives/ _documents/patient_physician_email.pdf/

http://med.fsu.edu/informatics/Articles/Smart% 20Practices%20Making%20the%20Most% 20of%20Physician-Patient%20E-mail.htm/

http://www.medem.com/node/1153/

http://www.medscape.com/viewarticle/504947_4/

http://www.aans.org/library/Article.aspx?ShowMenu =false&ShowPrint=false&ArticleId=9940

http://www.jabfm.org/cgi/reprint/18/3/180/

http://www.amia.org/mbrcenter/pubs/email _guidelines.asp/

33

RISK MANAGEMENT FOR RESEARCH

Jennifer Ruocco, PhD, CIP

INTRODUCTION

A variety of federal and state regulations cover the review, approval, and conduct of research, placing a considerable burden on investigators and the research enterprise of any organization. In addition to reconciling discrepancies between regulations and determining applicability of regulations to specific activities, one of the primary challenges in research compliance is applying regulations written years ago to today's science. Despite the ongoing debates about the currency of research regulations, they remain our society's national standards for the protection of research participants and maintenance of the integrity of the research. Non-compliance carries monetary and reputational penalties to investigators and institutions, as well as risk to research participants.

Risk management must proactively manage the most significant risks related to research in order to mitigate losses surrounding research-related injuries, deficiencies in informed consent, and issues that meet the so-called *New York Times* test for their negative impact on an institution's reputation, such as conflicts of interests. Risk management in research is also additionally challenged by the culture of investigators, who are reluctant to realize that research is a regulated activity and may have more rigorous requirements than clinical care. Any risk management program needs to strike a careful balance between preserving investigator autonomy necessary for scientific advancement with ensuring regulatory compliance and risk reduction for research participants and the institution.

What are the risk management issues inherent in research? From a risk management perspective, research-related injury poses the greatest area of exposure from the claims and patient safety perspectives. Case law in this area, however, is sparse and reveals mixed success for research participants, investigators, and institutions. This is in part due to the difficulty in determining whether a violation of the regulations governing research with human participants has occurred and which regulations were violated. In addition, courts traditionally rely on the more-relaxed standards of clinical informed consent when evaluating cases that involve injury to research participants. In all likelihood, many cases are settled out of court or before even reaching the courts. More than anything, case law highlights significant gaps in the current system of protecting human subjects in addition to a concerning lack of understanding about the research process within the judicial process. Institutions should incorporate mechanisms for identifying and resolving injury to research participants within their patient safety programs so that those programs truly encompass a clear understanding of the potential sources of injuries and the most effective manner in which to prevent them.

FEDERAL REGULATORY SUPERVISION OF RESEARCH INVOLVING HUMAN PARTICIPANTS

There are two distinct sets of federal regulations that apply to research involving human participants: the Food and Drug Administration (FDA) regulations and the "Common Rule" set of regulations. Both sets of regulations are based on the ethical principles in The Belmont Report (see Table 33–1);[1] however, each defines "research" and "human subjects" differently, with distinct applicability criteria. Even when grouped together, they do not cover all human-research activities that occur at every institution.

The FDA regulations apply to research subject through to supervision of the FDA itself, because the research involves drugs, devices, or data to be submitted to the FDA. The "Common Rule" regulations represent a set of equivalent regulations, policies, and executive orders that apply Subpart A of 45 C.F.R. 46 to research that is conducted, supported, or otherwise subject to regulation by 19 federal departments and agencies. In addition, several of the departments and agencies that follow the "Common Rule," such as the Department of Health and Human Services (DHHS), have additional subparts that apply to research that is conducted, supported by, or otherwise subject to, regulations by that department or agency.

The federal wide assurance (FWA) is the process by which institutions engaged in federally funded human-subjects research certify to the DHHS and other federal agencies compliance to Subpart A 45 C.F.R. 46 and all applicable subparts. By default, the FWA requires the institution to apply Sub-

Table 33–1 Ethical Principles as Established in The Belmont Report

Respect for Persons	Beneficence	Justice
Acknowledge and respect an individual's autonomy.	Do no harm.	Risks associated with research are distributed across groups.
Individuals with diminished autonomy are entitled to additional protection.	Maximize possible benefit. Minimize harm.	One group will not solely bear the risks of developing therapeutic interventions that will ultimately benefit a different group.

The Belmont Report. (1979). The National Commission for the Protection of Human Subjects of Biomedical and Behavioral Research. Available at http://ohsr.od.nih.gov/guidelines/belmont.html. Accessed May 8, 2010.

part A of 45 C.F.R. 46 and all applicable subparts to all research that is conducted, supported by, or otherwise subject to regulation by a federal department or agency subject to the "Common Rule." In the FWA, institutions can optionally check one of two boxes to extend the jurisdiction of the FWA. The options are to apply all subparts of 45 C.F.R. 46 to all research involving human subjects as that term is defined in the DHHS regulations,[2,a,3,b] regardless of funding, or to apply just Subpart A of 45 C.F.R. 46 to all research involving human subjects regardless of funding source. Selecting one of the options is the source of using the phrases "checking the box," meaning to extend the jurisdiction of the FWA to all research involving human subjects, and "unchecking the box," meaning to not extend that jurisdiction to the FWA.

---

[a] "[Research] means a systematic investigation, including research development, testing and evaluation, designed to develop or contribute to generalizable knowledge."

[b] "[Human] subject means a living individual about whom an investigator (whether professional or student) conducting research obtains (1) Data through intervention or interaction with the individual, or (2) Identifiable private information. Intervention includes both physical procedures by which data are gathered (for example, venipuncture) and manipulations of the subject or the subject's environment that are performed for research purposes. Interaction includes communication or interpersonal contact between investigator and subject. Private information includes information about behavior that occurs in a context in which an individual can reasonably expect that no observation or recording is taking place, and information which has been provided for specific purposes by an individual and which the individual can reasonably expect will not be made public (for example, a medical record). Private information must be individually identifiable (i.e., the identity of the subject is or may readily be ascertained by the investigator or associated with the information) in order for obtaining the information to constitute research involving human subjects."

Institutions are also free to customize their FWA with other obligations that range between applying all or none of 45 C.F.R. 46 to all research involving human subjects regardless of funding source. For example, some institutions agree to apply 45 C.F.R. 46 and all subparts to all research involving human subjects regardless of funding, with the exception of applying Subpart B (pregnant women) protections to social and behavior research or with the exception that reportable problems (unanticipated problems involving risks to subjects or others, serious or continuing non-compliance, and suspensions or terminations of approval of the institutional review board) in non-federally funded research will not be reported to agencies. The Office for Human Research Protections (OHRP), under DHHS, has asserted this oversight to be based on the occurrence date rather than the allegation date. For example, if an institution had opted to extend the FWA to all research between 1990 and 2007, dropped this extension in 2008 ("unchecked the box"), and an allegation was made in 2009 about an occurrence in 2006 related to non-federally funded research, OHRP would claim jurisdiction. Many institutions have unchecked the box as a way to mitigate the reputational risks associated with OHRP supervision of all human-subjects research at their institution, especially since the FWA cannot be retroactively restricted.

While unchecking the box prevents OHRP supervision of all non-federally funded research, courts have recognized 45 C.F.R. 46 as the national standard for protection of human subjects in research. If institutions do not elect to apply the FWA to all human-subjects research, the organization sets forth the appearance of having multiple standards for research depending on the funding of the research. This sends the message to potential research participants, regulators, and collaborators that the standards for protection and ensuring safety vary by type of research, funding source, and governing regulations. The best response to the disparate requirements is to have policies and procedures that apply equal protections to all research based on the requirements of 45 C.F.R. 46 but limit OHRP's authority by "unchecking the box" in the FWA. As always, the underlying ethical foundation behind any human-research protection program should embody those principles set forth in The Belmont Report.[4]

Regardless of whether the box is checked, any activity that meets the regulatory definition of a clinical investigation (21 C.F.R. § 50.3(c))[5,c] must comply with FDA regulations (regardless of funding source), which include protections that are equivalent to 45 C.F.R. 46, with some minor differences. If a human-subjects research protocol is a federally funded clinical investigation, then both the DHHS and FDA regulations apply. Many institutions also provide internal funds for research, whether through departmental support or competitive internal grants. As previously stated, institutions should have policies and procedures that protect all human subjects involved in research, regardless of funding source. It is important for institutions to establish equivalent protections for all human-subjects research regardless of funding source within their policies and procedures.

One way that institutions can assure that they are effectively protecting all human subjects is to seek accreditation of their human-research protection programs through the

Association for the Accreditation of Human Research Protection Programs (AAHRPP).[6] The process of accreditation helps organizations to develop and focus their programs around participant safety and consolidating compliance with multiple regulations into policies and procedures. Finally, the overriding message from an integrated safety program should be one that makes clear the priorities around injury prevention and expedient, thoughtful resolution when an injury does occur.

INNOVATION VERSUS RESEARCH

When an activity meets the regulatory definition of research, certain DHHS and FDA regulations govern the activity, including institutional review board (IRB) review of the protocol and informed consent document (unless the activity qualifies for an informed-consent waiver). The Belmont Report differentiates "practice" and "research" by stating:

> The purpose of medical or behavioral practice is to provide diagnosis, preventive treatment or therapy to particular individuals. By contrast, the term "research" designates an activity designed to test a hypothesis, permit conclusions to be drawn, and thereby to develop or contribute to generalizable knowledge (expressed, for example, in theories, principles, and statements of relationships). Research is usually described in a formal protocol that sets forth an objective and a set of procedures designed to reach that objective.

The design of an activity is a crucial aspect to distinguishing research from medical practice. Research about therapeutic interventions, for example, a comparison between two standard practices, constitutes research subject to IRB review and supervision when human subjects are also involved. The line between research and medical care becomes blurred

---

[c] Clinical investigation means any experiment that involves a test article and one or more human subjects and that either is subject to requirements for prior submission to the Food and Drug Administration under section 505(i) or 520(g) of the Act, or is not subject to requirements for prior submission to the Food and Drug Administration under these sections of the Act, but the results of which are intended to be submitted later to, or held for inspection by, the Food and Drug Administration as part of an application for a research or marketing permit. The term does not include experiments that are subject to the provisions of part 58 of this chapter, regarding nonclinical laboratory studies.

when benefit may be derived from experimental interventions within a research project, or when a physician wants to understand why successive patients improve after receiving an innovative treatment. The IRB is in the best position to determine whether an activity meets the regulatory definition of human-subjects research. One of the reasons for this conservative approach is so that participants are fully informed of the risks and receive all of the protections afforded to them under the regulations, which is more rigorous than what they would receive as patients receiving an innovative treatment as part of their clinical care. For innovative treatments that are determined by the IRB to not meet the regulatory definition of human-subjects research, the IRB and risk management should coordinate on an alternative review mechanism.

The most relevant recent case that highlights the court perspective on the distinction between innovative treatment and research was *Ancheff v. Hartford Hospital.*[7] In this case, the plaintiff suffered severe side effects from a once-daily high dosage of gentamicin following back surgery. To the hospital's own admission, this dosage represented a radical departure from accepted standard of care at the time and the FDA's own recommended dosage. The plaintiff claimed that he was a research subject and did not receive full *research* informed consent and submitted the regulations in 45 C.F.R. 46 and The Belmont Report to support his position. The hospital argued that the practice "constituted the implementation of a program or practice of medical therapy, which, in turn, was aimed, not at validating an untested theory or hypothesis, but at using the available literature, including prior research and clinical data, for the improvement of patient care and safety."[7] On appeal, the court affirmed the lower court's decision to exclude from evidence The Belmont Report and from instructing the jury on the definition of medical research because "there were . . . several different versions presented to the jury of what research involved and did not involve."[7]

This is the problem with quoting The Belmont Report: it is not regulation.

Everything the court decided here was consistent with the regulations and the protection of human subjects. If patients are not protected from their doctors, that is an important issue, but not a research issue. The court did not seem to wrestle with regulatory jurisdiction of the activity from DHHS or FDA perspectives and instead adopted the somewhat arbitrary approach, based on expert testimony that because there were no control groups and the program was based on a review of the literature, it did not constitute medical research. Is there a doubt that the court did not make the right decision? From a regulatory perspective, courts do not seem to follow the same algorithm followed by IRBs to determine whether an activity meets the regulatory definition of research involving human subjects (or clinical investigation).

Why should courts apply the DHHS and FDA regulations? They do not apply here. There is no federal funding. This was the use of an approved drug in the course of medical practice, which is excluded from FDA jurisdiction. Specifically, that algorithm entails considering whether the activity is subject to DHHS regulations and/or FDA regulations. Neither of these regulatory definitions draw upon the existence of control groups. Despite the fact that the hospital collected data and published the results in the academic literature (suggesting that the intent of the activity was to contribute to generalizable knowledge), the hospital prevailed on appeal.

A troubling conclusion was reached in *Moore v. Regents of University of California.*[8] In this case, multiple blood and tissue samples were taken from Moore while he was undergoing treatment for hairy cell leukemia over a number of years. His treating physician, David W. Golde, told Moore that the samples were necessary for his treatment. In fact, Golde used those samples for research and eventually to commercialize a cell line. While this case focused primarily on property rights associated with donated samples, the California Court of Appeals did consider the issue of informed consent in relation to the research intent and held that "a physician who is seeking a patient's consent for a medical procedure must, in order to satisfy his fiduciary duty and to obtain the patient's informed consent, disclose personal interests unrelated to the patient's health, whether research or economic, that may affect his medical judgment."[9]

Although Moore was successful under the breach of fiduciary duty and informed consent actions, the court's conclusion is unsatisfying from a regulatory perspective. One of the primary additional protections that research participants receive above patients is a more robust informed consent process, including a presentation of the risks and benefits of participating in the research, a clear statement that participation is *voluntary,* and an explanation that the purpose of the research is to benefit science (and not their own medical care, although they may receive benefit in the process of participating in research).[10] Moore did not receive these enhanced protections and the court was satisfied with a physician meeting any fiduciary duties through disclosure of external interests. Although Moore prevailed in principle, this case provides another example of how case law is not fully aligned with the regulatory framework for protecting research participants.

Regulations that govern the protection of human subjects are based on the long history of conducting research on unwilling (or unwitting) subjects. In addition, concerns have been raised about the willingness of a subject to consent to any interventions if they have a terminal or untreatable disease and thus may not question the risks attendant in the research or thoroughly assess the potentiality of the benefits. (This issue frequently arises in the case of children as research subjects when parents, so consumed with trying to cure their child's disease, consent to research without a comprehensive understanding of the risks involved.) In response to these abuses, the regulations provide increased protection by way of supervision and enhanced informed consent for research participants. Although courts may lack an understanding of how to interpret these regulations from a claims perspective, patients (and research participants) are still entitled to these additional protections.

From a patient safety perspective, risk management needs to consider the threshold between innovative treatment and research so that the institution can proactively provide these additional protections to its patients and research participants. The institution should have a process that applies standards of accepted medical care to innovative treatment and maintain those standards separate from IRB review. The IRB review process should be used to determine which activities meet the regulatory definition of human-subjects research, but they should not be used as a mechanism to review innovative medical care that is not research. Similarly, IRB approval of research does not necessarily indicate that the procedures in the research are consistent with the organization's accepted practices. It is completely within risk management's authority under the regulations to disapprove research that has been approved by the IRB when that research conflicts with the organization's risk management policy or for any other reason.

INCOMPLETE INFORMED CONSENT FOR RESEARCH PARTICIPANTS

It is important to keep in mind that research participants are volunteering for the advancement of science. This differs from the physician–patient relationship where the intent of an intervention is to benefit the individual person.[11] Because research participants agree to relinquish this relationship for the greater good, they are afforded certain additional protections, including supervision by an IRB of the protocol and informed consent. In addition, per federal regulations, the informed consent process and document must contain specific statements related to the risks, benefits, and alternatives (unless waived by the IRB).[12] The investigator is responsible for implementing the protocol as it is approved by the IRB. The ongoing relationship between the IRB and investigator is primarily one of trust—that is, the ability of an IRB to fulfill its supervisory functions after the initial approval of the research is almost entirely dependent upon the investigator providing current and accurate information to the IRB. Risk reduction and participant safety are therefore embedded in this complicated web of regulation, communication, responsibility, and trust, making the establishment of appropriate controls a considerable challenge.

A number of cases highlight the difficulties in adequately informing research participants of risks. In *Whitlock v. Duke University,*[13] Whitlock, an experienced diver, enrolled in the Atlantis III study, a simulated deep-dive experiment that took place in a hyperbaric chamber. The court affirmed that a higher standard for informed consent applied to "non-therapeutic research" as set forth in the Nuremberg Code. This includes the duty to disclose all reasonably anticipated risks and not just the "usual and frequent" risks that apply in consent for treatment. The fact that the court distinguished therapeutic from non-therapeutic is troubling from a regulatory perspective because it insinuates that there are some types of research ("therapeutic research") where the purpose is to treat disease. Yet, as previously discussed, the intent of research is entirely different from clinical care. Although research participants may benefit from research interventions, the purpose of the interventions in the first place is not to provide treatment to individual subjects.

This phenomenon is called "therapeutic misconception"[14] and is pervasive in many discussions about research, including in case law. Yet, the distinct intent between clinical care and research is one reason why the regulations that govern the informed consent process and documentation requirements are so detailed. In fact, both 45 C.F.R. § 46.116 and 21 C.F.R. § 50.116 require informed consent to include "a statement that the study involves research, an explanation of the purposes of the research and the expected duration of the subject's participation, a description of the procedures to be followed, and identification of any procedures which are experimental." The informed consent document and process are also scrutinized by IRBs; in contrast, clinical-care informed consent has no similar supervisory mechanism, except the physician and patient.

The IRBs spend an inordinate amount of time requiring (and/or striking) specific language from consent documents so that potential research participants are fully informed of the risks, and the overall tone is factual and not coercive. The IRBs struggle with which risks to include in the informed consent document and where to delineate between risks related to research interventions and standard of care. There is, however, a pervasive feeling throughout the profession that informed consent documents are too long and complex to be meaningful to a research participant, and that litigation is the reason why longer informed consent documents are the norm.

Courts, on the other hand, inconsistently reference the research regulations when presented with a case involving research informed consent. To illuminate this point, here is a sample of recent court cases regarding informed consent in research and their outcomes:

- *Wright v. The Fred Hutchinson Cancer Center*:[15] Families of deceased participants in Protocol 126 claimed lack of full informed consent regarding the risks of the research and investigator financial conflicts of interests. Protocol 126 sought to prevent graft-versus-host disease in leukemia patients undergoing bone marrow transplants by using monoclonal antibodies against T-cells, considered a highly experimental method at the time. The court ruled that under a "reasonably prudent patient" standard, research participants knowingly entered the study and were fully informed of the risks.

- *Darke v. Estate of Isner*:[16] Darke enrolled in a research study that examined the effects of VEGF2 gene therapy on coronary artery disease. After his death, Darke's spouse claimed that the investigators failed to reveal their financial conflicts of interests, intentional battery, and breach of duty to the patient (among other claims). The court denied summary judgment for the plaintiff on these counts because Darke knowingly consented to enroll in the clinical trial.

- *Stewart v. Cleveland Clinic Foundation*:[17] Klais enrolled in a clinical trial, after being diagnosed with stage-IV squamous cell carcinoma, that examined a preoperative chemotherapy. In this unblinded study, Klais was randomized to receive surgery and radiation only, which was considered standard treatment at the time. Although there was evidence in the medical literature that chemotherapy improved chances of survival, Klais' physician felt that this was "speculative." After his death, his estate brought a motion against Cleveland Clinic, including the failure to inform Klais of available alternative treatments. Although expert testimony showed that

the informed consent document did not meet the regulatory criteria set forth in 45 C.F.R. 46, the court referenced the tort of informed consent established by the Ohio Supreme Court[18,d] in reversing the trial court's summary judgments for the defendants.

The gap in the current system for human-subjects protection may be that the IRBs are too focused on administration and not enough on the identification and management of risks to improve participant safety. As an example, the regulations outline specific documentation requirements for meeting minutes and establishment of quorums. At the same time, IRBs struggle with implementing a reporting procedure that makes sense to investigators regarding unanticipated problems posing risk to subjects or others (UPIRTSO).[19] This is in part due to a lack of clear, harmonized guidance from the FDA and DHHS regarding how institutions should identify and manage UPIRTSOs, serious adverse events, and non-compliance (serious or continuing). Resnik notes that harm generates lawsuits, not paperwork:[20]

> Between trying to avoid lawsuits and attempting to comply with federal regulations, IRB members will be held accountable to the public. The threat of a lawsuit adds an important dimension to public accountability: the goal of minimizing harm to human research subjects. Many of the other regulatory pressures exerted on IRBs emphasize compliance with rules not directly related to subject welfare, such as voting procedures, meeting minutes, certifying a quorum, adequate record-keeping, and other "paperwork" activities. A negligence lawsuit, on the other hand, cannot get off the ground if the subject is not harmed. Moreover, paperwork errors, by themselves, cannot generate a negligence law-

---

[d] "The tort of lack of informed consent is established when: (a) the physician fails to disclose to the patient and discuss the material risks and dangers inherently and potentially involved with respect to the proposed therapy, if any; (b) the unrevealed risks and dangers, which should have been disclosed by the physician, actually materialize and are the proximate cause of the injury to the patient; and (c) a reasonable person in the position of the patient would have decided against the therapy had the material risks and dangers inherent and incidental to treatment been disclosed to him or her prior to the therapy."

suit. Thus, the added emphasis on subject safety and welfare provided by the threat of a lawsuit is important and appropriate.

This is where risk management can play an important role in human-participant protection, specifically in facilitating institutions to adopt a program that is focused on participant safety rather than on administrative compliance. Evaluating the human-research protection program for both accurate implementation of the regulations as well as identifying and eliminating areas of administrative burden and inefficiency would also greatly facilitate a focus on safety. It is also clear that IRBs and investigators need to increase collaboration around the informed consent *process,* rather than the document, so that when participants are injured in a research study, the groundwork for the claims to which they are entitled has been laid.

The most important point in that communication process is around the intent of research as differentiated from medical care, as well as the role of benefit in research. It is important for research participants to know that intent of medical care is to specifically increase the probability of a cure for a specific patient, whereas the intent of research is to increase the probability of a cure for unspecified future patients. Despite the gap between the current regulatory system of protection of research participants and case law, institutions and investigators should still hold patient-participant safety as an important goal in research.

ACCESS TO EXPERIMENTAL INTERVENTIONS AFTER RESEARCH CONCLUDES

In *Abney v. Amgen,*[21] patients living with Parkinson's disease enrolled in a research study that examined the effects of a protein, glial cell-line-derived neutrotropic factor (GDNF), on dopamine production. Although Amgen anticipated a significant improve-ment in motor skills of research subjects, the preliminary results were underwhelming. The research participants, however, experienced marked improvement in memory and motor function. Many of them elected to continue receiving GDNF for up to 24 months after the study ended, as outlined in the informed consent document. While the research participants continued to experience benefit from GDNF, Amgen identified several safety concerns and ceased all clinical uses of GDNF. The participants filed suit against Amgen, claiming that the company had effectuated a breach of contract, and demanded that the company continue to provide the drug. In a related case, *Suthers v. Amgen,*[22] the plaintiff suggested that the informed consent document itself was a binding contract between the participants and the company.

Ultimately, the court determined that the patients did not have a right of action against the company, because the Clinical Trial Agreement had been signed between Amgen and the University of Kentucky, not with the participants themselves. The court clarified as follows:

> Thus, while the plaintiffs' arguments have little merit against Amgen, they may have merit against the University and its Institutional Review Board. . . . Moreover, the litigation in this case indicates that the University, through its Informed Consent Document, and its other representations to the plaintiffs did a poor job informing the plaintiffs as to the grounds upon which the study would terminate and their access to GDNF would be denied. We urge the University's Institutional Review Board, and other review boards throughout the Circuit, to take additional measures to ensure that patients fully understand that even if they or their physicians believe an experimental treatment to be safe

and efficacious there may [be] circumstances under which they will be denied continued access to treatment. If this fact had been properly explained to the plaintiffs in this case prior to the outset of the clinical trial (and spelled out clearly in the Informed Consent Document) perhaps the litigation in this case could have been avoided.

Cases like this could also be avoided with improved education for potential research participants about therapeutic misconception, specifically the fact that while benefit may be derived from experimental interventions, those interventions are *not the same as medical treatment*. As previously discussed, although research participants are afforded additional protections under the regulations, they do not have rights that extend beyond the scope of the study itself. Additionally, from a risk management perspective, *Abney v. Amgen* establishes the trinity of fiduciary duty between sponsor, institution, and participant. Specifically, the university is an independent contractor for the sponsor, and therefore the sponsor does not have any "flow-through" responsibilities, except as documented in the contract. It is the institution, by way of the investigator and informed consent document, that is ultimately beholden to participants, a fact that this case clearly underscores.

INSTITUTIONAL AND INVESTIGATOR NON-COMPLIANCE

Due to the unique position of IRBs in an institution and a general lack of understanding of the scope and responsibilities of IRBs, there have been relatively few cases against IRB members. In the same way that the Clinical Trial Agreement shelters IRBs from litigation, because these agreements are signed between institutions and sponsors, IRBs may also be too remote from the informed consent process to be held liable for informed consent discrepancies. In *Robertson v. McGee*, however, IRB members from the University of Okla-

homa Health Science Center, Tulsa, were individually named in a suit brought by former participants and family members of deceased melanoma participants. The plaintiffs cited numerous complaints all revolving around allegations that the IRB had failed in its duties under 45 C.F.R. 46 to fully protect research participants. Ultimately, the court determined that the regulations do not establish a private right of action and dismissed the case for lack of jurisdiction.

There are a variety of reputational risks for research institutions, particularly emanating from investigator and IRB conduct. The OHRP routinely cites institutions for failure to follow federal regulations, including citing institutions based on failure to follow documentation requirements, as well as those that are more directly related to the protection of human subjects, such as supervision of the informed-consent process. The OHRP periodically halts research operations at institutions due to violations of the federal regulations, which certainly has a financial impact (although there are no fines associated with OHRP findings).

The FDA reviews IRBs every 5 years and specific protocols on a more frequent basis. Like OHRP, the FDA uses public notification in the form of warning letters to alert others of alleged regulatory violations, but there are also no fines or other financial penalties associated with FDA findings. The FDA also has a debarment list for the most egregious cases. Debarment usually includes suspension from conducting all or certain types of research, either permanently or for an extended period of time. It is important to note that under the FDA regulations, investigators who are also considered sponsors[23,e]

---

[e] Sponsor-investigator means an individual who both initiates and conducts an investigation, and under whose immediate direction the investigational drug is administered or dispensed. The term does not include any person other than an individual. The requirements applicable to a sponsor-investigator under this part include both those applicable to an investigator and a sponsor.

assume additional responsibilities and are often the focus of FDA investigations. Due to the synergistic effect of non-compliance in this area, institutional risk management strategies should pay particular attention to these activities. The DHHS Office of Research Integrity investigates allegations of scientific misconduct in federally funded research and also notifies the public of administrative actions on their Web site. Finally, findings of non-compliance from either the FDA or OHRP may lead to a more extensive investigation from the Department of Justice or Office of Inspector General, particularly regarding the use of federal research funds under the False Claims Act.

RISK MANAGEMENT FOR RESEARCH

It is important to recognize that risk management in research is a shared responsibility across the institution. A research program is one where investigators, leadership, and IRBs collaborate on managing the risks and following written policies and procedures that are compliant with the federal regulations. There are several areas of focus for a research risk management program. Those areas are as follows:

- Educating physicians regarding the differences in intent between clinical care and research, and the additional protections afforded to research participants
- Ensuring that the process of informed consent during research is comprehensive and dispels the notion of therapeutic misconception (investigator and IRB), and that the IRB reviews and approves the informed consent process as required by 45 C.F.R. 46.111(a)(4), 21 C.F.R. 46.116, 21 C.F.R. 56.111(a)(4), 21 C.F.R. 50.20, and 21 C.F.R. 50.25, rather than assuming that the consent document is the consent process
- Ensuring that IRB members as a committee understand and systematically apply the entire set of regulatory criteria for approval to all research

- When research subjects are injured, establishing procedures similar to those found in patient safety, where patients are dealt with honestly and fairly; specifically, honest disclosure to patient-participants regarding the cause of the injury, what the organization is doing to prevent this type of event from recurring, and, if appropriate, discussion of some type of compensation
- Reviewing approved research for risk management issues not covered by IRB review
- Establishing an easy, clear process for investigators and research staff to disclose financial interests; systematically reviewing disclosed interests for conflicts of interests and managing, reducing, or eliminating all conflicts of interests
- Ensuring that the IRB procedures identify "clinical investigations" under the FDA regulations, as well as those activities that require an Investigational Device Exemption (IDE) or Investigational New Drug (IND)

Institutions and physicians should partner on minimizing exposure to claims from patients who feel that they were the unwilling recipients of a research project. Objective criteria for distinguishing between medical care and research are sparse and thus add a layer of complication to an awareness campaign. Although increasing awareness around the various regulatory definitions of research might mitigate some of the exposure, clearly communicating throughout the institution the difference between medical care and research according to The Belmont Report, regarding intent, can be foundational for risk management in research. In any discussion around the differences between research and medical care, it is important to also note the FDA definition of clinical investigation because it is considerably more conservative and straightforward.

Risk management can also work directly with the IRB on their supervision of informed consent. Specifically, institutions may provide indemnification for IRB members in order to mitigate concerns about liability within the IRB. Risk management and IRBs may also focus their supervision of informed consent on the process and less on the document. The IRBs should require investigators to provide more information about the informed consent process, specifically:

- Who will be conducting the informed-consent visit?
- Who is funding the research? What is the study hoping to learn and how will the information be used?
- How much time will transpire between the informed consent visit and the first study intervention?
- Where will informed consent take place and how will it be coordinated with clinical visits?
- How long after initial diagnosis will potential participants be approached to participate and who will be making the first recruitment contact?
- Will the informed consent discussion include a clarification of the intent of the research project and the intent to provide potential benefit to *future* patients?

Institutions should also establish a coordinated mechanism for investigators and research coordinators to identify and report safety concerns in research. Research involving humans spans two supervisory bodies in an institution: the IRB and the institutional biosafety committee (IBC). The IBC is charged with reviewing research involving recombinant DNA, which includes gene-transfer research. Patient safety events that occur in gene-transfer research may therefore span FDA and DHHS regulations, as well as the National Institutes of Health Guidelines for Research Involving Recombinant DNA Molecules.[24] Institutions can coordinate policies and procedures across reviewing entities and regulations, which include clear definitions to help investigators and research coordinators report the most important

events from a patient safety perspective, through a single reporting mechanism. In addition, institutions should be able to easily identify those protocols where an investigator has disclosed a significant financial interest related to the research, as well as any management plans for identified conflicts of interests.

When participants are injured, institutions should have clear procedures for identifying which patients are also enrolled in research studies (and in which study they are enrolled). It may be difficult, particularly in large academic medical centers, to identify an incoming patient as a research subject and then link that subject to a particular protocol. Although this would require a large-scale coordination effort between patient-registration systems, medical records, and research protocols, it would be an important one from research-participant-safety and risk management perspectives. Institutions would then have a first line of defense to discuss the injury with the family in light of the particular research protocol and begin the important process of healing and remuneration without litigation. Institutions may also provide insurance to participants in high-risk research as an additional risk management strategy.

RISK FINANCING FOR RESEARCH

Although it may not make sense to transfer the speculative risk associated with clinical research (where limited data might make underwriting difficult and prices disproportionate to expected losses), an organization may wish to self-insure the types of events for which they might consider offering some form of compensation. This might include offers to cover medical expenses for patients who develop complications from the research, or actual out-of-pocket expenses for research subjects who experience problems associated with provider error, as opposed to complications that are a result of the clinical trial or research study but had not been anticipated in the study design. If research is being conducted on behalf of a third party (for example, a drug or device manufacturer), the risk manager or contract administrator may wish to negotiate with the company to either assume the losses associated with these types of injuries or to contribute a sum that the organization can use to compensate for specific types of losses. Of course, in some cases research subjects could bring claims for negligence if the study is not performed in a manner consistent with the agreed-upon protocol. These claims would be handled in the same manner as all other negligence claims.

CONCLUSION

There is a clear gap between case law and the regulatory infrastructure designed to protect research participants. From a safety perspective, precedents set in case law have been unsatisfying to date and not the preferred route for resolving research-related injury. It is clear that both, the regulations and case law, lag behind scientific advancement. Due to the complex intersection between science and the various research regulations, case law may not provide the ideal paradigm for research risk management; yet, institutions must confront the reality that research is an activity that car-

ries risk for patient-participants, the institution, as well as investigators and research coordinators.

Institutions can adopt a programmatic approach to identifying research that carries a higher likelihood of injury to research participants and innovative medical interventions that may need the increased authority of the research regulations. Coordination of policies and procedures for injury reporting, investigation, and resolution within a patient-participant safety program that includes research may also mitigate research risk. A patient-participant program should coordinate with the IRB, IBC, and Conflict of Interest (COI) in policies, procedures, and investigations so as to gain a complete picture of the factors contributing to the injury. Education for investigators and research participants about the differences between research and clinical care may improve the overall informed-consent process in research. A research risk management program that coordinates policies, procedures, and education across the institution, and focuses on the preservation of patient-participant safety, ultimately preserves the public's trust in research and the institution while mitigating financial and reputational losses stemming from research activities.

References

1. The Belmont Report. (1979). The National Commission for the Protection of Human Subjects of Biomedical and Behavioral Research. Available at http://ohsr.od.nih.gov/guidelines/belmont.html. Accessed May 8, 2010.
2. 45 C.F.R. 46 § 102(d).
3. 45 C.F.R. 46 § 102(f).
4. The Belmont Report. (1979). The National Commission for the Protection of Human Subjects of Biomedical and Behavioral Research. Available at http://ohsr.od.nih.gov/guidelines/belmont.html. Accessed May 8, 2010.
5. 21 C.F.R. § 50.3(c).
6. Association for the Accreditation of Human Research Protection Programs, http://www.aahrpp.org/. Accessed May 8, 2010.
7. *Ancheff v. Hartford Hospital,* 799 A.2d 1067 (Conn. 2002).
8. *Moore v Regents of the University of California,* 51 Cal. 3d 120; 271 Cal. Rptr. 146; 793 P.2d 479. (CA 1990).
9. Ibid, p. 132.
10. 45 C.F.R. § 46.116. Also at 21 § C.F.R. 50.25.
11. Morreim, E.H. (2003). Medical research litigation and malpractice tort doctrines: Courts on a learning curve. *Houston Journal of Health Law and Policy,* 4(1), 7.

12. 45 C.F.R. § 46.116. Also at 21 § C.F.R. 50.25.

13. *Whitlock v. Duke University,* 829 F.2d 1340 (4th Cir. N.C. 1987).

14. Applebaum, P.S., Roth, L.H., Lidz, C.W., Bensen, P., & Winslade, W. (1987, April). Hastings Center Report, p. 20.

15. *Wright v. Fred Hutchinson Cancer Research Center,* 269 F. Supp. 2d 1286 (W.D. Wash. 2002).

16. *Darke v. Estate of Isner,* 20 Mass. L. Rep. 419 (Mass. Super. Ct. 2005).

17. *Stewart v. Cleveland Clinic Foundation,* 136 Ohio App. 3d 244 (Ohio Ct. App., Cuyahoga County 1999).

18. *Nickell v. Gonzalez* (1985), 17 Ohio St. 3d 136, 17 Ohio B. Rep. 281, 477 N.E.2d 1145.

19. 45 C.F.R. 46.103(b)(5)(i); 21 C.F.R. 56.108(b)(1).

20. Resnik, D.B. (2004). Liability for institutional review boards: From regulation to litigation. *Journal of Legal Medicine, 25,* 131–184.

21. *Abney v Amgen, Inc.*, 443 F. 3d 540 (6th circuit 2006)

22. *Suthers v. Amgen Inc.,* 441 F. Supp. 2d 478 (S.D.N.Y. 2006).

23. 21 C.F.R. 312.3(b).

24. National Institutes of Health. (2009). *NIH guidelines for research involving recombinant DNA molecules.* http://oba.od.nih.gov/oba/rac/guidelines_02/NIH_Guidelines_Apr_02.htm/. Accessed May 10, 2010.

Index